INTRODUCTION TO
ANESTHESIA
The Principles of Safe Practice

SIXTH EDITION

ROBERT D. DRIPPS, M.D.

Late Vice-President for Health Affairs and
Professor, Department of Anesthesia,
The University of Pennsylvania School of Medicine,
Philadelphia

JAMES E. ECKENHOFF, M.D.

Dean and Professor of Anesthesia,
Northwestern University Medical School,
Chicago

LEROY D. VANDAM, M.D.

Professor of Anesthesia, Emeritus, Harvard Medical School;
Anesthesiologist, Peter Bent Brigham Hospital
and The Hospital at Parker Hill,
Boston

W. B. SAUNDERS COMPANY
PHILADELPHIA · LONDON · TORONTO · MEXICO CITY · RIO DE JANEIRO · SYDNEY · TOKYO

W. B. Saunders Company: West Washington Square
Philadelphia, PA   19105

1 St. Anne's Road
Eastbourne, East Sussex BN21 3UN, England

1 Goldthorne Avenue
Toronto, Ontario M8Z 5T9, Canada

Apartado 26370—Cedro 512
Mexico 4, D.F., Mexico

Rua Coronel Cabrita, 8
Sao Cristovao Caixa Postal 21176
Rio de Janeiro, Brazil

9 Waltham Street
Artarmon, N.S.W. 2064, Australia

Ichibancho, Central Bldg., 22-1 Ichibancho
Chiyoda-Ku, Tokyo 102, Japan

Library of Congress Cataloging in Publication Data

Dripps, Robert Dunning, 1911–1973.

Introduction to anesthesia.

Includes index.

1. Anesthesiology.   2. Anesthesia.   I. Eckenhoff, James
E.   II. Vandam, Leroy D.   III. Title. [DNLM: 1. Anesthesia. WO 200 D781i]

RD81.D7 1982   617′.96   82–47680
ISBN 0–7216–3194–0   AACR2

Listed here is the latest translated edition of this book together
with the language of the translation and the publisher.

French (*5th Edition*)—Doin Editeurs, S.A.,
            Paris, France

Portuguese (*5th Edition*)—Editora Interamericana Ltda,
            Rio de Janeiro, Brazil

Introduction to Anesthesia: The Principles of Safe Practice   ISBN   0–7216–3194–0

Last digit is the print number: 9   8   7   6   5   4   3   2

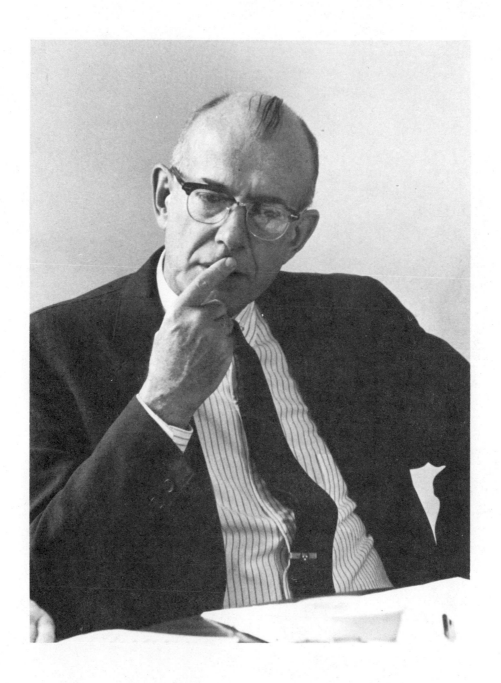

This book is dedicated to the memory of

ROBERT D. DRIPPS,

our tutor, colleague, and cherished comrade.
He remains very much alive in these pages.

Contributors

HONORIO T. BENZON, M.D.
Assistant Professor of Clinical Anesthesia, Northwestern University Medical School

The Therapy of Pain

JAMES R. BERRYMAN
Technical Director Respiratory Care, Brigham and Women's Hospital

Inhalation Therapy and Pulmonary Physiotherapy

DAVID L. BRUCE, M.D.
Professor of Anesthesiology, New York University Medical Center

Pharmacologic Principles and Drug Interactions

EDWARD A. BRUNNER, M.D., Ph.D.
Professor of Anesthesia, Northwestern University Medical School

Fundamentals of Inhalation Anesthesia
Inhalation Anesthetics
Evaluation of the Response to Anesthetics: The Signs and Stages

LEE J. DUNN, Esq.
General Counsel, Northwestern Memorial Hospital

Medicolegal Considerations

VLADIMIR FENCL, M.D.
Associate Professor of Medicine, Harvard Medical School

Inhalation Therapy and Pulmonary Physiotherapy
Respiration and Respiratory Care

BRETT B. GUTSCHE, M.D.
Professor of Anesthesia and Obstetrics and Gynecology, University of Pennsylvania School of Medicine

Obstetric Anesthesia and Perinatology

STEVEN C. HALL, M.D.
Assistant Professor of Clinical Anesthesia, Northwestern University Medical School

Pediatric Anesthesia

RONALD C. HARRISON, M.D.
Associate Professor of Clinical Anesthesia, Northwestern University Medical School

Intravenous Fluids and Acid-Base Balance
Blood Component Therapy

ANTOUN H. KOHT, M.D.
Associate of Anesthesia, Northwestern University Medical School

Neurosurgical Anesthesia

HARRY W. LINDE, Ph.D.
Professor of Anesthesia, Northwestern University Medical School

Anesthesia Equipment
Electric Hazards, Fires, and Explosions

FRANK L. MURPHY, M.D.
Associate Professor of Anesthesia, University of Pennsylvania School of Medicine

Education in Anesthesia

ANDRANIK OVASSAPIAN, M.D.
Associate Professor of Clinical Anesthesia, Northwestern University Medical School

Intubation of the Trachea

JAMES H. PHILIP, M.D.
Instructor in Anesthesia, Harvard Medical School

Monitoring of Physiologic Function

STEPHEN J. PREVOZNIK, M.D.
Professor of Anesthesia, University of Pennsylvania School of Medicine

Intravenous Anesthesia

TOD B. SLOAN, BSEE, Ph.D., M.D.
Assistant Professor of Anesthesia, Northwestern University Medical School

Electric Hazards, Fires, and Explosions

BARBARA E. WAUD, M.D.
Professor of Anesthesia, University of Massachusetts Medical School

Neuromuscular Blocking Agents

CAROLYN J. WILKINSON, M.D.
Assistant Professor of Anesthesia, Northwestern University Medical School

Cardiopulmonary Anesthesia

JAMES E. WHISSLER
Assistant Technical Director Respiratory Care, Brigham and Women's Hospital

Inhalation Therapy and Pulmonary Physiotherapy

Preface to the Sixth Edition

An apology for issuance of a sixth edition of Dripps, Eckenhoff, and Vandam *Introduction to Anesthesia* may be warranted, since we expressed uncertainty as to future plans in the preface to the fifth edition. After all, this continuity of effort began conceptually at Pennsylvania in 1949, followed by publication of the first hard-covered volume in 1957. With the 1982 publication of the present work, 33 years have elapsed — a span equivalent to the professional lives of most physicians. Nevertheless, Eckenhoff and Vandam remain active in all phases of the specialty: mainly teaching and writing, administering anesthetics, and perceiving the broader problems confronting anesthesiology and medicine. The virus of authorship is still alive and contagious in our blood streams.

Aside from the mere will to proceed, we sense the usefulness of this work through the response of novitiates — medical students, residents in training, nurse anesthetists, workers in allied fields, and to be sure the anesthesiologist who would keep abreast of the times. We are also the recipients of encouragement from the staff of W. B. Saunders Company who, between editions of the work, keep a finger on the pulse of the reading public and try to define the needs of anesthesiology.

Our basic philosophy remains unaltered. We present conceptually sound procedure, stripped of adipose tissue and the myriad of alternative considerations that comprise the everyday practice and preferences of the experienced anesthetist. In actuality ours is not a multiauthored text, for the majority of the writing has been accomplished by the senior authors, with the other sections edited to conform to our beliefs and literary style. Our coworkers all stem from or are members of the original staff at Pennsylvania and the Departments of Anesthesia at Northwestern University and Harvard Medical School. As in the past, we have attempted to eliminate from our discussions superannuated agents and techniques. Too much space can be occupied by nostalgia. However, we do cite older theory now grown factual and clarify many of the older bones of contention. Furthermore, in response to demand, we now present sections on neuroanesthesia, geriatrics, treatment of pain, and other items that have become special facets of practice. All of this we attempt within a volume of modest size, published at reasonable cost in this era of inflation. Perhaps continuity needs no apology.

JAMES E. ECKENHOFF
LEROY D. VANDAM

Preface to the First Edition

This book is a descendant of a smaller work privately printed in 1949 and circulated in the Department of Anesthesiology of the Hospital of the University of Pennsylvania. It was called "Organization and Procedures." A second and larger edition appeared in 1953. The third lineal descendant is now being made available to others.

Much of the teaching of anesthesia is by word of mouth. Beginners seek to learn countless details that cannot be found in general texts. This is the lore of anesthesia that must be passed on from individual to individual. A good bit of the material gathered in this volume might be classified as being in this rather shadowy area, including such topics as the philosophy of records, surgeon-anesthetist relations, the value of death reports, hazards of the immediate postoperative period, the treatment of immediate postoperative pain and excitement, and the determination of the depth of general anesthesia.

The subjects and the manner of their presentation represent the thinking and ultimate distillation into teaching practice of the senior staff at Pennsylvania, augmented and refined by all who came within teaching range. One who contributed much to the early editions and whose influence may be discerned in the present volume is Austin Lamont. We mention him with respect and give thanks to others who will find bits of their practice and philosophy in print.

Chapters dealing with fundamental aspects of certain techniques and with basic considerations of the drugs used in anesthesia have been included in the hope that such material can contribute to the safer practice of anesthesia. These are guides; they contain what we believe to be established precepts, but they are not covered in detail nor can they be regarded as complete.

We have intentionally omitted discussion of most of the specialized aspects of anesthesia such as hypothermia, deliberate hypotension, hypnosis, the technical considerations of regional anesthesia, and problems of the treatment of pain. These constitute advanced study in the field. We believe that the students for whom this book is intended should not be confronted by them until later in their training.

We trust that this book will be instructive for all students of anesthesia and those in other fields who would learn a little something of this specialty. We hope that it may be a useful introductory volume of interest before one proceeds to wider reading. Although we have listed only a few references as guides for further study, it has not been our intention to slight individuals who have made important contributions. Doubtless, omissions and reasons for disagreement will be found.

Dr. Henry L. Price, Dr. Ronald Woolmer, and others of our associates have contributed valuable suggestions. Miss Sally Van de Water has performed yeoman service as our secretarial assistant. We acknowledge these contributions with gratitude.

ROBERT D. DRIPPS
JAMES E. ECKENHOFF
LEROY D. VANDAM

Contents

Chapter 1
THE BROAD REALM OF ANESTHESIOLOGY

Anesthesia is recognized as a major American contribution to medicine. News of the first successful demonstration of ether in Boston, in 1846, spread rapidly to Europe, where leading surgeons were quick to try this remarkable substance. Within a year another general anesthetic, chloroform, was used in England; the introduction of the two agents set the stage for the development of the specialty of anesthesia. Chloroform was introduced by an eminent obstetrician, James Y. Simpson. It was both a respiratory and circulatory depressant, requiring great skill in administration, and it could be lethal in unskilled hands. After several years, a large number of deaths attested to the potency of chloroform; therefore only physicians were judged competent to administer it.

In the United States, dentist William T. G. Morton, who had publicly introduced ether, was challenged for the priority by his collaborator, scientist Charles T. Jackson; by dentist Horace Wells, who had earlier introduced nitrous oxide; and finally by physician Crawford W. Long, who had first given ether in 1842 but without audience or publication. The attempts at establishing patents and the controversy over who should receive recognition for the discovery discredited anesthesia. In contrast to chloroform, ether stimulated both respiration and circulation; it was therefore thought to be a built-in protection for the patient and the reason why a skilled person did not have to administer it. Students, nurses, newly graduated physicians, specialists in other fields, and even custodians were called upon to be "etherizers." When, toward the end of the century, nurses were encouraged to become full-time anesthetists, patients received better care because professionals with continuing experience were anesthetizing them.

Some 60 years elapsed before the first American physician devoted full time to anesthesia. Although the strides made by surgery around the turn of the century were great, little change occurred in anesthesia, even though some surgeons pleaded for anesthesia specialists. Two separate series of events sparked the development of anesthesia as a discipline. The first comprised the two world wars, which created a need for large numbers of anesthetists to care for battle casualties. The second was the increasingly complex nature of operations, which resulted in a demand for more qualified help. In 1931 there were already enough specialists on hand to form the American Society of Anesthetists, and in 1937 the American Board of Anesthesiology began to certify specialists. New agents and equipment appeared, and the older agents were studied anew in the laboratory and clinic. Training programs arose throughout the

1

country, the better ones attracting many trainees at the conclusion of World War II. The introduction of tubocurarine, with the accompanying need for control of pulmonary ventilation during and after operation; and the organization of postanesthesia recovery rooms provided further breadth for the fledgling specialty. By 1950 anesthesiologists' activities began to spread beyond the confines of the operating room.

For more than 100 years after the introduction of ether surgeons dominated the operating room, everyone bowing to their authority. This dominance now began to wane. Operating teams evolved consisting of several surgeons, anesthetists, and highly competent nurses. The development of new agents, adjuvants, equipment, and techniques had changed anesthesia into a discipline beyond the training of surgeons who had formerly supervised technicians or had given the anesthetics themselves. Therefore most surgeons readily welcomed physician anesthetists as full partners in the surgical team.

Over the past decades, anesthesiology has emerged as a clearly defined specialty recognized and respected throughout the country. In every medical school anesthesiology functions mostly as an autonomous academic department, in some as a division of surgery. There are approximately 2520 physicians in training in 162 anesthesiology residency programs in the United States. The American Board of Anesthesiology to date has certified over 10,000 specialists, and the Board has been recognized as a leader among specialty boards in setting standards and improving techniques of qualifying examinations. Approximately 4 per cent of all physicians practicing in the United States are anesthesiologists. There are more than a few national societies, and an impressive number of journals and texts on the subject is published each year.

NURSE ANESTHETISTS AND ANESTHESIOLOGISTS

About one half of the estimated 20 million anesthetics given annually in the United States are administered by nonphysicians. Thus the public is confused as to the difference between a nurse anesthetist and an anesthesiologist. To become certified as a registered nurse anesthetist (CRNA), the nurse must have had a high school education, an average of three years of nursing training, plus two additional years of anesthesia training followed by an examination. To become an anesthesiologist, after college and award of the medical degree a physician must have had four years of postgraduate training in an approved residency program, with one year devoted to medicine, surgery, or another clinical discipline. Two years are then spent in clinical anesthesia and the optional fourth year in a specialized area of choice. Some engage in practice for two years in lieu of the optional fourth year. Those who are qualified take an examination to become diplomates of the American Board of Anesthesiology. In the United States, neither a nurse nor a physician has to pass certification to administer anesthesia, nor indeed, to practice any specialty if a hospital will accept the lack of credentials.

It is apparent that the anesthesiologist offers greater depth of training than the nurse anesthetist, but this does not necessarily qualify the physician as a better anesthetist. By achieving the technical skills and the appropriate experience and knowledge, a conscientious nurse can easily surmount the gap in training. An anesthesiologist, acting as a technician, who fails to keep abreast of advances in medicine soon loses the advantage.

In general, the CRNA is an employee of a hospital; a few practice on a fee-for-service basis. The cost of their malpractice insurance is less than that of physicians (see Chapter 6). For the most part their activities are confined to the operating room; they usually do not participate in pre- or postoperative care and are not in a position by virtue of their background to exercise medical judgment. In the eyes of the law they function under the medical direction of physicians, either the surgeon or an anesthesiologist.

In most large hospital departments nurse anesthetists, anesthesiologists, and technicians work in harmony. Cases are assigned by anesthesiologists who evaluate the patients preoperatively, write preoperative notes and preanesthetic orders, assist as necessary during anesthesia and then remain available for consultation, and care for patients postoperatively in the event of complications. Considering the extensive national demands for anesthesia care it is unlikely that all anesthetics will ever be given solely by physicians. As paralleled by the trend toward midwifery in obstetrics, there is and always will be a need for nurse anesthetists.

FUNCTIONS OF THE ANESTHESIOLOGIST

The principal tasks of the anesthesiologist are to provide relief from pain for patients during operation and optimal operative conditions for surgeons, both in the safest possible manner. To do this the anesthesiologist must be a competent physician and a clinical pharmacologist, with a broad knowledge of surgery and the ability to utilize and interpret correctly a variety of monitoring devices.

In addition to anesthetics, drugs employed by anesthesiologists include opioids and antagonists, antisialagogues, barbiturates, tranquilizers, vasoactive substances, antiarrhythmics, cardiotonics, antihypertensives, neuromuscular blocks and antagonists, analeptics, antibiotics, and steroids — to cite just a few. In recent years the interaction of drugs and their pathways of elimination have assumed increasing importance, not only from the viewpoint of widespread drug usage by patients but also because inhalation anesthetics, once thought inert, are now known to undergo metabolic transformation, interacting with other drugs and body components.

Anesthesiologists must combine a knowledge of the patient's disease, the drugs taken, the demands of the operation, and the patient's concerns to arrive at a proper choice of agent and technique. Most monitoring devices used in intensive care units today are modifications and extensions of equipment used by anesthesiologists in operating suites. Recovery rooms arose out of the need for continued individualized patient care, while today both surgical and medical intensive care units extend such attention to all critically ill patients. Blood pressure via direct or indirect recording, heart and breath sounds, blood gas analysis, central venous pressure, body temperature, and pulmonary wedge pressure commonly are measured during anesthesia and an electrocardiogram recorded, sometimes an electroencephalogram as well.

Fluid replacement during operation is supervised by the anesthesiologist, who establishes the routes of administration and the kinds of fluids given while keeping track of blood loss and therefore determining blood or blood component therapy as needed. In this sphere, consultation between surgeon and anesthesiologist is essential.

Anesthesiologists spend more time in the operating room than any other group of physicians. It is logical, therefore, that many institutions have appointed an anesthesiologist chief of the operating room, responsible for day to day scheduling and overall supervision of activities.

In the United States, prior to the introduction of tubocurarine, the principal anesthetic used was ether. Because of its stimulant effect on respiration, control of ventilation was of little importance. Cyclopropane depressed respiration in light planes of anesthesia, allowing for easier control of respiration, but failed to provide good abdominal relaxation. Tubocurarine altered all of this; with muscle relaxation came respiratory paralysis. Not only was the patient unconscious, he was unable to breathe as well. By necessity, anesthesiologists became respiratory physiologists and experts at managing ventilatory inadequacy. New mechanical ventilators were devised, monitoring equipment was introduced to ensure ventilatory exchange, and blood gas analysis was perfected. Again, such expertise could not be restricted to the operating room. Anesthesiologists began to be consulted in intensive and respiratory care units, in the care of traumatized patients and those with neurologic deficits. In many hospitals today, anesthesiologists manage respiratory and inhalation therapy services; an appreciable number are solely involved in these endeavors (see Chapters 37 and 38).

SPECIALIZED ANESTHESIA SERVICES

Some anesthetists allied with general surgical services have found the field too broad and have preferred to specialize. Although a few have elected neurosurgical or cardiothoracic involvement, others have opted for pediatric and obstetric anesthesia. Management of the critically ill child, infant, or neonate is quite a challenge, as is made evident in Chapters 24 and 25; techniques used, responses to agents, monitoring, and the rapidity with which physiologic changes take place differ from those in the adult. Only recently have anesthetists chosen to care for obstetric patients. Anesthesia remains a leading cause of maternal mortality, and fetal monitoring is a developing field (see Chapter 24). Nevertheless, the problems of pain relief during labor, opportunities for the selection of regional or general anesthesia, the anesthetic care of two lives simultaneously, neonatal resuscitation, and the not uncommon emergencies that arise all add up to a challenging and rewarding activity.

Anesthesiologists have been in the vanguard in establishing ambulatory or day care surgical services. Operations performed on an ambulatory basis minimize costs and reserve available hospital beds for the critically ill and those requiring major procedures. Anesthesiologists arrange the schedule, interview and instruct patients before the day of operation, admit and examine them, anesthetize, supervise recovery, and discharge them (see Chapter 29). Anesthesia for the outpatient is quite different from that for in-hospital care; only reasonable risks for anesthesia can be accepted, and only agents that are dissipated rapidly are administered.

Relief of pain during operations can be provided by means other than general anesthesia. Regional anesthesia, without loss of the patient's consciousness, is afforded by injection of local anesthetics either into the subarachnoid or the epidural space, in proximity to nerve trunks, or infiltrated into areas where the incision will be made. Skill with the needle need not be confined to operation. Various neurosurgical and circulatory syndromes are amenable to nerve blocks, which are of value therapeutically, diagnostically, and prognostically. Anesthesiologists have established pain clinics, evaluated the newer local anesthetics, and published detailed observations on pain and its relief. Others have been concerned with major investigations into the actions and effectiveness of opioids and their antagonists as well as analgesics, sedatives, and tranquilizers.

Every day, anesthetists face cardiorespiratory emergencies in and out of the operating room. It is only natural that they should have organized cardiopulmonary resuscitation teams in hospitals, evolved rescue and transport systems for cases of cardiac arrest and drowning, and instructed firemen, the police, and civilians in emergency procedures.

RESEARCH

The opportunities for research in anesthesia are boundless. After all, the mechanism by which general anesthetics act is still unknown, 136 years after their discovery.

Tubocurarine was a laboratory curiosity for nearly 90 years until anesthetists put it to use in clinical anesthesia. Every patient to whom anesthesia is administered presents the opportunity to record clinical observations and accumulate data, provided that the ethics of research are observed. Standard monitoring equipment is of better quality than that used in most laboratories several decades ago.

Nearly all academic departments of anesthesia support laboratories for fundamental investigations. In the two decades following World War II, most basic studies on anesthesia largely involved the respiratory or circulatory systems. Now we have moved in the direction of biochemical and metabolic research, with emphasis on the pharmacokinetics of anesthetics, enzyme induction, toxicology, and cellular and immunologic effects. There is opportunity for full-time research in anesthesia, and many departments have one or more people so engaged. Many residency programs offer one or two years of training in research techniques during the years required for board certification. Moreover, more than a few anesthesiologists spend part of their time engaged in clinical activities and the remainder either in laboratory or clinical investigation.

TEACHING

Anesthesiology bridges the gap between basic and clinical science. Of all the disciplines, it is most suited to reinforcement of information learned in the basic sciences in the context of a patient's disease. Anesthesia practice is the ideal setting in which to teach ventilatory control and adequacy of respiratory exchange, circulatory monitoring, care of the comatose, assessment of levels of consciousness, and fluid replacement. Tracheal intubation, insertion of arterial and venous cannula, and spinal tap are also logically taught on an anesthesia service. Postgraduate training in anesthesia differs from that in other fields because it must be individualized. In considering the breadth of the surgical and obstetric fields, the specialty has wide exposure to many disciplines and offers the advantage of receiving information from all. Practically all university departments of anesthesia are in need of qualified anesthesiologists who are interested in teaching and research as well as in clinical practice.

SURGEON-ANESTHETIST RELATIONS

Surgeons and anesthetists constitute a team of physicians dedicated to the welfare of the surgical patient, whose interest is best served if members of the team recognize their individual responsibilities yet remain aware of the problems faced by colleagues. The anesthetist's position on the team is clearly defined, requiring a thorough knowledge of the patient's medical history, the operation proposed, and the risks involved. The stresses placed upon the bodily systems by the contemplated anesthesia and surgical procedure must be understood. There should be discussion with the surgeon and other consultants concerning unfamiliar aspects of the patient's disease. The surgeon should be informed of the patient's progress, not by routine recitation of vital signs but by instant transmission of important information. A multitude of details which would distract the surgeon's attention from the technical problems of operation, must be constantly monitored. Care of the patient in the crucial immediate postoperative period must be closely supervised while the surgeon is engaged elsewhere.

A surgeon should consult with the anesthetist before operation and discuss the details of surgical management. It is unwise to insist upon unnecessary speed in induction of anesthesia, since this can be detrimental to the patient. A particular anesthetic or technique rarely should be demanded, as the surgeon may not know the limits of an anesthetist's capabilities or the potential for harm of certain anesthetics and techniques. Cadaveric relaxation never is needed and cannot be produced with genuine safety under any circumstance. Problems peculiar to anesthesia must be realized and time allowed for their solution. On occasion the surgeon must agree to rapid conclusion of the operation if the anesthetist believes that the patient's condition is deteriorating; development of malignant hyperthermia is a good example (see Chapter 33).

A team is at its best when its members have worked together repeatedly. It takes time for individuals to learn where they fit into the scheme of things and how associates perform their particular tasks. Good teamwork arises from mutual respect. A new member of the team must be proved worthy before acceptance on the same basis as the others.

Surgical teams work under a variety of circumstances. In most operations there should be little tension, but in difficult operations or those in which complications arise, tempers may flare and harsh words may be exchanged. The care of the patient may suffer as a result. Surgeon and anesthetist must visualize each other's predicament. Technically simple operations may be performed under trying anesthetic conditions, whereas an intricate, difficult operation may be performed without anesthetic incident. If irritability is displayed by any member of the team, the others must assess the situation and minimize friction if possible. The operating room is no place for verbal battle. Words spoken in anger can be withdrawn later on, but if the patient has suffered, irreparable damage may ensue.

Perhaps the greatest sources of conflict among anesthetists, surgeons, and operating room nurses today are delay in initiating anesthesia and excessive deliberateness in establishing anesthesia so that the surgical procedure can begin. This is especially true between operations and involves the so-called turnaround time. Any one of the three disciplines may contribute to delay, members of all three must be conscious of their part. In a world where both consumer and provider are concerned about health care costs, all members of the surgical team must realize that delay and inefficiency in the operating room contribute significantly to the costs of surgical care.

The inexperienced observer sometimes believes that the anesthetist occupies a position subordinate to that of the surgeon. This feeling often arises from lack of experience with the team performance of complex operations, although the anesthetist may contribute to subordinate status by failing to participate fully in medical care. Evidence that an anesthetist is first a physician and then a competent specialist will assure acceptance as an equal in the overall care of patients.

Confusion once existed in the minds of both surgeons and anesthetists as to medicolegal responsibility in anesthesia. Court rulings confirm that surgeons are responsible for the anesthetic only if administered by a nurse or technician under their medical direction. Anesthetics given by anesthesiologists constitute their individual legal responsibility.

One might summarize the essentials of successful surgeon-anesthetist relations as comprising mutual professional confidence, understanding, frankness, honesty, courtesy, and fair-mindedness.

APPRAISAL

Anesthesiology is now a mature specialty, but its limits have not yet been clearly defined. We are unable to fill all the academic and clinical positions available, some in eminent institutions. Because of the intimate association with so many other medical specialties, a discerning anesthetist is more likely than not to stay abreast of advances in medicine. The relationship with the basic sciences is close, perhaps more so than in other specialties. Some have charged that the practice of anesthesiology is too routine and lacks intellectual challenge. This is a matter of individual opinion, for certainly the authors of this text have not lacked for challenge. Every branch of medicine has its share of routine. How much of a pediatrician's day is spent in examining normal infants and children, in giving prophylactic injections, or in treating respiratory infections? Obstetricians deal mostly with normal women who will deliver without incident, and a day in an internist's office has more than its share of routine work. So it is with anesthesia. Most patients will be healthy and will undergo elective, uncomplicated operations, recovering from anesthesia without incident. Few specialists, however, encounter such a high ratio of stressful moments in which a wrong or a tardy decision may spell disaster.

REFERENCES

Beal JB: Surgeons and "the captain of the ship" doctrine. *In* Eckenhoff JE (ed): Controversy in Anesthesiology. Philadelphia, WB Saunders Co, 1979.

Bunker JP: The Anesthesiologist and the Surgeon. Partners in the Operating Room. Boston, Little, Brown Co., 1972.

Eckenhoff JE: Anesthesia from Colonial Times. Philadelphia, JB Lippincott Co, 1966.

Eckenhoff JE: A wide-angle view of anesthesiology. Anesthesiology 48:272, 1978.

Freeark RJ: Current relations between surgery and anesthesiology: A look at the other side. Surgery 90:565, 1981.

Greene NM: Anesthesiology and the University. Philadelphia, JB Lippincott Co, 1975.

Vandam LD: Early American anesthetists: The origins of professionalism in anesthesia: Anesthesiology 38:264, 1963.

Vandam LD: Anesthesiologists as clinicians. Anesthesiology 53:40, 1980.

Chapter 2
EDUCATION IN ANESTHESIA

Over the past two decades innovations in educational techniques, along with forces such as governmental regulations and an increasing supply of medical graduates, have led to important changes in medical education. Professional educators who describe a systematic design for teaching programs have outlined what the good teacher has always intuitively known.

1. Objectives must be explicit, attainable, and capable of being tested.

2. The student must be made aware of the goals at the outset of a program and may participate in a pretest. Appropriate tests determine whether the goals have been attained.

3. Teaching techniques must be appropriate to the material being taught.

4. Testing following completion of the program serves three purposes: to correct deficiencies in learning, to alter teaching techniques, and to certify the graduate's competence.

These principles apply equally to the training of medical students, residents, practitioners, and nurses in anesthesia. Local logistics dictate the exact form of a teaching program, so we do not pretend to prescribe an exclusive formula, rather we propose a general approach.

THE MEDICAL STUDENT

An anesthesiologist is uniquely qualified to teach the properties and clinical uses of anesthetics and adjuvants, as well as exercises in respiratory and circulatory physiology, during a student's preclinical years. Correlations between basic science and clinical medicine can be provided and a scientific but compassionate approach to the patient simultaneously inculcated. Every medical student should be trained in cardiopulmonary resuscitation (CPR); anesthesia faculty and residents are uniquely qualified to teach this exercise. The American Heart Association defines cognitive and motor goals for courses in CPR and uses a progressive program of teaching and testing, which can serve as a model for academic teaching programs. We teach CPR to all incoming students during orientation week and advanced life support at the end of the second year.

In the clinical years students receive a brief required course (one to two weeks) that presents material pertinent to anesthesiology but equally relevant to all physicians, regardless of specialization. This includes care of the unconscious patient; airway maintenance; recognition and treatment of ventilatory and circulatory failure; proper use of sedatives and opioids; techniques of monitoring and placement of intravenous, intra-arterial, and central venous catheters; the techniques and hazards of lumbar puncture; and the application of pharmacokinetic principles to the rational use of intravenous drugs. As most students do not plan on careers in anesthesiology, the goals should be stated in terms relevant to all physicians; frequent mention of problems confronted beyond the operating room helps to maintain student interest. Senior anesthesia residents may well act as instructors for this course, as programmed instruction in teaching techniques improves their performance as teachers and maintains an interest in teaching. A simple test at the end of the course identifies strengths and weaknesses of the program and whether the goals of the course have been reached.

For students with special interests, whether in anesthesia, surgery, or a related field, more extensive elective courses in anesthesia are offered (four to ten weeks). With appropriate emphasis, these students may participate in the course of instruction offered beginning residents: the ability to perform a simple preoperative evaluation and to safely administer an anesthetic to a healthy patient for an uncomplicated operation. Time spent in more specialized areas, such as obstetric or pediatric anesthesia, or an intensive care or cardiac surgical unit enlarges the student's appreciation of the specialty, as does attendance at scheduled anesthesia conferences.

THE RESIDENT AND THE CRNA

OBJECTIVES

Trainees in anesthesiology seek to acquire a body of facts (perhaps, at first, too extensive for one person to master), habits of study that will serve well in the future, a set of attitudes reflected in a salutary behavior toward patients and colleagues, and finally the skills necessary to practice the specialty. Listing these goals in detail at the beginning of training facilitates both learning and testing; if goals are not apparent the resident must guess what to do to satisfy the anesthesia faculty. A relevant statement comes from the American Board of Anesthesiology (ABA).

One of the major concerns of the American Board of Anesthesiology is the certification of competent anesthesiologists. The Board believes it timely to present the criteria on which its judgment of competence is based. These include:
1. Technical facility. Facility in providing all technical services likely to be required in the practice of the specialty.
2. Medical judgment. Ready availability of mature medical judgment applicable to solution of medical problems associated with a patient's care as they arise in the practice of the specialty.
3. Scholarship. The talent, training and habits of study necessary for evaluating and applying appropriately new knowledge.
4. For the present the Board accepts the definition of anesthesiology as submitted to the United States Department of Labor, recognizing that this definition is likely to change with time:
   "Anesthesiology is a practice of medicine dealing with: (1) the management of procedures for rendering a patient insensible to pain during surgical operations; (2) the support of life functions under the stress of anesthetic and surgical manipulations; (3) the clinical management of the patient unconscious from whatever cause; (4) the management of problems in pain relief; (5) the management of problems in cardiac and respiratory resuscitation; (6) the application of specific methods of inhalational therapy; (7) the clinical management of various fluid, electrolyte, and metabolic disturbances."

Broad statements such as these do not meet all the needs of teacher or student, as they do not promote the design of either tests or teaching methods. A limited but more specific statement of goals is contained in the content outline of the *In Training Examination of the ABA and American Society of Anesthesiologists* (available from ASA).

Much less has been done to define the specifics of attitudes and noncognitive skills. Checklists describing the proper performance of spinal anesthesia or CVP catheter placement have improved both learning and testing. Anesthetists in training discern attitudes by observing the attending staff who serve as role models; well-defined lists of behavioral objectives are uncommon. Nonetheless, a potential for harm exists in listing objectives. Student and teacher must realize that personally motivated education never ceases, extending beyond mastery of limited sets of objectives; such lists should not stifle the growth of the individual or the specialty.

TESTING PROCEDURES

The practices of professional educators have been applied to testing in medical education; examinations have become more definitive, more related to realistic goals, and more likely to seek out reasoning ability rather than pure recall of facts. Testing of knowledge in anesthesia has improved recently with the advent of the ABA/ASA In Training Examination; a subset of these questions constitutes the written phase of the ABA examination. This test, based on objectives described in the content outline, is taken by residents at all levels of training. Both the score and an inventory of incorrect answers are returned to the examinee and to the teaching program for future mutual guidance. A subsequent oral examination probes areas of judgment not readily revealed through written exercises.

Just as the goals for attitudes and noncognitive skills are poorly defined, so is their evaluation. Certification of competence in these areas now depends on evaluation by the candidate's individual training program. Some useful techniques for examining practical skills have been described: self-assessment via videotape, use of checklists, and the establishing of outcome criteria for procedures. However, judgments concerning residents' attitudes are open to bias; methods such as criterion-referenced evaluation, in which resident behavior is compared with well-defined standards, may add a degree of objectivity.

TEACHING TECHNIQUES

Anesthesia residents learn from many sources: teaching in the operating room; independent study of texts, journals, audiovisual materials, computer–assisted programmed learning and the like; didactic programs such as lectures, seminars, conferences, and professional meetings. An approved teaching program incorporates all these in proper measure.

Supervision during anesthesia must ensure the patient's safety as the first concern, while simultaneously enhancing skills and attitudes, a difficult assignment at best. Instructors must be both experienced and competent, mindful of patient and surgeon, sensitive to residents' needs and emotions, in control of their own attitudes, and able to maintain their interest in teaching and learning despite the daily demands and stresses of the operating room. Good lectures can be recorded, good bedside teaching cannot; the wisdom of a bedside teacher is more elusive than that of a lecturer. The methods of instruction noted here place an equal burden on the resident, who must maintain a good demeanor and continue to learn despite being a novice and an urge to conceal a lack of skill from the patient and the scrutiny of the surgeon. Both instructor and pupil should exercise tact to permit learning to proceed under operating-room conditions. Obviously the situation is similar on both sides of the anesthesia screen, with some surgeons and anesthetists unwilling to be involved in instruction.

Good operating-room teaching extends beyond a simple apprentice-master relation, for an integrated program of study with clearly stated objectives is required. Instructor and resident should discuss problem cases beforehand to evolve a plan for conduct of the anesthesia in the individual patient. Increasing specialization in anesthesia requires a corps of teachers, implying that specialty rotations are essential in obstetric, neurosurgical, cardiac, regional, and pediatric anesthesia, as well as intensive care, to cite several.

No didactic or bedside program can substitute for independent study, which comprises the core of education — the most effective method of acquiring the limitless knowledge relating to anesthesiology. Study is based on current and recent volumes of relevant journals, introductory texts, major reference works, selections from the many monographs on specific subjects, and locally contrived teaching materials. The resident is well advised to make the investment necessary to acquire a personal library early in a training program. A departmental library houses not only relevant books, journals, and audiovisual aids but facilities for photocopying and literature searches.

A teaching program should guide the resident in the orderly study of available materials in connection with stated objectives, as well as providing the necessary time for study. Residents should not work for so many hours in an operating room that they cannot attend lectures or seminars and do not have the interest or the energy required for study.

A didactic program consists of an organized lecture series, including an introductory program for new residents, visiting professors, seminars, programs organized by residents as well as faculty, and finally case discussions. Regularly held morbidity and mortality conferences offer residents the opportunity to profit from the misadventures of others, so that each resident is not obliged to experience every possible error. The didactic content of the subspecialties is best taught during subspecialty rotations, reserving department-wide lectures for topics of broader interest.

Lectures have garnered a bad reputation largely because they are so often poorly executed. A good lecture should not transmit information already available in texts, journals, or monographs but should provide new information or present the old in a novel manner. Senior department faculty should teach their colleagues how to lecture, audit their performances, and provide constructive criticism. A lecture should incorporate objectives as in any teaching exercise so that all involved are able to judge their success or failure.

Success in teaching depends on competent instructors. Too often medical teaching is viewed as an obligation imposed on faculty. The rewards to many seem limited to self-satisfaction and the manifest esteem of students and peers; many a teacher believes that there is little return in the way of promotion or financial gain in teaching. Teaching programs of the kind outlined here require that there be both organized programs of instruction in teaching methods and a means of recognition and reward for teaching.

COUNSELING AND GUIDANCE

When the numbers of faculty and residents are large, counseling and guidance programs for residents should replace the close relations possible only in smaller departments. A project of this sort must reach residents early so that impediments to learning are not compounded and discovered only when the resident nears completion of training. Counseling may be needed by a resident who fails to make progress, who experiences financial problems, who has difficulty in dealing with patients or staff, or who is ensnared in personal hardship or is undecided in a career choice.

THE PRACTITIONER

Although continuing medical education programs offered to practicing anesthetists steadily increase in number, they remain rudimentary. Most programs providing pre-

and post-teaching, recertification, home study with evaluation, audiovisual aids, programmed learning, lectures, workshops, and refresher courses offer promise but lack direction and, often, satisfaction afterward. There are no articulated educational objectives, no agreed upon procedures for evaluating practice, and consequently no educational program upon which either anesthetist or society can rely to guarantee competence.

There is much to be learned upon completion of formal training. New drugs, new techniques, recent basic science information, and important advances in related clinical fields must be integrated into the body of knowledge needed to practice contemporary and safe anesthesia. In this respect the individual must be self-reliant. Lifelong study habits, with regular reference to journals and texts, careful selection of educational programs based on the quality and reputation of instructors, and an inquiring mind willing to analyze problem cases and discuss them with colleagues, constitute the foundations of continuing education.

REFERENCES

American Board of Anesthesiology: Quality anesthesia care: a model of future practice of anesthesiology. Anesthesiology 47:488, 1977.
Miller, GE: Educating Medical Teachers. Cambridge, Harvard University Press, 1980.
Segall, AJ, Vanderschmidt H, Burglass R, Frostman T: Systematic Course Design for the Health Fields. New York, Wiley, 1975.

Section 1
PRELIMINARY CONSIDERATIONS

Chapter 3
PREANESTHETIC CONSULTATION AND CHOICE OF ANESTHESIA

At one time the crucial phase of a surgical illness was thought to be the operation — the chance of survival depending on the patient's response to anesthesia. A question often posed was whether a patient in poor physical condition could tolerate the anesthetic; this concern has now undergone modification. Anesthesia is still of major importance, to be given with skill and good judgment, but it is the quality of pre- and postanesthetic care that largely determines whether the outcome will be satisfactory. This overall approach to anesthesia has led to a decrease in the number of intraoperative complications and a reduction in postoperative morbidity and mortality despite the extremes of age and the greater severity of disease in patients coming to operation.

Participation by anesthetists in preparation of patients for operation improves the outcome because they are knowledgeable in the pathophysiology of disease as it pertains to the action of anesthetics. Anesthetists must establish their reputations with the expectation that they will be asked to consult on operability and to help prepare the patient for the procedure. The attitude that these are "their" patients goes a long way toward dispelling the notion that anesthetists lack responsibility in patient care. Surgeons and referring physicians should avail themselves of anesthetists' advice and should acquaint them with specific aspects of the illness as well as the procedure planned.

GUIDELINES FOR THE PREANESTHETIC VISIT

Every patient should be seen by an anesthetist before operation. For this reason patients should be admitted to the hospital early enough to permit a complete examination. Past and present hospital records should be reviewed with attention focused on prior experiences and the physiologic alterations induced by disease. The ability to tolerate the adverse effects of anesthesia and operation depends largely on the normality of respiration and circulation, and the homeostatic functions of the liver, kidneys, endocrines, and central nervous system.

There is no substitute for talking to patients, listening to their problems, and acquainting them with the procedure planned. Thus, the visit is a subtle educational process for both patient and anesthetist; the patient learns what anesthesia has to offer, and if misconceptions exist they can be dispelled. The interview should be unhurried and tactful; if the patient is eating or receiving special therapy it is better to return at another time. If visitors are present they should be asked to leave before the examination.

If a patient has not yet been informed of the decision to operate, anesthesia can be described as though it were to take place in the future. It is best to avoid discussing matters in the surgeon's domain. Questioning should proceed along lines of past anesthetic experiences, familial problems with anesthetics, routine use of drugs, and unusual reactions to drugs and the concurrent illness (see Chapter 4).

While assessing the patient's emotional state, one should look for physical characteristics that may cause technical difficulties during anesthesia. The individual with a short, stout neck readily develops respiratory obstruction once unconscious; the athlete requires more medication than the asthenic. If there are loose or carious teeth or delicate dental work, the patient should be warned that dislodgement or damage may occur upon airway insertion, and a note to that effect should be written on the chart. Patients should be told to remove dentures and leave them in their rooms so that they will not be broken or misplaced.

The anesthetist should perform those elements of a physical examination deemed necessary. Simple tests of pulmonary function may be done and reserves of the cardiopulmonary system ascertained by questioning the patient about tolerance to exercise. A patient may be asked to walk in the corridor or up a flight of stairs to detect shortness of breath or claudication. In a patient with a history of myocardial infarction, presence or absence of angina pectoris provides an essential but not always conclusive index of sufficiency of coronary blood flow. Adequacy of digitalization can be determined by counting the pulse after exercise; a rise in rate from 72 to 120 beats per minute as a result of walking 20 to 30 feet suggests the need for a higher dose. A history of palpitation or the appearance of premature atrial or ventricular beats or left bundle block on the electrocardiogram may be the only clue to myocardial disease. If regional anesthesia is planned it is essential to inspect and palpate the site selected for injection of spinal or caudal anesthesia. It helps to test the effect of the operative position on circulation and respiration; for example, the arthritic patient may not tolerate the lithotomy position.

Once the preliminaries are over, the patient is told of the plans for anesthesia. Reactions will vary; some patients will accede readily, whereas others who fear the face mask or needle puncture will wish to be unconscious before going to the operating room. Still others will be concerned about postoperative vomiting or pain. Many object to spinal anesthesia, having heard that headache or paralysis may follow. Explanation and reassurance usually settle most of these problems, but the anesthetist should not be unyielding in choice of agent or technique. Finally, a plan is selected in the patient's best interest, bearing in mind the surgeon's needs. Most patients accept a physician's advice when confidence is inspired.

Special examinations and laboratory work should be carried out when necessary. If the patient has been admitted to the hospital late in the afternoon it may be necessary to wait until the morning of operation for a complete record, but there should be no compromise in quality even at this late time.

Patients should have a good night's sleep. They should be told when medications will be given and warned not to eat or drink during the six to eight hours preceding anesthesia; the reasons for this should be made explicit. The time and manner of transport to the operating room should be discussed, as well as the plan for postoperative observation in the recovery or intensive care area.

When the anesthetist leaves the patient, preliminary data are recorded on the anesthesia chart, a physical status category assigned, preanesthetic orders written, and a note made in the patient's record summarizing the results of the visit and the proposed anesthetic management. From a medicolegal point of view, this summary is more meaningful than a signed anesthesia permit, although an operative permit must be signed, particularly for minors and those incompetent to make judgments. Anesthetists in training should discuss their plans with the supervising anesthetist.

Anesthetists should develop enough judgment of their own to make a surgical diagnosis and to predict the effect of the surgical position and operation on physiologic processes. Occasionally an operation must be postponed, as when the patient has contracted a respiratory infection or digitalization is inadequate. Rarely should there be disagreement over the proper preparation of a patient for operation. On the other hand, standard practice may have to be abandoned in an emergency. Operation may be necessary even though a full stomach or an exceptionally low hematocrit reading would otherwise dictate delay. Immediate operation is the primary resuscitative measure in uncontrolled hemorrhage, rapidly increasing intracranial pressure, or a perforated viscus. We believe that an anesthetist can hardly ever refuse to give anesthesia if surgical opinion suggests that immediate operation offers a patient the best chance for survival.

PHYSICAL STATUS AND RISK

Questions are often raised concerning the chance of survival or the risk involved in undergoing anesthesia. The disparity in statistics on anesthetic-related deaths arises in part from the difficulty in defining death caused by anesthesia and in making a distinction between the effects of the patient's disease, the operation, and the anesthetic. From the standpoint of the individual, "risk" encompasses many variables. In addition to factors already mentioned, risk might involve the technical skills of the anesthetist or surgeon, socioeconomic factors in the home or hospital environment, extremes of atmospheric conditions, or duration of operation. Too often a patient is called a "poor risk" only after a catastrophe has taken place; this may represent a conscious or subconscious effort on the part of the physician to conceal errors in diagnosis or management. From a statistical or prognostic standpoint, therefore, the term "risk" is untenable, and improvement in patient care does not lie in attempting to establish the degree of risk.

One solution to the problem is found by categorizing the relative physical condition of the patient as representing a constant among the many variables of the surgical experience. For example, when physical status is quantified, prognosis and evaluation of therapy for heart disease are aided immeasurably by a functional classification. Thus, the classification of the American Heart Association has relevance to anesthetic problems. Such a classification is helpful in designating the resilience or reserves of the cardiac patient approaching operation, but it does not quite apply to other types of disease. For the purposes of anesthesia, therefore, the classification of physical status adopted by the American Society of Anesthesiologists is most useful. This is a practical system based on the presence of disease, but it suffers from a lack of scientific precision. Much inconsistency is found in ratings supplied by anesthetists.

Class 1. The patient has no organic, physiologic, biochemical, or psychiatric disturbance. The pathologic process for which operation is to be performed is localized and does not entail a systemic disturbance. Examples: a fit patient with inguinal hernia; fibroid uterus in an otherwise healthy woman.

Class 2. Mild to moderate systemic disturbance caused either by the condition to be treated surgically or by other pathophysiologic processes. Examples: non- or only slightly limiting organic heart disease, mild diabetes, essential hypertension, or anemia. Some might choose to list the extremes of age here, either the neonate or the octogenarian, even though no discernible systemic disease is present. Extreme obesity and chronic bronchitis may be included in this category.

Class 3. Severe systemic disturbance or disease from whatever cause, even though it may not be possible to define the degree of disability with finality. Examples: severely limiting organic heart disease; severe diabetes with vascular complications; moderate to severe degrees of pulmonary insufficiency; angina pectoris or healed myocardial infarction.

Class 4. Severe systemic disorders that are already life-threatening, not always correctable by operation. Examples: patients with organic heart disease showing marked signs of cardiac insufficiency, persistent anginal syndrome, or active myocarditis; advanced degrees of pulmonary, hepatic, renal, or endocrine insufficiency.

Class 5. The moribund patient who has little chance of survival but is submitted to operation in desperation. Examples: the burst abdominal aneurysm with profound shock; major cerebral trauma with rapidly increasing intracranial pressure; massive pulmonary embolus. Most of these patients require operation as a resuscitative measure with little if any anesthesia.

Emergency Operation (E). Any patient in one of the classes listed previously who is operated on as an emergency is considered to be in poorer physical condition. The letter E is placed beside the numerical classification. Thus, the patient with a hitherto uncomplicated hernia now incarcerated and associated with nausea and vomiting is classified as 1E.

Although there may be problems in assigning the appropriate physical status (usually because of the implications of the operation to be performed), an estimate should be made in every instance. Other factors being equal, one might anticipate that the patient with poor physical status would not fare as well as the patient in good condition. The role of physical status in relation to anesthesia mortality as found in several studies is shown in Table 3–1. Similar experiences have been reported by anesthesia commissions — groups formed on a voluntary basis to investigate the causes of anesthetic death. Almost as a rule, death in the better physical categories was deemed preventable from the standpoint of anesthetic management. Several reports also suggest that intraoperative cardiac arrest is more frequent in the poorer physical status categories.

Physical status, therefore, provides us with a common language and a method of examining anesthetic morbidity and mortality. Here is a means of assessing the relative safety of new techniques or anesthetics on an unchanging background of the patient's physical competence. A poor classification should alert the surgical team to employ greater safeguards. Lastly, physical status provides a means whereby one anesthetist's experience can be compared with others against a common background.

TABLE 3–1. Anesthesia Mortality (Primary and Contributory) and Physical Status *

Authors	Total Anesthetic Deaths	Percentage of All Anesthetic Deaths by Physical Status Class					Incidence by Physical Status Class				
		1	2	3	4	5	1	2	3	4	5
Beecher and Todd	384	56			44		1:2,426		1:599		
Edwards et al†	586	17	21	46	16						
Dripps et al	80	0	15	34	41	10	0	1:1,013	1:151	1:22	1:11
Boba and Landmesser†	44 (cardiac arrests)	32			68						
Clifton and Hotten†	52	33			67						
Memery†	64	5	19	44	23	9					

*Reprinted with permission from Goldstein A Jr, Keats AS: The risk of anesthesia. Anesthesiology 33:130, 1970.

†Breakdown of total population at risk not available.

EXAMPLES OF PREANESTHETIC CONSULTATION NOTES

A well-written consultation note provides instruction for all involved, likewise serving to illustrate the anesthetist's concern regarding all phases of the patient's illness.

Physical Status 1E.   First admission to hospital for this 16-year-old unmarried woman with complaint of profuse vaginal bleeding. Several episodes of pneumonia in infancy but no other major illnesses. She has not had anesthesia before, takes no drugs, and knows of no allergy to medications either familial or personal. She last ate and drank about ten hours prior to admission. On examination she is anxious, blood pressure 110/80, pulse 96, temperature 37°C. No airway problem. Teeth in good repair. Heart and lungs normal on percussion and auscultation. Urine shows many red blood cells. Hematocrit 29 per cent, BUN 11 mg per 100 ml, and blood glucose 122 mg per 100 ml. Chest x-ray normal. Physical status 1E. Immediate dilation of cervix and evacuation of uterus contemplated. Plan: induce anesthesia with thiopental followed by nitrous oxide by mask and meperidine (Demerol) intravenously as supplement. Patient accepts plan. Operation and anesthesia permits have been signed by mother. Please crossmatch two units of blood.

Physical Status 3.   Fourth admission to hospital of this 73-year-old woman with massive hematemesis ten days before admission followed by weakness and lethargy. Prior admissions for saphenous vein ligation, performed with spinal anesthesia, and for urinary tract infection and hematemesis. Other operations include tonsillectomy and adenoidectomy, appendectomy, and ovarian cystectomy many years ago; anesthesia tolerated well. On last admission diagnosis of Laennec's cirrhosis of liver made and esophageal varices demonstrated by barium swallow. Heavy alcohol intake for years, does not smoke, and knows of no drug allergy. Present medications include digitalis leaf daily, iron for anemia, and Maalox. Weight steady at 67 kg. She becomes short of breath after one flight of stairs. Prominent family history of arteriosclerotic heart disease. During the ten days in the hospital the following studies are of note: hematocrit, at first 31 per cent, has risen to 38 per cent with transfusion of whole blood and packed RBC; BUN 50 mg per 100 ml; urine loaded with RBC. Intravenous pyelogram showed slight bilateral decrease in dye density; total protein within normal limits; LDH 264 U per ml; SGOT 20 U per ml; bilirubin 1.5 to 2.0 mg per 100 ml; ECG normal sinus rhythm, left ventricular hypertrophy, no changes since prior tracing. Chest x-ray compatible with mild obstructive lung disease.

She is obese, somewhat anxious. Blood pressure 180/80, pulse 96, temperature 37.0°C. No airway problem. Mouth edentulous. Distant breath sounds, no rales. Heart not easily percussed. At apex and base, grade II over VI systolic murmurs, former transmitted to left sternal border. Liver 7 cm below costal margin, spleen just palpable. Neurologic examination normal.

Anesthesia problems in this woman for portacaval shunt: arteriosclerotic, cardiac, and renal disease, probable aortic stenosis, well compensated on digitalis. Borderline liver failure with corrected anemia. Obesity and possible pulmonary emphysema. Physical status 3. She will do best with light general anesthesia with nitrous oxide–oxygen (at most 2:1) and thiopental supplemented by tubocurarine. She accepts this plan, and consent is granted. Management: tracheal intubation, followed by controlled respiration; monitor blood pressure, pulse, respiration, central venous pressure, pulmonary artery wedge pressure, urine output, and body temperature. Give warm intravenous fluids and blood. Crossmatch about 10 units and have several units of fresh blood available. Very likely postoperative ventilatory assistance will be necessary. Continue to measure blood gases and to monitor progress as intraoperatively.

CHOICE OF ANESTHESIA

The evolution of anesthetic practice is mirrored in the present-day choice of agents and techniques. Originally the choice was among ether, nitrous oxide, and chloroform, given with simple devices. It is remarkable that ether lasted until modern times and that nitrous oxide is at present the most frequently used inhalation anesthetic. A second phase was marked by the introduction of cocaine, then procaine (Novocain) for regional anesthesia, most techniques in use today having been developed at the turn of the century. Synthesis of new inhalation agents, notably cyclopropane, and discovery of the short-acting barbiturates for intravenous use marked the 1930s. At this time the practice arose of giving combinations of agents in a "balanced" technique, each agent for a specific purpose — regional anesthesia for analgesia and muscle relaxation, thiopental intravenously for loss of consciousness, and an inhalant for maintenance of unconsciousness. Neuromuscular blocking agents added another dimension, providing muscle paralysis, whereas pain was relieved with nitrous oxide and opioids and unconsciousness was afforded by thiopental. Artificial hibernation and neuroleptanalgesia are modifications of balanced anesthesia. The provision of deliberate hypotension or hypothermia offers certain advantages in addition to the main anesthetic techniques. Over the last 20 years new halogenated hydrocarbons have come upon the scene — nonflammable halothane (Fluothane) and methoxyflurane (Penthrane), and slightly flammable fluroxene (Fluoromar). Although halothane survives, methoxyflurane is rarely used today, and fluroxene is no longer manufactured. The most recent additions are enflurane (Ethrane) and isoflurane (Forane).

An anesthetist skilled in a variety of techniques and well versed in the pharmacology of anesthesia can solve the problem of choice of anesthesia in many ways. But choice is dictated by several considerations: the patient as an individual (age, prior anesthetic experience, and complicating disease); the operation to be performed; the habits and experience of the surgeon; and the position required for the procedure. Thus it is illogical to state categorically that there is only one agent or technique for a specific situation. This does not imply that there are not definite contraindications to some methods of management (see chapters on agents and techniques). An ancillary concern is the avoidance of an agent or technique that could unjustifiably be implicated if a complication were to arise; for example, not using halothane when blood levels of liver enzymes are elevated.

THE PATIENT

If a patient has had a bad experience with anesthesia in the past, this will be evident in the reaction to the suggested choice of anesthesia. Not infrequently, relatives of the patient will have opinions on anesthetic choice contrary to those of the anesthetist, thus influencing the patient's response. In these situations analysis of the reasons for the choice, presented in a confident manner, usually saves the day. Nevertheless, a patient's preference ought to be considered. The law, under the doctrine of assault, dictates against imposing the anesthetist's will on a patient.

Emotional status must be taken into account in planning for anesthesia. Almost all patients have some degree of anxiety; the nature and extent of these feelings must be evaluated. A woman emerging from anesthesia following the performance of biopsy for possible cancer often shows agitation or delirium because of preoperative apprehension. In some, emotional instability or apprehension may require heavy premedication, which can predispose to circulatory and respiratory depression intra- and postoperatively. Under trying emotional conditions intravenous induction of anesthesia is preferred, as is avoidance of regional techniques. Even in the stolid person, a long operative procedure for which regional anesthesia can provide good pain relief may be quite trying.

Certain pathophysiologic changes justify exclusion of specific agents or techniques. For example, choosing to avoid the pharmacologic action of an anesthetic that could enhance an underlying abnormality, one might avoid halothane in the presence of increased intracranial pressure because of the cerebrovascular dilation produced. When coronary arteriosclerosis is present, addition of epinephrine to a local anesthetic solution can increase the work of the heart.

Body habitus must be considered. The asthenic, elderly, or chronically ill generally require minimal anesthesia. Conversely, the robust often need sustained higher concentrations of anesthetics. The obese patient presents special problems. Among other things, pulmonary ventilation will require careful attention because the short, thick-necked, obese individual readily develops soft tissue airway obstruction and may require tracheal intubation even for a minor operation.

Elsewhere we shall touch upon other matters that influence choice of anesthesia, such as drug therapy and physical status. It is worthwhile, however, at this point to delve deeper into the matter of complicating disease.

Circulatory Abnormalities

In general, the goals during anesthesia are to avoid an increase in myocardial irritability that can result in tachyarrhythmias and to prevent serious degrees of circulatory depression, both leading to hypotension and even cardiac arrest. These aims entail a comprehension of circulatory abnormalities already present, knowledge of the drugs used in the treatment of heart disease, and a thorough understanding of the circulatory effects of anesthetics. The rule has always been to ensure adequate oxygenation, elimination of carbon dioxide, and maintenance of a safe blood pressure. But a modest decrease in the mean arterial pressure will decrease the afterload and the work of the heart, thereby lessening oxygen consumption, whereas an increase in pulse rate and myocardial inotropic action also increases heart work and the demand for oxygen. Therefore, during anesthesia, an appropriate balance must be struck between avoiding a low blood pressure and avoiding those factors that increase the myocardial need for oxygen.

Respiratory Insufficiency

Respiratory abnormalities, arising at either the central or peripheral level, raise the possibility of the development of respiratory failure when anesthetics are superimposed. Commonly encountered pulmonary problems are bronchitis, bronchospastic states, emphysema, and restrictive defects. Central depression of respiration owing to intracranial disease, carbon dioxide retention, or drugs may be encountered as well as neuromuscular disability secondary to poliomyelitis, muscular dystrophy, myasthenia gravis, arthritis, or kyphoscoliosis. With the resulting diminution in pulmonary function and the relative inefficiency of defense mechanisms, alveolar ventilation and cough, patients with these problems are highly susceptible to development of postoperative atelectasis and bronchopneumonia. The approach to these problems is more or less as follows: tests of pulmonary function and determination of blood gas values preoperatively to define the extent of respiratory insufficiency; treatment of bronchospasm and infection by eliminating smoking and use of bronchodilating drugs with intermittent positive pressure breathing (IPPB); practice for the patient in pulmonary physiotherapy; and administration of antibiotics for known infection. IPPB serves to accustom the patient to the kinds of postoperative treatment given to encourage deep breathing and cough. Several days or more are required to arrive at full benefit when lung disease is severe. Opioids should be avoided because of diminution in the respiratory response to carbon dioxide and depression of cough. During anesthesia, controlled ventilation is carried out to maintain gas exchange as indicated by repeated blood gas analyses. Postoperatively, a stir-up regimen of deep breathing and physiotherapy is used, particularly if opioids are required for relief of pain. If inadequate pulmonary exchange is found, tracheal intubation and assisted or controlled ventilation are continued until a patient can be weaned from this regimen.

Liver Disease

The many homeostatic functions of the liver are readily influenced by anesthetics through their effects on splanchnic blood flow, their potentially hepatotoxic properties, and the role of the liver in biotransformation of anesthetic compounds, Parenchymatous disease must be severe before influencing biotransformation of drugs such as the short-acting barbiturates, succinylcholine (Anectine), and opioids. Acute stages of serum or infectious hepatitis, terminal phases of portal or biliary cirrhosis, advanced hemochromatosis, and extensive replacement of the liver by primary or metastatic neoplasms are associated with a high surgical death rate.

Thus, maximal improvement in liver function should be sought preoperatively. In portal cirrhosis, for example, prothrombin and serum albumin should at least be at minimally acceptable levels, as should liver function tests — Bromsulphalein excretion, alkaline phosphatase, plasma cholinesterase, and serum glutamic oxalic transaminase (SGOT), to mention just a few that are used as guidelines. Drugs used to treat the liver failure of cirrhosis (e.g., cortisone and neomycin), as noted elsewhere, may complicate anesthetic administration.

Kidney Disease

Excretion of anesthetic drugs and their metabolites by the kidney and its role in acid-base and water metabolism are essential considerations in anesthetic management. In a patient with minimal renal reserves, compounds excreted by the kidneys — the long-acting barbiturates, gallamine (Flaxedil), and succinylcholine given by constant infusion — are best avoided. Problems have been encountered in the reversal of the actions of pancuronium (Pavulon) given in the presence of renal failure. Before the era of hemodialysis, which maintains the patient with renal failure in a reasonable state of biochemical balance, such patients presented a formidable array of problems: high serum potassium levels, low sodium and calcium, metabolic acidosis, and increased susceptibility to infection. Drugs used to treat these conditions added to the problems of anesthesia — antihypertensive medications, digitalis, antibiotics, and cortisone. In preparation for nephrectomy or renal transplantation, chronic dialysis returns physiologic and biochemical abnormalities toward normal values, and the risks of anesthesia and operation are consequently lessened. But optimal conditions must be attained before operation. Starting with a borderline high serum potassium level, from 5.5 to 6.0 mEq per liter, several events during anesthesia may elevate potassium levels to the point of cardiac standstill or ventricular fibrillation: use of succinylcholine with attendant release of potassium; transfusion of large volumes of cold bank blood of low pH and high serum potassium; and use of sympathomimetic drugs. Hypoxia, hypercarbia, and low flow states also add to the K^+ load. Low flow states with concomitant blood transfusion or release of myoglobin from traumatized tissues and the use of sympathomimetic drugs that cause renal vasoconstriction predispose to postoperative acute tubular necrosis or vasoconstrictive nephropathy.

Endocrine Disease

Each endocrine abnormality calls for a specific anesthetic approach, problems becoming more complicated as new hormones are discovered (aldosterone, angiotensin, 5-hydroxytryptamine [serotonin], prostaglandins). Further, certain neoplasms may exhibit endocrine activity. Carcinoma of the lung or thyrotoxicosis may be accompanied by a myasthenic state; in a few instances new growths have been shown to secrete adrenocorticotropic hormone (ACTH). Diseases of the pituitary-adrenal axis may require correction of electrolyte imbalance, replacement therapy with steroids, and the use of nonstressful anesthetics. Although thyrotoxicosis can now be controlled by specific therapy affecting the release of thyroxine at one of several levels, the possibility of thyroid storm calls for elimination of atropine as a preanesthetic medication. Resection of a pheochromocytoma is now approached with alpha- and beta-adrenergic blocking drugs on hand and the prior use of alpha blockers to correct the known plasma volume deficit. Choice of anesthesia in this disease entails use of nonautonomic stimulating agents.

APPRAISAL

In this chapter we have sketchily depicted the many facets of the preanesthetic visit to patients: how best to approach the patient, how to categorize physical status, and how to write a consultation note. Using as background the information thus obtained, the anesthetist must then take into account complicating ailments, particularly those involving the vital organs and homeostatic systems, when determining the choice of anesthesia. As experience is gained the anesthetist will find that the preanesthetic visit, above all else, sets the stage for a safe course both before and after operation.

REFERENCES

American Society of Anesthesiologists: New classification of physical status. Anesthesiology 24:111, 1963.
Goldstein A, Jr, Keats AS: The risk of anesthesia. Anesthesiology 33:130, 1970.
Keats AS: What do we know about anesthetic mortality? Anesthesiology 50:387, 1979.
Vandam LD (ed): To Make the Patient Ready for Anesthesia: Medical Care of the Surgical Patient. Menlo Park, CA, Addison-Wesley Publishing Co., 1980.

Chapter 4
PHARMACOLOGIC PRINCIPLES AND DRUG INTERACTIONS

During preoperative visits, it is common to discover that patients are taking drugs either prescribed for medical conditions or purchased over the counter. Development of a rational plan for anesthesia requires that the anesthetist understand the actions of these drugs, the pathophysiology of the diseases for which they are given, and how these drugs interact with anesthetics and adjuvants such as neuromuscular blocking agents. In this chapter, drug uptake, biotransformation, and excretion will be reviewed, followed by consideration of concurrent drug therapies of interest. Figure 4–1 provides an overview of the pharmacokinetic phases.

BASIC PHARMACOLOGIC PRINCIPLES

DRUG UPTAKE

Uptake is influenced by route of administration, tissue blood flow, physical-chemical factors such as molecular size and ionization, binding by proteins in plasma and tissues, and availability of "receptors" at target cells. The uptake and distribution of inhaled and intravenous anesthetics are discussed in Chapters 11 and 14. Uptake entails delivery of an agent to the circulation, a process that occurs instantaneously when the drug is given intravenously and quite rapidly when an aqueous solution is injected intramuscularly. Oral and rectal absorptions are slower and less predictable.

The vehicle in which the drug is dissolved relates to its solubility, relevant in absorption from any site but of particular importance for drugs given orally. Volume and acidity of gastric juice may alter absorption. Some drugs are precipitated in acid solution and are thereby absorbed slowly; others dissolve more easily at low pH. The presence of food slows absorption of most drugs but improves absorption of lipid-soluble drugs taken with fatty foods. Drugs are also absorbed from the intestine and bowel, with motility governing the rate of delivery to absorption sites and, in irritable states, limiting absorption. High concentration favors absorption, but circulation to the site must be adequate for the process.

Once in the circulation, regardless of route of administration, the drug molecule behaves according to principles dictated by structure. The compound may exist in a free state, but most drugs are inactivated functionally to some extent by plasma protein binding, principally to plasma albumin. Once attached to a large protein molecule in the circulation, drugs are unable to reach extravascular target cells. Binding is influenced by pH; the higher pH is above the isoelectric point of the protein molecule, the more negative the net charge on that molecule. This is the principle underlying serum electrophoresis, wherein proteins migrate in an electric field at pH 8.8. With an isoelectric point of 4.7, albumin travels farthest because its charge is most negative at this pH, whereas gamma globulin migrates little since its isoelectric point is near pH 7.0. At the pH of blood, 7.4, albumin has a negative charge, greater than that of other proteins; drugs with a positive charge are thereby protein bound. Nonelectrostatic binding also may occur as a result of covalency or van der Waals' forces, perhaps accounting for binding of pancuronium to gamma globulins.

Ionization of a drug is likewise important not only in protein binding but also in determining lipid solubility and speed in crossing cell membranes. Most drugs are weak electrolytes present in aqueous solution in ionized and non-ionized forms, the proportions depending upon the pH of the solution, the pK_a of the drug, and whether the drug is an acid or base. The relationship is defined by the Henderson-Hasselbalch equation:

$$pH = pK_a + \log \frac{Salt}{Acid}$$

pK_a is the negative logarithm of the dissociation constant of a weak acid, HA, which ionizes to H^+ and A^-. The equation may be rewritten:

$$pH = pK_a + \log \frac{A^-}{HA}$$

Many drugs, local anesthetics for example, contain a tertiary nitrogen to which a hydrogen atom attaches reversibly. By pharmacologic convention, their dissociation is also described by pK_a and the equation becomes:

$$pH = pK_a + \log \frac{B}{BH^+}$$

Since an acid acts as an H^+ donor, dissociation of both acids and bases is described by the equation:

$$pH - pK_a = \log \frac{A^-}{HA} \text{ or } \log \frac{B}{BH^+}$$

FIGURE 4–1. Schematic representation of the interrelation of the absorption, distribution, binding, biotransformation, and excretion of a drug and its concentration at its locus of action. (From Goodman AG et al (eds): Goodman and Gilman's The Pharmacological Basis of Therapeutics. 6th ed. New York, Macmillan Publishing Co, 1980.)

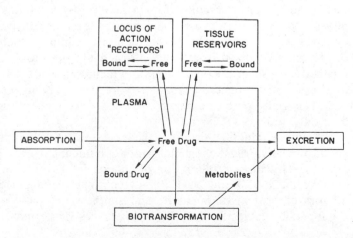

Thus, for a given pK_a, as pH increases the ionized form of an acid increases, whereas the ionized form of a base decreases. Which is the active form of the drug? The drug must penetrate lipid cell membranes to act. Uncharged species of the molecule penetrate membranes more easily than the ionized form. Thus, acidic drugs are easily absorbed from gastric juice where the pH may be 1.4; an acid drug with pK_a of 4.4 exists in a ratio of 1000 parts HA to 1 part A^- and is readily absorbed. At the pH of blood, 7.4, the ratio is reversed. Concentration gradients across cell membranes for one drug form can be produced simply by changes in pH. In addition, carrier-mediated membrane transport occurs as an active process. Drugs eventually reach not only their sites of action via the circulation but loci of metabolic degradation and elimination as well.

The effects on regional blood flow produced by anesthetics will be described elsewhere, but a few general remarks are relevant. Of greatest concern are the cerebral, coronary, pulmonary, splanchnic, and renal circulations. Each depends on cardiac output and vascular resistance, although there is some autoregulation in the cerebral, coronary, and renal circulations that maintains perfusion in the face of changes in perfusion pressure. Of these, splanchnic blood flow is most directly related to drug metabolism since it is by this route that orally administered drugs eventually reach the liver. Splanchnic flow is compromised directly or indirectly by most general anesthetics.

BIOTRANSFORMATION

Once carried to the liver, a drug is subject to biotransformation both for inactivation and elimination. Drugs that exist in a nonpolar, lipid-soluble form cross cell membranes easily and tend to remain in the body, since such molecules are easily reabsorbed by renal tubular cells. Modification of molecules by oxidation, reduction, or hydrolysis to polar compounds renders them less lipid soluble and thus more easily eliminated in urine.

Drug metabolism is mediated by both microsomal and nonmicrosomal enzymes. Hepatic drug-metabolizing microsomal enzyme systems have been the most thoroughly studied. First, it should be noted that "microsomes" are a laboratory product, not a biological reality. Liver cells contain a system of membranes or endoplasmic reticulum (ER), divisible into smooth and rough varieties. Upon differential ultracentrifugation, the smooth ER is fragmented into tiny structures that assume spherical forms called microsomes. These are rich in enzymes and contain cytochrome P-450, the terminal enzyme of the mixed function oxidase system. Cytochrome P-450 is a hemoprotein with iron in an oxidized (Fe^{3+}) or reduced (Fe^{2+}) form. Drugs combine with the oxidized form, and the drug complex is then reduced by a nicotinamide adenine dinucleotide phosphate (NADPH)–cytochrome c reductase reaction, with NADPH as the primary electron donor. The drug-Fe^{2+}-cytochrome complex then combines with molecular oxygen, the oxidized drug splits off, and the Fe^{3+} form of the cytochrome P-450 is regenerated. Several isoenzymes of cytochrome P-450 exist; their relative concentrations doubtless depend on genetic factors and on chemicals to which the individual has been exposed. Some isoenzymes may cause chemical reduction of the molecule rather than oxidation.

Enzyme induction describes the increased activity of microsomal enzymes brought about by many drugs, chemicals, or environmental agents. The prototype is phenobarbital, which causes proliferation of endoplasmic reticulum and increased synthesis of cytochrome P-450 and NADPH–cytochrome c reductase, reactions blocked by inhibitors of protein or nucleoprotein synthesis. Hepatic protein synthesis increases; Figure 4–2 shows the differing appearances of normal and enzyme-induced livers.

There are also nonmicrosomal enzyme reactions in drug metabolism, for example, conjugation of salicylates with glycine, N-methylation of catecholamines, hydrolysis of procaine and lidocaine, and oxidation of ethanol. Nonmicrosomal enzyme systems are not inducible.

EXCRETION

The kidney is largely responsible for elimination of drugs and their metabolites. Nonpolar compounds are eliminated slowly owing to reabsorption by renal tubular epithelium. Water-soluble polar drugs or metabolites are readily eliminated. Volatile anesthetics are for the most part exhaled via the lungs, but significant quantities of polar metabolites are produced from several inhalation agents.

If drugs are not bound to plasma protein, their elimination is proportional to the glomerular filtration rate. In the proximal renal tubules, certain organic cations and anions are added by active tubular secretion. Reabsorption of non-ionized substances occurs chiefly in the distal tubules in proportion to the rate of water and sodium reabsorption. The pH effect is important since, in the presence of alkalinized urine, weak acids are ionized and rapidly excreted. However, weak bases become less ionized as pH rises. Some drug metabolites are excreted in bile and either reabsorbed in the bowel for eventual renal clearance or excreted in feces, not an important mode of elimination.

DRUG INTERACTIONS

In the broadest sense, this topic includes every way in which one drug affects another. Cephalothin (Keflin) and thiopental form a precipitate in solution; cardiac output depression by thiopental slows the uptake of halothane; echothiophate iodide (Phospholine) inhibits plasma cholinesterase and may prolong neuromuscular blockade induced by succinylcholine. These examples represent, respectively, in vitro, pharmacokinetic, and pharmacodynamic kinds of interactions described in a recent monograph by Smith and associates. The following discussion of concurrent drug therapy will be restricted to the pharmacodynamic effects of preoperative medications on intraoperative anesthetic actions. Drugs to be discussed are those given for cardiovascular or psychologic effects, as they more directly affect anesthetic safety and efficacy. For greater detail and range of examples, the reader is encouraged to consult the references.

CARDIOVASCULAR DRUGS

Patients with cardiovascular disease may be treated with drugs of the following families: cardiac glycosides, antiarrhythmics, diuretics, and antivasoconstrictors or vasodilators (antihypertensives). Within each of these categories several drugs and, in some instances, several mechanisms of action exist. The addition of anesthetics and adjuvants increases the possible number of interactions, as can be seen in Figure 4–3, in which a hypothetical halothane anesthesia is used to illustrate the complexity of a routine case. The lines connecting the drugs denote possible interactions, and in the illustration total 17. If lidocaine were atomized into the trachea before intubation and morphine given at the end of operation for postoperative analgesia, there would be many more interactions to consider. The task of memorizing all interactions is overwhelming. Perhaps it is better to learn in detail the pharmacology of each drug than to appreciate intuitively the interactions possible.

Cardiac glycosides (digitalis) are given for their positive inotropic effect in treating heart failure and for their negative dromotropic effect in treating atrial flutter or fibrillation. Digoxin is the most commonly prescribed cardiac glycoside, and its serum concentration can be measured. The negative inotropy of general anesthetics can cause cardiac failure if the digoxin level is inadequate. On the other hand, digitalis toxicity causes myocardial irritability. Ventricular automaticity may be further enhanced during light anesthesia, as a result of hypercarbia caused by inadequate ventilation, with large doses of ketamine or cocaine, both of which may increase circulating catecholamines,

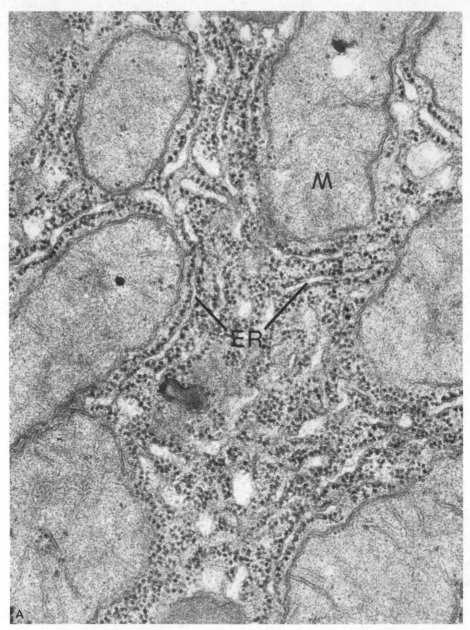

FIGURE 4–2.   Electron micrographs ($\times 42{,}500$) of mouse liver. Control (A) animal given saline injections daily for five days; induced (B) animal given 40 mg/kg phenobarbital intraperitoneally daily for five days. Both animals fasted 24 hours prior to sacrifice. Livers fixed in 1 per cent OsO_4. Symbols: M, mitochondria; ER, rough endoplasmic reticulum with attached ribosomes appearing as black beads; SER, smooth endoplasmic reticulum, seen best in transverse views, where it circumscribes vacuolar (cisternal) spaces. (Micrographs courtesy of Dr. RM Hinkley.)

Illustration continued on opposite page

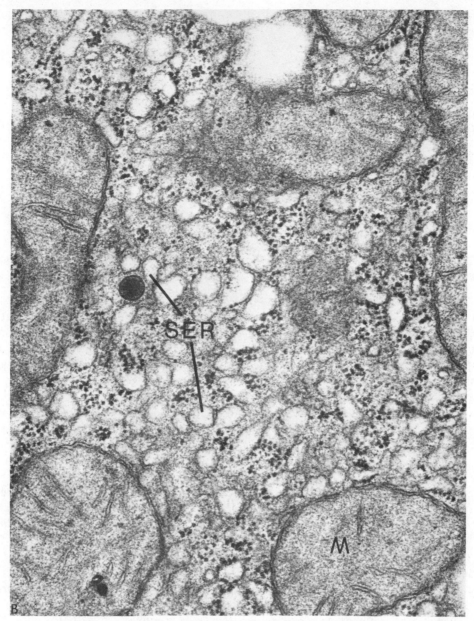

FIGURE 4–2 *Continued.*

or from hypokalemia attending hyperventilation sufficient to produce marked alkalosis. In the dog, volatile anesthetics diminish digitalis toxicity. Phenytoin (Dilantin) is considered by some to be the drug of choice for treating ventricular arrhythmias resulting from digitalis, whereas potassium infusion will counteract digitalis toxicity on a more chronic basis.

The *antiarrhythmic* drugs given to most patients include quinidine, procainamide, and propranolol (Inderal). The first two work on excitable cell membranes to block sodium influx during depolarization, whereas propranolol is a beta-adrenergic blocker. Newer beta blockers, more cardioselective (beta-1), are beginning to appear, but propranolol is presently the drug usually given. These drugs depress cardiac conduction and contractility and enhance the neuromuscular blockade produced by tubocurarine as do potent inhalation anesthetics. The potential for additive effect is obvious.

PREOPERATIVE DRUGS   INTRAOPERATIVE DRUGS

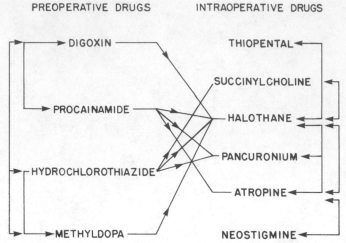

FIGURE 4–3. Drug interactions possible in a patient receiving cardiovascular drugs preoperatively and a routine halothane anesthesia intraoperatively. Lines connecting drugs denote possible interactions.

Diuretics contract the extracellular fluid space, of which plasma volume is a part. The patient may thus border on being hypovolemic, and therefore, may be subject to severe circulatory depression when anesthetized. On the other hand, if diuretic dosage is inadequate with resulting hypervolemia, anesthetic depression of myocardial contractility can cause cardiac failure. Clinical assessment of circulatory status is necessary preoperatively, and measurement of central venous and/or pulmonary artery wedge pressure may be indicated. Some diuretics decrease serum potassium concentration, notably the thiazides and "loop" diuretics, e.g., furosemide (Lasix) and ethacrynic acid (Edecrin), which are also the diuretics most commonly prescribed. Measurement of serum potassium is therefore critical, since both hypo- and hyperkalemia can cause cardiac contractility and rhythm disturbances that add to, or compound, adverse anesthetic and digitalis actions. Since potassium depolarizes the neuromuscular junction, abnormal serum levels also alter the action of all neuromuscular blockers. Furosemide also augments nondepolarizing blockade by a direct action independent of any change in potassium level. Spironolactone (Aldactazide), triamterene (Dyazide), and amiloride (Midamor) conserve potassium but still reduce plasma volume.

The third class of drugs is designated as *antivasoconstrictor* because that is its mode of action in treating hypertension. By impairing sympathetic nervous system function at sites ranging from the brain to vascular smooth muscle, these drugs depress the chronic vasoconstriction that characterizes essential hypertension. Since one in six adult Americans is hypertensive, the anesthetist will frequently find that a patient is taking one or more antihypertensive drugs preoperatively. Diuretics are usually given first. In addition to causing a reduction in plasma volume, the thiazide diuretics and possibly furosemide have direct vascular actions that are dilatory, perhaps related to a decrease in vascular smooth muscle sodium content. Other drugs are added if hypertension persists. Methyldopa (Aldomet) is metabolized to methylnorepinephrine, which stimulates inhibitory brainstem neurons to mimic an alpha-2 agonist action normally performed by CNS norepinephrine. Methyldopa also acts presynaptically at the sympathetic nerve–smooth muscle interface. Newer drugs with similar actions are clonidine (Catapres) and prazosin (Minipress).

Reserpine and guanethidine (Ismelin) deplete norepinephrine stores in the sympathetic nerve terminals, reserpine also acting in the brain, which is impermeable to circulating guanethidine. Propranolol acts in more than one manner. It has an immediate sedative CNS action, a probable blocking action, subsequently at sympathetic nerve terminals; and an eventual diminishing action on renal renin release, which in turn causes circulating angiotensin II levels to decrease. Hydralazine (Apresoline) acts directly to relax vascular smooth muscle. Further anesthetic interactions include additive depressant effects of potent inhalants given to patients taking CNS-active antihypertensives (reserpine, methyldopa, propranolol, clonidine, prazosin), antagonist effects of anesthetics (ketamine, cocaine, possibly nitrous oxide) with CNS adrenergic agonist action, and hypotensive effects of most anesthetics in the face of peripheral antiadrenergic and direct vasodilating actions of almost all antihypertensive drugs. It is better to continue antihypertensive drugs up to the time of operation than to discontinue them and deal with anesthetic reactions in the uncontrolled hypertensive state.

PSYCHOTROPIC DRUGS

Many drugs are prescribed for patients with affective, behavioral, or cognitive disorders. The CNS actions of levodopa (Larodopa) and agents such as ethyl alcohol, marijuana, cocaine, and amphetamines are also important, as patients consuming any of these compounds may present for operation, particularly in the emergency situation. One could predict that all such drugs will interact with anesthetics that also affect the brain, but specific effects vary from one class of drug to another.

Affective disorders include mania and depression. The most effective drug for mania is lithium. This monovalent cation substitutes for sodium and enters the cell during depolarization but is extruded very slowly, thus accumulating intracellularly. The neuromuscular block produced by succinylcholine or pancuronium is thereby prolonged but not that resulting from tubocurarine.

Depression, at the other affective pole, is a common complaint for which many drugs are available. The two major categories are the tricyclic antidepressants and the monoamine oxidase (MAO) inhibitors. *Tricyclics* block catecholamine uptake at presynaptic nerve terminals, and most of them also exert anticholinergic effects. Among these drugs are imipramine (Tofranil), amitriptyline (Elavil), desipramine, nortriptyline (Aventyl), and doxepin. They enhance opioid analgesia and respiratory depression in mice as well as barbiturate-sleep time. They also potentiate the actions of anticholinergic drugs and direct-acting vasopressors such as norepinephrine, epinephrine, and phenylephrine (Neo-Synephrine). Cocaine and ketamine can produce considerable vasopressor responses if given to such patients, and local anesthetics containing epinephrine should be avoided. *MAO inhibitors* have been almost entirely replaced by the tricyclic antidepressants. Many interactions occur among anesthetics and MAO inhibitors such as pargyline (Eutonyl), phenelzine (Nardil), and tranylcypromine. The most serious problem occurs when meperidine causes a hypertensive crisis characterized by muscle rigidity, restlessness, hypertension, hyperpyrexia, convulsions, and death. A similar crisis can occur if vasopressors or vasoactive drugs such as cocaine are given. Phenelzine reportedly inhibits plasma cholinesterase, thus prolonging the succinylcholine effect.

Many drugs are given for states ranging from sleeplessness and anxiety to frank psychosis. The *phenothiazines* include promethazine (Phenergan), perphenazine (Trilafon), prochlorperazine (Compazine), chlorpromazine (Thorazine), and trifluoperazine (Stelazine). They vary in potency and side effects but share the ability to produce sedation, central anticholinergic effects, reflex circulatory depression, and vasodilation. These phenomena are also seen with the *butyrophenones*, the one most commonly taken chronically being haloperidol (Haldol). Phenothiazines and butyrophenones interact with potent volatile anesthetics to favor hypotension. They exert a mild to modest alpha-1 adrenergic blocking action peripherally and increase sedation and respiratory depression caused by opioids. *Benzodiazepines* are the prototypes of the antianxiety and sedative drugs. They include chlordiazepoxide (Librium), diazepam (Valium), and lorazepam (Ativan). These drugs are less apt to cause hypotension when anesthesia is superimposed than are the phenothiazines and butyrophenones, but an adverse interaction does occasionally occur. In addition, opioid sedation and respiratory depression may be enhanced.

In the therapy of parkinsonism, levodopa crosses the blood-brain barrier and is converted to the dopamine normally present in the brain but absent in patients with Parkinson's disease. The liver converts circulating levodopa to dopamine, which can cause cardiac and peripheral vascular stimulation. Interactions with anesthetics are minor, confined to a theoretical propensity toward dysrhythmias in patients receiving halothane and ventilating insufficiently to maintain a normal P_{CO_2}, hence causing a rise in circulating catecholamine levels.

Socially consumed drugs can interact significantly with anesthetics if present in effective concentration at the time of operation. Alcohol depresses brain and heart function, adding to concurrent general anesthetic depression. Tricyclic antidepressants as well as most of the other drugs used to treat affective and behavioral disorders potentiate the alcohol effect. The person acutely intoxicated with alcohol may be seriously hypoglycemic. Even the combative, seemingly alert patient may actually be quite depressed by alcohol; anesthetic drugs should be given cautiously. Marijuana is not associated with serious drug interactions when taken alone, but the singularity of use should be verified in the history of the emergency patient on an obvious "high." If the marijuana, a very slight adrenergic stimulant, were smoked while cocaine or amphetamines were inhaled or ingested, the anesthetic requirement might be increased owing to CNS stimulation. If wine or another alcoholic beverage were ingested concurrently, the problem would be further compounded by the depressant effects of alcohol.

Ultimately, the anesthetist must rely on careful conduct of an anesthetic, being aware of the drugs used preoperatively and of their pharmacology and that of the anesthetics given. The same can be said about *any* anesthetic, but the dictum is particularly important when concurrent drug use complicates the clinical situation.

OPIOIDS AND ADDICTION

Anesthetists often encounter patients receiving opioids preoperatively for pain. The hazard of opioids lies mostly in postoperative morbidity. During surgical stimulation, the respiratory depressant action of opioids is offset by painful stimuli, but these are absent after operation. Thus, depression of respiration may last for many hours after therapeutic doses of morphine, particularly in the presence of hepatic or renal failure.

Additional problems are posed by the opioid addict. If in a treatment program, the addict is often unaware of the maintenance dose and tends to exaggerate drug needs; thus the unwary physician may inadvertently prescribe an overdose. Too small a dose of opioid is equally hazardous, since withdrawal symptoms may occur. Hospitalization for operation is not the time to alter maintenance programs or otherwise treat addiction. The maintenance plan should be continued and if treatment of pain is required, additional opioid should be given. Pentazocine (Talwin), butorphanol (Stadol), and nalbuphine (Nubain) should not be given because they are opioid antagonists and may precipitate the withdrawal syndrome. Many opioid addicts are dependent on other drugs as well, notably the barbiturates and alcohol. Withdrawal symptoms may result from withholding any of these agents. Obtaining a preoperative history is important in the event that problems arise during the postoperative period when information cannot be obtained.

Other drugs used illegally for mood and behavior alteration have not been as well studied in relation to anesthesia. Amphetamine, a sympathomimetic agent, exerts CNS excitatory actions; anesthetic requirements are higher when this drug is taken acutely as one dose but lower when taken chronically. This probably relates to the increased turnover rates of norepinephrine and dopamine. Anesthetics sensitizing the myocardium would seem to be contraindicated. Even less clear are the additive effects of lysergic acid diethylamide (LSD), mescaline, and marijuana on the actions of anesthetics. All these drugs, in the acute stage, are sympathomimetics resulting in tachycardia and hypertension.

REFERENCES

Cullen BF, Miller MG: Drug interaction and anesthesia. Anesth Analg 58:413, 1979.

Diagnosis and management of reactions to drug abuse. Med Letter 22:73, 1980.

Frohlich ED: Newer concepts in antihypertensive drugs. Prog Cardiovasc Dis 20:385, 1978.

Gifford RW: A guide to the practical use of diuretics. JAMA 235:1890, 1976.

Havdala HS, Borison RL, Diamond BI: Potential hazards and applications of lithium in anesthesiology. Anesthesiology 50:534, 1979.

Jenkins LC, Graves HB: Potential hazards of psychoactive drugs in association with anaesthesia. Can Anaesth Soc J 23:334, 1976.

Kopriva CJ, Brown ACD, Pappas G: Hemodynamics during general anesthesia in patients receiving propranolol. Anesthesiology 48:28, 1978.

Mason DT, De Maria AN, Amsterdam EA, et al: Antiarrhythmic agents: Therapeutic considerations. Drugs 5:292, 1973.

Smith NT, Miller RD, Corbascio AN: Drug Interactions in Anesthesia. Philadelphia, Lea and Febiger, 1981.

Chapter 5

PREMEDICATION, TRANSPORT TO THE OPERATING ROOM, AND PREPARATION FOR ANESTHESIA

During preanesthetic rounds the anesthetist should observe the mental and physical condition of a patient and, after due consideration for the patient's problems, the surgeon's requirements, and the anesthetist's own skills, make a decision on the conduct of anesthesia. Premedication can be given rationally only after these considerations have been taken into account. Selection of preanesthetic drugs should be the prerogative of the anesthetist, since anesthesia may be said to begin when these drugs are given. Wise choice of medication can pave the way for an uncomplicated anesthetic and postoperative course; improper choice can lead to an unsatisfactory experience for all concerned.

The kinds and amounts of preanesthetic drugs chosen depend on the anesthetist's goals. As will be noted, some agents are meant to diminish salivary secretions and vagal effects on the heart; others to eliminate the possibility of awareness during light planes of anesthesia; still others to act as basal analgetics when intravenous barbiturates and nitrous oxide are administered. We prefer that patients come to the operating room awake though drowsy, free from apprehension, and fully cooperative. If confidence has been gained by the patient during the preanesthetic visit, apprehension will usually be less and the need for sedation reduced. This contention had long been based on clinical impression until Egbert and coworkers (1963) and later Leigh and colleagues (1977) evaluated the comparative calming effects of a placebo, pentobarbital (Nembutal), and an informative, reassuring preoperative visit. The interview involved a frank discussion of the patient's fears, analysis of problems, statement of the time required for the operation, the nature of the anesthetic, and a description of immediate postoperative effects. Their findings, summarized in Table 5–1, clearly indicate that instruction, suggestion, and encouragement are useful nonpharmacologic antidotes to anxiety.

It should be emphasized that drowsiness or sleepiness does not guarantee freedom from apprehension. For many genuinely frightened patients, relief of anxiety comes only with considerable dulling of consciousness. One may be tempted, therefore, to agree to the frequent request that the patient be unconscious before leaving the hospital

TABLE 5–1. Premedication vs. Preoperative Visit by Anesthetist *

	No Visit No Drug	Visit Alone	Drug Alone	Drug and Visit
	Per Cent			
Feel nervous	58	40	61	38
Feel drowsy	18	26	30	38
Judged adequately sedated	35	65	48	71

*Comparison of effects of pentobarbital 2 mg per kg intramuscularly, one hour before induction of anesthesia, with those of a reassuring, informative preoperative visit by the anesthetist. (Modified from Egbert LD, Battit, GE, Turndorf, H, et al: JAMA 185:553, 1963.)

room. However, if unconsciousness is induced before the journey to the operating room additional hazards are created, resulting not only from central depressant effects of the drugs but also from complications such as respiratory obstruction and circulatory instability. A word to the patient that the practice is unsafe usually settles the issue.

The physical and mental condition of the patient determines both the need for as well as the dosage of premedicants. The more ill, the more elderly, and the less robust and active the patient, the smaller is the requirement for sedatives and analgetics. A degree of physical depression difficult to define is already present in these individuals, and, in general, the greater the body mass, the larger is the distribution volume for the drugs given.

THE PREMEDICANTS

In general, drugs used for premedication include sedatives, opioids, tranquilizers, and anticholinergics.

SEDATIVES

The term sedative or hypnotic does not connote a specific kind of action, because the wide variety of drugs used for these purposes produces a spectrum of effects ranging from mere sedation through general anesthesia and deep coma, terminating in death with gross overdose. The relation between sleep-producing properties and chemical constitution is not well defined. Few of these drugs mimic the action of natural sleep in terms of rapid eye movement (REM) activity. To a large extent the efficacy of a drug depends upon the pharmacokinetics involved, that is, the rate and extent of absorption, distribution in the body fluid compartments, degree of protein-binding, and speed and nature of metabolism and excretion. For passage across the blood-brain barrier, a matter of high lipoid solubility, a sedative should offer a low degree of ionization at body pH.

Barbiturates

Most patients scheduled for operation do better when given a hypnotic the night before operation, since apprehension, the newness of surroundings, and the disturbances in a hospital all cause insomnia. When used for this purpose, the barbiturates offer a long record of safety. There is no known teratogenic effect when they are given during pregnancy. In general, pentobarbital (Nembutal) or secobarbital (Seconal) in a dose from 100 to 200 mg is given orally at bedtime and repeated once if necessary. These drugs produce maximal sedation in one to one and one-half hours, the action largely dissipating after three to four hours. Although duration of action is an intrinsic property of the barbiturate chosen, classification of these drugs into short- and long-acting compounds has not been supported by controlled studies. Large doses of any of the barbiturates will result in a prolonged action. It is best to inquire whether a patient has been taking a sedative; if accustomed to a particular kind, this may be repeated, remembering that tolerance may have developed and that a larger dose may be required. Barbiturates can induce hepatic microsomal enzymes involved in the metabolism of other drugs as well as the barbiturates themselves (see Chapter 4).

We often give a barbiturate as the principal drug for premedication and favor secobarbital or pentobarbital in doses from 75 to 200 mg for the adult. Doses for infants and children are discussed in Chapter 25. Barbiturates offer an advantage over opioids in that sedation is the principal action. In usual amounts they rarely depress respiration (Fig. 5–1) or circulation. Allergic responses are not uncommon, and an occasional subject may become excited and confused rather than quieted. A barbiturate may be given orally two hours before operation with a sip of water, a convenient route of administration, with the duration of action as stated. When injected intramuscularly, an effect is usually noted within 30 minutes, disappearing in two to three hours. The intramuscular route is more certain and necessary when a gastric tube is in place. Barbiturates cause pain when injected because of the glycol solvent.

Depending on the barbiturate chosen, metabolism and excretion may differ. The so-called short-acting drugs are metabolized and conjugated principally in the liver, and

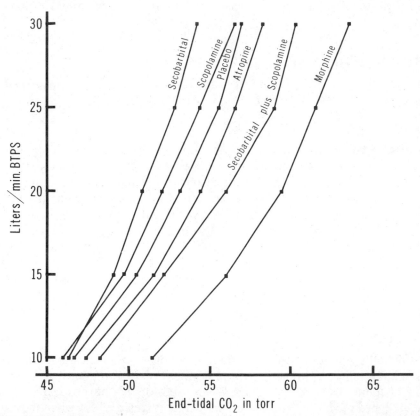

FIGURE 5–1. Effects of premedicant drugs upon respiratory response to carbon dioxide in man. Ten subjects rebreathed carbon dioxide in a closed system. Average end-tidal carbon dioxide tension required to produce minute ventilations of 10, 15, 20, 25, and 30 L/min are plotted. Secobarbital and scopolamine individually are mild respiratory stimulants (although clinically insignificant), whereas in combination they are depressant (although not so severely as 10 mg of morphine). (Reproduced with permission from Smith TC, Stephen GW, Zeiger L, et al: Anesthesiology 28:883, 1967.)

they therefore are useful in the patient with advanced renal disease in whom excretion of another kind of barbiturate would be delayed. In the presence of severe hepatic disease, however, the effects may be exaggerated and prolonged. Phenobarbital is excreted mostly by the kidney, hence the barbiturate of choice in patients with liver failure. High doses of barbiturates cause respiratory depression, and the drugs should not be given in the presence of acute intermittent porphyria because a crisis may be precipitated.

The central stimulating properties of local anesthetics such as muscle tremor, agitation, and convulsions can be treated with low doses of barbiturates, although diazepam is deemed more effective. Either one is given intravenously, together with inhalation of oxygen (see Chapter 18). The belief has long been held that administration of a barbiturate before regional anesthesia would minimize toxic reactions. There are no data to support this contention, and some claim that a higher mortality may result from additive circulatory depression. Diazepam given prophylactically does increase the median lethal dose of local anesthetic in laboratory animals.

If barbiturates rather than opioids are given preoperatively, the anesthetist might anticipate that the patient will awaken more quickly from general anesthesia, experience pain earlier, and exhibit restlessness as consciousness is regained, which is believed to reflect an antianalgetic action of barbiturates. The incidence of postoperative nausea and vomiting can be expected to be lower when these drugs are given for premedication, as compared with opioids. For several reasons, the chronic alcoholic may show cross tolerance to the barbiturates.

Nonbarbiturate Sedatives and Major Tranquilizers

Under a number of circumstances other sedatives are preferable to the barbiturates, as when allergic reactions have been experienced or when hyperactivity rather than sedation is anticipated. It is believed that when barbiturates are given to the elderly a higher incidence of disorientation, agitation, and transient psychoses may result.

In addition to promethazine, sometimes given with an opioid, other phenothiazine derivatives, tranquilizers such as hydroxyzine (Vistaril), and certain butyrophenones (droperidol) may be given for premedication. Hydroxyzine, in particular, has been shown to potentiate the analgetic effect of opioids without an increase in major side effects. The use of all these is predicated on a number of pharmacologic effects: sedative action *per se*, potentiation of the effect of opioids and general anesthetics, alpha-adrenergic blockade, blockage of certain autonomic reflexes, and antiemetic and antihistaminic activity. The major differences between these drugs and the barbiturates are that they are not anticonvulsants and do not lead to respiratory depression or physical dependence, although a few produce extrapyramidal effects. Some of these substances offer considerable antiemetic activity, but we believe it unwise to prescribe drugs routinely preoperatively for this purpose. If there is a history of protracted postanesthetic vomiting, an antiemetic can be given intramuscularly 15 to 20 minutes before the end of the operation or to treat nausea or vomiting already present. According to some, promazine (Sparine), triflupromazine (Vesprin), and propiomazine (Largon) also exert a mild analgetic action. Other phenothiazines such as promethazine (Phenergan) appear to increase sensitivity to pain if used independently of the opioids.

The benzodiazepines are among the most widely prescribed drugs in clinical medicine today. As a group these compounds are used as sedative-hypnotics for the treatment of anxiety (chlordiazepoxide), behavioral disorders, neuromuscular disease, seizures, and the alcohol withdrawal syndrome. Diazepam, used in 5 to 10 mg doses either orally or intravenously (the intramuscular route results in poor absorption), is employed before cardioversion and for both prevention and treatment of the central stimulant properties of local anesthetics. The drug is also used as a sedative alone for endoscopic procedures, to ease labor and delivery, and for intravenous induction of general anesthesia. The pain experienced upon intravenous injection probably results from precipitation of drug crystals from the glycol solvent. A localized sterile thrombophlebitis is, therefore, not an uncommon complication. In general, these remarks about diazepam also apply to another benzodiazepine, lorazepam (Ativan).

Excessive dosage of any of the benzodiazepines can result in respiratory and circulatory depression in addition to coma. However, in contrast to the barbiturates, the addiction liability may be less, and hepatic enzyme induction does not seem to occur. For these reasons, in addition to the fact that REM sleep is more closely approximated, flurazepam (Dalmane) rather than a barbiturate is used as a sleep medicine, in doses of 15 to 30 mg orally.

OPIOIDS

This group of drugs comprises the potent analgetics, which are classified as follows: (1) natural alkaloids of opium (morphine, codeine) and mixtures of the alkaloids (omnopon [Pantopon]), (2) semisynthetic modifications of these compounds (dihydromorphinone [Dilaudid]), (3) synthetics (meperidine [Demerol]), and (4) the agonist-antagonists (pentazocine, butorphanol, and nalbuphine). Although pain is not common prior to operation, it has been customary to prescribe the analgetics in part for sedation but mostly to diminish the amount of general anesthetic subsequently required. The efficacy of the analgetics in reducing the concentration of general anesthetic needed to produce a given depth of anesthesia is evidenced by a lowering of the minimum alveolar concentrations (MAC) (see Chapter 11).

It is common practice to give an analgetic to patients who are to be anesthetized with less potent combinations of general anesthetics like nitrous oxide and thiopental and to combine an opioid with a barbiturate or diazepam for regional anesthesia. Under these circumstances, the action of the opioid is probably more like that of a basal anesthetic. The respiratory depressant action of analgetics may be useful, since most volatile anesthetics increase the respiratory rate in the light planes; tidal volumes may become inadequate and respiratory acidosis may result. An analgetic may counter this tendency by maintaining a more satisfactory rate and depth of breathing. On the other hand, uptake of the anesthetic may be slowed by respiratory depression and respiratory assistance may be required.

Undesirable Effects of the Analgetics

All analgetics decrease alveolar ventilation, as shown by a diminished response to a carbon dioxide challenge. The degree and duration are dose-related but with approximately the same effect in equianalgetic doses. The duration of effect is longer than is generally appreciated. Figure 5–2 illustrates this response, showing that fentanyl (Sublimaze), a potent opioid with relatively brief analgetic action, continues to exert an effect on breathing for a matter of hours. A single dose of morphine has been shown to be active for 12 hours or more after intramuscular injection. Respiratory depression is also evident in the newborn as a result of placental transfer of an opioid. For the same reasons, the use of analgetics is associated with a higher incidence of postoperative pulmonary complications: atelectasis may result because of elimination of spontaneous intermittent sighing and depression of the cough reflex.

A reduction in the ability of the circulation to react to stress is evidenced by an increased incidence of hypotension and fainting following head-up tilt; this is the result of a direct vasodilating action on peripheral vascular smooth muscle, possibly owing to

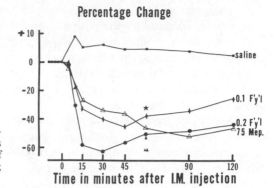

Percentage Change

FIGURE 5–2. Prolonged respiratory action of narcotic analgetics. The end-tidal carbon dioxide was kept at 46 torr by addition of variable amounts of carbon dioxide to inspired gas. F'y'l = fentanyl; Mep = meperidine. Doses in mg.

Time in minutes after I.M. injection

release of histamine. When cyclopropane was a popular anesthetic, the addition of morphine caused a reduction in cardiac output over a normal or increased state resulting from endogenous output of catecholamines. However, morphine given intravenously in high doses, 0.5 to 3.0 mg per kg, usually has little adverse effect on circulatory dynamics in the supine individual, except for the occasional person who develops profound hypotension. In this way morphine and fentanyl have been used as major analgetics supplemented by moderate concentrations of nitrous oxide and neuromuscular blockers for the performance of cardiac operations during extracorporeal circulation. Respiratory depression is profound, requiring ventilatory assistance well into the postoperative period. Meperidine may cause tachycardia and in rare instances may convert auricular fibrillation to flutter with a correspondingly higher ventricular rate.

So far as the bowel is concerned, after initial duodenal spasm and decreased gastric emptying time, peristalsis and intestinal tone diminish and constipation results. Analgetics can cause nausea and vomiting prior to induction of anesthesia, and they contribute to postoperative nausea and vomiting, either through an effect on the vestibular apparatus leading to motion sickness or through stimulation of the chemoreceptor trigger zone in the medulla. Sphincteric tone is increased and smooth muscle is constricted in other areas such as the biliary tract, ureter, and bronchioles. Release of antidiuretic hormone by opioids has been shown in the dog; in humans this may contribute to dilutional hyponatremia.

New opioids are introduced from time to time, each purporting to produce the same degree of analgesia provided by morphine but with fewer undesirable side effects. As a rule, these contentions are unfounded because the drugs in question have not been compared in controlled clinical studies with the analgesia produced by morphine in a standard dose of 10 mg per 70 kg body weight.

Attention has focused on the opioid antagonists as useful analgetics because they may be nonaddictive and some produce analgesia in their own right. Nalorphine (Nalline) is a satisfactory analgetic, but accompanying hallucinatory effects preclude its use. Pentazocine (Talwin), a benzomorphan related to phenazocine (Prinadol), is both a weak opioid antagonist and an analgetic in humans, a dose of 30 to 60 mg corresponding to 10 mg of morphine. However, in equianalgetic dosage, respiratory and other adverse effects differ little from those of the other opioids. Likewise, the belief that the drug is nonaddictive is incorrect, although the dependence potential is minimal; in certain individuals unpleasant hallucinatory phenomena occur.

The newest generation of opioid antagonist analgetics includes nalbuphine (Nubain), butorphanol (Stadol), and buprenorphine (Temgesic), each offering certain advantages over pentazocine or morphine. However, differences exist in the balance of their analgetic and antagonist potencies, their onset and duration of action, and their reversibility induced by the pure antagonist naloxone; their cardiovascular and central nervous system profiles may be important clinically. Although referred to as agonist-antagonist analgetics, the recent postulation of multiple opiate receptor sites in the brain challenges the concept that this class of compounds acts on the same receptors for both agonist and antagonist activity. Perhaps they are agonists on one or more types and antagonists on others.

During the preanesthetic visit, patients sometimes ask that a particular analgetic not be given because of allergy. Questioning usually reveals that the symptoms consisted of nausea, vomiting, or vertigo — common side effects rather than allergy. However, a history of protracted vomiting, excitement, urticaria, or wheezing suggests that the offending opioid should be omitted. If analgesia is required, an analgetic of different chemical configuration should be given. When time permits, a small test dose can be given several days beforehand.

Analgetics are given before anesthesia by the subcutaneous or intramuscular route. In the former, the optimal effect is reached in approximately 45 to 60 minutes; intramuscular injection provides a more rapid onset but shorter duration. Medication may also be given intravenously just before induction of anesthesia; under these conditions injection is made slowly and the dose reduced since respiratory depression may follow. A schedule for preanesthetic use of opioids in children is provided in Chapter 25. The dose of morphine in the adult varies from 5 to 10 mg per 60 to 70 kg body weight, with corresponding doses of meperidine from 50 to 125 mg. When an analgetic is combined with a barbiturate, the dose of analgetic is reduced.

Elderly patients, those in poor physical condition, or patients with circulatory instability should be given lower doses of the analgetics because of the higher incidence of side effects, particularly those relating to circulation and respiration. In the presence of liver failure, opioids should be used cautiously lest coma result. Patients with pulmonary emphysema, bronchial asthma, kyphoscoliosis, or cor pulmonale may react poorly to analgetics because diminished respiratory reserves and lack of compensation may result in respiratory failure. Therefore, a sharp reduction in dosage is indicated when pain relief is necessary. Preferably some other means of relieving pain should be tried, for example, intercostal or epidural nerve block postoperatively for thoracic or abdominal incisional pain.

ANTICHOLINERGICS

The copious respiratory tract secretions seen during open drop administration of ether anesthesia suggested the prophylactic use of a parasympatholytic agent, and atropine came to be used routinely for this purpose. As new, less irritating inhalation anesthetics were introduced, the need for antisialogogues diminished. Routine use of atropine or scopolamine certainly causes uncomfortable dryness of the mouth. More than a few studies describe the apparently safe administration of general anesthesia without prior use of anticholinergics. Although atropine or scopolamine is still given preoperatively by many anesthetists, we suggest that these drugs should be used only for specific indications.

There are other uses for these drugs, such as the prevention or treatment of severe reflex slowing of the heart during anesthesia. When this follows intrathoracic manipulation, traction on abdominal viscera, or stimulation of the carotid sinus, intravenous injection of atropine should restore heart rate and arterial pressure to normal. Prophylactically, to block reflex vagal effects on the heart, a dose of atropine of at least 1.0 mg per 60 kg body weight is required. Bradycardia may also be seen in association with increase in intraocular pressure, with traction on extraocular muscles during operation for squint, or when a dose of succinylcholine is repeated within a short period of time. Bradycardia is also common in infants and children after injection of succinylcholine and inhalation of halothane. Although the drying effect of scopolamine is superior to that of atropine, the former is not as effective in preventing reflex bradycardia during general anesthesia.

The sedative action of scopolamine is marked and useful for preanesthetic sedation, amnesia, and lack of awareness during balanced anesthesia. However, many patients become restless and irritable — even disoriented — after its use and the incidence of agitation during emergence from general anesthesia is high, a reaction commonly seen in response to pain. These reactions can be controlled by the intravenous injection of physostigmine (Antilirium), which crosses the blood-brain barrier to counteract the central anticholinergic action of several kinds of drugs. Physostigmine should be given slowly in 1 mg doses, not exceeding 3 mg, to avoid dangerous degrees of cholinergic activity peripherally, as seen with neostigmine (Prostigmine).

Atropine and scopolamine are usually ordered in doses of 0.4 to 0.6 mg per 60 kg body weight. However, if major vagal blockade is needed prior to use of neostigmine or to treat organophosphate poisoning, much higher doses are needed (1 to 3 mg). The effects of atropine or scopolamine on heart rate differ to some extent, of some importance when digitalis has produced slowing of the rate in auricular fibrillation or flutter or when neostigmine is given for reversal of neuromuscular blockade. Both atropine and scopolamine given intravenously in low doses may slow the heart rate for a matter of seconds. Atropine thereafter causes more prolonged tachycardia, whereas scopolamine is associated with bradycardia. Scopolamine, then, would seem to be the choice for the digitalized patient. In children who are febrile and dehydrated or in the presence of tachycardia or in patients with thyrotoxicosis, the dose of anticholinergic drug should be reduced or eliminated. Some anesthetists avoid these drugs in the presence of bronchial asthma or bronchitis, fearing inspissation of secretions and inability to eliminate them through cough. Both drugs, however, are bronchodilators and increase the physiologic dead space. Except for the narrow-angle variety, glaucoma does not contraindicate the use of anticholinergics since a rise in intraocular pressure does not occur unless the usual clinical doses are exceeded. Moreover, an effect on smooth muscle of the iris can be counteracted by pilocarpine instilled locally. The concept that an anticholinergic drug can prevent laryngospasm in light planes of general anesthesia is not tenable; the striated muscles of the larynx do not respond to drugs that in ordinary doses have no effect on neuromuscular transmission.

In spite of their universal acceptance, the belladonna alkaloids, atropine and scopolamine, have shortcomings in their relatively brief duration of action, their central nervous system stimulating properties, and their varying effects on pulse rate. For these reasons the quaternary ammonium compound, glycopyrrolate (Robinul), an anticholinergic drug long used in the treatment of gastrointestinal disorders, merits consideration as a premedicant. On a milligram for milligram basis, this drug is twice as potent an antisialogogue as atropine, in both adult and child, and the duration of action at least three times as long. Although the tachycardia produced is less, protection against vagal-induced bradycardia is greater than with atropine. Because the blood-brain barrier is not crossed, the central stimulation and confusion are lacking. Glycopyrrolate also offers the advantage of decreasing the volume and acidity of gastric secretions.

PREPARATION FOR ANESTHESIA

Anesthesia is given safely only if thoughtful preparations are made beforehand, beginning with the preanesthetic visit when the anesthetist envisions the problems that may be encountered and then orders premedication. Planning presupposes a thorough understanding of the surgical procedure contemplated and the anesthetic selected. If the anesthetic techniques are complex, it is helpful to follow detailed descriptive protocols, for example, use of deliberate hypotension or management for implantation of a cardiac pacemaker or for extracorporeal circulation. Sound practice would call for departments of anesthesia to convene on the afternoon before surgery or at the start of the day's schedule to discuss problems and management of patients to be anesthetized. Larger training programs can make "block assignments," placing staff and resident anesthetists in the same specialty area of an operating suite for weeks or months. This facilitates preoperative discussion, preparation, and supervision during anesthesia as well as postoperative teaching rounds.

Transport of the Patient

A patient should be brought to the operating area in sufficient time so that anesthesia need not be hurried. Rapid induction is not in the best interests of the patient nor is it conducive to instruction of beginners. Careful transport to the operating room is essential, if possible under the supervision of a nurse or nurse's aide. Detailed instructions for transfer are written when needed; for example, one should specify that the orthopneic patient should be in a head-up position or the desperately ill patient accompanied by a physician. Upon arrival, the patient must be identified. Preparation may proceed in either a holding room or the operating room proper. Use of anesthesia induction rooms is no longer recommended because some believe it unsafe to anesthetize patients in one area and then move them to another, although others believe better operating room utilization is achieved this way and that the practice is not a hazardous one. However, an induction room can be used when intra-arterial or pulmonary artery catheters are inserted for the more complicated operations. Regardless of opinion, patients should await anesthesia in a quiet area where an intravenous infusion can be started and a blood pressure cuff applied. They should not be subjected to the sights and sounds of the operating room as they lie strapped to a litter in a busy corridor. The purposes of premedication are defeated by this practice.

Immediate Preanesthetic Care

The patient should be assisted in the transfer from litter to operating table. Care in movement is important in the extremely ill, the patient in pain, the osteoporotic, and for those whose circulation is precarious. Intravenous infusions, drainage catheters, and traction apparatus must be protected. The patient should be covered with a clean bed sheet or cotton blanket for modesty and warmth. A lifting sheet should be present beneath the back and a broad restraining strap above the knees. The arms and legs should be comfortably restrained to protect against peripheral nerve injury, and the legs should not be crossed. Some patients find that flexion of the operating table provides more comfort. When there is a potential explosion or electric hazard, the patient should be grounded to the table by means of a conductive pad. An operating room cap should be applied to protect the hair and promote asepsis. Whether every patient should wear a mask is a matter of opinion, although this should be the case when virulent pulmonary infections are present. Once placed on an operating table or litter, a patient should not be left unattended.

The beginner tends to concentrate on technical matters, although obviously assessment of the patient's condition should be the first consideration. The patient is asked when he or she last ate or drank and whether medication was given. The nurse's record is consulted for preoperative vital signs and temperature, to be sure dentures have been removed, and for dosage and time of administration of medicines. The latest recordings of laboratory data are noted. Of particular interest here are serum electrolyte levels, coagulation defects, hematocrit reading, the electrocardiogram, the chest x-ray, and sickle cell prep in blacks. These are recorded on the anesthesia record with the assessment of the degree of sedation and other changes in physical or mental condition. Cancellation of the operation may be necessary if preparation has been inadequate.

Stethoscope and blood pressure cuff are applied to the arm and a stethoscope may be taped to the chest; these remain in place throughout the operation. The blood pressure cuff can be protected against contact at the side of the operating table by a tobogganlike device. Baseline blood pressure, pulse, and respiratory rate are recorded. Monitoring devices such as electrocardiograph leads may be applied or a central venous catheter inserted at this time, with care taken not to cause pain or alarm the patient (see Chapter 9). When there is a deviation from the expected, in symptoms or signs, an explanation must be sought. The supervising anesthetist, surgeon, and consulting internist should then determine whether to proceed.

Technical Procedures

An intravenous infusion is usually started before anesthesia so that drugs can be injected quickly in an emergency. Complicated venipunctures and venous or arterial cutdowns may be less disturbing to the patient after consciousness has been lost and peripheral vasoconstriction abolished through the action of general anesthetics. Likewise, bladder catheterization or passage of a gastric tube or esophageal stethoscope is better completed after the patient is asleep. Present-day anesthesia practices may require several infusions for giving drugs and for fluid and blood replacement. For some operations, such as major vascular or radical cancer procedures, an important part of anesthetic management lies in the anticipation, measurement, and replacement of blood loss, for which large cannulas are inserted.

Artificial airways, endotracheal tubes, laryngoscope, and suction catheters and apparatus are arranged neatly on the anesthetist's work table. Each piece of apparatus should be clean and working properly. Dirty equipment is placed in a container kept separate from clean supplies. A source of suction is at hand. Drugs used for induction, such as neuromuscular blockers, are drawn into labelled syringes beforehand.

A second person can be of considerable help during induction to restrain the patient when there is excitement, aid in positioning for operation, observe the pulse at crucial times, prepare injections, start an intravenous infusion, or seek additional help when necessary. Anesthesia for complicated operations may require the continuous attention of two or more anesthetists.

The value of a prescribed routine in the preparation of the patient is appreciated only after the beginner has encountered difficulties during induction. Extra time set aside for preparation permits one to deal with the unexpected. Anesthetists should be prompt; if tardy, they take unnecessary chances and perform poorly under the scrutiny of an impatient operating team. Calm, unhurried activity, neatness, cleanliness, and punctuality mark the skilled clinician.

APPRAISAL

After reading the contents of this chapter, both anesthetists and other physicians will understand why the prescription of premedication is so much an essential part of anesthetic administration *per se*. Premedication was once a routine practice, consisting for the most part of the administration of atropine and morphine. Today it entails a knowledge not only of the pharmacology of many compounds but of the patient's characteristics, the complicating ailments, drugs concurrently given, and the anesthetic technique planned. Trite as the dictum may seem, preanesthetic medication may very well set the stage for all that follows, both good and bad.

REFERENCES

Conner JT, Bellville JW, Wender R, et al: Morphine, scopolamine and atropine as intravenous surgical premedicants. Anesth Analg 56:606, 1977.

Egbert LD, Battit GE, Turndorf H, et al: The value of the preoperative visit by an anesthetist. JAMA 185: 553, 1963.

Giuffrida JG, Bizzari DV, Saure AC, et al: Anesthetic management of drug abusers. Anesth Analg 49:272, 1970.

Greenblatt DJ, Shader RI: Drug therapy. Anticholinergics. N Engl J Med 288:1215, 1973.

Greenblatt DJ, Shader RI: Drug therapy. Benzodiazepines. N Engl J Med 291:1011, 1239, 1974.

Koch-Weser J, Greenblatt DJ: Editorial — The archaic barbiturate hypnotics. N Engl J Med 291:790, 1974.

Lasagna L: Drug therapy. Hypnotic drugs. N Engl J Med 287:1182, 1972.

Leigh JM, Walker J, Janaganathan P: Effect of preanaesthetic visit on anxiety. Br Med J 2:987, 1977.

Ostheimer GW: Comparison of glycopyrrolate and atropine during reversal of non-depolarizing neuromuscular block with neostigmine. Anesth Analg 56:182, 1977.

Vandam LD: Drug therapy. Butorphanol. N Engl J Med 302:381, 1980.

Section 2
ESSENTIAL PREANESTHETIC CONSIDERATIONS

Chapter 6
MEDICOLEGAL CONSIDERATIONS

The last 15 years have seen a precipitous rise in malpractice actions. A report of a national commission studying medical malpractice recommended that the problem be managed at the state level, and state legislatures have responded with a multiplicity of new malpractice laws, most of which are now being challenged in the courts. Meanwhile, costs of insurance premiums have risen to the point of having appreciable influences on physicians' manner of practice, kinds and location of practice, patient fees, and early retirement plans.

What is the explanation for this change in attitude of the American public toward its health care system? Many reasons come to mind, and the list that follows is by no means all inclusive. (1) Medicare, Medicaid, and third party insurers have brought millions of people into the health care system who were not involved before; more insured individuals mean more lawsuits. (2) As a result of civil rights legislation in the 1960s, individuals are more aware of their rights than previously, and they are more willing to litigate if they feel those rights have been abridged. (3) As a result of the consumer movement, people are far more apt to challenge and question medical products or services received, just as they question any other goods or services. (4) Specialization in medicine has led to a deterioration of traditional doctor/patient relations. Major problems are inherent in the hospital system. (5) Hospitals are innately unsafe places; no other industry deals with a consumer population that presents so many difficulties and so many possibilities for failure or adverse results. (6) A degree of malpractice does exist in the health care profession.

This chapter deals with the character and causes of medical law suits; the legal responsibilities of medical students, residents, and nurse anesthetists; how to minimize legal risk; and what is to be done in the event of an accident or untoward medical outcome.

THE CHARACTER OF LAW SUITS

What is malpractice? Conditions of law under which suits may be filed and the judgments awarded vary among the states. An excellent defense in one state may constitute no defense in another. Legal precedent may even be reversed and new principles of law established. Although generalizations can be made, anesthetists should be familiar with procedures in their own areas.

Malpractice is a theory arising from tort law. A tort is a civil wrong for which an

47

individual can seek compensation through legal action. Malpractice itself is not a criminal act, although a given act or omission that constitutes malpractice can constitute a criminal act separately.

Malpractice implies negligence in the care of a patient or failure to employ methods, agents, or skills ordinarily considered appropriate, but to characterize all malpractice cases as negligence is an injustice to the medical profession. One judge has observed that "persons undertaking to administer anesthetics in the course of medical or dental treatment . . . are neither insurers against harm or guarantors of a favorable result, but are required only to exercise ordinary or reasonable care or skill under the circumstances, that is, . . . the skill and diligence of the ordinary person engaged in similar practice at the time, and in the locality where the defendant undertook to act." That the hoped-for result does not follow or that complications occur does not imply liability unless the physician has promised a specific result or the complication arises from improper care.

Generally speaking, a physician does not have a contractual relation with a patient to provide care but does have an obligation to provide reasonable care. If a promised result does not occur, then the physician is liable on the theory of breach of contract, not malpractice. The usual professional liability policy excludes claims based upon a warranty of cure or guaranteed result. A physician is not responsible for an error in judgment unless it is so gross as to be inconsistent with the skill expected of every physician. Liability and negligence cannot be avoided by pleading that one was engaged to attend more patients than could properly be cared for, a point of importance to anesthetists who attempt to supervise two or more anesthesias simultaneously. The title of physician implies an awareness of medical literature and conformity of practice to medical standards. However, if one proposes to be a specialist in medicine, then judgments on practice are made in terms of national, not local, standards.

A court trial is society's way of peacefully resolving a dispute. A patient claims injury by a physician, obtains legal counsel, and files a malpractice suit; depositions are taken by attorneys for both sides to elicit plaintiffs', defendants', and various witnesses' opinions as to what actually transpired; a court hearing is arranged, usually with a jury present; plaintiffs, defendants, and witnesses including experts testify at this time; the attorneys sum up their cases; the presiding judge explains to the jury points of law involved; and the jury then makes a decision and recommendation of compensation for damages. This chain of events may be interrupted at any point: the plaintiff may learn through counsel's advice that there is no legitimate basis for a suit; the defendant may be forewarned that there is liability without question and that a settlement might be made on behalf of the plaintiff; after hearing depositions, the plaintiff may drop the suit or the defendant may be advised by counsel to make settlement; sometimes a suit is dropped because the plaintiff cannot find experts who can testify that there was malpractice; finally, a settlement can be arranged with the aid of the judge at any time during the trial prior to the jury verdict. Only a small proportion of malpractice suits are settled through court verdict.

Proof of malpractice can be established in several ways. Most commonly, the plaintiff and defendant produce expert testimony establishing the standard of care applicable to the specialty involved. Physicians once reluctant to testify against a colleague are less reluctant today, especially in significant departures from standard patient care; thus the complaint of "conspiracy of silence" may no longer be applicable. It is obvious that expert witnesses called by the plaintiff may provide evidence in favor of the defendant and vice versa. The matter is complicated in that courts usually apply a liberal interpretation of what may constitute an "expert" witness, and the jury is left to decide upon the expert's qualifications. Many physicians harbor preconceived notions, frequently not well founded, concerning their obligation to testify.

Because physicians were once reluctant to participate, the law recognizes the doctrine of *res ipsa loquitur,* which for practical purposes eliminates the need for expert testimony. Literally, the doctrine means "the act speaks for itself." This has usually been applied in situations in which harm could not have occurred except through negligence and the technique or treatment causing the harm was under the control of the physician. The doctrine is seldom applied today except when foreign objects are left in the body after a surgical or diagnostic procedure.

CAUSES OF MALPRACTICE ACTIONS

Failure of physicians to establish rapport with their patients is the principal cause of suits. Anesthetists are frequently negligent in this regard. While having worked hard for recognition of the specialty as an independent discipline, they have failed to appreciate the responsibility of closer identification with their patients. Unfortunately, custom and tradition have not required the usual patient-physician relations. Opportunities for contact with patients outside the operating room are less than those afforded most other specialists, and too often visits are hastily completed. When a preoperative examination has been omitted and postoperative visits are not made, the only recollection the patient may have of the anesthetist is receipt of a bill for services. Obviously under these circumstances a bond of understanding between patient and physician had not been established. With the patient usually unconscious during the time when the anesthetist makes a major contribution, the stage is set for resentment against a physician unknown.

Failure to obtain adequate informed consent for a surgical procedure has become an increasingly important cause of malpractice actions. Informed consent is discussed subsequently.

Other factors render anesthetists susceptible to suits. They work as a team, some members of which are even more liable to suit, and the present tendency in malpractice actions is to name all members of a team as well as the hospital.

Some patients are "suit conscious," believing that they should receive compensation for anything other than a perfect result and for inadvertent accidents, unexpectedly long periods of convalescence, and even hurt feelings. An attorney described this attitude as follows: "The present philosophy of the bulk of American people is that they are entitled to absolute protection from someone for every misfortune of human life, regardless of whether caused by divine providence, human frailty, or their own improvidence or misconduct." The emotional component of a medical malpractice case may be strong. In the ordinary personal injury action unrelated to medical practice, plaintiffs wish to be compensated for the injury and the damage caused, but they believe that the award will be paid by an insurance company and they may harbor no ill will or malice toward the person or organization thought to be responsible. However, in medical malpractice suits, although the source of payment is again thought to be an insurer, bitterness is likely to arise if an illness or deformity is unsuccessfully treated. The patient may have regarded the doctor as a last hope, and treatment failed to measure up to expectations.

RESPONSIBILITY OF MEDICAL STUDENTS, RESIDENTS, AND NURSE ANESTHETISTS

Medical students and resident physicians are not immune to court action and should be protected by malpractice insurance. Rarely are they named as sole defendants but more likely as one of several, including the supervising anesthesiologist, the surgeon, perhaps, and the hospital. Medical students pursuing courses for credit and registered with a university or college are usually protected against suit through the institution, sometimes by the hospital and occasionally by both provided that they act under supervision of a faculty member on staff at the hospital. However, students on preceptorships or in elective courses not approved by the medical school or those training in hospitals or working with physicians unaffiliated with a medical school should inquire as to their protection rather than assume that they are protected and carry no risk. House staff likewise are protected through the hospital or medical center in which they are training, but they should inquire as to insurance protection and, if need be, secure it for themselves. Residents who indulge in "moonlighting" should recognize that they are not protected outside the parent institution unless they have made prior arrangements with an insurance carrier.

A nurse anesthetist can be held liable for negligence in the administration of anesthesia. This person is assumed to be responsible for the technical administration of the anesthetic, for the observation and recording of vital signs, and for the well-being of the patient. Most certified registered nurse anesthetists avail themselves of malpractice protection. However, the likelihood is that legal responsibility for the actions of the nurse will be shared at least in part by others. If a surgeon or anesthesiologist supervises a nurse in the administration of an anesthetic, under the "borrowed servant" doctrine the nurse is the assistant of the physician and the latter must assume responsibility. If an anesthesiologist or surgeon employs the nurse or advises the hospital as to the qualifications or conditions of employment, the anesthesiologist is responsible even though not directly concerned in supervision at the time of an alleged act of negligence.

The last 15 years have seen an important expansion of two theories of law, *respondeat superior* and "corporate liability," into the doctrine of hospital liability. The impetus for change came from the Darling v. Charleston Community Hospital case (1966), in which hospital liability was extended to include failure, through control of staff membership and clinical privileges, to monitor the care provided by attending physicians. To hold a hospital liable on a corporate liability theory, a plaintiff must show that the hospital knew, or should have known, that the physician (and presumably the resident or nurse) whose negligence caused the plaintiff's injury was providing substandard care. The implications of this doctrine are fairly obvious and include the need for hospitals, through their responsible physicians, to routinely survey the clinical privileges of professional staff. No longer can hospitalized patients be treated in isolation from the remainder of the community, since suits against only one member of a hospital staff will likely become a rarity.

HOW TO MINIMIZE LEGAL RISK

Preparation for Anesthesia. Anesthetists' responsibilities commence before the patient arrives in the operating room; they should conduct themselves after the manner suggested in Chapter 3. Pertinent points of the history should be summarized on the patient's chart with results of the physical examination and interview including a statement of any unusual risk involved and the type of anesthesia planned. If such a procedure were always followed, many a law suit would be avoided.

The problem of "informed consent" must be considered at the time of the interview with the patient, and notation made on the chart. Not only must patients sign a statement authorizing operation and anesthesia, but they must thoroughly understand what is to be done. The surgeon explains the operative procedure and anesthetists what they propose to do. The patient should be given the opportunity to ask questions or to make a choice if any is to be made. Choice should not be interpreted to mean that the anesthetist presents the patient with a "shopping list" of agents and techniques; few patients have the competence to make such selections. The choice is more likely to involve regional versus general anesthesia, intravenous induction versus inhalation induction, and so on.

What constitutes an adequate *informed* consent? The various states have different interpretations, some insisting that every possible complication be described to the patient, others recommending speaking only of likely complications and tempering what is said. A reasonable approach to the problem is presented from Natanson v. Kline in the Kansas Supreme Court.

"A physician violates his duty to his patient and subjects himself to liability if he withholds any facts which are necessary to form the basis of an intelligent consent by the patient to the proposed treatment. Likewise the physician may not minimize the known dangers of a procedure or operation in order to induce his patient's consent. At the same time, the physician must place the welfare of his patient above all else and this very fact places him in a position in which he sometimes must choose between two alternative courses of action. One is to explain to the patient every risk attendant upon any surgical procedure or operation, no matter how remote; this may well result in alarming a patient who is already unduly apprehensive and who may as a result refuse to undertake surgery in which there is in fact minimal risk; it may also result in actually increasing the risks by reason of the physiological results of the apprehension itself. The other is to recognize that each patient presents a separate problem, that the patient's mental and emotional condition is important and in certain cases may be crucial, and that in discussing the element of risk a certain amount of discretion must be employed consistent with the full disclosure of facts necessary to an informed consent."

The anesthesiologist should go into detail about possible complications if an unusual technique is to be used, a new drug employed, or the physical condition of the patient renders him particularly complication-prone, such as the possibility of dislodgement of loose or diseased teeth during laryngoscopy. The note on the record should include a statement that the anesthetist has described the proposed anesthesia and that the patient understands. When new drugs or techniques are to be used or when patients are in critical condition or are to undergo prolonged, involved operations, it is best to have them sign for both approbation and consent.

In the Operating Room. Anesthetists are responsible for the immediate preoperative preparation and care (Chapters 5 and 7). While it is their duty to see that gas cylinders are properly attached to the anesthesia machine, adequately filled, and identified by color and label, they are not charged with the manufacturer's responsibility of providing correctly identified gases of acceptable purity. They must identify all drugs injected and assure themselves that the materials used for injection satisfy sterility requirements. Protective devices such as suction, airways, and the like must be provided. Although there is no law requiring that all safety devices such as a defibrillator be immediately at hand in every operating room for every procedure, this equipment should be available in the operating suite.

Transport of patients is a shared responsibility, but the hospital should provide the means for safe transportation. Once a patient has been delivered into the hands of the anesthetist, the anesthetist assumes control except when this is shared by the surgeon. If surgeons supervise positioning of the patient for operation, complications arising therefrom may be wholly their responsibility.

The surgeon is not responsible for the conduct of the anesthetic; the anesthesiologist is in effect an independent contractor. During anesthesia, care is exercised to protect the patient against injury as outlined in subsequent chapters. In the event that new techniques, equipment, or agents are employed, anesthetists should be able to substantiate familiarity with these methods and an understanding of any complications that may arise from their use.

Electric and Combustion Hazards.   Anesthetists are not ordinarily responsible for maintenance of equipment in operating rooms insofar as electric and combustion hazards are concerned. They should, however, point out to the hospital administration any inadequacies in flooring, lack of explosion-proof electric connections, improper control of humidity and ventilation, inadequate disposal of waste gases, and explosion and electrocution hazards associated with the electrocautery, the electrocardiograph, and other devices. If anesthetists find that equipment is defective, continue to use it, and an accident involving that equipment occurs, they are liable. The surgeon should inform the anesthetist of the intended use of electric equipment. Prevention of electric accidents, fires, and explosions is discussed in Chapter 34. If anesthetists choose to administer flammable anesthetics, they should observe necessary precautions and should be able to defend the choice, showing that they were aware of the hazard and that steps to avoid an accident were taken.

Records.   The best protection an anesthetist can have is an accurate and complete anesthesia record with written observations at regular intervals as operation and anesthesia progress. A record should never be altered *post facto*. If items of information are subsequently recorded, these must be clearly indicated as additions.

Blood Transfusion.   The kinds and quantities of parenteral fluids given during operation are best determined by consent between surgeon and anesthetist. The physician who starts a transfusion is responsible for identifying each unit of blood given and determining that it has been properly crossmatched. The anesthetist must be aware of the hazards of blood transfusion and must be certain that indications for transfusion are valid.

Postoperative Care.   Responsibilities of the anesthetist do not cease when the patient is transported from the operating room. Observation continues until care is assigned to another competent person. If dissatisfied with the patient's condition, the anesthetist should remain in attendance. In most institutions the recovery room is supervised by anesthesiologists. A detailed record of the patient's progress in the recovery room is essential.

During postoperative visits, discussion of the anesthesia experience should be encouraged; if the patient is dissatisfied, this is usually apparent. It is the disgruntled patient not given the opportunity to express dissatisfaction who may ultimately sue.

WHAT SHOULD BE DONE IN THE EVENT OF AN ACCIDENT?

It is inconceivable that medicine can be practiced without accident or complication. Most patients are understanding and are satisfied by frank discussion of problems. If, however, the physician belittles or ignores a complication or fails to impart sympathetic understanding, the stage is set for malpractice action.

In the event of an accident or complication definitely or possibly related to anesthesia, the anesthetist should document the facts on the patient's chart in chronological order during or immediately following administration of anesthesia. Treatment should be noted and consultative opinions included. Subsequent notations should be made on the chart periodically during the remainder of the hospital stay and a record of treatment kept.

The physician should immediately provide the hospital and the insurer with a complete account of an accident. Should a suit be threatened or legal inquiry made concerning a patient, the physician should immediately notify the carrier and, where appropriate, seek legal assistance. Many large hospitals now retain attorneys full time, whose advice should be sought. Failure to carry out these requirements within a reasonable period has resulted in loss of protection in more than a few instances.

APPRAISAL

The attitude of the courts toward malpractice suits undergoes continuous revision. The body of law lies between the tradition that liability must be predicated upon fault and that calling for reimbursement of those who suffer injury. When care may have been improper, malpractice or negligence can be accepted as descriptive of the defendant's action, and the traditional concepts of law apply. In such cases, physicians should be willing to testify on behalf of a plaintiff.

More perplexing problems involve those instances in which the physician's conduct has been blameless according to accepted standards, but the patient has had a poor result and seeks compensation. When the terms malpractice and negligence are used in this context, they are not applicable. There is increasing pressure to settle out of court, as a large judgment may be made when a jury views a poor result and is unable to understand the situation facing the physician at the time of treatment. At present, few courts seem willing to recognize that there is an irreducible risk in the practice of medicine. Nonetheless, when fault is not involved, settlement should not be made and the case should be brought to trial.

The filing of a malpractice action against a physician should not lead to hysteria. Approximately four out of five such suits are settled out of court, and of those that go to court, physicians win more than they lose.

Meanwhile, the best protection against medicolegal action lies in the thorough and up-to-date practice of anesthesia, coupled with sympathetic interest in the patient and compilation of detailed records of the course of anesthesia. One must keep in mind that sickness does not deprive the patient of legal rights and that physicians cannot impose what they think is advisable simply because they know what is in the patient's best interest. Patients or their families must be given the information on which to base decisions.

REFERENCES

Curran WJ: Malpractice insurance. N Engl J Med 292:1223, 1975.
Curran WJ, Shapiro D: Law, Medicine, and Forensic Science. Boston, Little, Brown and Co, 1970.
Dornette WHL: The medical malpractice problem, and some possible solutions. Anesthesiology 44:230, 1976.
Hayt E, et al: Law of Hospital, Physician and Patient. Berwyn, Il, Physicians Record Co, 1972.
Kramer C: Medical Aspects of Negligence Cases. New York, Practising Law Institute, 1970.
Kramer C: Medical Malpractice. New York, Practising Law Institute, 1972.
Morris C, Moritz AR: Doctor and Patient and the Law. St. Louis, C V Mosby, 1971.
Report of the Secretary's Commission on Medical Malpractice (DHEW Publication No OS 73–88), Washington DC, US Government Printing Office, January 16, 1976.
Shapiro D, et al (eds): Medical Malpractice. Ann Arbor, Institute of Continuing Legal Education, 1965.
Waltz JR, Imbau FE: Medical Jurisprudence. New York, The Macmillan Company, 1971.
Wecht C (ed): Exploring the Medical Malpractice Dilemma. Mt. Kisco, NY, Futura Publishing Co, 1972.

Chapter 7

ANESTHESIA EQUIPMENT

ANESTHESIA MACHINES

Every anesthetist should be conversant with the mechanisms and physical principles governing use of an anesthesia machine. There are various makes of machine, all with the same basic elements. These include a source of oxygen and anesthetic gases; the means for measuring and controlling their delivery; a means to volatilize and deliver liquid anesthetics; and safety devices. The anesthetic-oxygen mixture delivered from the machine is administered to the patient through a breathing system. One system, the circle absorber, is shown in Figure 7–1. Others are described in Chapter 13. Anesthesia machines are often equipped with a gas-driven mechanical ventilator and devices to monitor the electrocardiogram, blood pressure, and inspired or expired gas oxygen tension. Alarm systems to signal apnea or disconnection of the breathing circuit are also in common use. Standards for the design and performance of anesthetic equipment have been developed by the American National Standards Institute.

COMPRESSED GASES

In the first few decades after the introduction of anesthesia, there was little need for compressed gases or anesthesia machines, for ether and chloroform were given as vapors in atmospheric air. When nitrous oxide was used, the gas was supplied from a generating apparatus. Although the vital importance of oxygen was known, it was not until 1868 that Andrews introduced mixtures of nitrous oxide and oxygen. This created an interest in apparatus for simultaneous administration of the gases. In 1872 the Johnston Brothers Concern began to supply liquid nitrous oxide in metal cylinders, thus requiring measurement of pressure and flow rate of gases; this, in turn, led to the development of anesthesia machines.

Gases used in anesthesia are available in cylinders mounted on the machine (Fig. 7–1), or, for oxygen and nitrous oxide, they may be piped in from a central container or bank of cylinders. Precautions are necessary in both systems, some specific for one or the other. Because a central supply may fail, it is essential to mount cylinders on machines for emergency use.

In the United States, specifications for identity and purity of medical gases are established by the United States Pharmacopeia and supervised by the Food and Drug Administration. Safe practice for manufacture, packaging, shipping, handling, and storing of gases is set by the Department of Transportation (DOT), the Compressed Gas Association (CGA), and the National Fire Protection Association (NFPA). Among

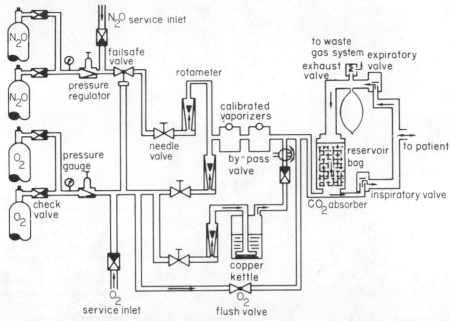

FIGURE 7–1. Anesthesia machine circuit. Oxygen and nitrous oxide enter the machine from cylinders or from the hospital service supply. Pressure regulators reduce cylinder pressure to about 50 psi. Check valves prevent transfilling of cylinders or gas flow from cylinders to service line. The fail-safe valve prevents flow of nitrous oxide if the oxygen supply fails. Needle valves control flows to rotameters. Calibrated vaporizers provide a preselected concentration of volatile anesthetics. An interlock allows only one vaporizer to be on at a time. The Copper Kettle delivers the saturated vapor of any agent; thus the effluent must be diluted. The bypass valve vents vapor from the Kettle when it is not in service. Gases are delivered to the circle absorber, where unidirectional valves assure flow from patient through carbon dioxide absorber. Excess gas is vented through the exhaust valve into a waste gas scavenger system. The reservoir bag compensates for variations in respiratory demand.

other things, these organizations regulate safety devices and markings on cylinders, uniformity of valve threads on large cylinders, and the pin-indexing system (Fig. 7–2) for post-type valves on small medical cylinders. Manufacturing and testing data can be discerned from the markings on a cylinder shoulder (Fig. 7–2). Manufacturers and distributors of medical gases are required to maintain cylinders and valves in good condition, to insure the purity and identity of gases, and to periodically test the effect of high pressures on the container.

Compressed gases should be handled carefully to minimize the risk of fire or explosion. Oxidizing gases, oxygen and nitrous oxide, are stored away from flammable gases. All gases must be stored at temperatures below 52° C. Detailed specifications are given in "Inhalation Anesthetics" and "Nonflammable Medical Gases" published by the NFPA, as well as in publications of the CGA.

The following recommended practices are based on those of the CGA.
1. Never permit oil, grease, or combustible material to come in contact with cylinders, valves, regulators, gauges, or fittings. Oil may react with oxygen or nitrous oxide with explosive violence.
2. Never lubricate regulators, fittings, or gauges.
3. Open the high pressure valve on the cylinder before connecting the apparatus to the patient.
4. Open cylinder valves slowly, with the face of the gauge on the regulator pointing away from personnel.
5. Never drape a cylinder with sheets, hospital gowns, masks, or caps.
6. Never use gas fittings, valves, regulators, or gauges for service other than for the purpose intended.

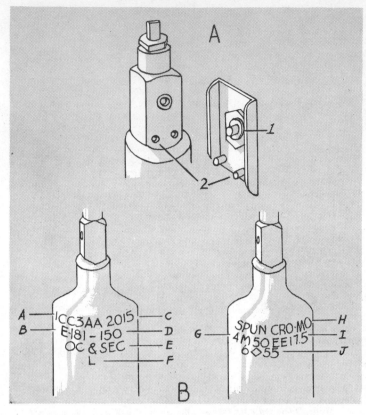

FIGURE 7-2. Features of gas cylinders. *A*, Cylinder valve and yoke connection: *1*, washer; *2*, pin-index system specific for each anesthetic gas. *B*, Cylinder markings: *A*, Interstate Commerce Commission (now Department of Transportation, DOT) specifications; *B*, cylinder size; *C*, maximum working pressure in pounds per square inch; *D*, manufacturer's serial number; *E*, ownership; *F*, inspector's mark; *G*, manufacturer's mark and date of original test; *H*, chrome-molybdenum (steel); *I*, elastic expansion in ml at 3360 psi; *J*, retest dates.

7. Never mix gases in cylinders. Never refill cylinders.
8. Always use oxygen from a cylinder equipped with a pressure regulator.
9. Do not use regulators in need of repair or cylinders with valves not operating properly.
10. Defective equipment should be repaired or replaced by the manufacturer or an authorized agent.

Additional precautions are taken when cylinders are placed in service. Paper wrappings are removed so that identifying labels are clearly visible. Valves are opened completely when the cylinder is in use and closed tightly when idle, an economic as well as a safety measure. The flowmeter valve on the anesthesia machine is closed before a cylinder valve is opened; if the valve is open, a high gas flow may damage the flowmeter or cause the bobbin to stick at the top. Compressed gas cylinders are connected to the machine by means of yokes with hand screws and washers of nonflammable material. Pin-indexed cylinders and yokes prevent attachment of a cylinder to the wrong yoke (Fig. 7-2).

The gauges indicate cylinder pressures (Fig. 7-1). Before anesthesia is induced, the cylinder or supply system is tested to be sure that sufficient gas is available. Anesthesia machines usually have double yokes so that two cylinders of oxygen or nitrous oxide are at hand. Check valves prevent one cylinder from transfilling the other. Metal tubing conducts the gases from cylinders to pressure-reducing valves.

The physical properties of commonly used medical gases are given in Table 7-1. Compression of gas to a liquid state offers the most economic supply and smallest volume, but the physical properties limit the conditions under which this may be accomplished. Compressed oxygen can only be supplied as a gas because the critical temperature, above which liquefaction cannot occur, is below ambient temperature.

TABLE 7–1. Properties of Medical Gases

	Oxygen	Nitrous Oxide	Carbon Dioxide
Symbol	O_2	N_2O	CO_2
Molecular weight	32	44	44
Cylinder color	Green*	Blue	Gray
Physical state in cylinder (20°C)	Gas	Liquid	Liquid
Specific gravity of gas (Air = 1)	1.11	1.53	1.53
Critical temperature (°C)	-118.8	36.5	31.3
Boiling point (°C)	-183.0	-89.5	-78.4§
Cylinder contents (L) E	625	1590	1590
G	5300	12,110	12,110
Gas weight (kg)† E	0.8	3.0	3.0
G	7.0	22.7	22.7
Cylinder pressure (psi)‡	2200	745	838
(100 × kPa)	152	51	58

*The World Health Organization specifies that medical oxygen cylinders be painted white, whereas U.S. standards require green.

†Empty E cylinder including valve weighs approximately 7 kg.

 Empty G cylinder including valve weighs approximately 45 kg.

‡Nominal filling pressures at 21°C. Values for nitrous oxide and carbon dioxide are their vapor pressures at 21°C. One psi = 6.89 kPa.

§Sublimes.

black – N_2 air – black + white

Liquid oxygen, however, is now in common use and is vaporized for supply throughout a hospital. It is stored in large, insulated containers under pressures of 5 to 10 atm, with corresponding temperatures from $-160°$ to $-150°$ C. Unlike oxygen, nitrous oxide is compressible to a liquid at temperatures up to 36° C. Compressed carbon dioxide is also a liquid at ordinary temperatures.

As compressed oxygen is used from a cylinder a gradual decrease in pressure occurs. Thus, cylinder contents are judged by pressure levels on the gauge: at a given temperature when the original pressure is reduced by half, the cylinder will be half full. For example, an E cylinder containing 625 L of oxygen when full will have 312 L remaining when the pressure decreases to 1100 psi. With nitrous oxide, as long as some liquid remains, that is, until the cylinder is about 75 per cent exhausted, cylinder pressure is equal to the vapor pressure of nitrous oxide, about 745 psi at room temperature. The pressure, therefore, does not indicate the amount of gas remaining. Carbon dioxide behaves similarly. Vaporization of liquefied gases as well as the expansion of compressed gases absorbs heat, which is extracted from the metal cylinder and the surrounding air. For this reason atmospheric water vapor may condense or freeze on cylinders and in valves during high gas flows; to prevent internal icing, liquefied and compressed gases must be free of water vapor.

PRESSURE-REDUCING VALVES

Pressure-reducing valves or regulators serve to lower cylinder pressure to a less hazardous and more easily controlled level (Fig. 7–1). Oxygen pressure in a full cylinder at 2200 psi is reduced to about 50 psi before delivery to the needle valves on flowmeters. Reducing valves also maintain a constant outlet pressure, providing a constant pressure at needle valves and a stable flow for a given valve setting.

Fail-Safe Devices. To eliminate the possibility of administering an hypoxic gas mixture resulting from failure of the oxygen supply, systems have been developed to regulate the flow of other gases in proportion to oxygen pressure. The essentials of one such system are shown in Figure 7–3. A master oxygen regulator supplies a reference

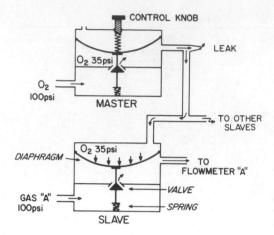

FIGURE 7-3. Master-slave fail-safe system. Master oxygen reference pressure on slave diaphragm permits gas "A" to flow.

pressure to slave regulators controlling the pressure of other gases. If the reference oxygen pressure decreases, so will oxygen flow, but the reference pressure in other slave regulators will also decline, thus resulting in a proportionate reduction of all gas flows. Incorporation of a fixed-ratio gas mixer for oxygen and nitrous oxide downstream from the master-slave regulators provides additional safety. The mixer delivers a constant 25 per cent oxygen at variable gas flows. Higher concentrations are provided by adding oxygen through a supplementary flowmeter.

FLOWMETERS

Rotameters measure the flow of a gas based on the principle that flow past a resistance is proportional to pressure. In a rotameter (Fig. 7-1), gas flows from below through a tapered tube, raising a bobbin or float. The channel through which the gas flows varies in diameter according to the height of the bobbin: the higher the flow, the larger the channel. The bobbin comes to rest when the force of gravity is balanced by the fall in pressure caused by the bobbin. Proportionality between pressure and flow is determined by the shape of the resistance and the physical properties of gases. If the resistance is an orifice, density is the controlling factor; if the resistance is tubular, viscosity becomes dominant. At low flow rates a rotameter acts as a tube; at high flow rates as an orifice. Since few gases have the same viscosity and density, rotameter calibrations are not interchangeable.

RESERVOIR BAG

Flows having been adjusted, gases are then delivered to the patient. Most anesthetics are administered by means of a system that permits at least partial rebreathing of the gases. A reservoir bag (Fig. 7-1) is needed to compensate for variations in respiratory demand. At peak inspiration, gas flows of 30 to 60 L per minute may be required, whereas during respiratory pause and exhalation, no gas flow is required. In the former instance, the larger quantity of gas needed is obtained from the reservoir bag, and in the latter, gas accumulates in the reservoir. In addition, the reservoir bag permits manual assistance or control of ventilation. Movement of the bag is unreliable as an index of adequacy of respiration. However, if the bag does not move, the cause must be sought immediately. The patient may be apneic, the airway obstructed, a faulty connection present, or there may be a poor mask fit.

VAPORIZERS

VAPORIZATION OF VOLATILE LIQUIDS

The first volatile anesthetics, ether and chloroform, were inhaled from masks or containers in which the anesthetic was vaporized by air drawn over the surface of the liquid. This simple method is still utilized in open drop techniques, in portable vaporizers, and in vaporizers placed within the breathing circuit, especially in under-developed countries. With ether and chloroform the vapor concentrations obtained were erratic; sudden high concentrations led to overdosage, whereas at other times the concentrations were insufficient to maintain anesthesia. An understanding of the physics of vaporization led pioneers like Snow and Clover to devise apparatus that provided predictable concentrations. The surface area for vaporization was increased and the metal containers were surrounded by warm water to maintain constant temperature and vapor pressure. These lessons were largely forgotten when compressed gas came to be used as the carrier for anesthetic vapors. Although oxygen was used instead of atmospheric air, the high flow of gases over liquid surfaces or bubbling through the liquid produced vapor concentrations that were hardly predictable.

An ideal vaporizer should yield a constant concentration of anesthetic under varying conditions of gas flow, liquid volume, and ambient temperature. Vapor concentration should be controlled with an accuracy equal to that for gases metered by flowmeters. Three physical characteristics are fundamental to the design of vaporizers: dependence of vapor pressure on temperature; latent heat of vaporization; and intimacy of the gas-liquid contact. The maximum partial pressure (concentration) of a volatile liquid that can be obtained in the vapor phase is limited by the vapor pressure at the existing temperature. If the temperature of the liquid fluctuates, vapor concentration changes proportionately. The relation between vapor pressure and temperature for some of the volatile anesthetic agents is given in Figure 7–4. Heat is required for the change to a gaseous state. If heat is not provided by the surroundings, it is derived from the liquid itself, with cooling as a consequence. Finally, to vaporize a liquid by a stream of gas, the two must be brought into contact. Since contact time is limited, a large gas-liquid interface, such as that provided by many small bubbles, assures more efficient vaporization.

VAPORIZERS

These physical concepts were incorporated by Morris in his design of the Copper Kettle vaporizer (Fig. 7–5). To provide a relatively constant temperature, a heavy

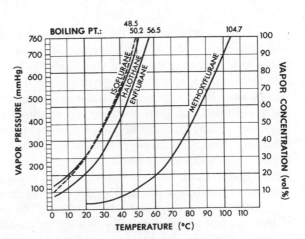

FIGURE 7–4. Vapor pressure curves of liquids commonly used for anesthesia.

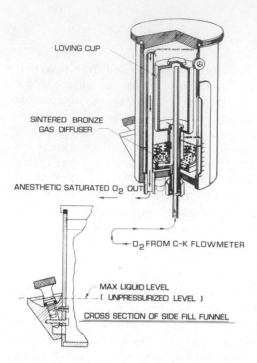

LOVING CUP

SINTERED BRONZE
GAS DIFFUSER

ANESTHETIC SATURATED O₂ OUT

O₂ FROM C-K FLOWMETER

MAX LIQUID LEVEL
(UNPRESSURIZED LEVEL)

CROSS SECTION OF SIDE FILL FUNNEL

FIGURE 7–5. The Copper Kettle. The copper container plays an important role as a source of heat and in transfer of heat from room air and metal parts of the gas machine to the liquid to be vaporized. Gas flowing through the liquid is finely dispersed by passing through a sintered bronze (Porex) disc. The tiny bubbles produce maximal vaporization efficiency by providing a large surface for the liquid-gas interface. The disc conducts the heat required for vaporization directly to the liquid. Filling port is placed on the side to prevent overfilling. (Reproduced with permission of Air Products and Chemicals, Inc.)

copper container with its high heat capacity and good conductivity is employed. A separately metered flow of oxygen passes through the container while intimate gas-liquid contact is assured by dispersing the gas through a sintered bronze disc to form streams of fine bubbles. Gas exiting from the vaporizer is nearly saturated with anesthetic vapor, the concentration equal to its vapor pressure at that temperature divided by atmospheric pressure.

$$\text{per cent vapor} = \frac{\text{vapor pressure}}{\text{atmospheric pressure}} \times 100 = \frac{\text{ml vapor} \times 100}{\text{ml oxygen} + \text{ml vapor}}$$

The concentration of vapor delivered to the breathing system is the volume of vapor delivered per minute divided by the total gas flow.

$$\text{per cent delivered} = \frac{\text{ml vapor}}{\text{total gas flow}} \times 100$$

Total gas flow includes the flow from the Kettle as well as the direct flow of oxygen and nitrous oxide. A rapid means of calculating the delivered concentration of halothane or isoflurane uses the vapor pressure of these agents, which is about one-third atmosphere at room temperature. One third of the gas exiting from a Kettle will be anesthetic vapor and two thirds oxygen; that is, each 2 ml of oxygen that enters the Kettle will add 1 ml of vapor, delivering 3 ml of gas. Similar calculations can be made for enflurane, with the vapor pressure about one-fourth atmosphere, or methoxyflurane, with the vapor pressure about one-thirtieth atmosphere. The delivered percentage of vapor may also be read from a graph or slide rule that provides values for liquid temperature, metered oxygen, and total gas flow; from a specially calibrated flowmeter; or from a pocket calculator programmed to calculate concentrations.

Although the Copper Kettle antedated the introduction of the halogenated agents, it was readily adapted to vaporization of these volatile liquids. The Vernitrol is of similar design, incorporating a separate oxygen flow, which is saturated on passage through the vaporizer. Other vaporizers (Fluotec, Pentec, Fluomatic, Pentomatic, Dräger Vapor) are made for specific agents and provide relatively constant vapor concentrations over wide variations in flow rate (Fig. 7–6). These vaporizers, which function outside the breathing circuit, divert a portion of the total gas flow into a vaporizing chamber, where a wick saturated with anesthetic provides a large gas-liquid interface for vaporization. The gas-vapor mixture exits from the chamber and rejoins the main gas stream. The proportion of gas diverted to the chamber is controlled by a calibrated dial, the settings of which are accurate only within the flow range specified for the device. Calibration should be verified periodically in a laboratory or by the manufacturer. Unless a protective device is incorporated, back pressure from the breathing circuit may build up and alter pressure in the vaporizing chamber, causing surges of anesthetic-laden gas. The vaporizers mentioned minimize change in temperature both by having a large heat capacity (mass) and by compensation with temperature-sensitive ports that alter the proportion of gas flows.

Although some agent-specific vaporizers (Fluotec Mark III) have an indexed filling port that accepts a tube specific for a flask of that anesthetic, many vaporizers can inadvertently be filled with any agent. For this reason, vaporizers should be filled with the same care used in handling other potent drugs and clearly labelled to indicate their contents.

When two or more vaporizers are mounted in series, the vapor delivered upstream can condense and contaminate that in the downstream vaporizer. To prevent this, an interlock should be provided so that only one vaporizer may be turned on at a time. If the vaporizers are not so equipped, care should be taken to see that only one vaporizer at a time is in use. All vaporizers should be turned off fully when not in use. Since the downstream vaporizer is contaminated, it should contain the more potent agent; addition of a less potent agent is a lesser risk.

Preservatives such as the thymol in halothane accumulate in a vaporizer with time because of their low volatility. While these residues do not appear to be harmful, excessive quantities may interfere with the functioning of the vaporizer. Some recommend that the contents of vaporizers be drained and discarded every two weeks, but we consider this wasteful. A more rational approach is to discard the liquid if it is

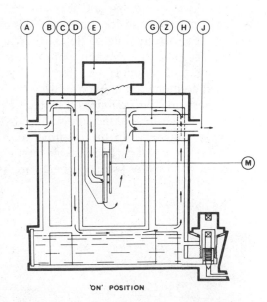

FIGURE 7–6. Fluotec Mark III agent-specific vaporizer. When control knob E is rotated clockwise, the vaporizer is ON. In this position, oxygen enters at A, passes through channel B into the vaporizing chamber at the bottom, and thence through channels H and Z to outlet J. Wicks saturated with halothane in the vaporizing chamber assure a large gas-liquid interface for efficient vaporization. Oxygen also flows through temperature-sensitive valve M and joins the halothane-laden stream from H to exit at J. The position of the control knob regulates the size of the opening of channel H and thus the flow through it. In the OFF position, with knob E fully counterclockwise, oxygen flows directly from A to J and ports D and H are occluded. Indexed filler port and drain are lower right. (Reproduced with permission of Cyprane-North America, Inc.)

'ON' POSITION

discolored. The vaporizer can be rinsed with a fresh charge of the agent. Ether can also be used to rinse vaporizers, taking the usual precautions for flammable agents and thoroughly airing the vaporizer before returning it to service. Neither enflurane nor isoflurane have preservatives added.

CARBON DIOXIDE ABSORBERS

In a rebreathing system, an absorbent is necessary to remove exhaled carbon dioxide (Fig. 7–1). To ensure that all of the exhaled gas passes through the absorber, directional valves are incorporated (Fig. 7–1). Before anesthesia is begun, the valves should be tested to assure unidirectional flow through the absorber. Thus, the anesthetist should inhale and exhale through the system to determine competency and during anesthesia should observe the action of the valves as well as the patient for signs of carbon dioxide accumulation. Among other things, duration of efficient action of an absorber depends on carbon dioxide output, tidal volume, respiratory rate, flow rate of fresh gases, capacity and shape of the canister, surface area, water content, porosity of the absorbent granules, and the chemicals used for absorption. When used with high fresh gas flows, modern canisters may be efficient for 16 to 18 hours of use. Some clinicians change absorbents on a weekly or biweekly schedule. Others prefer to rely upon color change. In any case, the anesthetist should observe any change in color of the indicator dye or any accumulation of heat as a rough index of carbon dioxide absorption. Fresh granules of soda lime crumble easily, whereas the exhausted material is quite hard.

CHEMICAL ABSORPTION OF CARBON DIOXIDE

Carbon dioxide combines with the hydroxides of alkali or alkaline earth metals. Two mixtures are commercially available.

1. Soda lime (NFXV) is a mixture of calcium hydroxide with sodium and/or potassium hydroxides, containing 12 to 19 per cent water.

2. Barium hydroxide lime (USPXX) is a mixture of barium hydroxide octahydrate, $Ba(OH)_2 \cdot 8H_2O$, and calcium hydroxide. It may also contain potassium hydroxide.

For practical use, the combined substances are supplied in granules sufficiently hard to resist crumbling and formation of dust, which is a respiratory tract irritant. Water is incorporated for the neutralization reaction; barium hydroxide lime contains water as the octahydrate of $Ba(OH)_2$. Water constitutes 12 to 19 per cent of the total weight of soda lime. When not present in chemical combination the water can evaporate, thus reducing the effectiveness of the soda lime. Soda lime should be stored in sealed containers and exposed to some degree of moisture when in use.

Absorbents incorporate dyes which change color as the reaction of neutralization proceeds. Regardless of the color of the absorbent, carbon dioxide can still be channeled through a canister into the inspired gas. Since the color change is not completely reliable, evidence of carbon dioxide retention in the patient must be sought. Neutralization reactions for the two absorbents are as follows:

Soda lime:

$$H_2CO_3 + 2\,NaOH \rightarrow Na_2CO_3 + 2H_2O \text{ (rapid)}$$
$$H_2CO_3 + Ca(OH)_2 \rightarrow CaCO_3 \downarrow + 2H_2O \text{ (slower)}$$

Barium hydroxide lime:

$$H_2CO_3 + Ba(OH)_2 \rightarrow BaCO_3 \downarrow + 2H_2O \text{ (fairly rapid)}$$
$$H_2CO_3 + Ca(OH)_2 \rightarrow CaCO_3 \downarrow + 2H_2O \text{ (slower)}$$

In each case the fundamental reaction is that of neutralization:

$$H^+ + OH^- \rightarrow H_2O$$

The heat of neutralization, 13.7 kcal per mole of water formed, is liberated during this reaction. As carbon dioxide is absorbed, therefore, the canister becomes warm to the touch. The reaction itself does not require addition of heat, for canisters at 0, 28, or 100° C absorb effectively.

The larger the surface area of absorbent exposed to expired gas, the more rapid and efficient is the absorption of carbon dioxide. An irregular granule offers a larger surface area than a cylindrical pellet. Whereas surface area also increases as granule size decreases, granules that are too small increase resistance to gas flow. The common soda lime granule is approximately 8 mesh, 2.5 mm, in size.

Optimal absorptive conditions provide that at least one tidal volume be accommodated entirely within the void space of the canister. When flow of expired gases ceases during inspiration, the tidal volume remains in contact with the absorbent. About half the volume of a properly packed canister consists of intergranular space or voids.

CARBON DIOXIDE ABSORPTION SYSTEMS

As gas passes through the system, absorption first takes place near the inlet, next along the sides of the canister, and finally at the outlet. With obstruction to gas flow, or because of areas of lesser resistance, channeling can occur; the gas follows the path of least resistance, bypassing the bulk of absorbent. The absorbent should, therefore, be tightly packed and held in place with screens, and baffles are used to disperse gas flow uniformly. Because of these variables, only about half of the theoretical capacity will have been used at the time of failure of a single charge of absorbent.

Soda lime and barium hydroxide lime are both strongly alkaline and corrosive to skin and mucous membranes; barium hydroxide is toxic if ingested. If granules of these substances remain in contact with tissues for any length of time, chemical burns result. The water of exhalation, which condenses and accumulates in a canister, dissolves alkali, forming a caustic solution that has caused burns in both patient and anesthetist.

CONDUCTING TUBES AND FACE MASK

Gases are led from the machine to the breathing system, which incorporates a circle absorber as shown in Figure 7–1 or some other kind (Chapter 13). Tubing carrying gas from the machine to the breathing system is of small bore, but tubing through which the patient breathes must be nonkinkable and of wide bore to minimize resistance. Corrugated, black conductive rubber tubing with an inside diameter of 22 mm is commonly used. However, sterile disposable sets containing breathing tubes, face mask, Y-connector, and reservoir bag are available in both conductive and nonconductive materials. Some sets incorporate a bacterial filter, although their value is questionable. Disposable sets are appropriately used in bacteriologically contaminated patients or in those unduly susceptible to infection.

An appropriate face mask is chosen; the best fit is attained by testing prior to induction. Poor fit delays induction of anesthesia and thwarts application of positive pressure breathing when needed. In applying the mask, excessive pressure on the face, nose, or eyes must be avoided.

ESCAPE VALVES AND SCAVENGER SYSTEMS

Techniques that supply gases in amounts larger than those required to meet the metabolic need for oxygen and uptake of anesthetic result in an excess of gas, which must be vented through an escape (pop-off) valve (Fig. 7–1). For example, during nitrous oxide anesthesia, to provide a safe concentration of oxygen yet give an effective percentage of nitrous oxide, gas flows of 4 liters or more per minute are often used; this also facilitates denitrogenation of the lungs and body tissues. Unless nitrogen can escape from the system, the anesthetic effect of nitrous oxide will not be achieved. High gas flows also assist in carbon dioxide elimination and avoidance of heat retention. If the gas volume supplied exceeds the minute volume of ventilation, there is little likelihood of carbon dioxide retention.

Formerly, excess gas was vented through an escape valve into the surrounding atmosphere; now there is evidence suggesting that long-term exposure to traces of anesthetic gases may cause an increase in spontaneous abortions, fetal malformations, and malignancies in female operating room personnel. Cognitive and motor skills may also be impaired during exposure. Many anesthetists use total gas flows of 3 to 7 L per minute, far in excess of the amount taken up by the patient. When a mixture of nitrous oxide, oxygen in 50 per cent concentration, and halothane, 1 per cent, is used at such flows in an air-conditioned operating room, the atmosphere may contain 10 parts per million (ppm) (0.0001 vol per cent) of halothane and 500 ppm of nitrous oxide. By the use of scavenger equipment and avoidance of leaks, these concentrations can be reduced more than tenfold.

Waste gases from the escape valve must be eliminated without increasing risk to the patient or others. Gases may be vented to an air-conditioning exhaust duct, but only if all exhaust air is vented to the outside. Alternatively, the gases can be drawn into the suction system or removed via a separate pump. Finally, the gases can be directly vented to the outside if an exterior wall is adjacent. Gas must be removed from the escape valve without pressure buildup or without causing negative pressure in the breathing circuit. The scavenger valve, tubing, and system must accommodate maximal flows used. Finally, the exhaust tubing must be protected against kinking or occlusion.

The kind of scavenger system used depends on the anesthetic technique; systems have been adapted to the open, semi-open, and circle techniques. A scavenger valve to replace the escape valve of an anesthesia circle is shown in Figure 7–7. Others are described in Chapter 13.

Additional pollution of the operating room atmosphere occurs while vaporizers are being filled and if there are leaks from breathing circuit connections as well as high and low pressure gas leaks within the machine. Mechanical ventilators may cause the same kind of contamination.

USE OF MECHANICAL VENTILATORS ON ANESTHESIA MACHINES

The use of a mechanical ventilator during anesthesia to control respiration allows the anesthetist to attend to parenteral fluid therapy, monitoring, and other matters

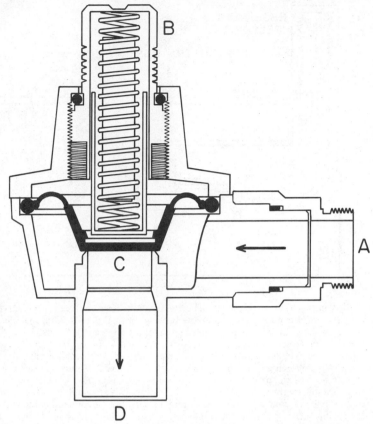

FIGURE 7–7. Waste gas scavenger valve. The waste gas scavenger valve is a modification of the exhaust valve that allows the excess gases to be collected and removed from the operating room. The valve replaces the exhaust valve and is fitted to the machine via the thread at (*A*). Gases in excess of those needed by the patient enter at (*A*), raise the diaphragm (*C*), and exit at (*D*). The pressure required to raise the diaphragm is adjusted by rotating knob (*B*). The exiting gases are led through wide-bore tubing to the outside atmosphere through the air-conditioning exhaust duct or hospital suction or directly through an outside wall. Appropriate precautions must be taken to avoid pressure or vacuum buildup in the exhaust line. (Redrawn, with permission from Ohio Medical Products, Airco Inc.)

essential to the care of patients. However, their use can also divert attention from the patient and lead to complacency. A ventilator powered by a compressed gas supply can be mounted directly on the anesthesia machine, the bellows of the ventilator replacing the reservoir bag in the breathing circuit. A simplified diagram of a compressed gas-driven ventilator is shown in Figure 7–8. Ventilators for adult use should be able to deliver tidal volumes up to 1500 ml at pressures up to 50 torr with controls to vary rate and volume of respiration. Other controls for inspiratory and expiratory flow rate and for an expiratory pause are useful in providing a ventilatory pattern with minimal circulatory depression. Safety devices should be incorporated to prevent overpressurization of the lungs (pressure relief valve) and should include a bypass to permit the patient to breathe should the bellows empty. The ventilator should also permit rapid change to manual control of respiration with a reservoir bag.

Assisted or controlled respiration during anesthesia is best conducted by manual compression of the reservoir bag. By this means, changes in pulmonary compliance can be detected instantly, periodic hyperinflation of the lungs is more readily accomplished, and the anesthetist's attention is constantly focused on the patient. Mechanical ventilation is of greatest value to the anesthetist who must work without assistance.

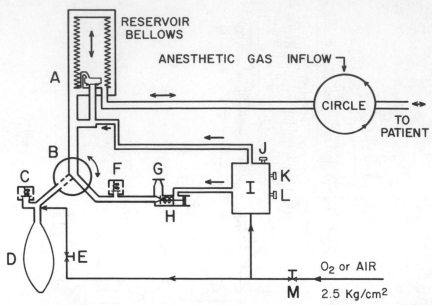

FIGURE 7–8. Gas-driven mechanical ventilator. The **Reservoir bellows** replaces the reservoir bag of the anesthesia breathing system. Respired gases enter the bellows from the anesthesia machine, through the anesthesia **circle.** The bellows, contained in a transparent closed vessel, is compressed by oxygen (or compressed air) entering the vessel from the respiratory cycle controller (*I*). At the end of inspiratory phase, this oxygen flow ceases, the exhalation valve (*H*) is opened by a second flow from the controller, and the oxygen exits at valve (*G*). Following exhalation, the cycle repeats itself. Volume of respiration as well as inspiratory and expiratory times and pauses are governed by the settings (*J, K, L*) of the controller. Excessive positive pressure is prevented by the relief valve (*F*). The overflow valve (*A*) dumps excess gas if the bellows is overfilled. Manual-assisted or controlled respiration may be selected by connecting the manual bag (*D*) to the exterior of the bellows using the selector valve (*B*), after filling the bag through the valve (*E*). Alternatively, the ventilator may be disconnected from the machine and replaced by a reservoir bag. The ventilator is turned on by opening valve (*M*). The oxygen (or compressed air) used to drive the ventilator serves only that purpose and does not enter the breathing system. The Venturi negative expiratory pressure generator and the airway pressure sensor for assisted respiration are not shown. (Redrawn from the Ventimeter/Ventilator circuit with permission of Air-Shields, Inc., a Narco Health Company.)

HAZARDS OF ANESTHESIA MACHINES

In spite of many advances in the design and incorporation of safety features in anesthesia machines, hazards are still associated with their use. The two greatest dangers are inadvertent administration of an hypoxic gas mixture and overdose of anesthetic. Either of these errors may result from carelessness on the part of the anesthetist, improper mechanical design or malfunction of the machine, or a combination of both. Delivery of an inadequate amount of oxygen may be caused by many faults: an empty oxygen cylinder or failure to open the valve, loose connections, clogged lines, sticking flowmeters, or failure or faulty installation of the service oxygen supply. Prior to use, newly installed or repaired oxygen or nitrous oxide supply lines should be tested to ensure the identity and purity of the gases as well as the adequacy of flow. Central supply systems must be checked regularly by the hospital engineering service. Overdose of anesthetic can result from unobserved changes in oxygen flow, failure to add diluting oxygen when using a Kettle vaporizer, sticking flowmeters, inadvertent use of several agents caused by leaking valves or malfunctioning flowmeters, failure to turn off the Kettle vaporizer, use of a wrong agent or a mixture of agents in the vaporizer, or an overfilled Kettle vaporizer. Steps have been taken in machine design to reduce the possibility of human error or mechanical failure. The pin-index system prevents incorrect installation of cylinders. Fail-safe systems should eliminate the possibility of administering hypoxic gas mixtures. Most machines now incorporate color-coded flowmeters, scales, needle-valve knobs, distinctively shaped knobs, and other features calculated to reduce error. Newer agent-specific vaporizers offer indexed filling ports. Ultimately, however, proper use of an anesthesia machine rests with the anesthetist; there is no mechanical substitute for vigilance.

Machines should be checked routinely for leaks, sticking or cracked flowmeters, defective needle valves, loose or worn components, and other evidence of wear or breakage. Although every anesthetist should understand the principles, parts, and functioning of these machines, unless technical personnel in the hospital are skilled in the maintenance and repair of such equipment, all but minor repairs should be left to trained servicemen. The best policy is to have the machines serviced by the manufacturer or a qualified technician on a regular basis.

ANESTHESIA CHECKLIST

Prior to induction of anesthesia, the anesthesia machine and its contents should be readied for use. All parts of the machine should be in good working order and all accessory equipment and necessary supplies on hand. After completion of anesthesia, the gas tanks should be turned off, expended items replaced, and the machine cleaned and readied for use. The following checklist is useful in preparing for anesthesia.

ANESTHESIA MACHINE CHECKLIST

Prior to Induction

A. Inspection for presence of
   1. Tank wrench
   2. Reservoir bag
   3. Breathing tubes
   4. Mask and connector
   5. Scavenger system
   6. Head strap
   7. Vaporizers filled, caps and drains closed
B. Gases
   1. Tanks on proper yokes
   2. Central oxygen and nitrous oxide lines properly connected
   3. Turn on nitrous oxide, check pressure; turn on nitrous oxide flowmeter (if gas flows, fail-safe is not functioning); turn off flowmeter
   4. Turn on oxygen, check pressure; turn on oxygen flowmeter, check flow
   5. Turn on nitrous oxide flowmeter — gas should flow; turn off nitrous oxide cylinder, turn on flowmeter and vent
C. Carbon dioxide absorber
   1. Soda lime: present? functional?
   2. Replace if necessary and secure canister properly
D. Breathing circuit
   1. Fill bag with oxygen, occlude outflow, and compress bag; investigate cause of leaks
   2. Breathe through circle filter, investigate
      a. Undue resistance
      b. Presence of irritating gas
      c. Competence of directional valves
E. Ventilator
   1. Turn on gas supply
   2. Check for function
F. Monitors
   1. Oxygen analyzer: does it indicate PO_2 of approximately 150 torr on room air and 760 torr on 100 per cent oxygen?

2. Electrocardiograph
   a. Turn on and standardize
   b. Apply leads to patient: does the ECG appear on the scope? Does the recorder function?
G. Alarms
   1. Turn on, and disconnect system: does the alarm function?

After Anesthesia

A. Turn off gas cylinders; allow pressure gauges to come to zero
B. Close flowmeter knobs gently so that valve seats are not damaged
C. Replace empty cylinders; disconnect central oxygen and nitrous oxide lines
D. Remove face mask, breathing tubes, and reservoir bag for cleaning
E. Turn off ventilator, monitors, and alarms; replace used supplies
F. If machine, ventilator, monitors, or alarms are defective, remove machine from use and notify responsible individual

REFERENCES

American National Standards Institute, 1430 Broadway, New York, NY 10018. Anesthetic Equipment Standards: Anesthetic Machines for Human Use, ANSI Z79.8-1979.
   Anesthetic Reservoir Bags ANSI Z79.4-1974.
Bancroft, ML, duMoulin, GC, Hedley-Whyte, J: Hazards of hospital bulk oxygen delivery systems. Anesthesiology 52:504, 1980.
Bruce, DL, Bach MJ, Arbit J: Trace anesthetic effects on perceptive, cognitive and motor skills. Anesthesiology 40:453, 1974.
Compressed Gas Association, 500 Fifth Avenue, New York, NY 10036. Pamphlets:
   C-9: Standard Color-Marking of Compressed Gas Cylinders Intended for Medical Use in the United States (1973).
   G-4: Oxygen (1972).
   P-2: Characteristics and Safe Handling of Medical Gases (1978).
   V-1: Standard Compressed Gas Cylinder Valve Outlet and Inlet Connections (1977).
   V-5: Diameter Index Safety System. Non interchangeable low pressure connections for medical gas applications (1978).
Compressed Gas Association, Handbook of Compressed Gases. 2nd ed. New York, Reinhold Publishing Corporation, 1981.
Cooper JB, Newbower RS, Long CD, et al: Preventable anesthesia mishaps. A study of human factors. Anesthesiology 49:399, 1978.
Cooper JB, Newbower RS, Moore JW, et al: A new anesthesia delivery system. Anesthesiology 49:310, 1978.
Dorsch JA, Dorsch SE: Understanding Anesthesia Equipment. Baltimore, Williams & Wilkins Company, 1974.
Lecky JH (ed): Waste Anesthetic Gases in Operating Room Air: A Suggested Program to Reduce Personnel Exposure. Park Ridge, Ill. American Society of Anesthesiologists, Inc, 1981.
Macintosh RR, Mushin WW, Epstein HG: Physics for the Anaesthetist. 3rd ed, Philadelphia, F. A. Davis Company, 1963.
Morris LE: A new vaporizer for liquid anesthetic agents. Anesthesiology 13:587, 1952.
National Fire Protection Association, 470 Atlantic Avenue, Boston, MA 02110. Pamphlets:
   NFPA No. 56A: Inhalation Anesthetics, 1978.
   NFPA No. 56F: Nonflammable Medical Gases, 1977.
   NFPA No. 76A: Essential Electrical Systems for Health Care Facilities, 1977.
Occupational Disease Among Operating Room Personnel: A national study. Report of an ad hoc committee on the effects of trace anesthetics on the health of operating room personnel. Anesthesiology 41:321, 1974.
Rendell-Baker L: Some gas machine hazards and their elimination. Anesth Analg 55:26, 1976.

Chapter 8

THE ANESTHETIST'S ROLE IN THE CONTROL OF INFECTION

After the introduction of anesthesia in 1846, surgery made little progress until two main issues were resolved: revision of the traditional humoral theory of disease so that surgery could be accepted as a mode of therapy, and prevention of postoperative wound infection. Both problems were solved around the turn of the century, in the former case by the contributions of pathologic anatomy and in the latter by the acceptance of aseptic technique. But the operation is only one phase of the surgical experience, and today many other factors, pre-, intra-, and postoperative, bear upon the possibility of the development of infection. Although the problem of wound sepsis is still not fully controlled, the majority of postoperative infections are systemic in nature, mainly involving the lungs, urinary tract, and entry sites for diagnostic and therapeutic procedures.

Anesthetists generally hold themselves blameless for infection, more or less content with gross cleansing or sterilization of the obvious elements of equipment. Without strict surveillance and epidemiologic study, anesthesia's role in the development of perioperative infection is hardly obvious. There are no hard data, but Walter, has graphically described several epidemics of sepsis clearly traceable to anesthetists. Such occasional occurrences are expected, as anesthetists take care of patients not only in the operating room but in respiratory and intensive care units and in the course of respiratory care and resuscitation. Thus, anesthetists themselves and the patients with whom they come in contact, whether overtly infected or healthy carriers of disease, can easily act as vectors of infection for others.

In the ensuing discussion antiseptics are defined as agents that destroy microorganisms on animate surfaces, and sterilization implies death of all forms of microbial life.

THE ANESTHETIST

Operating room garments should be changed and shoes cleaned with disinfectant after exposure to infection. Operating room clothing and shoes should not be worn outside of the operating area. Face masks saturated with exhaled vapor should be discarded after several hours of use and not continually worn about the neck. Conversation during operation should be minimal, since droplet nuclei containing bacteria multiply with talking. A physician with an acute respiratory infection should not enter the operating room; the presence of virulent bacteria can be determined by throat culture. The hands must be kept clean. Repeated washing throughout the day with detergent bactericidal soaps reduces transient bacterial flora. These precepts are of more than theoretical significance as anesthetists in the course of their work are at risk for contraction of several diseases: tuberculosis, viral hepatitis, Creutzfeldt-Jakob disease, herpes, and gonococcal infection.

THE PATIENT

Theoretically, the patient should wear a cap and mask, as should any other person in the operating room. Although a mask is seldom worn, a cap is useful to contain the hair and any shed products of the scalp. A patient with sepsis should be masked until the anesthesia face mask is applied, the anesthetist in turn being protected by a gown and gloves. Bedding on litters and bed clothes should be clean and not agitated unnecessarily, as bacterial flora in the air will be increased. Upon return to the recovery area, a patient with infection is placed in isolation so as not to endanger others. Similar precautions are followed for those at high risk for infection: the premature infant, the tracheostomized or burned patient, a patient with uremia, and a patient with bone marrow suppression. Ultraviolet light barriers help to protect these people and should be used in any area where airborne infection must be kept at a minimum. The wavelength of ultraviolet light emanating from a cold cathode low pressure mercury lamp is 2537 Å. The optimal intensity at the level of an operating table is 25 μw/cm^2, which results in an intensity at eye level of 46 μw/cm^2. Unless the patient and the anesthetist are protected by an antisunburn lotion or cream, a painless skin erythema appears at six to ten hours after ten minutes of exposure. Although the retina is not affected, an annoying conjunctivitis and photophobia appear after exposure. Thus, a protective eye shield should be worn. Another approach in the high-risk situation is the use of laminar flow techniques whereby potentially contaminated air currents are directed away from the patient.

Prophylactic antibiotics are now given before many kinds of operation. For example, bacteremia may result from oral procedures in patients with dental or gingival disease. Those patients with coincident cardiac valvular disease should be treated with antibiotics for prevention of bacterial endocarditis.

ANESTHESIA TECHNIQUE

There is nothing more indicative of a poor clinician than a chaotic, unclean anesthesia table and machine. Equipment should be arranged in an orderly manner and waste containers used for disposable objects; contaminated equipment such as endotracheal tubes and suction catheters should be kept separate from clean material. A disinfectant is used to clean the surface of the anesthesia machine and work table upon completion of each procedure. Any piece of apparatus used in conjunction with anesthesia, whether a blood pressure cuff or a cooling blanket, should be scrupulously cleaned.

INJECTIONS AND INTRAVENOUS THERAPY

This subject is discussed in Chapters 22 and 23. The infection hazard of these procedures lies not only in careless preparation of the injection site but in the contamination of equipment and fluids used. Multiple dose vials should be carefully handled to avoid contamination. When closed liquid containers have been autoclaved, a vacuum should be demonstrable upon opening, an index of sterility. Dates of sterilization and sterilization indicators are checked, even though the latter are not infallible. In administering whole blood or its products, the possibility of massive bacterial contamination or transmission of serum hepatitis must be borne in mind. An excellent preventive against infection is the use of disposable sterilized equipment whenever practicable.

PREPARATION FOR NERVE BLOCKS AND PERCUTANEOUS PROCEDURES

Although needle puncture is not the equivalent of a surgical incision, preparation of the skin should be done carefully, especially in spinal and peridural anesthesia. Although there is no such thing as sterilization of the skin without destruction of the skin, a bacteriologically clean surface can be prepared. Transient bacterial flora can be removed by washing with soap and water and the bacteria killed with antiseptics. Resident flora, consisting for the most part of *Staphylococcus albus* and about 5 per cent other pathogenic bacteria, require scrubbing and chemical treatment for removal. Deep or hidden bacteria in hair pits and orifices of sebaceous glands cannot be removed, but these are mostly nonpathogenic. Because transient and resident bacteria multiply after the skin is injured, it is best to shave the skin just before a procedure rather than the night before.

The bactericidal activity of an antiseptic depends on its concentration, the temperature of the solvent, and the degree and duration of contact. Dirt and grease are removed beforehand with a detergent or triethylene glycol. The most effective skin antiseptics are ethyl or isopropyl alcohol in 70 per cent concentration by weight and the iodophors. Iodine 2 per cent in 70 per cent alcohol is likewise effective but has the disadvantage of causing burns and allergic reactions. All these are bactericidal if sufficient contact and duration of action are allowed. Alcohols and the iodophors (Betadine, Wescodyne) are nontoxic to skin, nonallergenic, relatively inexpensive, and easily stored. For asepsis, one of the alcohols, suitably colored to indicate the area covered, is effective with one application. If the skin is obviously contaminated, a more thorough surgical scrub is employed.

STERILIZATION OF EQUIPMENT FOR ANESTHESIA AND INHALATION THERAPY

Equipment used for inhalation should be cared for so that the possibility of transmission of infection from one patient to another is avoided. The esthetic aspects of providing clean equipment require no comment; deterioration of equipment that can result from cleaning must be a secondary consideration in the important matter of preventing the spread of disease. Reports concerning transmission of disease via anesthesia apparatus are confusing at best; to our knowledge a complete epidemiologic study has not yet been done. However, it is well known that mechanical ventilators and humidifiers used in respiratory therapy can be responsible for crossinfection. It is also important to note that pathogenic bacteria have been cultured from equipment at the termination of anesthesia in infected persons. For this reason we follow the practice of treating anesthesia apparatus as if it were always contaminated. A corollary of this approach is that sufficient equipment must be on hand so that apparatus can be properly cleaned while others are in use. Disposable equipment has come into vogue as a possible means of preventing transmission of disease from one patient to another. However, at least two recent reports indicate that sterile anesthesia breathing circuits and bacterial filters do not prevent or decrease the incidence of postoperative pulmonary infection.

Infective organisms comprise the nonsporulating vegetative bacteria, fungi, tubercle bacillus, viruses, protozoa, and bacterial spores. The method of sterilization chosen depends on the nature of the material to be sterilized and the degree of sanitation sought. The following procedures are applicable to anesthesia apparatus.

HEAT STERILIZATION

Moist heat is the most dependable means of killing pathogenic organisms. Moisture increases cell permeability, and heat destroys by coagulating protein. Elevated pressures permit utilization of higher temperatures; no living organism can withstand 10 to 15 minutes exposure at a temperature of 105° C and 6.8 kg pressure as applied in an autoclave. Material thus treated is properly wrapped beforehand to allow penetration of heat and subsequent handling and storage without contamination. The package is considered sterile for up to four weeks. Dating of a package and sterilization markers indicate that the material has been treated but is not necessarily sterile. Although autoclaving eliminates the hazard of allergic reactions and irritation from chemical germicides, deterioration of rubber and plastics is hastened and sharp instruments become dull and discolored.

Other methods of heat sterilization include boiling in water for 15 minutes, offering only a bactericidal effect, and dry heat treatment at 160°C for one hour, useful for powders, greases, oils, and glass syringes.

CHEMICAL STERILIZATION

Solutions or gases are used for sterilizing objects that cannot be treated with heat, the incorporated chemicals killing organisms by coagulation or alkylation of protein. The time required for action depends on the nature of the material to be sterilized; the degree and nature of the contamination; and the temperature, concentration, and effectiveness of the chemical as a bactericidal agent. Nonsporulating vegetative bacteria, common viruses, the tubercle bacillus, and spores are increasingly resistant to destruction, in the order named. The disadvantage of most chemicals is that they act only at exposed surfaces, some reacting with metals, whereas others impregnate materials and remain as a source of irritation. Rubber is particularly susceptible to deterioration because of its adsorptive porosity and the chemicals used in its manufacture. Mineral and vegetable oils, ethers, esters, oxidizing acids, and hydrocarbon solvents cause swelling, tackiness, and a more or less rapid destruction of rubber. Phenols and cresols are not only destructive but may cause cutaneous burns if the rubber becomes impregnated. Water, alkalis, and salts of mercury do little harm. Plastics are especially susceptible to destruction by strong chemicals. The agents discussed in the next section are commonly used for sterilization.

Liquid Germicides

Phenols. These are tuberculocides and viricides but not sporicides, ordinarily used in 1 to 3 per cent concentrations to clean surfaces of furniture and apparatus. Some of the proprietary phenols are Staphene, Amphyl, and O-Syl. These should never be used on equipment that comes in contact with patients.

Halogens

Chlorine. Agents incorporating chlorine usually provide only a light tuberculocidal and sporicidal action; they are often used in the operating area to clean floors. Metals are corroded by chlorine-containing agents. Clorox is a commonly used proprietary preparation.

Iodine. When used in 0.5 to 2.0 per cent concentration in alcohol, iodine is bactericidal and tuberculocidal. Disadvantages in cleansing skin are staining of fabrics, irritation, burns, and allergic reactions. The combination of iodine with detergents, quaternaries, and macromolecules to form iodophors eliminates these faults; Wescodyne and Betadine are nonirritating, do not stain, and are nonallergenic. Iodophors can be used instead of aqueous and alcoholic solutions of iodine, being useful for topical application and for irrigation of mucous membranes and on surfaces of apparatus as well as for cleaning floors and walls.

Alcohols. Ethyl and isopropyl alcohol in 70 to 90 per cent concentration not only kill vegetative bacteria readily but are tuberculocidal as well. These solutions have been underrated for sterilization purposes. The combination of alcohol and other germicides renders the latter more effective.

GAS STERILIZATION

Ethylene Oxide

The trend toward use of disposable equipment has led manufacturers to seek nondestructive methods of sterilization. Ethylene oxide (EO), a colorless gas with a pleasant ethereal odor, is an excellent bactericidal agent for this purpose. Major advantages include excellent penetration and the fact that few materials are harmed; practically any object or piece of apparatus can be treated without damage. However, EO lacks rapidity of action even though it is effective against all organisms. The gas is extremely flammable so that mixture is necessary with carbon dioxide or Freon, both flame-quenching substances. Humidification, elevated temperature, increased pressure, creation of a vacuum beforehand, and thorough airing afterward are essential steps in the sterilization procedure. The inhalation toxicity of EO is approximately equivalent to that of ammonia, and a vesicant action is demonstrable if it is allowed to remain in contact with skin. The long time for sterilization (8 to 24 hours for the complete process), the special equipment required, and the need for dilution with carbon dioxide or Freon result in a time-consuming and costly method of sterilization. The major hazard is inadequate aeration. Residual EO and its by-products, ethylene glycol and ethylene chlorohydrin, are highly irritating to tissues and have caused tracheal inflammation as well as facial burns after contact with endotracheal tubes and masks sterilized with EO. A properly designed aerator supplies adequate aeration upon 12 hours' exposure at 50° C. Plastic or rubber materials, if stored at room temperature, should perhaps not be used until a minimum of several days has elapsed after sterilization.

PRACTICAL POINTS IN CLEANING EQUIPMENT

Contaminated anesthesia apparatus includes face masks, airways, laryngoscope blades, suction catheters, breathing tubes, reservoir bags, and, in the anesthesia machine, directional valves, the carbon dioxide absorber, and certain types of vaporization bottles. Before sterilization, apparatus should be washed with soap and hot water to remove gross debris, although ordinary soap is not bacteriostatic. Immediate immersion of apparatus in cleaning solutions prevents crusting and drying of secretions that are difficult to remove. Scrubbing of equipment is a hazard to personnel if pathogenic bacteria are present. For this reason we suggest that disinfection of apparatus be carried out initially with a solution of Wescodyne, a detergent-iodine complex (1½ oz in a pail of water), which is tuberculocidal and viricidal. Immersion in this solution should be complete and should last at least three minutes. Scrubbing can be performed in the solution without hazard. An alternate antiseptic is Cidex, an activated buffered solution of glutaraldehyde, which is bactericidal, sporicidal, and viricidal. Fortunately this solution is good for treatment of metal objects and instruments, offering rust-resisting properties as well. The interior of tracheal and pharyngeal airways should be cleaned with tight-fitting, stiff-bristled malleable brushes. Pipe cleaners can be used for finer apertures. Other equipment is scrubbed with a brush, particular attention being paid to crevices and angles that accumulate dirt and secretions. This is probably the single most important aspect of equipment sterilization. Brushes, too, should be sterilized periodically. Suction catheters and metal suction tips are rinsed with water under pressure; adhesive tape and oily lubricants are removed with acetone. At the termination of mechanical cleansing, the parts should be thoroughly rinsed in tap water. Certain pieces of apparatus, such as the reservoir bag, delivery tubes, and face masks, if not used for patients with obvious transmissible disease, may be hung to drain and dry, then used again.

Once equipment has been cleaned, sterilization can be performed in various ways. The best procedure is to package the items and then expose them to EO sterilization.

In a bacteriologic study performed by one of us, considerable contamination of presumably sterile tracheal tubes was found just before introduction into the trachea. Further study revealed that the method of handling equipment was just as important as the initial sterilization. Therefore, the following procedure has been followed: with the exception of the anesthesia machine, all items of equipment are sterilized with EO. Equipment must be handled properly to avoid transmission of disease. Breathing valves of the anesthesia machine are tested for competency by breathing through them, with corrugated tubing kept on each machine. Before removing sterile goods from containers, the hands are rinsed in a lubricating germicide provided in a plastic squeeze bottle. The breathing system, once assembled, is tested for leakage of gas without breathing through the apparatus. Oral and nasal airways are placed in a basin of sterile saline. Endotracheal cuffs are tested for leakage without removing them from the plastic sheath. The tracheal tube is removed just prior to intubation and lubricated with sterile saline from the basin. Suction catheters are kept packaged until ready for use.

SPECIAL PRECAUTIONS IN VIRULENT INFECTIONS

In the presence of tuberculosis or other infection with virulent pathogens, everything used during the anesthesia procedure must be sterilized. If closed system anesthesia is selected, disposable equipment, a to-and-fro technique, or nonrebreathing system is used because a circle filter is difficult to sterilize. If the patient has a pulmonary infection, a mask should be worn before induction of anesthesia. At the termination, the patient is then isolated from others. The anesthetist should wear a gown, and some may wish to wear gloves as well. At completion of the procedure the anesthetist's gown is placed in a "dirty linen" bag to be sterilized in the autoclave along with other material from the operating room. Gloves and soda lime are decontaminated in O-Syl solution and the soda lime then discarded. All metal parts of the anesthesia equipment are autoclaved. Rubber and plastic parts are boiled in water for 15 minutes; the rubber cushion on the face mask is deflated before subjecting it to heat. The anesthesia machine is scrubbed with a sporicidal chemical. The following disinfectants have been shown to be effective against the tubercle bacillus: ethyl alcohol, 70 per cent; isopropyl alcohol, 70 per cent; cresol solution saponated, N.F. XIII; orthophenyl phenol; p-tert-amylphenol, 2 per cent (O-Syl); and Cidex.

REFERENCES

Feeley TW, Hamilton WK, Xavier B, et al: Sterile breathing circuits do not prevent postoperative pulmonary infection. Anesthesiology 54:269, 1981.

Gajdusek DC, Gibbs CJ Jr, Asher DM, et al: Precautions in medical care of, and handling materials from patients with transmissible virus dementia (Creutzfeldt-Jakob disease). N Engl J Med 297:1253, 1977.

Laufman H: The control of operating room infection: discipline, defense mechanisms, drugs, design and devices. Bull NY Acad Med 54:465, 1978.

Symposium on infection. Br J Anaesth 48:1, 1976.

Walter CW: Cross infection and the anesthesiologist. Anesth Analg 53:631, 1974.

Walton B: Effects of anaesthesia and surgery on immune status. Br J Anaesth 51:37, 1979.

Chapter 9
MONITORING OF PHYSIOLOGIC FUNCTION

To monitor is to watch and warn. Physiologic monitoring involves continuous assessment of a patient's condition, with special emphasis on detection of change. The task of physiologic monitoring is accomplished in two ways. First, anesthetists qualitatively assess the patient's condition continuously by monitoring with their senses — touch, hearing, and sight. Second, they quantitatively assess the patient's condition by periodically making specific measurements.

Most anesthetics depress the cardiovascular and respiratory systems. If not corrected, anesthetic depression can progress to circulatory or respiratory arrest. Likewise, inadequate replacement of blood lost during surgery can lead to a decrease in cardiac output and cardiovascular collapse. Should cardiac or respiratory arrest occur, recognition and treatment must be immediate to avoid irreversible neurologic sequelae. If recognition is delayed because intermittent rather than continuous monitoring is practiced, vital time may be lost in resuscitation. Cardiovascular and respiratory function must, therefore, be monitored continuously.

At the second level of monitoring, i.e., quantitative assessment, the anesthetist periodically measures cardiorespiratory and other system functions, measurements designed to detect physiologic trends that could otherwise go unnoticed. Intermittent measurements serve, therefore, as calibration points for continuous qualitative monitoring, providing the anesthetist with the quantitative information needed to interpret the qualitative changes detected.

CIRCULATORY MONITORING

The most common techniques for monitoring the circulatory system comprise palpation of a superficial artery and auscultation of the heart. Blood flow and rate, rhythm, and strength of heart contraction can be evaluated qualitatively with either of these techniques.

A superficial pulse can be palpated over the temporal, carotid, radial, or brachial artery. Alternatively, a plethysmograph, which senses tissue blood volume by attenuating transmitted light, can be placed over a digit. As blood enters and leaves the finger following each heart contraction, infrared or visible light, which varies in intensity with the contraction, is transmitted through the finger from source to detector. The intensity received is converted to an electrical signal and then displayed on an oscilloscope. Amplitude is proportional to pulsatile blood flow in the finger and is continuously monitored to indicate cardiovascular change. Constant, quantitative circulatory moni-

76

toring can be obtained with an indwelling arterial catheter connected to a transducer and display. This is reserved for a special class of patients as later discussed.

COMBINED CIRCULATORY AND RESPIRATORY MONITORING

Continuous auscultation of the chest allows the anesthetist to monitor the cardiorespiratory system as unitary. The quality of heart sounds provides data on strength of cardiac contraction; during hypovolemia, cardiac sounds may become muffled, and with hypervolemia or congestive heart failure, extra cardiac sounds (S3 gallop rhythm) may be heard. Obviously, heart sounds are not heard during asystole or ventricular fibrillation. The onset of extrasystoles, tachycardia, or bradycardia is immediately apparent even to the inexperienced listener. Attention to breath sounds during continuous chest auscultation also provides data on the quantity and quality of ventilation. Changes in breath sounds may reveal the development of bronchospasm, upper airway obstruction, or airway circuit disconnection. However, because respiratory rate is relatively slow, a decrease in rate and even total absence are difficult to detect, even for the experienced listener.

During induction of anesthesia, a weighted stethoscope bell placed at the suprasternal notch or anterior chest provides adequate combined cardiopulmonary monitoring (Fig. 9–1). If the quality of sounds is inadequate, an esophageal stethoscope may be substituted if the trachea is first protected against aspiration by a cuffed tracheal tube. An esophageal stethoscope consists of an 18-inch #16 catheter sealed at one end with perforations at the distal 2 cm, covered with a low pressure balloon; a Luer fitting is at the other end. The balloon end is inserted through the mouth into the esophagus to the level of the heart. Here both pulmonary and cardiac sounds can usually be heard clearly. Either of the two stethoscopes can be connected by plastic tubing to a snug-fitting earpiece worn for monitoring purposes at all times. A monaural earpiece allows the anesthetist to communicate freely with operating room personnel while monitoring cardiopulmonary status. Esophageal monitors are preferred during thoracic or abdominal operations when movement of the surgical team interferes with auscultatory monitoring.

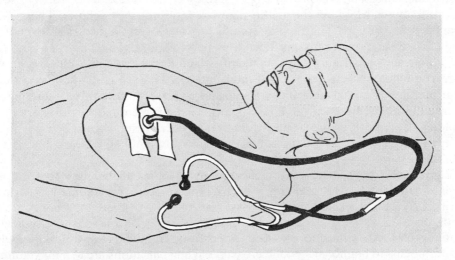

FIGURE 9–1. The precordial stethoscope, an excellent monitor of cardiac rate and rhythm in infants, children, and adults. If desired, the binaural stethoscope attachment can be replaced by a single hearing aid consisting of an individually molded carpiece or the wide, soft proximal end of a Foley, catheter.

NONINVASIVE BLOOD PRESSURE MEASUREMENT

In addition to constant qualitative monitoring of the circulation, quantitative assessment of systemic arterial blood pressure is suggested at least every five minutes. Blood pressure values, along with cardiac and respiratory rates, are then recorded on the anesthetic record.

Arterial blood pressure is usually measured indirectly using a sphygmomanometer, originally introduced by Riva-Rocci in 1896 and then used during anesthesia by Cushing, a neurosurgeon, in 1903. The sphygmomanometer consists of a compression bag surrounded by an unyielding cuff, which applies even pressure to the encircled arm. The compression bag is connected to two other devices: a hand-operated inflation bulb equipped with a valve that allows rapid inflation and slow deflation of the cuff and an aneroid (dry, gauge type) or mercury manometer. Before use, either kind of manometer must be examined to ensure that the indicator or mercury level is within the designated zero range. Aneroid manometers with a mechanical stop near the zero indicator should not be used because zero verification is obscured.

Proper use of the sphygmomanometer requires that the full cuff pressure be transmitted to the brachial artery. To ensure this, the cuff width must be at least 20 per cent greater than the mean diameter of the arm. If too narrow, the pressure obtained will be higher than the true arterial pressure; if too wide, artifactually low pressures sometimes result. Standard and large arm cuffs, thigh cuffs, and various pediatric cuffs are available.

A blood pressure cuff should be placed on the arm contralateral to the intravenous line to permit adequate infusion despite frequent measurement. When only one arm is available because of surgical constraints, both intravenous infusion and blood pressure cuff may be placed on the same arm with due caution. Alternatively, blood pressure can be measured with a blood pressure cuff of appropriate width applied to the thigh.

Auscultation of Korotkoff sounds is the standard technique for blood pressure measurement. The Guidelines of the American Heart Association should be followed. A stethoscope is placed over the antecubital space just distal to the pressure cuff. The cuff is then manually inflated until pressure reaches 30 torr above the previous systolic pressure measurement; cuff pressure is then released at a rate of 2 to 3 torr per second. Korotkoff sounds heard via the stethoscope are interpreted as follows: Phase 1 is the first appearance of faint clear tapping sounds that mark systolic pressure, even if these sounds disappear as cuff pressure decreases (auscultatory gap); Phase 2 is the period when a murmur or swishing sound is heard, which then blends into Phase 3, in which the heart sounds become crisper and more intense. Phase 4 is marked by a distinct, abrupt muffling of sounds that indicates diastolic pressure. As cuff pressure is further decreased, sounds disappear at Phase 5, occasionally recorded as an alternate (less desirable) diastolic pressure value. Sounds are occasionally heard even when cuff pressure arrives at zero. If so, the value at which slight muffling is heard is recorded as diastolic pressure.

Blood pressure can also be measured using other techniques that employ a sphygmomanometer. The technique of oscillotonometry (oscillometry), originally described by von Recklinghausen in 1904, is utilized by some. A second pressure-sensing bladder within the compression cuff is connected to a sensitive indicator of pulsatile pressure. As the cuff pressure is decreased from above systolic, the pulsatile indicator begins to bounce at systolic pressure. When pulsations are at a maximum, cuff pressure equals mean arterial pressure, and when pulsations suddenly diminish or cease, cuff pressure is equal to diastolic pressure.

A third technique for blood pressure measurement uses a flow detection device, described by Franklin and Rushmer in 1961. They applied the Doppler principle whereby the frequency of sound waves is increased or decreased by reflection from a surface that is moving toward or away from the sound source, respectively. The sound is of ultrahigh frequency (approximately 8,000,000 cycles per second or 8 MHz) and is known as ultrasound. The difference between the transmitted and received frequencies is converted to audible swishing sounds, which are interpreted as the blood pressure. This ultrasound energy is transmitted and received by piezoelectric crystals mounted in a plastic housing. In the original description, the ultrasound beam was directed along the axis of the artery. Frequency changes in the signal depended mostly on reflection from interfaces between red blood cells and plasma, hence detecting blood flow. Modification of the original technique, with the transducer now re-oriented perpendicular to blood flow, allows detection of vessel wall motion. With this orientation, placement of the transducer at the distal end of the blood pressure cuff permits determination of systolic and diastolic blood pressure. During cuff deflation, the listener first detects the onset of wall motion by a swishing sound, which is systolic pressure; deflation continues and the time between sounds decreases until the sounds coalesce at diastolic pressure, then separate again.

Systolic pressure can also be determined by monitoring the pulse distal to a sphygmomanometer cuff. The distal monitor might be an index finger placed over the radial artery, an "optical" finger plethysmograph, or an electronically transduced intra-arterial pressure waveform. Diastolic pressure cannot be assessed using any of these techniques.

AUTOMATED NONINVASIVE BLOOD PRESSURE MEASUREMENT

Automated devices are available that periodically measure blood pressure using one or more of the noninvasive methods described. Measurements of systolic, diastolic, and sometimes mean blood pressure in addition to heart rate can be made as often as every minute. Doppler and oscillometric units function well in noisy environments, whereas devices that interpret Korotkoff sounds are superior when the extremity is likely to be compressed or moved. Most commercial devices can measure blood pressure accurately even during circulatory shock.

When these devices are programmed to make frequent measurements and to sound an alarm at abnormal conditions, they act as true cardiovascular monitors. Their routine use would no doubt reduce or eliminate many incidents of undetected hypotension. They are most useful for monitoring the circulation of patients who do not meet the criteria for invasive pressure monitoring but in whom manual blood pressure determinations every five minutes are inadequate.

THE ELECTROCARDIOGRAM

The electrocardiogram (ECG) should be monitored during the administration of any anesthetic. Although yielding information only on the electric and not the mechanical activity of the heart, the ECG is useful in diagnosing and quantifying bradycardia, tachycardia, and extrasystoles. Proper diagnosis requires continual display on an oscilloscope. An audible indicator of QRS complexes is usually employed whenever the mechanical activity of the heart is not under continual surveillance with a stethoscope. This audible indicator allows the anesthetist to carry on other necessary activities while prepared to observe the ECG trace should an arrhythmia be detected.

The ECG is also a useful monitor of myocardial ischemia. As ischemia most often occurs over the anterior, lateral, or inferior cardiac surfaces, ECG leads to these areas should be utilized. A modified lead II, from right shoulder to cardiac apex, is most commonly used during anesthesia as it is equally and moderately sensitive to ischemia arising in various locations. An additional advantage is that both P waves and QRS complexes are of good amplitude and are upright because the cardiac and monitoring axes are similar. Better detection of ischemia is obtained if a true lead II and lead V_5 are simultaneously or alternately observed. Ischemia is diagnosed when the ST segment is depressed more than 0.1 mv in any lead. A definitive diagnosis can only be made when the ECG instrument used is of "diagnostic quality", i.e., it must have a band width as low as 0.05 Hz. Many ECG devices do not have this diagnostic ability but are better able to keep the ECG trace on the screen despite variations in electrode contact. These are "monitoring quality" instruments.

Most anesthetists employ pregelled adhesive-backed electrodes for routine ECG monitoring. For proper adherence of these electrodes, the underlying skin must be dry. Better electric conduction is provided if the skin is abraded slightly before the electrodes are applied. Information derived from ECG monitors should be recorded on paper to permit comparison of tracings obtained at various times during anesthesia and to provide a permanent record if needed.

Ideally, ECG monitors used in the operating room should be insensitive to electric interference. Specific interference in the operating room commonly occurs at power line frequencies, at electrosurgical frequencies, and at the sampling frequency of line isolation monitors.

The artifact caused by 60 Hz (50 Hz, UK) power line interference broadens the ECG trace line. Observation of a trace width greater than 0.2 mv should prompt a search for the source of the interference. In descending order of occurrence, the most common technical problems are poor lead contact, poor choice of monitoring axis, and fractured ECG leads.

Major interference is usually caused by electrosurgical units (ESU) operating at frequencies above 500 KHz, with artifacts produced by both cutting and coagulating modes. When the surgical electrode is energized but not in contact with the patient, energy is transmitted through the atmosphere from the electrode to the ECG lead, cable, and monitor per se. When the surgical electrode is energized and in contact with the patient, direct conduction also takes place through ECG leads and cable to the monitor. Radio frequency interference also travels through electric power lines. Most newly designed operating room monitors offer negligible ESU interference.

Line isolation monitors (LIMs) present in most operating rooms (see Chapter 34) monitor potential leakage currents in each of the two electric power wires. The device alternately samples the two power lines several times per second. Interference occurs at the frequency of the LIM sampling, usually 3.3/sec (200/min). On some ECG monitors, especially when lead contact is poor, artifacts that resemble supraventricular tachycardias appear on the waveform. Better lead contacts usually eradicate this artifact.

INVASIVE BLOOD PRESSURE MONITORING

All patients requiring blood pressure measurement more frequently than once every minute, as provided by manual or automated noninvasive techniques, require intra-arterial pressure monitoring. Rapid pressure changes might be expected as a result of decompensation in pre-existing cardiac disease; with the use of the deliberate hypotension technique; or during cardiopulmonary bypass, vascular procedures on major vessels, intracranial operations, or carotid sinus manipulation. Arterial cannulation is also indicated in the management of respiratory problems via frequent blood gas sampling. Whenever an indwelling cannula is present for respiratory measurement, blood pressure should be monitored by connection to a pressure monitoring system.

The intra-arterial pressure monitoring system usually consists of an intravascular catheter connected via fluid-filled tubing to a mechanical-electric transducer, attached electrically to an amplifier, which displays waveform and numerical measurement and sounds an alarm. Without an alarm, the waveform must be continually observed lest this medium be degraded to intermittent measurement.

Ideally, an invasive pressure monitoring system should faithfully represent true arterial pressure both graphically and numerically, measurements easily achieved for static (nonvarying) pressure as long as the system is "zeroed" and calibrated. A zero pressure location is first established with a stopcock near the transducer, at a water meniscus adjusted to the height of the right atrium. With the patient supine, this is taken as the midaxillary line or 5 cm posterior to the manubrium. With the weight of the small hydrostatic column of water applied to the transducer, the pressure monitor is electronically zeroed manually by turning a knob or automatically by the monitor after pressing the zero button.

If the transducer, pressure amplifier, or displays have an exposed sensitivity adjustment, the entire system must next be checked against a reference pressure, usually a mercury column. A mercury manometer and bulb are connected via a bacterial barrier at a convenient location, typically the stopcock used for transducer zero. The bulb is compressed, generating a pressure near the top of the selected pressure range; correct numerical values and waveform height are then verified. Care must be exercised to ensure that the hydrostatic measuring system is not contaminated, the transducer is not damaged, and that neither air nor mercury enters the tubing. When pressure monitoring systems lacking sensitivity knobs are combined with pressure transducers whose gains do not vary, calibration before use may be eliminated. Desirable accuracy for pressure monitoring systems is taken as 3 torr or 5 per cent of the reading, whichever is greater, throughout the useful range.

Transducers used for blood pressure measurement convert the force exerted on a diaphragm, crystal, or semiconductor to an electric signal, which is then processed by a pressure amplifier. The amplified signal is an almost perfect representation of the force imposed on the transducer. The signal is conveyed to electronic circuitry, which senses systolic and diastolic pressures as the peak and valley, respectively, of the electronic waveform. Numerical displays then offer the correct values for systolic, diastolic, and mean pressures at the pressure tranducer.

Unfortunately, the pressure sensed by a transducer may not be identical to that present in the cannulated vessel, because intervening tubing distorts the shape of the pressure waveform. The fidelity with which the pressure waveform is conducted is dependent upon physical properties of the fluid-filled system. During a single pulse wave if pressure changes slowly, the pressure pattern can be conducted without distortion. When pressures change rapidly, the fluid-filled tubing is unable to convey accurately the original pressure waveform. As the frequency of the waveform approaches a value called the resonant frequency, pressure values are distorted by inappropriately excessive amplification, and overshoot of the waveform occurs. The resonant frequency of the measurement system is proportional to tube diameter and is inversely proportional to the square root of tube length, fluid density, and system elasticity.

In practice, a high resonant frequency results in more accurate dynamic pressure measurement by utilizing short, stiff, wide-bore tubing while meticulously eliminating air bubbles, which contribute to system elasticity or bouncing. A large air bubble within the tubing or transducer causes severe waveform damping and results in incorrect measurement. If dynamic accuracy is needed, the transducer can be placed within inches of the arterial cannula. Transducers designed to be placed intra-arterially are also available.

The radial artery is usually chosen for blood pressure measurement for convenience and because both it and the ulnar artery perfuse the hand. To assure adequacy of circulation in the event of thrombosis of the radial artery, a modification of Allen's test is recommended to evaluate ulnar arterial blood flow. The patient makes a tight fist to partially exsanguinate the hand while the anesthetist occludes both radial and ulnar arteries with digital pressure. If release of pressure over the ulnar artery does not lead to postischemic hyperemia, the contralateral ulnar artery should be similarly evaluated. If ulnar circulation is insufficient bilaterally, the benefits of arterial monitoring should be re-assessed relative to the added risk. In the absence of adequate ulnar circulation, except in unusual circumstances, ischemia of the fingers is rare when #18 or smaller catheters are used.

Radial artery cannulation is preceded by positioning the wrist in slight hyperextension with a small folded towel behind it and taping the hand and forearm to a rigid arm board. The skin is prepared with antiseptic. Sterile gloves help prevent contamination of that portion of the cannula entering the artery. If the patient is awake, a wheal of local anesthetic is raised over the point of maximal arterial pulsation, usually 1 to 2 cm proximal to the crease at the wrist. The skin is incised with an 18-gauge steel needle to facilitate passage of the cannula. With the index finger of the operator's nondominant hand palpating the artery proximal to the site of puncture, an 18- or smaller gauge plastic cannula-over-needle is inserted parallel to the axis of the artery while angled 30 to 45 degrees to the surface. The operator's hypothenar eminence is supported on the palm of the patient's supinated hand, while the hub of the cannula-over-needle is grasped between thumb and index finger.

With the direct cannulation technique, the intent is to puncture the arterial wall cleanly with a single insertion. To help assure that the back wall of the artery is not inadvertently punctured, the bevel of the needle is held downward. When brisk spurting of blood is seen, indicating puncture, the steel needle is held firmly while the overlying plastic cannula is advanced full length (4 to 6 cm) into the artery. If arterial blood flow is not encountered during insertion, the inner needle should be withdrawn before the catheter is removed, because successful puncture is sometimes evident during withdrawal rather than insertion. In an alternate technique, the catheter-over-needle is rapidly advanced through both anterior and posterior vessel walls. The needle is then removed and the catheter slowly withdrawn. When the tip re-enters the vessel lumen the catheter is advanced. This technique appears to offer the same relative safety.

CENTRAL VENOUS PRESSURE

Right and left heart filling pressures provide useful indices of the adequacy of circulating blood volume and cardiac contractility. Central venous pressure (CVP) represents the hydrostatic pressure in the right atrium or intrathoracic vena cavae. Beyond the thorax peripherally and below the diaphragm, venous valves and external compression may cause peripheral pressures to differ from the central pressure. The normal CVP is 2 to 15 cm H_2O or 1.5 to 11 torr. The pressure rises and falls with changes in intrathoracic pressure, an effect particularly pronounced during positive pressure pulmonary ventilation. Therefore, CVP must always be measured at end expiration. The central location of the catheter must be verified by carefully observing the respiratory fluctuation of the CVP trace or by the use of an electronic transducer or a chest x-ray. When CVP is low, circulating blood volume may be inadequate or venous capacity excessive owing to sympathetic blockade or vasodilation. In patients with normal cardiac function, a high CVP suggests an elevated circulating blood volume or decreased venous capacity, owing to vasoconstriction or vasoactive drug therapy. CVP measurement is required whenever one is uncertain of the adequacy of circulating blood volume in relation to the need for fluid replacement.

Electronic transducer systems similar to those used for measurement of arterial pressure improve the reliability of CVP measurements, as artifacts resulting from changes in airway pressure can be visually removed. Indeed, with an electronic device, the venous pressure can be continuously monitored. A water column is commonly used to measure CVP but requires apnea to achieve a stable height (Fig. 9–2). For this reason, electronic monitors may be preferable. With either method, the sensor must be carefully zeroed at the height of the right atrium as described previously. Affixing the arterial or venous transducer to the patient's chest or the operating room table facilitates initial transducer alignment as well as later correction for table height adjustment. Alternatively, a fluid-filled tube can be attached at the zero port of the transducer and then to the patient's chest at right atrium height and the transducer electronically zeroed after each table adjustment.

Central venous or right atrial pressure is influenced by the degree of emptying of the right ventricle with the previous contraction, an effect combined with that of venous return. If the right ventricle fails to empty because of pulmonary hypertension or, more

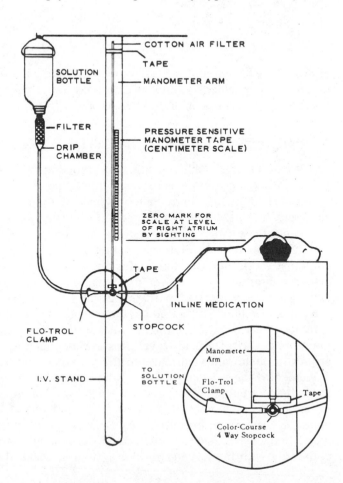

FIGURE 9–2. Constant monitoring of central venous pressure. Inset shows detail of circled area. (Reproduced with permission of the Fenwal Co.)

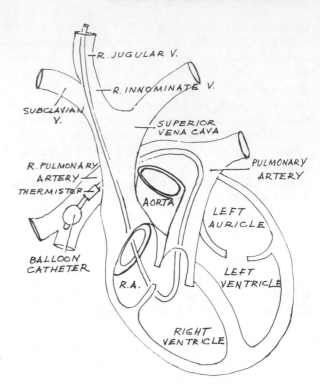

FIGURE 9–3. Representation of a balloon-tipped pulmonary flotation catheter traversing the right heart.

often, left heart failure, CVP will be elevated and one may draw the incorrect inference that the patient's blood volume is expanded. If left heart failure is suspected, additional monitoring is required as noted hereafter.

PULMONARY CAPILLARY WEDGE PRESSURE

When left heart failure is present preoperatively or when the potential for onset exists during anesthesia, left heart filling pressure should be measured. This is accomplished by use of a balloon-tipped pulmonary artery flotation catheter (PA catheter), first described by Swan and Ganz (Fig. 9–3).

A plastic sheath with introducer is inserted percutaneously into the internal jugular vein. The sheath has an internal diameter sufficient to pass a #7 French catheter and contains a side port for fluid infusion. A device permitting sterility at the sheath-catheter interface during later manipulation is placed over the sheath, and the PA catheter is then inserted with the distal port connected to a prezeroed electronic transducer system. The balloon at the catheter tip is then inflated with 1 ml air, and the catheter is advanced while the pressure waveform sensed at the catheter tip is visually monitored. Characteristic waveforms are identified as the catheter passes from right atrium through right ventricle into the pulmonary artery. The catheter is then further advanced to the wedged position, where display of a venous waveform with balloon inflated and a pulmonary artery waveform with balloon deflated is possible. Care must be taken to ensure that the balloon is not left in the wedged position except during actual measurement lest pulmonary ischemia or infarction result. A venous waveform with a and v waves is observed because the balloon places the catheter tip in direct fluid continuity with the left atrium in a system in which there is no flow; the pulmonary capillary wedge pressure (PCWP) therefore accurately represents mean left atrial pressure (LAP). Failure to obtain LAP occurs when fluid flows past the catheter owing to improper balloon placement or when obstruction to blood flow occurs in vessels between the pulmonary artery and left atrium and during positive end–expiratory pressure (PEEP) ventilation. To avoid respiratory artifacts, PCWP should always be obtained at ambient pressure, at end expiration, and an electronic pressure transducer should always be used.

If PCWP is high (above 12 torr), myocardial function is deemed inadequate regardless of CVP. If normal (less than 12 torr) and simultaneous with a normal CVP, circulating blood volume and myocardial function are probably adequate. With the balloon-tipped catheter deflated, pulmonary artery pressure can be monitored — a useful measurement in patients with elevated pulmonary vascular resistance or right heart failure.

CARDIAC OUTPUT

An overall quantitative estimate of cardiovascular performance is provided by measurement of cardiac output, as this represents total blood flow to all body tissues and associated vascular shunts. Although alterations in peripheral vascular resistance can result in regional ischemia despite normal cardiac output, total output is nevertheless a most useful guide in cardiovascular assessment.

As cardiac output cannot be monitored continuously with currently available methods, intermittent assays are done. A modification of the balloon-tipped pulmonary artery flotation catheter is used for this purpose. A bolus of 10 ml of iced, normal saline or dextrose solution is injected through the central venous pressure port of the catheter. Thus, a thermal indicator, quantified in negative calories, is carried through the right ventricle into the pulmonary artery and diluted by blood flow through the right heart. Temperature is sensed in the pulmonary artery by a thermistor located proximal to the deflated balloon. Cardiac output is inversely proportional to the area under the temperature-time curve, as blood flow is the source of "thermal dilution." An injectate can be used at room temperature, but measurement precision is degraded, especially when intravenous fluids are concurrently and rapidly infused. The thermodilution technique has virtually replaced other invasive techniques for clinical cardiac output measurement.

AIR EMBOLISM

When operation is performed in areas in which venous pressure may fall below atmospheric pressure, air embolism can occur owing to gas entrapment. This complication is detected with the greatest sensitivity by means of a Doppler ultrasound transducer placed over the heart. When air is present in the right atrium, the interface between air and blood in the heart results in an abnormal ultrasound reflection, uniquely apparent in the instrument's audible output. Air embolism can also be detected by observation of a sudden fall in respiratory end-tidal Pco_2. Continuous monitoring for air embolism is required whenever its occurrence is anticipated, as treatment must begin immediately (see Chapter 27).

RESPIRATORY MONITORING

Rate and quality of respiration should always be monitored during anesthesia. Observing chest movement combined with listening for the sounds of airway obstruction is adequate for monitoring sedated patients receiving regional anesthesia; however, auscultation of the chest provides a convenient and useful means of monitoring.

During general anesthesia, pulmonary ventilation is always monitored. Inhalation anesthetics typically cause shallow, rapid ventilation, whereas opioids induce breaths of apparently normal depth but of lesser frequency. Monitoring is usually accomplished via auscultation of the chest with a precordial or esophageal stethoscope, also used for cardiac monitoring as noted previously. With the stethoscope, depth and regularity of breathing as well as the presence of wheezing or rales can readily be detected. Additionally, direct observation of the chest and neck can reveal signs of respiratory obstruction, tracheal tug, use of accessory muscles of respiration, or asymmetric ventilation. Adequacy of ventilation can only be guaranteed through arterial blood gas analysis; this should be performed when inadequate ventilation is suspected.

During manual ventilation with a reservoir bag in the anesthesia circuit, the anesthetist can assess rate and depth of respiration qualitatively. Care must be taken not to overestimate the volume of exhalation when the reservoir bag fills with high fresh gas flows as well as during the patient's exhalation.

When mechanical ventilation is employed, additional monitoring is required. The human ear is unable to detect changes consistently when respiration is slow (less than 15/min). Auscultation is thus insufficient to detect even such gross abnormalities as disconnection of tubing or mechanical ventilator failure. For this reason, an additional monitor of ventilation is required. Most commercially available monitoring devices sense a cyclically varying positive pressure, sounding an alarm after 20 seconds of perceived apnea. Expiratory volume or flow monitoring devices would be better but are not yet clinically available. As a ventilator can malfunction and apply high pressure to the patient's airway, an overpressure alarm or relief valve should be incorporated therein. When waste anesthetic gases are scavenged using a closed reservoir connected to a vacuum system, monitoring and protection against application of negative pressures are also suggested (see Chapter 7).

Hypoxic gas mixtures can easily be delivered by anesthesia machines because of malfunction or flow control adjustment; therefore, inspired oxygen concentration should be monitored (see Chapter 7). This is done with an oxygen analyzer and alarm, the threshold of which cannot be set below 21 per cent oxygen. If, on occasion, the analyzer is to be used on the expired side of the circuit, the threshold can safely be as low as 18 per cent.

Most currently available oxygen monitors employ the Clark polarographic sensor, an electrode usually consisting of a precious metal cathode and an anode polarized with a 0.7 volt potential. The electrodes are separated by a KCl bath contained by an oxygen-permeable membrane. Reduction of oxygen occurs at the cathode, resulting in current flow proportional to the partial pressure of oxygen. The oxygen analyzer should be calibrated before each anesthetic; the electrode is exposed to 100 per cent oxygen and the reading adjusted to indicate 100 per cent. Calibration is confirmed by exposing the electrode to room air, which should result in a reading of 21 per cent.

RESPIRATORY VOLUME MEASUREMENTS

Measurements of tidal volume can be performed when adequacy of ventilation is questionable. A spirometer or volume meter in the expiratory circuit provides a convenient measure of tidal volume. Some devices also incorporate a timer to indicate minute volume. Care must be taken in interpreting the results of measurements in the expiratory anesthesia limb, as the volumes are artifactually elevated by elastic expansion of the materials of the anesthesia circuitry. To assess respiratory volumes without error, measurement must be made at a point between endotracheal tube and anesthesia circuit.

MONITORING OF RESPIRATORY GAS EXCHANGE

Analysis of exhaled gases can provide information on the function of both the respiratory and circulatory systems. This is performed only when specially indicated or when the special equipment required is easily available. A normal expiratory CO_2 curve displaying a sharp rise and flat plateau at approximately 40 torr suggests normal CO_2 production, adequate circulation, and adequate alveolar ventilation. An abnormal expiratory CO_2 pattern may suggest a problem in any of the three variables. Carbon dioxide percentage, or partial pressure, can be monitored with an analyzer whereby infrared light of a particular wavelength is passed through a minute sample of expiratory gas. The wavelength of infrared light is selected to coincide with maximum absorption by CO_2 plus the coincident minimum absorption by other gases. Absorption is thus accomplished, and CO_2 tension or concentration is displayed both graphically and numerically. Some CO_2 analyzers permit the infrared beam to pass directly through expired gas to avoid the sampling factor.

Physiologic and anesthetic gases can be monitored by mass spectrometry. Oxygen, nitrous oxide, carbon dioxide, and inhalation anesthetic gases and vapors can be monitored in both inspired and expired gas. In the mass spectrometer, gases are drawn into a vacuum and ionized, accelerated in a magnetic field, and finally measured at a detector based on their mass-to-charge ratio. Fixed field devices employ multiple locations for atomic mass sensing, whereas quadrapole devices accelerate ionized atoms in a variable fashion to be measured at a single detector. Because a mass spectrometer is an expensive piece of apparatus, the device is often programmed to make measurements in several operating rooms in rapid sequence.

Transcutaneous measurements of oxygen tension (T_cPo_2) can be made using a modified Clark electrode, which measures the combined effects of PaO_2, skin perfusion, and dermal oxygen consumption. In neonates and infants, measurements with this device closely approximate PaO_2, but in the adult the influences of perfusion and oxygen consumption are far greater, so that PaO_2 cannot be reliably predicted. However, monitoring T_cPO_2 as an indicator of combined tissue oxygenation and perfusion may be useful. Oxygen saturation can be monitored using an optical transducer applied to the ear lobe.

To assure the adequacy of carbon dioxide elimination and blood oxygenation, indwelling catheters employing Po_2 and Pco_2 electrodes have been developed for continuous arterial blood gas analysis and monitoring. Because of their great expense and precarious adjustment, they have not yet been adopted into clinical practice. Periodic sampling of arterial blood for gas analysis provides the ultimate verification of the adequacy of ventilation, recognizing that the data become available only after the fact.

Closed circuit anesthesia techniques can be useful in monitoring oxygen consumption when oxygen is administered at a rate that maintains both circuit oxygen concentration and reservoir bag volume at a constant. In a steady state, adjusted oxygen delivery is equal to the patient's oxygen consumption.

URINARY OUTPUT

The urinary bladder should be catheterized during most major operations to avoid overdistention of the bladder and to observe urine flow and as an indicator of adequacy of blood and fluid replacement. The collecting system must be capable of accurately measuring half-hour outputs of between 1 and 200 ml. Flows greater than 30 to 40 ml/hr usually reflect adequate intravascular volume. Oliguria can result from a reduced circulating blood volume, the antidiuretic effect of anesthetics, the stress of operation, or impending acute renal failure. If infusion of blood or fluid restores blood pressure and CVP to acceptable values but does not result in adequate urine flow, further inquiry is needed. First, the mechanical adequacy of the collecting system should be assured. Pulmonary artery catheterization may be indicated if congestive heart failure is suspected. If a diuretic such as furosemide (Lasix) or mannitol is administered, the value of urine volume in judging adequacy of volume replacement is lost. Monitoring urinary output also permits visual evidence of hemoglobinuria, sometimes the first and occasionally the only sign of incompatible blood transfusion.

TEMPERATURE MONITORING

Body temperature may change markedly during anesthesia (usually declining during general anesthesia) when the abdomen or thorax is open and because thermoregulatory function is depressed by most inhalation anesthetics and because operating rooms are air cooled. Body cooling also occurs when cold blood or fluids at room temperature are given intravenously. Infants, with their large surface area–to–body mass ratio, are particularly susceptible to hypothermia during anesthesia (see Chapter 25).

Hyperthermia, although less common, can occur in the anesthetized infant or adult because of the thermal insulation provided by sterile drapes and the pharmacologic loss of thermoregulatory capacity secondary to the use of anticholinergic drugs and inhalation anesthetics. Some patients are febrile prior to induction of anesthesia; in this situation, every effort should be made to lower body temperature beforehand. Malignant hyperthermia is a relatively rare complication of anesthesia (see Chapter 33). While the body temperature rises precipitously in this syndrome, tachycardia and tachypnea precede detection of fever.

During anesthesia, temperature is usually monitored in the esophagus, although the nasopharynx, axilla, rectum, and external ear canal adjacent to the tympanic membrane are alternate sites. Measurement in the esophagus records the average temperature of blood returning to the heart and permits early detection of changes in body core temperature. Unfortunately, the reliability of esophageal temperatures is influenced by pulmonary ventilation and local cooling of the heart. Tympanic membrane temperature approximates that in the regulatory centers of the brain, but the danger of eardrum perforation on insertion may be high when performed in an anesthetized patient unresponsive to pain. Rectal temperature measurement is not nearly as useful because of poor access to the site and the slow response to temperature changes in central organs.

Electronic thermometers containing thermistors or thermocouples are used for routine internal temperature measurement. Thermistors comprise tiny beads of semiconductor material, the resistance of which varies with temperature. The thermistor circuit incorporated in an esophageal probe produces a voltage that varies linearly with temperature and does not require calibration. These thermistor circuits form the basis of most digital electronic thermometers. Analog thermistor thermometers contain a single thermistor and utilize a nonlinear scale for temperature reading. In other electronic thermometers, a thermocouple composed of two dissimilar metals joined at the point of temperature measurement is used; the voltage derived from variations in temperature is produced at this junction.

Surface temperature monitoring with a temperature sensor applied to the forehead has been advocated because it is both noninvasive and convenient. Liquid crystal technology is useful for this purpose, with the appropriate temperature-sensitive chemicals compounded and laminated into a thin plastic sheet. As temperature varies, the mixtures of chemicals change crystalline structure and, hence, color. By geometric arrangement of various chemical mixtures, an interpretation through an overlying numerical display is possible. This technique is useful for forehead temperature monitoring when information on temperature trends is desired, as core temperature changes are fairly well tracked. Mercury thermometers are not useful during anesthesia because they fail to respond to decreases in temperature and are breakable.

CENTRAL NERVOUS SYSTEM

The central nervous system is traditionally monitored by the anesthetist, who carefully observes clinical signs of anesthetic depth (see Chapter 17). In addition, the electroencephalogram (EEG) can be monitored during anesthesia for procedures in which localized brain ischemia can be expected, as in carotid endarterectomy with surgical occlusion. For other than such specific purposes the EEG has proved of little value in anesthesia, as the brain wave patterns vary from agent to agent and are readily affected by changes in $Paco_2$ and Pao_2. When recording a multichannel EEG, read-outs are usually interpreted by a trained technician or neurologist. There are, however, new analysis and display techniques that can be utilized during anesthesia (see Chapter 11).

NEUROMUSCULAR BLOCKADE

A full discussion of neuromuscular blockade monitoring can be found in Chapter 15.

THE ANESTHESIA RECORD

The meticulous recording of measurements in the anesthesia record serves many purposes (see Chapter 10). In addition to recording information for permanent record, the ongoing anesthetic record is in reality a monitoring medium. Every time a new piece of information is added to the record in graphic form, an ongoing picture of the overall anesthetic course is extended so that anesthetists can observe the evolving trend. The five-minute interval suggested in the record format prompts anesthetists to make measurements at least at that frequency. Attention to the record assists in monitoring the progress of a patient's condition, thus guiding anesthetic management.

SUGGESTED FURTHER READING

Laver MB (ed): Symposium on Monitoring. Anesthesiology 45:113, 1976.
Newbower JS, Ream RS, Smith AK, et al: Essential Noninvasive Monitoring. New York, Grune & Stratton, 1980.
Sykes MD, Vickers MD, Hull CJ: Principles of Clinical Measurement. Boston, Blackwell Scientific Publications, 1981.
Uhl RR: Monitoring: present concepts and future directions. Curr Probl Anesth Crit Care Med 1:1, 1977.

Chapter 10
THE ANESTHESIA RECORD

Although anesthetics had been given since 1846 and many important clinical observations had been made by individuals like John Snow, the first formal records of anesthetic administration were not kept until 1895. At that time, Harvey Cushing and Amory Codman, then second-year Harvard medical students, began to keep "ether" charts. They recorded pulse rate, respiration, depth of anesthesia, and amount of ether given in an effort to give safer anesthesia; they realized full well the dangers involved. Subsequently, in 1902, Cushing introduced the Riva-Rocci method of measuring blood pressure, and this datum was added to the anesthesia record.

Anesthesia records are of undeniable value to patient, anesthetist, surgeon, and nursing staff. If pulse rate, respiration, blood pressure, and other pertinent findings are recorded at frequent intervals, the patient's condition can be assessed at any moment. A good anesthesia record is also of help if a patient must be re-anesthetized. There are cogent medicolegal reasons for keeping accurate records, since review can establish the course of events more convincingly than recourse to memory. In one article on prevention of malpractice claims, it was stated that in a 10-year experience of reviewing cases of alleged malpractice, the author had yet to see one in which a record of the anesthetic course was complete. If one engages in the simplest clinical research, anesthesia records are the key to the collection of data, but it must be emphasized that conclusions derived from data are only as reliable as the original records. Furthermore, governmental supervision of medical practice and reimbursement for services require the evidence provided by records.

A fine record is of little value if anesthesia is poor; in other words, care of the patient should never be sacrificed for the sake of a record. There are times when the patient demands complete attention; it would be foolhardy at these times to withdrawn one's attention to complete the record. In the majority of cases, however, one should be able to keep a full and detailed account of any procedure.

Examples of suitable records are shown in Figures 10–1 and 10–2. Records should be kept in duplicate — one for the hospital chart, the other for departmental files and analysis. A third copy is sometimes kept for the anesthetist's own files, and parts of the record may be used for billing purposes.

INFORMATION DERIVED FROM ANESTHESIA RECORDS

The instructions given here apply to any anesthesia chart and should improve the quality of information gained. Notations should be entered with a ballpoint pen, pressing firmly.

90

FACE OF THE RECORD

Name. The patient's name is printed legibly, family name first. Address and telephone number are useful for follow-up studies and for business purposes. These items are usually stamped on the chart with an addressograph plate.

Age. Age is written in years for adults and for infants in months, weeks, or days.

Height. Height is written in inches or centimeters; if not known, an estimate should be made.

Weight. Weight is given in pounds or kilograms; if not known, an estimate should be made.

Recent Meal. The patient is asked when last food or drink was ingested. "No" is entered if the patient has had nothing by mouth for at least six hours; otherwise, "yes" is written and a description given of oral intake. At the same time, the patient is asked about removal of false teeth and chewing gum or tobacco. Infants and young children usually will have been fed within four hours of operation; injury, shock, emotional tension, or alcohol ingestion almost always delays emptying of the stomach. Parturients are considered to have full stomachs.

Physical Status. See Chapter 3 for numerical rating.

Premedication. The amount, time, route of administration, and effect of preanesthetic drugs are recorded. Note is made as to whether sedation is adequate or if untoward effects have occurred. If no medication was given, "none" is written.

Information of Vital Importance. There should be a place at the top of an anesthesia record to call attention to information of special importance. If a patient has myasthenia gravis, active tuberculosis, or major allergy, this is of vital importance. Some may choose to indicate whether the patient has accepted or is a suitable candidate for the anesthesia planned.

Operative Permit. The patient should have granted permission in writing for performance of anesthesia and operation. This is essential in the case of minors, for whom the parent or legal guardian should grant permission. Individual states vary in their legal requirements, and anesthetists should be familiar with the law in their community.

Drug History. As indicated in Chapter 4, many therapeutic drugs adversely affect the course of anesthesia. Questions should be asked and notes made of any drugs the patient has been taking.

L. P. This refers to spinal or peridural anesthesia. In evaluating the cause of untoward sequelae of spinal anesthesia, it is important to have an idea of the trauma caused by lumbar puncture. One should record needle gauge; spinal level of insertion; kind of lumbar puncture, whether midline or lateral; number of insertions; absence of paresthesias or location when produced; character of cerebrospinal fluid (CSF), whether clear or bloodstained; ease of aspiration or flow of CSF. When using a catheter for serial spinal or peridural anesthesia, estimated length of catheter insertion is noted.

Induction: S.U. If induction is satisfactory, "S" is circled; if unsatisfactory, the "U," and reasons are given. Common components of unsatisfactory induction include vomiting, retching, cough, soft tissue obstruction, laryngospasm, excessive mucus, excitement, slow uptake of inhalation agents, apnea, respiratory depression, hypotension, cyanosis, and ECG irregularities.

Airway. Details of airway insertion during anesthesia are recorded in this space. When an airway is placed in the pharynx through the mouth or nose, "oropharyngeal" or "nasopharyngeal" is written. One should indicate whether insertion was accompanied by trauma such as bleeding from the gums or nose, damage to teeth, or injury to lips. Information regarding trauma is likewise recorded when a catheter is passed into the trachea. In addition, "endotracheal" should be circled and the following data supplied:

1. Route of intubation: orotracheal or nasotracheal (right or left).
2. Number of attempts at intubation: each insertion of the laryngoscope or each time the tube is passed beyond the epiglottis is counted as an attempt. When intubating blindly, an attempt is considered as each time the tube is advanced with the expectation of entering the larynx.
3. Diameter of tube; use of stylet.
4. Method of intubation; unless otherwise noted it is assumed that intubation was performed under direct vision with a laryngoscope. If a laryngoscope was not used, "blind" is written.
5. Note is made if the tube is cuffed (also when the cuff was inflated and how much air was used) or if a pharyngeal pack was placed.

Maintenance. This space is for recording important happenings during anesthesia. As experience increases, the anesthetist is better able to select which observations should be recorded. The simplest method is to number the observations 1, 2, 3 — chronologically, writing the same number below the graphic chart with the remark made. Here comments are made on aspects of the patient's condition other than pulse, respiration, and blood pressure; for example, excessive secretions, laryngospasm, hiccough, fever, tremor, muscle twitching, or convulsions. Notes are made concerning the conduct of anesthesia that cannot be shown on the graphic chart: respiratory obstruction, cyanosis, and wearing off of spinal or regional anesthesia. An

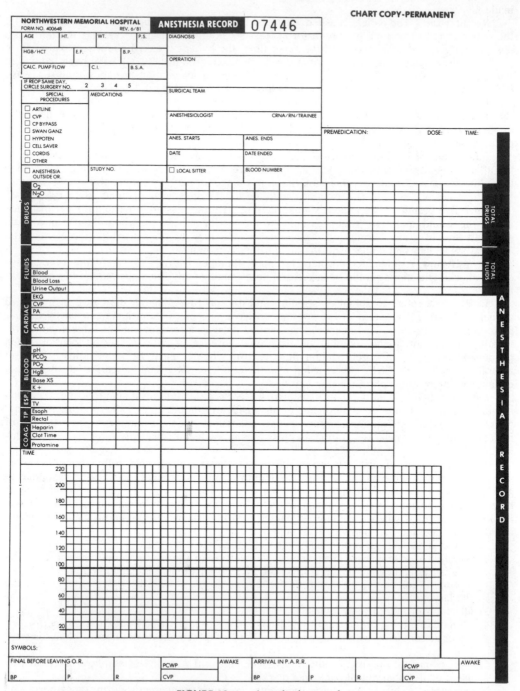

FIGURE 10–1. Anesthesia record.

THE ANESTHESIA RECORD

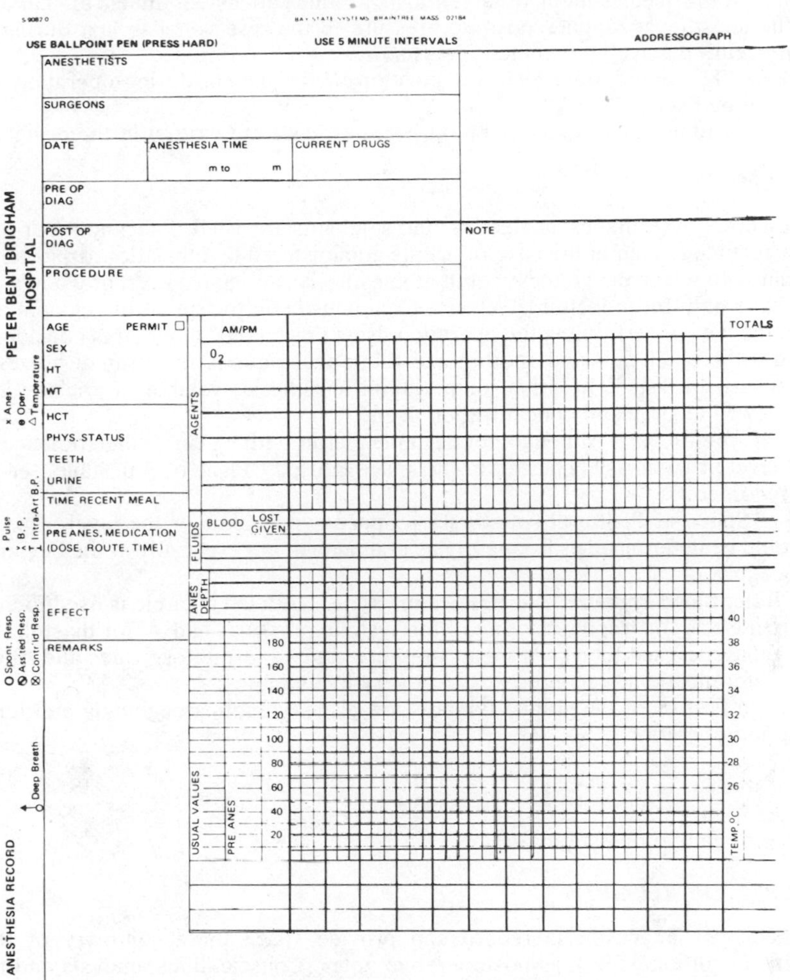

FIGURE 10–2. Anesthesia record.

anesthesia record should have a place for recording esophageal or rectal temperature, central venous and pulmonary artery pressure, blood loss, and fluid replacement. It is important to note reasons for changing the anesthetic or method of administration and to record the time at which the patient's position is changed, because alterations in respiration or circulation often appear.

Treatment given during the procedure that is not recorded elsewhere should be noted here: for example, tracheobronchial toilet (TBT); aspiration of mucus or other material from trachea or bronchi; dose and route of administration of drugs. When transfusion is given, positive identification of each unit of blood is made.

Details of surgical manipulation that may be significant physiologically or that may affect the conduct of anesthesia should be included in the record. For example, traction on the gallbladder may cause a fall in blood pressure.

Technique. The technique by which an anesthetic is given is written directly below the agent. More than one method may be used for the same agent during anesthesia; any change is recorded. The several techniques of inhalation anesthesia are described in Chapter 13.

Controlled Respiration (CR). This signifies that the anesthetist "breathes" for the patient, controlling both rate and depth of respiration after apnea has been produced by hyperventilation, administration of drugs that depress activity of the respiratory center, or administration of a neuromuscular blocker.

Assisted Respiration (AR).   This technique is used to improve ventilation and to minimize movements of the mediastinum or diaphragm as the patient continues to make respiratory efforts. The anesthetist supplies positive pressure to the reservoir bag just during inspiration; expiration occurs passively at ambient pressure.

Position.   The appropriate term for position of the patient during operation is indicated. Symbols may be used.

Fluids.   Amounts of solution given during anesthesia are written in the designated space.

THE CHART

Anesthetics.   Anesthetics, analgetics, and adjuvants are listed. The amount or concentration of agent is included, even in the case of agents administered by inhalation. In general, the main agent is that with which the greatest depth of anesthesia is obtained (except when a potent agent has been used only for induction). When a local anesthetic for spinal or regional anesthesia is given with the idea of performing the operation using this method alone, it is considered the main agent even if the block fails and another anesthetic technique is substituted; however, the new agent must also be listed. In spinal or peridural anesthesia, volume of anesthetic injected is recorded as well as drug and concentration used.

Depth of Anesthesia.   Although not a simple matter with modern inhalation anesthetics, the estimated level of narcosis is charted in the space labeled "Plane of 3rd Stage" each time vital signs are recorded.

Level of Spinal or Peridural Anesthesia.   Space is provided for the level of sensory block. Levels should be determined as frequently as practicable, but especially at the beginning and end of the procedure.

Pulse Rate, Blood Pressure, and Respiratory Rate.   A filled in circle is used to indicate pulse rate, an open circle for respiratory rate, v for systolic pressure, and $\wedge$ for diastolic pressure. A dash (—) may be used to record mean pressure. Pulse, respiratory rate, and blood pressure should be determined and recorded at least every five minutes.

Along the bottom of the graph, symbols are placed denoting beginning and termination of anesthesia and operation.

Start of anesthesia — X
Start of operation — ⊙
End of anesthesia and operation — ∧

REVERSE OF RECORD

The back of an anesthesia record can provide space for a summary of the patient's preoperative condition as well as postoperative notes. Conscientious analysis and recording of significant events of the postoperative course provide valuable data. It is common to hear expressions of opinion as to the incidence of a particular complication. Unless reliable data have been gathered, such opinions merit little credence.

Notes for the record are obtained from the patient and the hospital chart, the nurse's notes, the surgeon's notes, and the anesthetist's physical examination. Ideally, every patient should be seen within the first 24 hours of operation and again on the second, fourth, and sixth postoperative days, the frequency of visits relating to the patient's condition. Sufficiently close contact should be maintained during the patient's stay in the hospital to enable recording of such delayed phenomena as pulmonary embolism, wound disruption, and postlumbar puncture (LP) headache. Any of these complications may take place as late as the seventh to tenth postoperative day. The number of days of observation should be recorded.

Although the form of the anesthesia chart may vary, there are certain fundamentals of anesthesia and surgical convalescence that should be recorded. These are described according to systems.

Nervous System

Headache.   Adequate description of headache includes time of onset; when patient sat up or got out of bed; duration; location; severity; presence of nausea, vomiting, stiff neck, or dizziness; disturbances of hearing or vision; and relation to posture — a nonpostural LP headache with stiff neck suggests a meningeal reaction. Dimness, blurring of vision, or diplopia is noted. "Blocking of the ears," diminution in hearing, and tinnitus may relate to changes in CSF pressure transmitted to the internal ear. These details are important in describing LP headache.

Disturbance of Sensation. Under this heading one lists hyperesthesia or hypoesthesia, that is, increased or decreased perception of any sensory modality (touch, pain, temperature, vibration, or position sense). Patients given spinal or other kinds of regional anesthesia are questioned specifically about the presence of numbness, tingling, or paresthesia. Backache can be recorded under the heading of sensory disturbance.

Disturbance of Motor and Visceral Function. Paresis or complete paralysis should be recorded including any subjective or objective evidence of weakness, change in gait, or abnormalities of bowel or bladder function.

Mental State. One of the complications of general anesthesia and operation may be development of a toxic psychosis. The elderly are likely to show mental disturbance of varying degree in the early postoperative days. Disorientation may also occur as a result of administration of sedatives — a reaction common in the aged. Emergence delirium and excitement in the immediate postoperative period should be recorded in detail and treatment noted. Delayed recovery of consciousness or occurrence of convulsions is listed.

Respiratory Tract

Sequelae of Tracheal Intubation. These include evidence of trauma to nose, mouth, pharynx, or larynx. One also records presence of edema, obstruction to respiration, infection, subcutaneous emphysema, mediastinal emphysema, hoarseness, sore throat, or cough.

Major Respiratory Complications. Development of atelectasis is not uncommon. Diagnosis of pneumonia may be made if the clinical course is prolonged, if a febrile reaction subsides slowly, and if there are physical and x-ray signs of consolidation. Miscellaneous respiratory complications include hiccough, pleural effusion, pneumothorax, and aspiration pneumonitis.

Circulatory System

Complications such as shock, hemorrhage, cardiac arrhythmias, thrombophlebitis, pulmonary edema, and embolism are recorded. Sequelae related to anesthetic management, like low blood pressure and bradycardia, and prolonged hypertension or tachycardia related to vasopressor drugs should also be noted.

If cardiac failure and pulmonary edema occur, one evaluates the role of parenteral fluid therapy, hypoxia, respiratory obstruction, hypertension, or hypotension as causative factors. If signs of coronary insufficiency or infarction develop, similar evaluation is made.

Gastrointestinal Tract

Although it is difficult to analyze the causes of nausea or vomiting in the postoperative period, a beginning can be made in this direction if certain details are recorded. These are time of onset, duration, severity, presence of abdominal distention, relation to administration of opioids, or prior history of these sequelae.

Liver

Evidence of hepatic damage is recorded and the role of anesthetic management evaluated.

Kidney and Bladder

Prime concerns are oliguria, anuria, and urinary retention. Hypotension, incompatible transfusion, and drugs given are evaluated as possible causes. Treatment of sequelae is noted. The nature of retention can be evaluated best by recording the number of catheterizations. If an indwelling catheter is in place, this is stated.

NOTES ON THE PATIENT'S HOSPITAL CHART

In addition to the preoperative notes and data written on the back of the anesthesia record, notes should be made on the patient's permanent hospital record. Significant facts concerning the postoperative course are recorded over the signature of the anesthetist. Headache and pulmonary, cardiovascular, gastrointestinal, and urinary tract complications are analyzed from the standpoint of anesthesia.

USE OF RECORDS FOR STATISTICAL PURPOSES

If every anesthesia chart contained sufficient information, many aspects of anesthesia subject to erroneous impression might be described with reasonable accuracy. Even if this were accomplished, however, the ordinary anesthesia record could not lend itself readily to the gathering of facts for analysis. For this reason, several systems have been devised to facilitate accumulation of data of statistical value. We describe several techniques here because not all anesthetists have access to computer-based systems.

Perhaps the least complicated method of gathering data is the use of a punch card system. The chart is made of lightweight cardboard, with rows of holes at the edges of the card. Each group of holes pertains to an item of interest, such as anesthetic used or operation performed. During conduct of anesthesia the usual information is recorded on the chart. Subsequently, the holes at the edges are cut with a punch. For example, if halothane had been used the hole opposite "halothane" would be punched so that it extended to the edge of the card. Eventually, in obtaining data on halothane anesthesia, all records would be stacked and a sorting needle passed through the holes punched. All unpunched charts would be carried away, leaving only the halothane charts for counting and analysis. Such charts can be "combed" with one or two needles or a hand-operated mechanical device containing as many as six needles. This kind of card can be used for many purposes such as the study of nerve blocks or inhalation therapy.

In another system in increasing use, code numbers are substituted for items of interest on the anesthesia chart. Numbers may be printed directly on the chart for encirclement or printed on a second sheet. In either case code numbers are transferred to a final record card, a small oblong cardboard with vertical and horizontal spacings. This card, too, is punched, the perforations corresponding to code numbers of the variables studied. Initial punching and final sorting as well as duplication and checking for errors are accomplished by machine.

Data gathered from any system of record keeping can be used as input to a computer-based system and stored on permanent magnetic tape. Depending on the computer program adopted, hospital reports can be prepared, billing done, or research and case follow-ups accomplished with the data automatically recovered and assembled by the computer. In a variation of this approach, a computerized monitoring system has been described that can noninvasively obtain, process, display, and print out the vital signs contained on the standard anesthesia record.

A semiautomatic anesthesia keypad record system has also been devised. Special keys classifying drugs by physiologic effect and adaptive programming features minimize the number of keys needed, the entry time, and the need for drug codes or mnemonics. In comparison with typical handwritten records, the keypad records are more accurate and more legible and usable for subsequent patient management; and long delays between reading and recording are reduced.

We have presented this brief discussion of statistical systems because we believe this to be an important aspect of anesthesia. Obviously an anesthesia department will have to assess the advantages and disadvantages of the several anesthesia charts available before adopting one for use. Whatever the statistical system selected, the user should remember the dictum that the record is only as good as the individual who keeps it. Nevertheless, little progress can be made toward safer administration of anesthetics unless clinical practice is under continuous unbiased scrutiny. Record keeping and statistical systems discussed in this chapter represent a step in this direction.

DEATH REPORTS

The conscientious anesthetist will analyze carefully the circumstances surrounding the death of every patient who has received an anesthetic After discussion among supervising staff, a decision is reached as to whether a written summary of the events should be prepared. If anesthesia management as viewed in its broadest aspects appears not to have contributed to the death, a report is not written. In the United States the Joint Committee on Residency Training Programs insists on an analysis of every surgical death occurring within 24 hours of anesthetic administration. If anesthesia is judged to be an obvious contributing factor, detailed analysis is indicated. In some instances a cause-and-effect relation between anesthesia and death is less certain but suggestive. Examples follow.

1. A patient, having retched violently in the postoperative period, ruptures an abdominal incision and dies as a result of this complication.

2. Severe hypotension occurs during operation, and a cerebral or coronary vascular accident is responsible for death 24 to 36 hours later.

3. Hepatic failure follows a prolonged period of hypotension during or after operation.

4. Delayed death from pneumonia or lung abscess results from aspiration of gastrointestinal contents during or following anesthesia.

These cases deserve as careful an analysis as those in which death can be attributed directly to the anesthetic. Careful preparation of a report is of considerable educational value to the individual who administered the anesthetic. Discussion of reports at departmental conferences or by anesthesia study commissions is also enlightening. In the aggregate, such information can be used to assess the many factors that contribute to a fatal outcome. We believe that preparation of death reports is an essential feature of the teaching and practice of anesthesia. An anesthetist or a department not resorting to analyses overlooks an opportunity for self-appraisal and improvement. The death report should include:

1. Name — last, first; race; sex; age; physical status.
2. Date of admission.
3. Date of last anesthesia.
4. Date of death.
5. Hospital number.
6. Family and past history, including previous anesthesias.
7. Present illness, physical examination, and laboratory findings. Course in hospital prior to operation.
8. Surgical diagnosis and proposed operation.
9. Anesthesia — complete description including premedication, time given, effect, technique, course, and complications, and recovery.
10. Operation — surgeon, surgical procedure, and surgical complications. Anesthetist's opinion of surgical contribution to death.
11. Recovery room record (Chapter 36).
12. Postoperative course and treatment, including kind and amount of fluids, opioids, oxygen, and vasopressor drugs.
13. Death — date, time after operation, and description (if during anesthesia or operation, include under 19).
14. Discussion of probable causes of death.
15. Cause of death according to anesthetist who gave the anesthetic.
16. Cause of death according to supervising anesthetist and departmental staff.
17. Lessions to be learned.
18. Additional notes, with references.
19. Autopsy findings, autopsy number.

20. Cause of death according to pathologist.
21. Final decision on causes of death (anesthesia, condition of patient, operation, and so on).

Items 9 through 13 should be written within 24 hours of death and discussed with the supervising anesthetist as soon as possible.

APPRAISAL

To a beginning resident, an intern, or a student, record keeping may seem a mundane aspect of anesthesia. However, its importance is stressed by far too few. Problems that may arise as a result of inadequate record keeping are as follows.

1. A patient fails to recover as expected from anesthesia. Was there anything that happened during the operation to provide a clue as to when and how the problem arose?

2. The elapsed time between entry into the operating room, induction of anesthesia, and beginning of operation is long. Are there data available to prove that anesthesia preparation time was too slow?

3. A medicolegal suit against an anesthesiologist results in a court appearance. The court asks the defendant for the written proof on which the defense is based.

4. An anesthetist claims that his patients experience postlumbar puncture headache in only one of 100 cases. Where is the documentation for this statement?

Accurate record keeping is a discipline; if taught and mastered early it is likely to be followed throughout one's professional life. If not, it may never be practiced until a case discussion before peers requires proof of a statement that is not available, or a court of law seeks documentation that the defendant cannot produce; or a research project fails because of lack of acceptable data.

Learn from those who have experienced or witnessed all of the examples given. Accurate record keeping is necessary.

REFERENCES

Baetz WR, Schneider AJL, Apple H, et al: The anesthesia keyboard system. *In* Gravenstein JS et al (eds.): Monitoring Surgical Patients in the Operating Room. Springfield, Ill., Charles C Thomas, 1979.
Beecher HK: The first anesthesia records. Surg Gynecol Obstet 71:689, 1940.
Moore DC: Professional Data Anesthetic Record System. Seattle, Washington, 1972.
Shaffer MJ, Kaiser PR, Klingenmaier CH, et al: Manual record-keeping and statistical records for the operating room. Med Instrum 12:192, 1978.
Zollinger RM, Kreul JF, Schneider JL: Man-made versus computer-generated anesthesia records. J Surg Research 22:419, 1977.

Section 3
ANESTHESIA AND OPERATION

Chapter *11*

FUNDAMENTALS OF INHALATION ANESTHESIA

To produce a desired pharmacologic effect with any class of drugs, an adequate dose of a compound of sufficient potency must be administered and delivered to the effective site of action. Usually, the oral or parenteral route of administration is utilized in therapy. However, the inhalation anesthetics are unique in that the respiratory tract is utilized as a means of entry into the body. The special characteristics of this mode of administration are considered in the section on Uptake and Distribution. Factors altering dose requirements are considered under Minimal Anesthetic Concentration.

UPTAKE AND DISTRIBUTION OF INHALATION ANESTHETICS

Although the precise mode of action of anesthetics is not completely understood, it is clear that the primary site of action is located in some part of the brain. The aim in clinical anesthesia is to achieve an adequate partial pressure of anesthetic in the brain so that it may exert the desired effect, which will vary according to the concentration developed in the brain (Fig. 11–1). Concentration in tissues is the product of the solubility and partial pressure of the anesthetic in that tissue. The solubility of an anesthetic is, for all practical purposes, considered a constant. The partial pressure is changeable, therefore controlling the concentration of anesthetic present. The partial pressure of anesthetic in the brain is indirectly controlled by altering the composition of the inhaled gas mixture.

The concentration of a gas in a mixture is proportional to its partial pressure. The terms partial pressure (torr) and concentration (vol per cent) are used interchangeably to describe the dosage of inhaled anesthetics:

$$\frac{PP_A}{Total\ P} \times 100 = concentration,\ vol\ per\ cent$$

Where PP_A = partial pressure of anesthetic, and P = pressure

The term "tension" is used synonymously with partial pressure, applicable to both gas mixtures and body tissues.

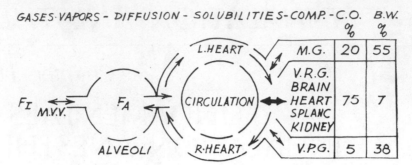

INSP. MIXT-VENTILATION-BLOODCARRIAGE-TISSUE UPTAKE

FIGURE 11–1. Schematic diagram of uptake and distribution of inhalation anesthetics. The inspired concentration, F_I or fraction inspired, of anesthetic is under direct control of the anesthetist. F_I is delivered to the alveoli by the minute volume of ventilation (*M.V.V.*). The alveolar concentration, F_A or fraction in alveoli, regulates tension (partial pressure) of anesthetic agent in arterial blood. The four tissue groups or compartments (*COMP.*), the vessel rich group (*V.R.G.*), the muscle group (*M.G.*), and the vessel poor group (*V.P.G.*) tend toward equilibration with anesthetic tension in arterial blood but reach that equilibrium at rates determined by the volume of blood flow to each tissue. The brain is the site of action. *C.O.* = cardiac output and *B.W.* = body weight, both expressed in per cent. *SPLANC* = splanchnic circulation.

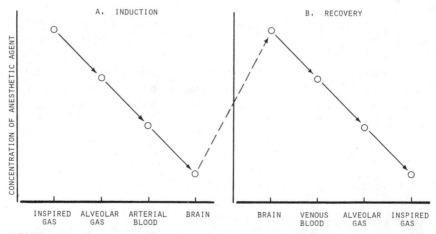

FIGURE 11–2. Pressure gradient of anesthetic agent during (*A*) induction and (*B*) recovery from anesthesia. Arrows indicate movement of anesthetic down the pressure gradient. With induction, the anesthetic agent moves into the brain and the brain anesthetic concentration rises as indicated by dashed arrow. An inspired gas mixture devoid of anesthetic agent is administered at the termination of the anesthetic, and there is a reversal of pressure gradients, allowing anesthetic agent to flow out of the brain until recovery occurs.

By controlling the composition of the inspired gas mixture, a pressure gradient is created between the inspired atmosphere and the blood circulating to the brain so that the anesthetic flows into or out of the brain, with the respiratory and circulatory systems as conduits. The difference in partial pressures is the driving force that causes anesthetic agents to move down the concentration gradient. During induction of anesthesia, a chosen concentration of anesthetic is added to the inspired mixture. A gradually decreasing pressure gradient is created between the inspired mixture and alveolar gas, then to arterial blood and the brain (Fig. 11–2A). During recovery, as the anesthetic is allowed to escape into the atmosphere, reversal of the pressure gradient occurs, and the anesthetic moves down the gradient from brain, to blood, to alveolar gas, and finally to the external atmosphere (Fig. 11–2B). During the period between induction and recovery, the partial pressure of anesthetic in the brain is controlled indirectly by discrete manipulations of the inspired concentration.

The brain and other body tissues tend to equilibrate with the partial pressure of anesthetic drug delivered to them by arterial blood; the blood, in turn, tends to equilibrate with the alveolar partial pressure of anesthetic. The alveolar tension of anesthetic is paramount because it determines the tension of anesthetic in blood perfusing the brain and other body tissues. Factors that indirectly affect the alveolar partial pressure therefore alter the concentration of anesthetic in blood, brain, and other tissues.

FACTORS AFFECTING ALVEOLAR TENSION

The partial pressure of anesthetic in alveolar gas represents the algebraic sum of factors that deliver and remove anesthetic from the alveoli. Increasing the inspired concentration and augmenting the minute volume of ventilation increase delivery of anesthetic and cause alveolar partial pressure to rise (Table 11–1). Conversely, decreased inspired tension or decreased minute volume of ventilation reduces alveolar tension. A high pressure gradient between alveolar gas and venous blood enhances removal of anesthetic and ultimately reduces alveolar tension. Similarly, an increase in cardiac output or in the solubility of an anesthetic tends to increase removal from alveolar gas and to reduce the partial pressure of anesthetic in the alveolus. Alternatively, reducing any of these variables reduces uptake and tends to cause a rise in alveolar partial pressure of anesthetic.

The effects on alveolar anesthetic tension of alterations in inspired tension, ventilation, and cardiac output are obvious and need no further explanation. The mixed alveolar-venous tension gradient of anesthetic relates to removal of the anesthetic from the circulating blood by tissues or to the addition of anesthetic to the blood from the tissues during recovery. Over a given period uptake of anesthetic from the lung must equal the total uptake by the various body tissues. An agent of high solubility is taken up rapidly from the lungs by the blood and from the blood by the tissues. This delays the rise of anesthetic partial pressure in both alveolar gas and blood. This in turn limits the rise in partial pressure in the brain and slows the rate of induction. Conversely, with

TABLE 11–1. Factors Promoting Increase in Alveolar Anesthetic Tension

Increased Delivery
  Increased inspired tension of anesthetic
  Increased minute volume of ventilation

Decreased Removal
  Decreased cardiac output
  Decreased alveolar–venous anesthetic gradient
  Decreased solubility of anesthetic

TABLE 11–2. Partition Coefficients of Anesthetics at
Body Temperature 37 ± 0.5°C* (Ostwald)

Anesthetic	Blood/Gas	Brain/ Blood	Muscle/ Blood	Fat/ Blood	Oil/Gas
		Tissue/Blood			
Ether	12.1	1.1	0.9	5	65
Halothane	2.3	2.6	2.5	60	224
Enflurane	1.8	2.6	1.7	105	98
Isoflurane	1.4	3.7	4.0	45	98
Nitrous oxide	0.47	1.1	1.2	3	1.4

*Average values gathered from the literature.

an anesthetic of low solubility not so much is removed from the lungs. Alveolar tension of anesthetic therefore rises quickly and alveolar gas, blood, and brain equilibrate rapidly, facilitating the onset of anesthesia.

The solubility of anesthetics is expressed in terms of blood:gas or tissue:blood partition coefficients. Anesthetic gases and vapors equilibrate between the two phases, according to pressure gradients. At equilibrium the partial pressure of anesthetic is the same in both phases. An agent with a blood:gas partition coefficient of 2 will reach twice the concentration (in vol per cent) in the blood phase as in the gas phase at equilibrium, but the partial pressure will be the same in both phases. Similarly, an agent with a brain:blood partition coefficient of 2 will reach twice the concentration of anesthetic in the brain as in the blood at equilibrium, but the partial pressure in brain and blood will be equal. Table 11–2 lists the currently employed anesthetics in decreasing order of blood solubility, hence according to increasing rapidity of induction of anesthesia. Also shown are the tissue solubilities of these agents. Tissue solubility regulates tissue uptake of anesthetic, thus governing depletion of anesthetic from capillary blood. As a result, the partial pressure of anesthetic is lowered, influencing the alveolar-venous concentration gradient and in turn affecting alveolar tension.

THE RELATION BETWEEN INSPIRED AND ALVEOLAR TENSION

At a constant inspired tension of anesthetic, alveolar tension tends to approach that inspired until total body equilibrium is reached. At equilibrium, the inspired alveolar, blood, and tissue tensions are equal and no exchange of anesthetic occurs across the alveolar-capillary membrane. This state is rarely reached. The curves describing the rate at which alveolar tension approaches equilibrium have a uniform shape, each divided into three portions: an initial steeply rising slope, a midportion where the knee of the curve occurs, and a final, relatively flat slope slowly rising toward ultimate equilibrium. The steep rise represents initial uptake of anesthetic from the alveoli; the midportion represents approaching equilibration of the rapidly perfused vessel-rich group of tissues — brain, heart, kidneys, liver; and the final portion represents the slower equilibration of the more poorly perfused tissues (Fig. 11–3). These curves lie in inverse order to the solubility of the anesthetic, that is, the least soluble approaches equilibrium most rapidly. These curves also faithfully represent the manner in which anesthetic in arterial blood approaches an ultimate steady state, since arterial blood is in equilibrium with the alveolar tension upon each perfusion of the lung. Also, these curves depict the partial pressures at which the brain approaches equilibrium.

To summarize, during administration of an inhalation anesthetic, alveolar tension at first rapidly rises toward that of inspired gas, then more slowly. Arterial tension

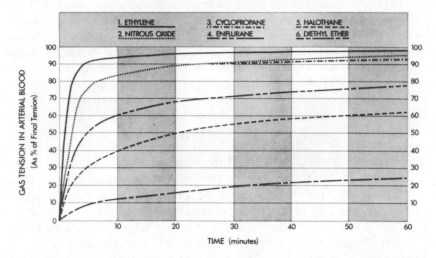

FIGURE 11–3. The rate of rise of tension of anesthetic in arterial blood with different agents administered at a constant inspired tension.

follows the alveolar tension as pulmonary blood equilibrates with alveolar gas. Then tissue tensions rise, approaching the arterial level. The vessel-rich tissues, including the brain, equilibrate most rapidly, the remaining tissues more slowly. As a rule, the administration of anesthesia is completed before alveolar gas tension has reached the inspired tension. When the anesthetic is removed from inspired gas, diffusion from the alveoli occurs, subsequently reflected in the blood and tissues. The same physical and biologic factors regulating uptake also affect the rate of elimination of anesthetics.

PHYSICAL CONSEQUENCES OF ANESTHETIC UPTAKE

Normally, gas is moved in and out of the lungs solely by the mechanical activity of ventilation, but this is not quite true during induction of and recovery from anesthesia. During induction, uptake by the blood of anesthetic from an inhaled gas mixture tends to reduce the volume of gas in the alveoli. This causes a mass movement of inspired gas into the alveoli from the tracheobronchial tree and into the tracheobronchial tree from the inspired source, in effect augmenting the volume of gas inspired. During recovery, anesthetic moves from blood to alveoli, increasing the volume of alveolar gas and inducing mass movement of gas out of alveoli into the air passages, thus augmenting the volume of gas exhaled. The consequences are of practical importance during administration of nitrous oxide, which is taken up in significant volume when inhaled at high concentrations even though poorly soluble. The more potent agents (halothane, enflurane, and isoflurane) are administered in such low concentrations that volume uptake is limited despite their high solubility.

The *concentration effect* is caused by two factors: the ventilatory augmentation action and the concentrating action, both of which operate when anesthetics are taken up in significant volume during induction. The higher the concentration of anesthetic administered, the greater the uptake and the greater the augmentation of inspired volume. Increased volume of ventilation promotes an increase in alveolar partial pressure (see Table 11–1) and tends to offset the fall in partial pressure induced by pulmonary capillary uptake; thus a more rapid induction of anesthesia results. A concentrating action also contributes to the concentration effect. Removal of half the volume of nitrous oxide from a lung filled with 50 per cent concentration (50 parts in 100 parts total) yields 33⅓ per cent nitrous oxide (25 parts in 75 parts total) instead of halving the concentration to 25 per cent. At lower concentrations, such as 1 per cent (1 part in 100 parts total), removal of half the volume of the anesthetic reduces concentration by nearly half (0.5 part in 99.5 parts total). Higher inspired partial pressures tend to concentrate the anesthetic and blunt the effect of uptake. The concentration effect implies that the higher the inspired concentration, the more rapid the rise in alveolar partial pressure and, consequently, induction of anesthesia.

The *second gas effect* occurs when two anesthetics are administered concurrently; this results from the two factors that produce the concentration effect — ventilatory augmentation and a concentrating action due to anesthetic uptake. Uptake of a large volume of a "first gas," usually nitrous oxide, in a gas mixture augments inspired volume and increases alveolar delivery of the "second gas" in the mixture, more than would be expected in the absence of the first gas. Moreover, uptake of the first gas tends to increase the alveolar concentration of a second gas by a concentrating phenomenon similar to that described for nitrous oxide. The result is a more rapid rise in alveolar partial pressure of the second gas in the presence of, rather than in the absence of, the first gas, thus a more rapid induction of anesthesia.

Augmentation of exhaled volume may occur as anesthetic gases are eliminated. Diffusion hypoxia may appear owing to rapid diffusion of nitrous oxide from pulmonary capillary blood into alveolar gas at the termination of anesthesia. The resulting reduction in partial pressure of both oxygen and carbon dioxide can be prevented and the patient protected from hypoxemia by administration of an enriched oxygen atmosphere for two or three minutes at the termination of nitrous oxide anesthesia.

MINIMUM ALVEOLAR CONCENTRATION — A MEASURE OF POTENCY

The relation between an administered dose and quantitative effect produced is an expression of drug potency. Per se, potency is a relatively unimportant property of an anesthetic, as the sole limitation placed on the inhaled partial pressure is the need for an adequate oxygen content in the inhaled gas mixture. Only in the case of nitrous oxide is potency a meaningful limitation. The ability to assess potency, however, is important in evaluating factors that alter patient response to anesthetics and in the study of mechanisms of anesthesia.

The pharmacologic concept of the median effective dose was adapted by Eger to fill this need. He defined *minimum alveolar concentration* (MAC) as the anesthetic concentration at 1 atm that produces immobility in 50 per cent of subjects exposed to a noxious stimulus (Table 11–3). The concept has been criticized because it measures only a single point — abolition of muscular response — on a continuum of responses

TABLE 11–3. MAC Compared with Anesthetic Concentration

Agent	MAC	Induction Concentration (Vol/%)	Maintenance Concentration (Vol/%)
Methoxyflurane	0.16	Up to 3	0.2–1.0
Halothane	0.76	2–4	0.5–2.0
Isoflurane	1.12	2–4	1.0–3.0
Enflurane	1.68	2–5	1.5–3.0
Ether	1.92	10–30	4–15
Cyclopropane	9.2	20–50	10–20
Nitrous oxide	105.0	Up to 80	Up to 80

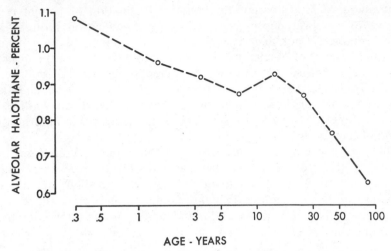

FIGURE 11–4. Halothane MAC (vertical axis) constantly decreases with age, with the possible exception of a slight increase at puberty. (From Gregory GA, Eger EI II, Munson ES: Anesthesiology 30:488, 1969.)

that represents a graded dose response curve to anesthetics. The concept neglects the importance of slope of the response curve.

Analysis of a second point in the anesthetic dose response curve, the point at which response to verbal command returns (MAC/AWAKE), permits the inference that the curves for methoxyflurane, halothane, ether, and fluroxene are parallel, since the ratios of MAC/AWAKE to MAC are constant. Moreover, the MAC concept is applicable to all inhalation anesthetics and no satisfactory alternate method is available. Thus, MAC has been used extensively to evaluate factors that influence anesthetic requirements.

The variability of MAC in a single species is small, and the correlation of MAC values in man with all other species studied shows a remarkable consistency. Based on measurements of MAC, it appears that patient susceptibility to anesthetics is not altered significantly by gender, duration of anesthesia, thyroid function, variations in Pa_{CO_2} between 10 and 90 torr, metabolic alkalosis or acidosis, variations in Pa_{O_2} between 40 and 500 torr, or moderate anemia or hypertension. A slight circadian variation has been demonstrated in the rat.

Increased susceptibility to anesthetic depression occurs with marked hypercarbia, severe anemia or hypoxemia, increasing age (Fig. 11–4), decreasing body temperature (Table 11–4), depletion of brain catecholamines, and exposure to other central nervous system depressants.

TABLE 11–4. Effect of Lowering Body Temperature on MAC

Agent	Number of Dogs	MAC at 37 C	Change in MAC/10C*	Decrease in MAC/10C(%)
Cyclopropane	6	15.9 ± 3.6	3.0 ± 1.5	20 ± 9
Diethyl ether	5	3.3 ± 0.7	1.2 ± 0.5	38 ± 11
Fluroxene	8	6.6 ± 0.8	2.8 ± 1.2	42 ± 15
Methoxyflurane	7	0.24 ± 0.03	0.13 ± 0.03	52 ± 11
Halothane	6	0.87 ± 0.11	0.44 ± 0.88	53 ± 8

*The change in MAC/10C indicates the decrease in absolute per cent gas concentration required to prevent movement in response to tail clamp per 10C lowering of body temperature from 37C. Values are the average ± one standard deviation. (From Regan MJ, Eger EI II: Anesthesiology 28:689, 1967.)

Measurement of MAC permits quantitative evaluation of patient responses to combinations of cerebral depressants. Opioid premedication reduces MAC in a dose-related manner. Each increase in dose is accompanied by a proportionate decrease in the amount of inhalation anesthetic required to reach the desired level of anesthesia. Diazepam also reduces anesthetic requirements. The additive effect of mixtures of inhaled anesthetics has also been documented. Antagonism of anesthetics by central stimulants, such as amphetamine, has likewise been verified. Thus, an awareness has developed among anesthetists of the quantitative nature of anesthetic potency and of factors that may alter it.

Anesthetists have long recognized the resistance of the infant and the relative susceptibility of the elderly to anesthetic depression. A progressive decrease in anesthetic requirement from infancy to old age, except for a slight increase at puberty, is now documented. The clinical impression that hypothermia reduces anesthetic requirements has also been verified, and the variability in the interaction of hypothermia with different anesthetics has been shown (see Table 11–4).

MECHANISM OF ACTION OF ANESTHETICS

The manner in which chemical compounds interact with living cells to produce the anesthetic state has intrigued scientists and clinicians ever since the phenomenon of anesthesia was first observed over 135 years ago.

Any theory of anesthetic action must be able to explain a perplexing series of facts relating to narcosis:

1. An extensive array of unrelated chemical structures produces general anesthesia. They seem to share no common structure-activity relation.
2. During narcosis, alterations of function occur in virtually all systems of the body. Physiologic, metabolic, and structural changes have been described and must be rationalized.
3. Lipid solubility of anesthetics seems to be of importance, as the wide range of effective concentrations is reduced to a small range when solubility in body lipids is calculated.
4. The phenomenon of pressure reversal of general anesthesia occurs and must be explained by any mechanistic theory.

Heretofore attempts at an explanation of narcosis based on chemical, physical, physicochemical, neurophysiologic, biochemical and neurochemical interactions have been wanting. Over the last decade, however, a revival of interest in and an application of newer techniques to this still unsolved problem have taken place. Approaches that hold promise focus on physicochemical interactions of anesthetics with biologic membranes and on resultant alterations in membrane function.

The interested reader is referred to any standard textbook on pharmacology for an extensive discussion of theories of historical interest as proposed by some of the outstanding biologic scientists of the last century. The following discussion focuses primarily on molecular interactions of current interest, although reference to older approaches is made when applicable.

PHYSICOCHEMICAL MECHANISMS

The basic principle postulated by Meyer and Overton (1899–1901) that lipid solubility of anesthetics controls anesthetic action remains viable. Specifically, the narcotic action of a drug correlates strongly with its solubility in biologic membranes. Interactions of anesthetics with biologic membranes causes expansion of the membrane. Membrane expansion by a critical volume of 0.4 per cent results in anesthesia, and both expansion and anesthesia are reversed by hyperbaric pressure (40 to 100 atm). Membrane expansion in protein-containing biologic membranes is ten times greater than that predicted solely on the basis of the amount of anesthetic present in the lipid phase, whereas the expansion of the pure lipid membranes of liposomes is of the predicted order of magnitude. This suggests an interaction between anesthetic molecules and membrane protein. Evidence is available to show that anesthetics selectively combine with hydrophobic groups in biologic protein, whether purified or membrane associated. Perhaps these alterations in membrane structure affect synaptic transmission in the brain, giving rise to anesthesia.

Eyring has postulated that anesthetics induce changes in the tertiary structure of membrane protein that could alter cation flux through membrane pores, thereby depressing membrane excitability. Long before this, Lillie, in 1909, demonstrated anesthetic-induced alterations in membrane permeability, but there is no reason to suspect that anesthetics selectively alter only plasma membranes. Membranes in mitochondrial and endoplasmic reticulum cannot be disregarded as potential sites of anesthetic action. Functions of mitochondria in regulating intracellular calcium levels and in metabolic and energy metabolism may be altered by anesthetic deformation of mitochondrial membranes. Consequently, mechanisms of anesthesia based on those functions have been postulated.

NEUROPHYSIOLOGIC AND BIOCHEMICAL MECHANISMS

The classic experiments of Larrabee and Posternak suggested assignment of the primary site of anesthetic action to the synapse. C. P. Richards has demonstrated synaptic inhibition by all anesthetics studied (halothane, ether, methoxyflurane, enflurane, trichloroethylene, and chloroform), but it is not clear whether the site of action is pre- or postsynaptic. If acting presynaptically, decreased release of the excitatory neurotransmitter, acetylcholine, or increased release of the inhibitory neurotransmitter, γ-aminobutyric acid, could be responsible. Both events occur upon experimental exposure to anesthetics. If the anesthetic is acting postsynaptically, reduced sensitivity to acetylcholine or hyperpolarization of the postsynaptic membrane could occur; both phenomena have been observed. Therefore, depressed excitation or increased inhibition in cerebral synaptic areas must be considered separate, viable mechanisms of anesthetic action.

Inhibition of synaptic transmission could result from several other kinds of metabolic actions of anesthetics. The anesthetized brain is rich in energy stores, but older theories of anesthetic action based on reduced cellular respiration or deficiencies in energy stores are inconsistent with current observations. Anesthetic inhibition of metabolism in mitochondria has been demonstrated but lacks linkage to a causative mechanism of narcosis. The concomitant depression of calcium uptake by brain mitochondria implies elevation of intracellular Ca^{++}, which should reduce release of transmitter and stabilize postsynaptic membranes. Both actions depress synaptic transmission and lead to depression of central nervous system function.

The several mechanisms discussed here are not necessarily exclusive of one another. It is possible that the basic underlying event in anesthetic action is an alteration of membranous structure within the cell by anesthetic molecules. Subsequent events may involve metabolic or neurophysiologic alterations that depress synaptic transmission, resulting in anesthesia. All other alterations associated with anesthesia could then take place. Alternatively, a unitary theory of anesthetic action may not explain the actions of the many drugs that give rise to anesthesia. In fact, there may be several ways in which the anesthetic state is induced.

PRACTICAL POINTS

INDUCTION

Induction of anesthesia is accomplished either by intravenous administration of a short-acting barbiturate or other intravenous agents or by inhalation of an appropriate mixture of anesthetic and oxygen. The anesthetic potency of the gas mixture initially administered nearly always exceeds that needed for maintenance, frequently approaching 5 MAC (see Table 11–3). This is called overpressure, a stratagem used to overcome the delays in induction imposed by anesthetic solubility in blood and the need successively to equilibrate alveolar gas and circulating blood to deliver anesthetic to the brain. If this is not done, induction may be prolonged and excitement may occur. When the expedient of overpressure is adopted, induction is relatively rapid.

As the mask is applied and unconsciousness approached, encouragement and gentle suggestion should lull the patient into a state of security. It is better not to concentrate attention on physiologic processes such as breathing but to explain quietly what is happening and suggest a tranquil induction and safe emergence from anesthesia. This kind of hypnotic suggestion adds considerably to the ease and smoothness of induction.

AIRWAY AND RESPIRATORY PROBLEMS

The most troublesome problems in inhalation anesthesia involve the airway and adequacy of respiration. In probable order of development, these may be encountered as follows.

Mask Fit

If a mask is poorly fitted to the patient's face, the effective concentration of anesthetic is diluted by admixture with room air. A good mask fit is not easily achieved in the edentulous, in the patient with a prominent nose or receding jaw, in the patient who has gastrointestinal drainage tubes, or in the patient with a heavy beard. A poorly fitted mask creates difficulty in applying positive pressure ventilation to the lungs. On the other hand, excessive pressure by the mask may injure the trigeminal or facial nerves, eyes, or skin.

Depressed Respiration

If during induction respiration is depressed by premedicants or inhalation agents, the alveolar concentration of anesthetic may not readily approach that needed to provide anesthesia. Opioids used for premedication are a common cause. Depression of respiration may not be evident until the first few breaths of anesthetic are taken. Large doses of intravenous barbiturates used for induction or the too early administration of a neuromuscular blocker, both of which reduce alveolar ventilation, also delay induction. Whenever respiration is depressed, assisted or controlled breathing is necessary not only to facilitate induction of anesthesia but to prevent hypoxia and hypercarbia.

Abnormal Respiratory Patterns and Pulmonary Disease

Rapid shallow breathing may not provide the alveolar ventilation required for uptake of anesthetic. Tachypnea is common during induction, not the result of stimulation of the Hering-Breuer receptors as once thought but probably a central effect of the anesthetic. Abnormalities of the lung characterized by poor mixing of gases and unequal distribution or slow diffusion of gases across the pulmonary membrane interfere with attainment of anesthesia, as do certain kinds of heart disease with associated diminution in respiratory function.

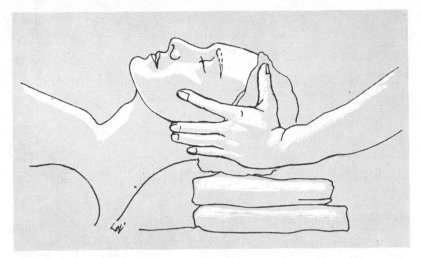

FIGURE 11–5. Technique of lifting jaw with fingers behind the mandible to overcome respiratory soft tissue obstruction.

Respiratory Obstruction

Almost as soon as a supine patient loses consciousness the lower jaw relaxes and recedes; or during excitement the jaws may be clenched tight. In either case the tongue may cause obstruction as it is sucked against the hard palate during inspiration or when it falls back into the pharynx; this is indicated by stertorous sounds. Such obstruction may be sensed by the hand holding the mask or detected by listening over the breathing tubes, but is best discovered by observing the rise and fall of the chest rather than the movement of the reservoir bag. In the presence of obstruction, the chest retracts as the diaphragm descends instead of expanding as it should; this gives rise to a characteristic rocking motion indicating that descent of the diaphragm is not followed by free inflow of air. Although movement of the reservoir bag does not indicate adequacy of pulmonary ventilation, failure of the bag to move with respiration implies that the anesthetic is not being breathed.

Respiratory obstruction must be corrected as soon as practicable. When obstruction is diagnosed the jaw should be lifted upward, moving the tongue with it. Extension of the cervical spine or turning the head to the side may help. The most effective means of lifting the jaw is to place the fingers behind the vertical ramus of the mandible (Fig. 11–5). This maneuver is one of the most difficult to teach a beginner; when applied it should be maintained for only a short time, as soreness and swelling may result. A pharyngeal airway should be inserted as soon as possible.

It is feasible beforehand to single out a person who may develop soft tissue obstruction when unconscious, usually the individual who has a short thick neck or who is obese. There are two kinds of airway, oropharyngeal and nasopharyngeal (Fig. 11–6). Their purpose is to displace the tongue anteriorly; the patient then breathes through or around the airway. The oral airway is more efficient, but if obstruction takes place before the jaw relaxes it may be impossible to open the mouth. In this situation, a soft, well-lubricated nasopharyngeal tube should be passed; care must be taken to avoid injury to the highly vascular mucous membrane of the nose. Similarly, the oral airway should be placed carefully to avoid injury to lips and teeth and is more easily inserted if lubricated. Placement of an airway must be done deftly; haste is essential so that the partial pressure of anesthetic in the lungs is not reduced while the face mask is

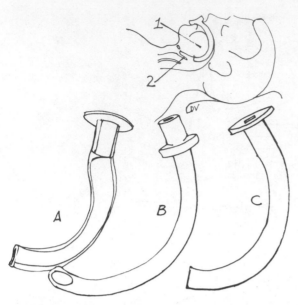

FIGURE 11–6. Pharyngeal airways. Oro-pharyngeal airway displacing tongue (*1*) forward and upward from the pharynx (*2*). A, Plastic oropharyngeal airway. B, Soft rubber nasopharyngeal airway. C, Hard rubber oropharyngeal airway.

removed. At the same time, the reservoir bag should not be allowed to empty because it will require refilling with oxygen, thereby offering a lower anesthetic concentration.

Cough and Laryngospasm

Cough sometimes follows placement of an airway, usually caused by pharyngeal irritation as a high concentration of anesthetic is delivered after the airway is cleared. Irritation can be avoided by temporarily decreasing the concentration of anesthetic after airway insertion, then increasing it slowly. Cough is overcome by gradually deepening anesthesia and assisting the inspiratory phase following cough by pressure on the reservoir bag.

Laryngospasm is a serious complication at any time but possibly of greatest consequence during induction of anesthesia. This occurs most frequently at light levels of anesthesia when there is direct pharyngeal, laryngeal, or peripheral painful stimulation. All manner of laryngospasm may occur, from a minor degree indicated by a high-pitched crowing sound to complete, impassible closure of the glottis. Sustained moderate pressure on the reservoir bag helps to facilitate ventilation and overcome the spasm, but should it persist an assistant should keep a finger on the pulse to detect signs of failing circulation when anoxia develops, often indicated by progressive slowing and loss of amplitude of the pulse. If laryngospasm is complete and lasts as long as a minute, an intravenous or intramuscular injection of succinylcholine, 20 mg, will relax the striated muscles of the larynx.

The halogenated hydrocarbons are associated with less cough and laryngospasm than those encountered with the older, more irritating anesthetics. Cough and laryngospasm are also more frequent in the heavy smoker or a patient with chronic bronchitis. The increased risk of laryngospasm in those with excessive secretions may be adequate justification for postponement of an elective operation.

Mucous and Salivary Secretions

Accumulation of secretions in the air passages can result in obstruction. Increase in secretions may be part of the initial neurologic stimulant phase of general anesthesia or the result of irritation from the anesthetic, further increased by hypoxia and retention of carbon dioxide during a difficult induction. The halogenated hydrocarbons pose fewer problems with secretions and pharyngeal irritability than the others; thus many clinicians now eliminate atropine from premedication when a halogenated anesthetic is to be administered. Diminution of parasympathetic activity with atropine or scopolamine eliminates the profuse, watery kind of secretion, leaving a sparse, viscid material. If secretions are troublesome, the patient's head can be turned to the side and lowered to allow their escape through the side of the mouth. When the problem is more serious, suction of the pharynx should be performed, preferably in a deeper plane of anesthesia to avoid laryngospasm or vomiting.

Retching and Vomiting

Stimulation of the vomiting center frequently occurs during induction and emergence from anesthesia. Opioid premedicants, movement of the patient, persistent attempts at pharyngeal suction, and too early placement of an airway contribute to this complication. Postoperatively, the incidence is higher in women, particularly during the third and fourth weeks of the menstrual cycle, after prolonged deep anesthesia, and following intra-abdominal operations.

Anesthetists should be on the alert for premonitory signs during induction such as repetitive swallowing. The sequence of swallowing, retching, and vomiting can sometimes be interrupted if care is taken to avoid partial respiratory obstruction, which seems to precipitate the problem. Unfortunately, fluid and particulate matter may well up into the pharynx without warning, and silent aspiration during general anesthesia of gastric material is more common than realized. So long as gastric contents are not carried into the respiratory tract, little harm is done. The head is lowered and turned to the side and vomitus sponged or suctioned. This should be done in stages, with intermittent administration of oxygen. Once assured that aspiration has not occurred, induction should then proceed rapidly, as the risk of vomiting is reduced at a deeper level of anesthesia. If regurgitation or vomiting occurs during recovery, the patient should be turned to the lateral position and closely observed until able to protect the airway. Treatment of aspiration of stomach contents is discussed in Chapter 33.

The aforementioned complications may be encountered in rapid succession during induction of anesthesia in addition to prolonged excitement with vigorous muscle movement and breath-holding. In the past, considerable experience was required to avoid these complications as well as manage them.

Today, some anesthetists avoid the problems of induction by substituting rapid intravenous induction and rapid tracheal intubation in every patient before administration of an inhalation anesthetic. They do not thereby reduce the risk from these problems; they merely substitute a different set of complications. There is still an important place in the practice of anesthesia for inhalation induction and management of the anesthetized patient by mask administration of anesthetics. The fluorinated hydrocarbon anesthetics make this task more pleasant than it was in the ether-cyclopropane era for both the patient and the anesthetist.

MAINTENANCE

Induction of anesthesia should be followed by the start of operation without delay. Patients fully anesthetized by the potent anesthetics in current use may become hypotensive when not stimulated surgically. Usually, the patient will show a mild response such as pupillary dilation, increase in heart rate or depth of respiration, or breath holding as incision is made. Slight movement, if it does not affect the surgical field, is not objectionable. If in doubt, it is better to reach a plane somewhat deeper than necessary before incision is made. It is easier to lighten anesthesia than to deepen it once the complications of light anesthesia appear. Subsequently, the inspired concentration of anesthetics can be decreased.

Once a satisfactory level has been reached, the lightest level of anesthesia compatible with good operating conditions is maintained. The smaller the amount of drug administered the better, but too little anesthesia defeats the purpose, prolongs operation, and often leads to more drug administration later on. When muscle relaxation is required, as during closure of the peritoneum, the need is anticipated and anesthesia deepened at the time.

An anesthetist can obtain valuable information by observing the surgical field throughout operation, for example: (1) Adequacy of oxygenation, as indicated by the color of arterial blood in the wound, is a valid means of detecting hypoxemia, especially in dark-skinned persons. (2) Comparison of the color of venous and arterial blood is of value in estimating cardiovascular function. Dark venous blood suggests inadequate tissue perfusion; continuous ooze may signify a clotting defect or transfusion reaction; continued brisk arterial or venous bleeding suggests the need for transfusion. (3) A competent anesthetist should observe surgical maneuvers, understand operative procedure, and be able to anticipate the surgeon's actions. Only then is one able to prepare for sequential events, essential because alterations in depth of anesthesia involve a certain time lag. Placement of surgical packs, traction on viscera, and rapid decompression of the abdomen all may lead to precipitous hypotension. (4) Degree of muscular relaxation should be watched carefully. More or less relaxation may be needed at different stages of the operation. The caliber and tone of the bowel and its extrusion from the peritoneal cavity are indicative of depth of anesthesia. Progressive loss of tone and dilation of bowel occur with deepening anesthesia; extrusion usually suggests inadequate muscle relaxation. A surgeon should not be expected to inform an anesthetist that better relaxation is needed; usually the anesthetist can anticipate the need by observing the field or by sensing chest wall compliance during manual ventilatory control.

EMERGENCE

A patient should be nearly awake at the termination of operation. When laryngeal and pharyngeal reflexes have recovered, the patient is less likely to develop respiratory obstruction or aspirate gastric contents. However, the need to have a patient awake should not lead to administration of so little anesthetic that restraint is necessary as the last sutures are placed or fascial closure is disrupted; this too, is hazardous.

During emergence, complications described under induction of anesthesia may re-appear. When it is considered safe to move the patient, transfer to bed or litter is done gently to avoid strain on ligaments and muscles in the relaxed individual. If still unconscious, the patient is placed in the lateral decubitus position to protect against airway obstruction and aspiration of vomitus. After transfer to the recovery room and before the anesthetist leaves, vital signs should be obtained and all information relating to treatment communicated to the recovery room nurse.

APPRAISAL

The theoretic and practical aspects of inhalation anesthesia have been treated in this chapter. Inhalation anesthesia is a controllable technique because the lungs act as the avenue of entrance and the principal route of escape for the anesthetic. The patient's respiratory efforts or the anesthetist's artificial control of respiration influence the level of anesthesia from moment to moment. Premedication must be chosen with a view to disturbing respiration and circulation least. Respiratory obstruction owing to soft tissue, excessive secretions, or laryngospasm must be avoided and treated promptly if induction of anesthesia is to be rapid and safe. Abnormalities of pulmonary ventilation and diffusion must be detected, because they markedly influence the course of anesthesia. The role of the circulation and the body tissues as relates to the partial pressure of anesthetic in the brain must be kept clearly in mind. Physical properties of the gases relating to solubility and diffusion must be understood. In spite of all the knowledge required, we believe that inhalation is still the best technique to teach the beginner.

REFERENCES

Eger, EI: Anesthetic Uptake and Action. Baltimore, Williams & Wilkins Co., 1974.

Fink BR (ed): Molecular Mechanisms of Anesthesia. New York, Raven Press, 1980.

Gilman AG, Goodman LS, Gilman A (eds): The Pharmacological Basis of Therapeutics. 6th ed. New York, MacMillan, 1980.

Halsey MJ, Miller RA, Sutton JA (eds): Molecular Mechanisms in General Anaesthesia. Edinburgh, Churchill-Livingstone, 1974.

Miller KW, Paton WDM, Smith RA, et al: The pressure reversal of general anaesthesia and the initial volume hypothesis. Mol Pharmacol 9:131, 1973.

Seeman P: The membrane actions of anesthetics and tranquilizers. Pharmacol Rev 24:583, 1972.

Chapter 12
INHALATION ANESTHETICS

Most classifications of neurotropic drugs include only two categories: the central nervous system depressants and the stimulants. Anesthetics are classified as depressants in this one-dimensional scale of neurophysiologic function. The actual properties of neuropharmacologic agents are inadequately described by this simplistic approach. Some drugs, including most anesthetics, combine neurodepressant and neuroexcitatory effects; others, such as pentylenetetrazol, exert only stimulant effects; still others, such as pentobarbital, are primarily depressants. Winters has examined the behavioral and neurophysiologic correlates of neurotropic drug action and postulated a two-dimensional continuum of central nervous system response to stimulants and depressants (Fig. 12–1). It is likely that each of these responses involves a different membrane site in the central nervous system and that drug exposure may promote either the activating site or the depressive site or both. Some anesthetics, such as enflurane, exert

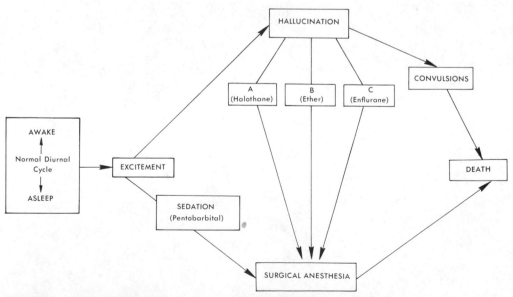

FIGURE 12–1. After Winters' scheme of drug-induced CNS excitation and depression as shown by gross behavior and EEG recordings. (Winters WD: Neurophysiological classification of psychoactive drugs. *In* Kales A (ed): Sleep: Physiology and Pathology. Philadelphia, JB Lippincott Co, 1969).

more prominent excitatory effects than others, for example, the barbiturates, but most activate both sites and result in an electroencephalogram (EEG) that progresses through successive stages toward a seizure pattern. Most anesthetics diverge from this pattern before seizure activity is manifest, while inducing a pattern of suppression and periods of electric silence.

GENERAL CHARACTERISTICS OF THE INHALATION ANESTHETICS

Ideally, one should be able to regulate the partial pressure or concentration of general anesthetic agent in the blood from moment to moment, as the central nervous system tends to equilibrate with the partial pressure of anesthetic in blood. If more is needed, the concentration should be amenable to prompt increase; if overdose is evident, one should be able to reduce the concentration just as promptly.

The three methods of producing anesthesia — rectal, intravenous, and inhalation — vary considerably in controllability. Blood levels following intravenous administration remain more or less under control, as injection is made directly into the circulation. Because of the enormous absorptive surface of the lungs, changes in alveolar anesthetic concentration are rapidly reflected in blood, but the residual gas volume in the lung serves as a buffer to retard changes in alveolar concentration when inspired anesthetic tension is altered. Absorption into the blood from the rectum and colon is highly unpredictable.

From the standpoint of elimination, the majority of drugs used for intravenous anesthesia undergo metabolic change in the body and are thus rendered inactive in varying degrees by oxidation, reduction, hydrolysis, or conjugation. The ultimate safety of these substances is therefore related to the totality of their metabolism. Although subject to careful titration, once an injected drug enters the circulation there are no means for prompt removal. Urinary excretion is both slow and unpredictable. On the other hand, although inhalation anesthetics also are metabolized in varying degree, their uptake and elimination are accomplished primarily by alveolar ventilation. This is therefore the most controllable method for inducing general anesthesia.

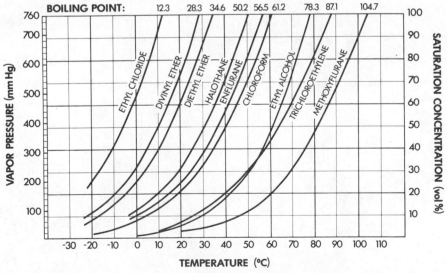

FIGURE 12–2. Vapor pressure curves of some volatile liquids. The vapor pressure curve for isoflurane is nearly identical to that of halothane.

TABLE 12–1. Some Physical and Chemical Properties of the Inhalation Anesthetics*

Agent	Formula	Boiling Point (°C)	Vapor Pressure (20° C-Torr)	Latent Heat of Vaporization (Cal/Gm)	Useful Inspired Concentrations (Per Cent)		
					Induction	Maintenance	MAC
Water†	H_2O	100.0	21	537			
Nitrous oxide	N_2O	–89		90	60–80	50–70	110
Cyclopropane	C_3H_6	–33		114	25–50	10–20	9.2
Diethyl ether	$(C_2H_5)_2O$	35	450	87.5	10–30	5–15	1.92
Halothane	$CF_3CHBrCl$	50.2	243	35	1–4	0.5–2	0.77
Methoxyflurane	$CH_3OCF_2CCl_2H$	104.6	22.5	49	3	0.25–1	0.16
Trichloroethylene	$CHCl:CCl_2$	86–88	60	57.2	2.5	1.0–1.5	
Enflurane	$CFHCl \cdot CF_2 \cdot O \cdot CHF_2$	56.5	175	42	2–5	1.5–3.0	1.68
Isoflurane	$CF_3 \cdot CHCl \cdot O \cdot CHF_2$	48.5	238	44	1–4	0.8–2.0	1.15

*In many instances the figures given are approximate, as data are lacking.
†Water is included for reference purposes.

PHYSICAL AND CHEMICAL PROPERTIES

VAPOR PRESSURE AND BOILING POINT OF LIQUIDS

The physical properties of anesthetic gases and volatile liquids determine how they are supplied by the manufacturer, suggest the systems used in their administration, and influence both uptake and distribution in the body after inhalation. The basis of these phenomena is the molecular nature of matter and the general laws of physics that govern diffusion, solubility in body fluids, and the relations among pressure, volume, and temperature. Anesthetists should bear these concepts in mind as they administer anesthesia. For this reason, the vapor pressure curves of some of the volatile liquids are shown in Figure 12–2 and various other physical and chemical properties are listed in Table 12–1. The ideal volatile liquid would be that compound easily vaporized at ambient temperatures with a low boiling point that would result in rapid evaporation. Heat of vaporization should be minimal so that the liquid is not markedly cooled as vaporization takes place, and the vapor pressure must be sufficient to provide enough molecules for anesthetic effect.

REACTIVITY AND STABILITY

Anesthetics are soluble in the conductive rubber parts of breathing systems in proportion to their concentration and the rubber-gas partition coefficient (Table 12–2). Not only may rubber undergo deterioration, but considerable amounts of anesthetic may be given to a second patient who breathes through the same apparatus. The solubility of these agents is less in polyethylene, but deformation of plastic equipment occurs after prolonged exposure. Halothane plus water vapor corrodes brass, solder, and aluminum. In the presence of heat, trichloroethylene reacts with the alkali of carbon dioxide absorbents to form dichloroacetylene and phosgene. Thymol is added to halothane. Enflurane and isoflurane are innately stable and require no added preservative. Most volatile anesthetics are now supplied in tinted glass bottles to minimize decomposition by light.

FLAMMABILITY

With few exceptions, the older anesthetics were flammable and therefore liable to be ignited and to cause explosions when mixed with oxygen or nitrous oxide. The emphasis in development of new agents has therefore focused on nonflammability. Advances in fluorine chemistry allowed the synthesis of partially fluorinated ethers and hydrocarbons, which are potent nonflammable anesthetics. This group of agents has virtually supplanted all of the older anesthetics with the exception of nitrous oxide.

TABLE 12–2. Solubility of Anesthetic Agents in Conductive Rubber and Blood

Agent	Rubber-Gas Partition Coefficient (25°C)	Blood-Gas Partition Coefficient (25°C)
Nitrous oxide	1.2	0.43
Diethyl ether	58	13.0
Isoflurane	62	1.4
Enflurane	74	1.9
Halothane	120	2.4
Methoxyflurane	635	12.0

BIOTRANSFORMATION

For many years it was assumed that, except for trichloroethylene, the inhalation anesthetics were inert, that is, excreted by the lungs and not metabolized in the body. Using radioactive-labelled compounds, Van Dyke and his colleagues (1975) found that inhalation anesthetics are converted to carbon dioxide and the metabolites excreted by the kidneys, suggesting that these agents may owe part of their pharmacologic properties to chemical reactivity. Subsequent studies have shown that the majority of inhalation anesthetics are metabolized, biotransformation being greatest with methoxyflurane (about 50 per cent), intermediate with halothane (about 10 to 20 per cent) and minimal with enflurane and isoflurane. Anesthetics are altered in the microsomal fraction of liver and other organs, where they may not only induce or accelerate their own rate of metabolism but likewise may be influenced by microsomal-inducing drugs such as phenobarbital (see Chapter 4). The metabolic products may be inert or toxic, perhaps causing destruction of hepatocytes or malfunction of renal tubular epithelium, as noted in the discussions on halothane and methoxyflurane, respectively.

PHARMACOLOGIC ACTIONS OF INHALATION ANESTHETICS

EFFECTS ON RESPIRATION

Anesthetics alter normal respiratory patterns and interfere with the normal mechanisms of gas exchange. Various respiratory patterns ranging from apnea through breath holding and irregular breathing to a predictable rhythmic pattern or tachypnea may be seen during anesthesia. Breath holding and irregular respiratory patterns are common during induction with most anesthetics, especially at presurgical levels. The onset of surgical anesthesia is often heralded by regular, rhythmic respiration. Tachypnea may be observed during attempts to increase the depth of anesthesia with any of the volatile anesthetics. With tachypnea, the tidal volume is sharply reduced, alveolar ventilation becomes inadequate, and respiratory acidosis results. Halothane, enflurane, and isoflurane induce significant degrees of hypoventilation during surgical depths of anesthesia.

An unmedicated individual at rest generally takes regular breaths of nearly equal tidal volumes, a pattern interrupted periodically by a breath two or three times the normal volume. This serves to prevent development of micro-atelectasis and is thought to be mediated by stretch receptors at the root of the lung. The opioids and general anesthetics depress this sighing mechanism and therefore predispose to development of atelectasis and hypoxemia.

Ventilation can be described in terms of removal of carbon dioxide from arterial blood. The relation between CO_2 and ventilation is a reciprocal one because ventilation is stimulated by CO_2 and CO_2 is eliminated by ventilation, best described by a CO_2 *ventilation diagram* (Fig. 12–3). Two kinds of curve, each representing one variety of the relation between CO_2 and ventilation, can be plotted on the V_E and Pa_{CO_2} axes: the CO_2 excretion hyperbola (curve A), and the CO_2 *ventilatory response curve* (curve B); these describe the spontaneous ventilatory response to alterations in Pa_{CO}. The latter curve is displaced to the right both by opioids (curve C) and anesthetics in a dose-related manner. Normally, curve B is nearly a straight line with the slope increasing about 2 L in terms of V_E for each torr increase in CO_2, with considerable variation among individuals. The slope becomes steeper with hypoxia and catecholamine stimulation and plateaus with loss of consciousness or onset of anesthesia. Thus it is reduced by one third to one half in light anesthesia (curve D) and reaches a plateau in

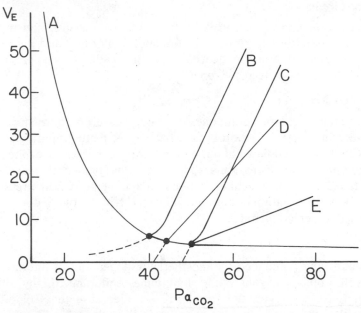

FIGURE 12–3. Ventilation—carbon dioxide diagram. *A* represents the CO_2 excretion hyperbola, *B* the CO_2 ventilatory response curve, and *C, D,* and *E* represent the shift of the CO_2 ventilatory response curve occurring with opioids and light and deep anesthesia, respectively.

deep anesthesia (curve E). Agents that stimulate the sympathetic nervous system (e.g., cyclopropane, diethyl ether, and nitrous oxide) do not result in as much of a depression of the slope.

The mechanisms responsible for the respiratory changes noted during general anesthesia are imperfectly understood, but all of these compounds diminish the ventilatory response to CO_2, presumably reflecting depression of the central nervous system response to the intracellular effect of H^+ on cells of the respiratory centers.

CARDIOVASCULAR EFFECTS

Effective concentrations of most anesthetics alter blood flow significantly. The actions on several vascular beds will be considered separately, as alterations in flow result from locally mediated mechanisms and cannot be predicted on the basis of changes in arterial pressure alone.

Cerebral Circulation

Anesthetics affect cerebral circulation both directly and indirectly, the indirect actions mediated by ventilatory depression and accumulation of CO_2, a potent cerebral vasodilator, and by depression of cerebral metabolism, which may affect local metabolic control mechanisms for cerebral perfusion. Anesthetics directly affect smooth muscle of the cerebral vessels. All inhalation anesthetics are direct cerebral vasodilators, but differences among them are not distinctive enough to justify further detail here. Increases in intracranial pressure taken as indices of cerebral vasodilation have been reported with all the commonly used inhalation anesthetics. It has been suggested that the direct effect on vascular smooth muscle may not be the principal cause of cerebral vasodilation but rather the result of uncoupling of metabolic control of the cerebral circulation. Cerebral autoregulation is depressed by all of the commonly used volatile anesthetics.

Coronary Circulation

The relations among coronary blood flow, blood pressure, and myocardial metabolism are discussed in Chapter 32. Halothane, isoflurane, and methoxyflurane all reduce coronary blood flow and myocardial oxygen consumption, apparently as a result of a decreased myocardial need for oxygen.

Splanchnic Circulation

The splanchnic circulation comprises the blood vessels of the gastrointestinal tract, pancreas, liver, and spleen. Cyclopropane, halothane, methoxyflurane, and isoflurane all reduce splanchnic blood flow but not by the same mechanism. Despite a rise in blood pressure, cyclopropane induces a marked increase in splanchnic vascular resistance. Halothane leaves resistance unaltered while reducing perfusion pressure. Methoxyflurane acts by a combination of both mechanisms. Nitrous oxide does not significantly alter splanchnic hemodynamics.

Renal Circulation

Renal blood flow is reduced by anesthetics independent of alterations in arterial pressure. Cyclopropane, nitrous oxide, halothane, enflurane, diethyl ether, and isoflurane all increase renal vascular resistance and decrease renal blood flow. These effects are easily explained for agents stimulating the sympathetic nervous system but hardly account for the renal vasoconstriction seen with halothane. Reductions in glomerular filtration rate (GFR, inulin clearance) ranging from 19 to 55 per cent and in renal plasma flow (RPF, PAH clearance) from 36 to 67 per cent have been reported at surgical planes of anesthesia. In general, higher reductions in GFR and RPF are associated with deeper levels of anesthesia. The filtration fraction (GFR/RPF) and calculated renal vascular resistance are consistently increased, suggesting that increased efferent arteriolar tone maintains glomerular filtration pressure. Changes in renal perfusion also activate the renin-angiotensin system, so that part of the vasoconstriction can be ascribed to the latter.

Circulation to Skin and Muscle

Diethyl ether, cyclopropane, isoflurane, halothane, and nitrous oxide all dilate cutaneous vessels, probably owing to a central inhibitory action on thalamic temperature-regulating mechanisms, thus allowing vasodilation to occur at onset of anesthesia. Increased flow persists at deep anesthetic levels of cyclopropane, ether, isoflurane, and methoxyflurane, but with halothane a return toward normal flow occurs as depth of anesthesia is increased. Neither nitrous oxide nor diethyl ether significantly alters muscle blood flow; however, both cyclopropane and halothane diminish it, the former by increasing muscle vascular resistance, the latter by decreasing perfusion pressure.

CARDIAC EFFECTS

All commonly used potent anesthetics exert a direct depressant effect on myocardial contractility (Fig. 12–4) (Table 12–3). In the isolated heart exposed to 1 MAC concentration of any potent anesthetic, this depression is approximately equivalent to that seen in uncompensated congestive heart failure. During clinical anesthesia with cyclopropane, diethyl ether, and isoflurane, cardiac output, stroke volume, and mean arterial pressure are maintained at or above normal owing to stimulation of sympathetic nervous activity. Halothane, methoxyflurane, and enflurane, by contrast, lack sympathetic stimulatory properties, and cardiovascular depression is evidenced by a dose-dependent decrease in arterial pressure, stroke volume, and cardiac output. Among the

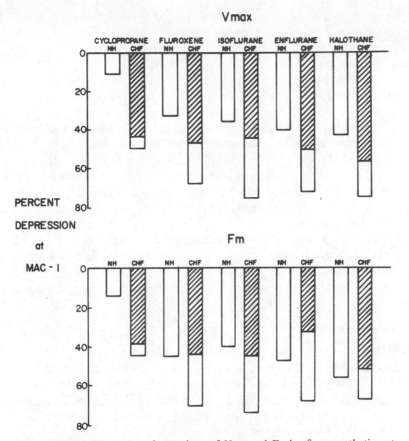

FIGURE 12–4. Percentage depressions of V_{max} and F_m by five anesthetics at equipotent concentrations (1 MAC) in muscles from normal hearts and muscles from hearts after congestive heart failure. Percentage depressions were calculated from the preanesthetic control values for normal hearts. Hatched areas of bars for cardiac failure values represent the depression caused by cardiac failure alone. (Reproduced with permission from Kemmotsu O, Hashimoto Y, Shimosato S: Anesthesiology 40:252, 1974.)

commonly used volatile anesthetics, isoflurane is unique in increasing cardiac index. Prolonged anesthetic administration partially reverses the depressant effect of halothane and increases the stimulant effects of agents activating the sympathetic nervous system. These changes may result from increased beta-sympathetic activity, since Price has shown that propranolol (Inderal) blocks the phenomenon.

RENAL EFFECTS

General anesthesia results in an antidiuresis characterized by a marked reduction in urine volume, 60 to 70 per cent, increased urine osmolality, and reabsorption of

TABLE 12–3. Δ Decreases in Myocardial Mechanics at MAC-1 (%)*

	V_{max}	F_m	Max Power	Max Work	Max dF/dt
Enflurane	12	36	44	50	37
Methoxyflurane	31	40	55	51	43
Halothane	39	35	51	52	45

*Reprinted with permission from Shimosato S: The effects of Ethrane (correspondence). Anesthesiology 31:386, 1969.

water by the renal tubules in excess of solute, resulting in negative free water clearance. Partial reversal of the antidiuresis by intravenous administration of ethanol suggests that antidiuretic hormone is released during general anesthesia, which is in part responsible for the antidiuresis. Reduction in GFR also contributes to the oliguria observed. Sodium and potassium excretion are reduced as a result of the reduction in GFR, possibly because of hormonal factors acting on the renal circulation. Increased amounts of renin sampled in the renal vein during cyclopropane and halothane anesthesia suggest that activation of the renin-angiotensin-aldosterone system may, in part, be responsible for renal vasoconstriction as well as sodium retention.

The antidiuresis resulting from anesthesia, together with that arising from operative trauma and the use of opioids, may result in persistent oliguria and postoperative fluid retention. Administration of large quantities of fluid in the immediate perioperative period may therefore result in dilutional hyponatremia and water intoxication, particularly in geriatric patients.

In most patients without renal disease, changes in hemodynamics and water and electrolyte excretion are transitory and return to normal in the postanesthetic period. Renal effects of general anesthetics in patients with pre-existing renal disease have not been thoroughly assessed. A toxic nephrogenic effect of methoxyflurane is discussed further on.

MUSCLE RELAXATION

Many of the inhalation anesthetics cause muscle relaxation. Diethyl ether provides excellent relaxation at doses that allow ventilatory volume and blood pressure to be maintained at near normal levels. The relaxant effect of ether may result in part from depression of sensitivity to acetylcholine at the postjunctional membrane of the neuromuscular junction and in part from depression of central nervous system and spinal reflex activity. Methoxyflurane demonstrates similar effects. At least part of the relaxant effect of halothane, ether, enflurane, and isoflurane is exerted beyond the acetylcholine receptor. Nitrous oxide does not produce muscle relaxation, and low concentrations of cyclopropane increase contractility of skeletal muscle. Halothane, enflurane, and isoflurane at anesthetic concentrations produce muscle relaxation but are often combined with nondepolarizing neuromuscular blockers. See Chapter 15 for a discussion of the interaction between general anesthetics and neuromuscular blockers.

ANALGESIA

It is not easy to assess the degree of analgesia produced by anesthetic levels of inhalation agents, for the anesthetized subject cannot report on the experience. One is tempted to interpret such signs as movement, rise in pulse rate or arterial pressure, tachypnea, or sweating as evidence of inadequate analgesia, but there may be other causes for these reactions. Nevertheless, the MAC at which a subject does not move in response to a painful stimulus is employed as a measure of analgetic potency, although MAC involves variables other than analgesia. Use of the tibial pressure method to assess subanesthetic doses of anesthetics suggested to Dundee that methoxyflurane produces minimal analgesia, whereas trichloroethylene and ether are more potent. Considerable analgesia is present in the first plane of ether anesthesia after some degree of tissue saturation has taken place. During early phases of anesthesia with halothane or enflurane in oxygen, analgesia may be inadequate even at inspired concentrations that result in cardiovascular depression. The addition of nitrous oxide frequently counteracts the cardiovascular depression, because it acts as a mild sympathetic stimulant while simultaneously providing the analgesia needed. A role for the endogenous opioid system in mediating analgesia produced by anesthetic agents has been suggested but not yet evaluated.

EFFECTS ON THE ELECTROENCEPHALOGRAM

The effects of anesthetics on the EEG of humans were first described in 1937. Since then much effort has been devoted to correlating EEG activity with blood concentrations of anesthetics, and attempts have been made to establish a characteristic progression of EEG tracings indicating sequential levels of anesthesia. However, the effects of anesthetics on the EEG differ widely. Cyclopropane stands at one end of a spectrum, causing progressive slowing with increasing depth of anesthesia until, at approximately 40 per cent inhaled concentration, a clocklike regularity is established at about 1 Hz. Enflurane falls at the opposite end of the scale, producing 14 to 18 Hz activity, then progressing to spike-dome complexes alternating with periods of electric silence, ultimately resulting in frank seizure activity. Nitrous oxide and ether provide intermediate patterns. The administration of combinations of anesthetic drugs, a common clinical practice, stamps identification of anesthetic depth by EEG as improbable.

A rigorous EEG comparison of agents at various levels of anesthesia is not possible because of differences in arterial pressure produced. Cyclopropane can be inhaled in concentrations five times greater than that required for surgical anesthesia without causing hypotension, but halothane and enflurane cause severe hypotension in much lesser amounts. Carbon dioxide accumulation alone can slow the EEG, and when respiratory acidosis develops during general anesthesia, slowing is also evident.

Alternative forms of recording EEG information have been developed over the last ten years and may find use, not for monitoring depth of anesthesia but for early recognition of cerebral hypoxia. Computer analysis of the EEG signal generates a frequency-power histogram plotted as a three-dimensional pictorial display with a compressed time scale. The decrease in power at fast frequencies (>8 Hz) that occurs with hypoxia is apparent and offers ready visual recognition of cerebral hypoperfusion, information that should be clinically useful in operations directly or indirectly involving the cerebral circulation.

TOXICITY OF INHALATION ANESTHETICS

The inhalation anesthetics are potential protoplasmic poisons, thus affecting cellular function. Nitrous oxide inhaled in subanesthetic concentrations over a period of several days results in depression of cell division in bone marrow granulocytes. Halothane inhibits both leukocyte motility and phagocytosis. Epidemiologic studies in both Europe and the United States indicate that women working in operating rooms have an increased incidence of spontaneous abortion and delivery of infants with a significant increase in congenital anomalies. Although the impact of stress on women working under these conditions has not been clearly delineated, exposure of pregnant rats to trace concentrations of halothane produces embryotoxic effects manifest as structural changes in brain, liver, and kidney. Both epidemiologic studies in humans and animal experiments provide presumptive evidence that some anesthetics may be carcinogenic. A committee of the American Society of Anesthesiologists has recommended control over anesthetizing locations to protect personnel (see Chapter 7).

RENAL TOXICITY

High dose methoxyflurane anesthesia causes nephrotoxicity characterized by vasopressin-resistant polyuria and azotemia. Methoxyflurane is metabolized in the liver to free fluoride and oxalate, both nephrotoxic. Inorganic fluoride inhibits some of the enzymes essential for fluid and electrolyte exchange in the loop of Henle, the proximal convoluted tubule, and the collecting ducts. At serum levels of fluoride greater than 50 μM, polyuria is usually evident and the tubular effect may become irreversible with prolonged high levels. The syndrome is further characterized by a high serum osmolality and low urine osmolality. In some patients renal failure has been irreversible, requiring chronic dialysis, whereas several patients have undergone renal transplantation. Enflurane and isoflurane both are metabolized *in vivo* to inorganic fluoride, but the resulting serum levels are much lower than those found with methoxyflurane; the risk of renal toxicity is probably nonexistent for isoflurane and minimal for enflurane.

LIVER TOXICITY

After widespread usage, even the diehards among anesthetists will admit that halothane, on rare occasion, may induce hepatic necrosis. Halothane was introduced to the U.S. around 1958, following rather limited studies on animals and similar circumscribed studies in man that revealed no evidence of hepatic derangement. Halothane was a major innovation after more than a century's use of nitrous oxide, ether, chloroform, and then cyclopropane. No doubt existed that "delayed chloroform poisoning" was an entity, but nearly 80 years elapsed before that knowledge resulted in abandonment of its usage. Halothane was said to be inert and nonflammable in ordinary anesthetic concentrations, affording a stress-free induction and emergence as well as maintenance. The circulatory depression was later accepted as benign, in that the work of the heart was reduced with a lesser demand for oxygen when coronary arterial disease was present.

Around the 1950s and 1960s a spate of case reports appeared in which halothane was linked to development of hepatic damage. Some patients were anicteric, some had transient jaundice, others fatal hepatic necrosis. Anecdotal case reports provided no acceptable explanation other than the association with halothane. Although viral hepatitis was suspect, there was no means to establish the diagnosis by serologic testing. Some patients incurred hepatitis after one exposure; others developed symptoms only after multiple administrations or in sequence with other halogens, such as methoxyflurane. More than a few of the patients were middle-aged women, a good many obese, with a high incidence of atopy in their histories. Unexplained fever appeared early, as did skin rash, arthralgia, and eosinophilia; liver function tests indicated hepatic necrosis. At postmortem examination the livers were almost totally necrotic; lesions arose in the central portion of the lobule, and pathologists were hard put to distinguish between viral and drug-induced lesions. For these reasons hepatitis was interpreted as a sensitivity reaction. However, despite many experiments and tests for sensitivity in man, the concept of sensitivity has not been substantiated.

The National Halothane Study was instituted in 1962 to settle the controversy. For both practical and ethical reasons, this was a retrospective project based on postmortem findings of hepatic necrosis in relation to halothane usage. However, in only 50 per cent of the deaths attributed to hepatic necrosis were there postmortem examinations. In many instances microscopic sections suggested postmortem autolysis; in others, poorly stained sections were unfit for diagnosis and the panel of pathologists could not distinguish the lesion of viral hepatitis from drug-induced disease because necrosis was so extensive. After completion of the study, an attempt was made to mount a multi-institutional prospective study, but this failed because of ethical problems involved in securing patients' informed consent.

Based on 865,500 anesthetics, the study showed that halothane-related hepatitis was a rare event, occurring about once in every 10,000 inductions of anesthesia, but that repeated exposure could well be a factor in development of the lesion. Compared with ether, cyclopropane, and the balanced anesthesia technique, halothane had the best overall safety record, based on mortality figures. Cyclopropane had the poorest record even though traditionally it had been reserved for the poor risk patient; statistical correction for physical status failed to exonerate cyclopropane. Without regard to anesthesia, most of the massive hepatic necroses developed in high risk operations, cardiac and neurosurgical, or in procedures involving massive trauma and shock. Then in 1965 inhalation anesthetics were shown to be reactive compounds metabolized in varying degree, forming potentially toxic intermediates. Methoxyflurane, which readily released its fluoride ion and formed oxalate crystals in the renal parenchyma, caused a unique kind of renal failure so that its use has now been virtually abandoned. Fluroxene, highly toxic in animals, has been withdrawn from the market. During and after halothane anesthesia free bromide ion is found in both plasma and urine, showing that the compound is metabolized to a considerable extent, but the chief metabolites have proved innocuous. Perhaps there is a unique kind of biotransformation. Biotransformation of any drug is not a one-stage, predictable kind of reaction but a complex process qualitatively and quantitatively, perhaps influenced by sex, age, amount of adipose tissue (leading to storage of this fat-soluble agent), hepatic blood flow, oxygenation, acid-base balance, unknown genetic factors, and hepatic microsomal enzyme induction. With many subtle atmospheric contaminants, there need be no prior exposure to other drugs to account for enzyme induction.

In 1975, Cohen and associates performed an analysis of the urinary metabolites of halothane and found that two were possibly reactive enough to combine with liver macromolecules, although the amounts of these compounds were small. Brown has listed several mechanisms by which an organic halogen such as chloroform might destroy hepatocytes. Lipoperoxidation is one possibility, for the endoplasmic reticulum of hepatocytes contains a variety of fatty acids (e.g., arachidonic and linoleic acids) coupled as esters with phosphatidylcholine and phosphatidylethanolamine, many of them long-chain unsaturated molecules. The unsaturated carbon bond decreases the binding energy of hydrogen so that only minimal energy is required to displace the hydrogen ion and replace it with oxygen in the form of a peroxidizing radical. The latter, being unstable, attracts another hydrogen ion from an adjacent fatty acid to form a carboxylic acid group. The resultant cleaving action leads to denaturation of the fatty acid and an autolytic chain reaction causing catastrophic destruction of cellular components, or lipoperoxidation. This is now accepted as the mechanism of chloroform and carbon tetrachloride toxicity. The trigger is biotransformation to a free radical. When biotransformation of chloroform is minimal, little lipoperoxidation occurs; if biotransformation is inhibited, cell necrosis does not occur. On the other hand, with hepatic microsomal enzyme induction, more free radicals are formed and massive hepatic necrosis may develop.

A second mechanism by which halogens may induce hepatic necrosis is the reduction of the hepatic content of free radical quenchers (antioxidants). Several compounds found in liver can act on the covalent electron of a free radical, thereby averting destruction; reduced glutathione, a polypeptide, is the most important of these. Vitamin E or alpha-tocopherol and certain ions such as zinc and selenium also act as antioxidants. If the glutathione content of liver is experimentally reduced to 25 per cent of normal, a nontoxic dose of chloroform (1% $CHCl_3$ for an hour) results in massive centrolobular hepatic necrosis. The central locus is the result of a higher content of microsomal enzymes in the central portion of the lobule, as evidenced by a high concentration of cytochrome P-450, the terminal oxidase in the system.

A third mechanism whereby halogens may destroy liver macromolecules lies in covalent bonding, by which reactive intermediates or metabolites couple with free fatty acids, proteins, phospholipids, and other macromolecules. Such coupling with free radicals alters both function and structure, and necrosis is part of the cascading reaction. Covalent binding is dose dependent, for if binding is extensive obvious changes are seen. Biochemists believe that during halothane anesthesia a degree of covalent binding takes place, but centrolobular necrosis does not develop and plasma enzyme concentrations do not increase.

In summary, all three mechanisms may coexist and the primary event would seem to be the formation of reactive, intermediate, or free radicals via biotransformation. When biotransformation is inhibited, hepatic necrosis does not appear, but when transformation is enhanced via enzyme induction (as with administration of phenobarbital or phenytoin) the possibility of toxicity is augmented.

Ordinarily, in man, biotransformation of halothane is innocuous, for the most part an oxidative reaction leading to the formation of trifluoracetic acid and bromide and chloride ions. Even if the enzymatic pathway is induced, few harmful effects are seen in animals, provided that hypoxia is avoided. But if animals are treated with the compound Arochlor to produce a reductive, non–oxygen dependent pathway, hepatic necrosis ensues. Does such an alteration occur in man? Even though phenobarbital induces the oxidative pathway, the rate of biotransformation is benign. However, there could be a genetic predisposition toward the reductive pathway, and environmentally encountered chemicals (e.g., ethanol, insecticides) may play ancillary roles. Chance exposure to such chemicals between successive halothane administrations might then lead to centrolobular necrosis on repeated exposure.

It seems, then, that development of hepatic necrosis after administration of chloroform, fluroxene, halothane, and Ethrane (in decreasing order of possibility) might depend on a chance combination of events: genetic background, exposure to other drugs, reduced hepatic blood flow or hypoxia, dose and molecular structure of the agent, and the physicochemical properties whereby it might be retained in tissues.

THE GASEOUS ANESTHETICS

NITROUS OXIDE

Nitrous oxide (N_2O) was first prepared by Priestley in 1776, and its anesthetic properties were described by Humphry Davy in 1799. Davy's suggestion that this inorganic gas might "be used with advantage during surgical operations" passed unheeded until 1844, when Gardner Quincy Colton administered nitrous oxide to Horace Wells while a fellow dentist extracted one of Wells' teeth. It was not until 1868 that Andrews combined oxygen with nitrous oxide to lay the foundation for present-day use. Nitrous oxide supports combustion, the combination with oxygen increasing the range over which the anesthetic explosion may occur. Although impurities inherent in the manufacturing process have largely been eliminated, the possible presence of nitric oxide and nitrogen dioxide, both of which are highly toxic to the lung, should be noted.

Today more techniques of general anesthesia are based upon the use of nitrous oxide than upon any other agent. This practice prevails despite the fact that the highest concentration of nitrous oxide that can be given safely for maintenance of anesthesia ranges from 75 to 80 per cent, concentrations that will not anesthetize a fit subject. However, lack of potency is overcome by the addition of drugs of various kinds.

Analgesia is enhanced by prior intramuscular injection, followed by intermittent intravenous use of opioids. Anesthesia is aided by the use of thiopental for narcosis, and skeletal muscle relaxation is provided by a neuromuscular blocker. In many instances anesthesia obtained with halothane or enflurane entails the use of low concentrations of these volatile liquids in conjunction with the analgetic property of nitrous oxide; if the latter were eliminated, anesthesia would prove to be inadequate. This is not to say that nitrous oxide must be given whenever the volatile liquids are used, but experience indicates that nitrous oxide can be combined with minimal amounts of other vapors for surgical anesthesia, a concept supported by measurement of MAC. One cannot claim that supplementation with nitrous oxide is preferable to administration of a potent, all-purpose anesthetic such as halothane, but clinical impression suggests that the combination provides a more satisfactory intraoperative and postanesthetic course. Excessive depth of anesthesia is avoided, while circulatory and respiratory depression with the more potent agents is lessened and even counteracted by the mild sympathetic stimulating effect of nitrous oxide. Finally, initial recovery is more rapid because of the low solubility of nitrous oxide, which is rapidly cleared from the circulation.

For the patient in profound shock or the debilitated or the desperately ill from a variety of causes, nitrous oxide in concentrations as low as 40 to 50 per cent may provide adequate anesthesia even for intra-abdominal procedures. The susceptibility of these patients to depressant drugs is reflected in serious signs of overdose when normal concentrations of the potent anesthetics are given.

Although it is commonly held that nitrous oxide in the absence of hypoxia has no adverse actions, this concept is not strictly true. Price and Helrich showed that 80 per cent nitrous oxide in oxygen exerts a mild, direct depressant action on myocardial contractile force. Inhalation of nitrous oxide after thiopental induction is associated with reduction in the respiratory stimulant response to carbon dioxide, more than that attributed to the barbiturate alone. Nitrous oxide, like all inhalation anesthetic agents, has a dilating effect on cerebral blood vessels. The incidence of nausea and vomiting after nitrous oxide–oxygen anesthesia is low but not negligible.

The high partial pressure of nitrous oxide in blood and its low blood-gas partition coefficient cause it to diffuse into air-containing body cavities until equilibrium is approached, the volume increasing because of the lesser solubility of nitrogen in blood. This can cause considerable distention of bowel during prolonged anesthesia at high inspired concentrations. Intrapleural gas volume likewise increases (Fig. 12–5), as will the volume of gas in other air pockets such as lung cysts or the middle ear; use of nitrous oxide has been shown to displace a tympanoplasty graft. During pneumoencephalogra-

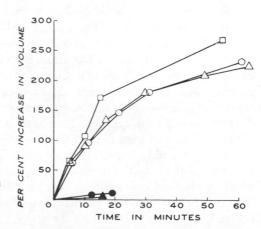

FIGURE 12–5. Increase in intrapleural gas volume on administration of nitrous oxide (*open squares, circles, and triangles*) as opposed to change in volume on administration of oxygen plus halothane (*filled circles and triangle*). (Reproduced with permission from Eger EI II, Saidman LJ: Anesthesiology 26:61, 1965.)

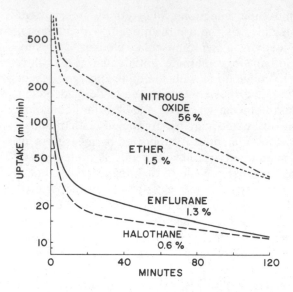

FIGURE 12–6. Total uptake of ether, enflurane, and halothane is illustrated here for alveolar concentrations (as indicated). When combined with 56% alveolar nitrous oxide (equals 60% inspired nitrous oxide), these are sufficient to produce surgical anesthesia. The shape of each curve is similar but their positions differ; a lower potency or higher solubility raises the position of the curve. Thus we see nitrous oxide (low potency) and diethyl ether (high solubility) as the uppermost graphs. (Reproduced with permission from Eger EI II, Uptake, Distribution and Elimination of Enflurane. Madison, Wisc, Ohio Medical Products, 1975.)

phy, inhalation of nitrous oxide can increase intracranial pressure through diffusion; however, if necessary, nitrous oxide can be used as the contrast medium. Lastly, nitrous oxide dissolved in blood can enlarge the volume of air emboli, increasing their lethality proportionately. These sequelae may occur after inhalation of any relatively insoluble agent given at high partial pressures.

During induction of anesthesia with nitrous oxide, the $P_{A_{O_2}}$ increases above the inspired pressure because, despite the relative insolubility of the anesthetic in blood, a large amount of the anesthetic is rapidly taken up (Fig. 12–6). This is the second gas effect (see Chapter 11) that offers a modest margin of safety for a few minutes if high concentrations (90 per cent) of nitrous oxide are given to healthy patients to facilitate induction. A large volume, as much as 30 L of nitrous oxide, may be taken up by the lungs over the first 20 minutes for distribution to body tissues. At termination of anesthesia, if the patient is abruptly permitted to breathe room air, a correspondingly large volume of nitrous oxide diffuses outward, thus lowering $P_{A_{O_2}}$ and temporarily causing hypoxemia (diffusion hypoxia). At the same time $P_{A_{CO_2}}$ is lowered, causing respiratory depression. The sequence is avoided by administration of oxygen for a few minutes before exhalation or removal of the face mask.

CYCLOPROPANE

Cyclopropane is a simple, cyclic hydrocarbon anesthetic introduced to clinical practice in 1934 by Waters and now almost entirely abandoned because of the explosive hazard. It is the most potent of the anesthetic gases, generally producing smooth, rapid induction of anesthesia. The substance was usually administered in a low flow, closed, carbon dioxide absorbing breathing circuit for safety and economy. Because it was a potent respiratory depressant, assisted or controlled ventilation was used to avoid respiratory acidosis. Maintenance was characterized by a mild elevation of blood pressure owing to drug-induced stimulation of sympathetic vasomotor control centers in the midbrain. A mild but definite slowing of heart rate reflected a pressure activated, vagally mediated increase in baroreceptor tone. Myocardial contractile force was well maintained as a result of increased sympathetic activity. Cardiac arrhythmias, including nodal rhythm and premature ventricular contractions, were not uncommon. Emergence delirium, postanesthetic nausea and vomiting, and headache on recovery commonly occurred.

VOLATILE LIQUIDS

HALOTHANE

During 1951 to 1956 halothane ($CF_3CHBrCl$) was synthesized by Suckling as the possible ideal anesthetic, conceived largely on theoretic principles. Primary features in the molecule are chemical stability, nonflammability, and potency. Toxicity is related to chemical reactivity, as an inert compound is unlikely to enter into, and therefore alter, metabolic processes. The CF_3 group is not only inert but confers stability on adjacent carbon atoms, decreasing the reactivity of chlorine and bromine. Halogenated hydrocarbons are also nonflammable if the percentage of hydrogen in the molecule approximates that in halothane.

In terms of theoretic criteria, preparation of halothane was successful, but there are deficiencies in terms of the ideal anesthetic. Halothane is overly depressant to the cardiovascular system; it requires stabilization against photochemical decomposition by both addition of thymol and storage in tinted glass bottles; it exerts undesirable effects on rubber, plastics, and some metals; and the initial costs are high. In spite of these failings, however, halothane represented a remarkable advance.

Induction of anesthesia is rapid but slower than for agents of lesser solubility in blood, e.g., nitrous oxide, enflurane, and isoflurane. Irritability of the larynx is reduced, spasm is rare, and respiratory tract secretions are not stimulated. Return to consciousness is not as rapid as with other substances of comparable blood-gas partition coefficients because of the higher blood-tissue solubility coefficient and the considerable uptake in fat, which delays elimination of halothane for many hours. Emergence from anesthesia is frequently accompanied by pyramidal tract signs and shivering, probably of neurologic origin rather than the result of the lowered body temperature commonly found. Shivering can be eliminated by administration of methylphenidate. Halothane produces relatively poor relaxation of abdominal muscles, hence it is usually given in conjunction with a neuromuscular blocker for abdominal operations.

Halothane decreases arterial blood pressure, myocardial contractile force, and heart rate. There is no predominant action to account for the circulatory depression produced by halothane. The combination of central autonomic inhibition, ganglionic blockade, and suppression of the peripheral response to norepinephrine effectively robs sympathetic mechanisms of their compensatory action, permitting unantagonized

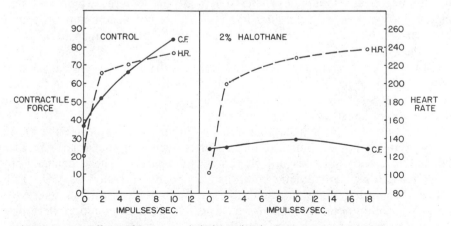

FIGURE 12–7. Effects of 2 per cent halothane (inspired) on responses of cardiac rate and contractile force in the dog to graded poststellate ganglionic stimulation. Contractile force is in arbitrary units, rate in beats per minute. (From Price HL, Price ML: Anesthesiology 37:764, 1966.)

depression of cardiac action and vasodilation peripherally. Muscle blood flow, therefore, decreases not as a result of vasoconstriction but as a result of reduction in perfusion pressure. The altered balance between pressure and perfusion also accounts for the diminution in splanchnic and renal blood flow. Cerebral circulation, on the other hand, increases because of vasodilation.

Ventricular arrhythmias are rare during halothane anesthesia if respiratory acidosis and hypoxia are avoided, but nodal rhythm is common, often accounting for episodes of hypotension. The drug sensitizes the heart to catecholamines; thus, indiscriminate injection of these substances is unwise. Local infiltration of epinephrine is permissible if ventilation is adequate and the total dose in the adult does not exceed 100 μg (10 ml of a 1:100,000 solution) over a 10-minute period or more than 300 μg per hour.

Halothane seems to cause bronchodilation, perhaps through stimulation of beta-adrenergic receptors, for in the dog the decreased airway resistance is eliminated by beta-adrenergic blocking drugs. However, there is little evidence for a direct broncho-dilating action in humans. Respiration is depressed at all anesthetic concentrations, the central effects unopposed by the peripheral reflex stimulation seen with ether. Whatever the mechanism, the drug is useful in the anesthetic management of patients with bronchial asthma.

ENFLURANE

Because of emerging disadvantages with all the available anesthetics, chemists continue to search for better compounds. Interest has focused on the ethers because the investigations of Krantz and others suggested the greatest rewards in that sphere. In 1963, Terrell synthesized enflurane (Ethrane) ($CFHClCF_2$-O-CHF_2) and in 1965 its isomer, isoflurane (Forane) (CF_3-CHClO-CHF_2). Enflurane was introduced to clinical trial in 1963 and released for general use in 1972.

Enflurane is a stable, nonflammable liquid, somewhat less volatile than halothane, that produces rapid induction of anesthesia, easy maintenance, and rapid recovery. Cardiac rhythm tends to be stable, and there is only mild sensitization of the heart to epinephrine. The occurrence of signs of motor hyperactivity, such as twitching of the muscles of the jaw, face, neck, or extremities, accompanied by the appearance of EEG seizure patterns, which were reported during initial clinical evaluations of this drug, has proved to be of little consequence in daily practice. The high blood levels of Ethrane and low levels of Pa_{CO_2} required for seizure production are beyond the ranges generally reached in practice. Nonetheless, the potential for seizure, which has not been associated with evidence of cerebral hypoxia and is not accompanied by untoward sequelae, exists. Still some recommend that enflurane not be given to a patient with a seizure disorder.

Ventilatory depression parallels anesthetic depth. The decrease in slope of the ventilatory response to CO_2 with both enflurane and isoflurane is similar to that seen with comparable MAC equivalents of halothane. Assisted or controlled ventilation at surgical depths of anesthesia is thus indicated.

Cardiac output is well maintained during enflurane anesthesia; the cardiac responses to hypercarbia are similar to those seen in awake persons (markedly increased cardiac output), and output is not altered by hypocarbia. These changes probably reflect intact cardiac sympathetic control mechanisms activated by CO_2. Enflurane depresses myocardial contractility (Table 12–3) in a dose-related and reversible manner. Arterial hypotension occurs as a result of a fall in peripheral vascular resistance. Cardiovascular reflexes remain intact.

Muscle relaxation also occurs in a dose-related manner, with surgical depths of anesthesia adding to the effects of the competitive-type neuromuscular blockers. In general, small doses of either tubocurarine or pancuronium are administered to permit lighter levels of general anesthesia.

Enflurane is metabolized in liver by defluorination to produce free fluoride, but serum fluoride levels are far lower than those found with methoxyflurane. The use of enflurane in patients with renal disease of minimal or moderate magnitude (creatinine clearance of 50 per cent or serum creatinine levels twice normal) may be acceptable.

ISOFLURANE

Isoflurane was synthesized in 1965 by R. C. Terrell, but its development lagged behind that of its isomer, isoflurane, because of difficulties in synthesis, purification, and now-refuted claims of carcinogenesis. It is a nonflammable fluorinated methyl ethyl ether with physical, pharmacologic, and clinical properties similar to those of halothane and enflurane, but with striking differences. This agent is a more potent muscle relaxant than halothane. Isoflurane has only recently been introduced to clinical practice.

Induction of anesthesia with isoflurane is relatively rapid and may be associated with excitement, coughing, breath holding, and laryngospasm. All are minimized if adequate premedication is given, and all are absent after thiobarbiturate induction.

Isoflurane is a superb muscle relaxant allowing tracheal intubation without the need for neuromuscular blocking drugs, but the concentrations needed severely depress respiration and arterial pressure. The action is potentiated by both competitive and depolarizing types of neuromuscular blockers, but this does not interfere with reversal of their action by anticholinesterase drugs. The decrease in ventilation that occurs is the result of a decrease in tidal volume. Although respiratory rate tends to increase, that effect is not sufficient to compensate for the depressed minute volume; thus, assisted or controlled ventilation is needed to avoid respiratory acidosis.

Cardiac contractility is decreased by isoflurane, but a concurrent rise in heart rate maintains cardiac output at normal levels. Blood pressure falls in a dose-related manner primarily because of decreased peripheral vascular resistance. Muscle blood flow increases. The stimulatory effects of carbon dioxide on the cardiovascular system are diminished by isoflurane; consequently, an excessive reduction in arterial blood pressure is a sign of relative overdose. Isoflurane protects the heart against catecholamine-induced arrhythmia, whereas cardiac rhythm remains stable. There is no evidence of central nervous system EEG activation and irritability, as are occasionally seen with enflurane. Intracranial pressure rises with isoflurane owing to cerebrovascular dilation. Uterine relaxation similar to that seen with halothane occurs in the pregnant uterus, and the safety of use of this agent during pregnancy has yet to be established.

VOLATILE ANESTHETICS NOW SELDOM USED

DIETHYL ETHER

Diethyl ether (C_2H_5-O-C_2H_5) is an excellent anesthetic, safer perhaps than any other although technically more difficult to administer and flammable. C. W. Long of Georgia first gave ether for a minor surgical operation in March of 1842, and W. T. G. Morton subsequently gave the definitive public demonstration in Boston on October 16, 1846. Today the average patient intuitively objects to ether because of the more pleasantly experienced induction with intravenous barbiturates but more so because ether as given decades ago was so unpleasant. Induction was difficult, with salivary secretions, vomiting, and laryngospasm; excessive depths were produced; and fluid and electrolyte disorders were untreated in those days, while the postoperative course was accompanied by headache, nausea, vomiting, and dehydration. Today, ether given to a patient otherwise well managed need not be followed by these grim events; nevertheless, the agent is seldom used in the Western hemisphere.

As with all other inhalation anesthetics, ether is a myocardial depressant, but in intact man or animal this effect is opposed by increased activity of the sympathetic nervous system. Cardiac output and arterial pressure usually remain at normal levels, with heart rate tending to remain elevated, in part related to vagal blockade. Ether does not sensitize the myocardium to the action of catecholamines. Early in the course of anesthesia cutaneous blood flow increases, as with other anesthetics. Splanchnic and renal blood flow decline, and a strong antidiuretic action is seen, owing in part to antidiuretic hormone secretion.

Ether provides profound muscle relaxation. The mechanisms responsible are several but primarily involve the central nervous system, revolving around depression at synaptic pathways in the spinal cord. However, the effects of curare are augmented, dictating a lower dose of that blocking agent. As part of the action on the autonomic nervous system, ether results in bronchodilation, which suggests its use both therapeutically and for general anesthesia in patients with bronchial asthma. Spontaneous respiration remains adequate throughout deeper levels of anesthesia, even though the response of respiratory centers to CO_2 is reduced.

METHOXYFLURANE

Methoxyflurane (CH_3-O-CF-$CHCl_2$) was synthesized in 1958 by Larsen and introduced to clinical practice in 1959 by Artusio. Effective anesthetic doses are well below the flammable range. It is the most potent and least volatile of the liquid anesthetics. In clinical practice, induction of anesthesia is slow and recovery prolonged because of the high solubility in blood. Myocardial contractile force and cardiac output are depressed without compensatory sympathetic stimulation. Respiratory depression and muscle relaxation are prominent, ventilatory assistance is required, and the dose of neuromuscular blockers should be reduced. Because of high fat solubility, methoxyflurane is retained over long periods in the body, and persistent analgesia prevails with recovery. Delayed elimination allows hepatic metabolism of over half of an absorbed dose of methoxyflurane, causing high serum levels of free inorganic fluoride ion, a major metabolite. This metabolite is nephrotoxic, and a dose-related nephrotoxicity occurs. The use of methoxyflurane is limited because of its nephrotoxicity, slow onset, and slow recovery from its effects.

FLUROXENE

Fluroxene (F_3C-H_2C-O-CH=CH_2) is a fluorinated combination of ethyl and vinyl ether, one of a series of compounds introduced to practice by Krantz in 1954. It has been withdrawn from the market because of limited use and its inherent toxicity. The drug is flammable at concentrations used for induction and lacks sufficient potency for rapid induction. Emergence is associated with a high incidence of nausea and vomiting. As with cyclopropane, it activates the sympathetic nervous system. Use of the drug was popular when clinicians were searching for an alternate to halothane to avoid "halothane hepatitis," but since the introduction of enflurane it has been little used.

TRICHLOROETHYLENE

Trichloroethylene (CHCl = CCl_2), first prepared by Fisher in 1864, was used as an industrial solvent and is associated with irreversible neurologic sequelae. In 1934 Jackson used the drug as a general anesthetic for minor surgical procedures and obstetric analgesia. Its use as an inhalation anesthetic has been superseded by the new generation of fluorinated hydrocarbon anesthetics.

APPRAISAL

We have adopted a historical approach in this discussion of the inhalation anesthetics. Of the older agents, only nitrous oxide enjoys widespread usage. Ether and cyclopropane have been abandoned not only because of the potential hazards of anesthetic explosion but because the effects of these agents, as the sole drugs for surgical anesthesia, were unpleasant for patients thus treated. It is probable, however, that if ether or cyclopropane were employed today with the balanced techniques used for the newer agents the effects would not be nearly as unpleasant.

The introduction of the fluoride atom into the anesthetic molecule led to the design, synthesis, and wide acceptance of halothane as a near ideal anesthetic, except for the threat of liver toxicity. Further studies have led to the release to practice of isoflurane, which, if it fulfills its promise, may come closer than any other anesthetic to ideal standards. For as long as intravenous agents have been administered, most of them have been given in combination with inhaled drugs to fulfill specific requirements such as rapid induction, analgesia, or muscle relaxation. Probably current research will provide continuing improvements in intravenous drugs used as anesthetic supplements, but it is unlikely that any manufacturer will be willing to undertake the expensive and tedious task needed to find a better inhalation anesthetic. The risk is too great to justify the effort.

REFERENCES

Bunker, JP, Forrest, WH, Mosteller F, et al (eds.): The National Halothane Study. A Study of Possible Association Between Halothane Anesthesia and Post-operative Hepatic Necrosis. Bethesda, Md, US Government Printing Office, 1969.

Cohen EN, Trudell JR, Edmunds HN, et al: Urinary metabolites of halothane in man. Anesthesiology 43:392, 1970.

Cohen EN: Occupational disease among operating room personnel: A national study. Report of an ad hoc committee on the effects of trace anesthetics on the health of operating room personnel. American Society of Anesthesiologists. Anesthesiology 41:321, 1974.

Dundee JW: Alterations in response to somatic pain associated with anaesthesia. II. The effect of thiopentone and pentobarbitone. Br J Anaesth 32:407, 1960.

Eger, EI II, Smith NT, Cullen DJ, et al: A comparison of the cardiovascular effects of halothane, fluroxene, ether and cyclopropane in man. Anesthesiology 34:25, 1971.

Eger EI II: Anesthetic Uptake and Action. Baltimore, The Williams & Wilkins Co, 1974.

Eger EI II, White AE, Brown CL, et al: A test of the carcinogenicity of enflurane, isoflurane, halothane, methoxyflurane, and nitrous oxide in man. Anesth Analg 57:678, 1978.

Fleming RA, Smith NT: An inexpensive device for analyzing and monitoring the electroencephalogram. Anesthesiology 50:456, 1979.

Linde HW, Dykes MHM: Evaluation of a general anesthetic, isoflurane. JAMA 245:2335, 1981.

Mazze RI, Cousins MJ: Renal toxicity of anaesthetics: With specific reference to the nephrotoxicity of methoxyflurane. Can Anaesth Soc J 20:64, 1973.

Mazze RI, Cousins MJ, Barr GA: Renal effects and metabolism of isoflurane in man. Anesthesiology 40:536, 1974.

McLane GE, Sipes, IG, Brown BR Jr: An animal model of halothane hepatotoxicity: Roles of enzyme induction and hypoxia. Anesthesiology 51:321, 1979.

Miletich DJ, Ivankovich AD, Albrecht RF, et al: Absence of autoregulation of cerebral blood flow during halothane and enflurane anesthesia. Anesth Analg 55:100, 1976.

Price HL, Helrich M: Significance of the competence index in the measurement of myocardial contractility. J Pharmacol Exp Ther 115:199, 1955.

Theye RA, Michenfelder JD: Individual organ contributions to the decrease in whole-body VO$_2$ with isoflurane. Anesthesiology 42:35, 1975.

Van Dyke RA: Metabolism of halothane (editorial). Anesthesiology 43:386, 1975.

Waud BE, Waud DR: The effects of diethyl ether, enflurane and isoflurane at the neuromuscular junction. Anesthesiology 42:275, 1975.

Chapter 13
TECHNIQUES OF INHALATION ANESTHESIA

Techniques of inhalation anesthesia are classified according to the presence or absence of a reservoir bag in the breathing circuit, rebreathing of expired gases, an absorber to remove expired carbon dioxide, and directional valves in the breathing circuit. The reservoir bag and absorber have been discussed in Chapter 7 and will be considered here only as they relate to the techniques described.

REBREATHING OF EXPIRED GAS

At end expiration, that part of the tidal volume remaining in the tracheobronchial tree, pharynx, and mouth is returned to the alveoli as inspiration begins; some rebreathing is therefore inevitable. Inhalation techniques may increase rebreathing in varying degrees. The least rebreathing is associated with insufflation, in which large volumes of fresh gas are continuously delivered to mouth or trachea. The higher the gas flow, the greater the displacement of expired air and the less rebreathing. Insufflation was used in the early days of thoracic surgery to provide positive pressure to counteract pneumothorax, but it was abandoned because it depressed blood pressure and because carbon dioxide accumulated through lack of expansion and contraction of the lungs.

In the "open" or, as it is often somewhat incorrectly called, the "nonrebreathing" technique, a valve directs expired gas to the atmosphere. At the beginning of inspiration, if the valve is competent, the only gas rebreathed, excluding that in the respiratory dead space, is the gas between the valve and the mouth or nose. At expiration all the gas is vented. The volume rebreathed increases if the valve is attached to a mask rather than a tracheal tube. Rebreathing increases with the semiopen and semiclosed techniques even though valves are used, whereas complete rebreathing characterizes a closed system.

Directional valves may be made of rubber, metal, mica, or plastic; they must seat properly to be competent and should offer minimal resistance to breathing. They should be tested periodically for competence and cleaned to hold resistance to a minimum. The presence and location of the valves are important. If they are absent in a closed system, a high inspired concentration of carbon dioxide will result even though a carbon dioxide absorber is present. If the valves are located close to the reservoir bag, inspired carbon dioxide levels will be higher than if they are near the mouth. Nonetheless, in most circle systems the valves are adjacent to the reservoir bag, on the expiratory side.

Various combinations of the four factors listed earlier are incorporated in the several techniques of inhalation anesthesia (Table 13–1); brief descriptions follow.

136

TABLE 13–1. Techniques of Inhalation Anesthesia

	Reservoir Bag	Rebreathing of Expired Gases	Chemical Absorption of Expired CO_2	Directional Valves
Insufflation	No	Least	No	None
Open (nonrebreathing)				
Demand (McKesson),	No	Minimal	No	Two
Leigh, Fink, Ruben, Stephen-Slater, or Frumin valve	Yes	Minimal	No	Two
Semiopen				
Open drop	No	Partial	No	None
Ayre technique	No	Partial	No	None
Magill attachment	Yes	Partial	No	One
Semiclosed	Yes	Partial	Yes	Two
Closed				
To-and-fro	Yes	Complete	Yes	None
Circle	Yes	Complete	Yes	Two

INSUFFLATION

With this technique, anesthetic gases and oxygen are delivered either to the mouth via a metal hook or directly into the trachea. Valves are not required nor is a carbon dioxide absorber or reservoir bag necessary. If 8 to 10 L of gas/min are delivered into the trachea at the level of the carina, there is little rebreathing. During inspiration the inhaled mixture is composed of gas coming from the delivery tube plus room air breathed through nose or mouth. Dead space in the tracheobronchial tree is minimal. The technique is rarely used today but offers the advantages of minimal resistance to breathing and simple equipment. Disadvantages include waste of gas; inability to assist respiration in the absence of a reservoir bag; variable dilution of the anesthetic by room air, highest during peak inspiratory flow rates (the composition of the inspired gases is thus unpredictable); drying of the tracheal mucosa with loss of water and heat; and difficulty in scavenging the expired gases or vapors. Some of these disadvantages characterize other techniques as well.

OPEN OR NONREBREATHING SYSTEMS

These systems permit the patient to inhale only the anesthetic mixture delivered from the machine (Fig. 13–1). The composition of the inspired mixture can therefore be determined precisely. Each expired breath goes directly into the surrounding air, as with the Ruben or Fink valves. With this technique and normal ventilation, residual nitrogen in the lungs can essentially be washed out in three minutes; this minimizes the dilutional effect of nitrogen and increases the partial pressure in the alveoli of anesthetics such as nitrous oxide. Induction of anesthesia is thus hastened. If a reservoir bag is not used, the inspiratory valve must be capable of supplying a high flow of gas upon demand.

The disadvantages of the technique are: high gas flows are necessary; water vapor and heat are lost; anesthetic gases are not confined to the breathing system; and resistance to breathing varies with the efficiency of the valves and both the diameter and total length of the delivery tubing. Unless the inspired gases are humidified, the technique is ill-advised in children or for lengthy operations in adults.

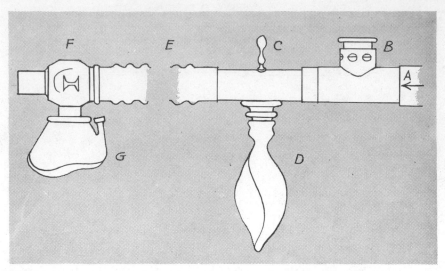

FIGURE 13–1. One type of nonrebreathing system: *A*, gas supply; *B*, pop-off valve; *C*, obturator for reservoir bag; *D*, reservoir bag; *E*, corrugated conducting tubing; *F*, nonrebreathing valve of the Ruben type; *G*, face mask.

SEMIOPEN SYSTEMS

The system that we call semiopen is characterized by the British as "semiclosed without carbon dioxide absorption." A semiopen system allows exhaled gas to be vented with some return to the inspiratory limb of the apparatus for rebreathing, the degree of return determined by the volume of fresh gas flow. If the flow is great enough, rebreathing can almost be eliminated. The rate of flow required to achieve this depends on the design of the system. There is little need for chemical absorption of carbon dioxide.

THE OPEN DROP METHOD

This is the simplest of the inhalation techniques, requiring the least equipment. A volatile anesthetic is dripped on gauze stretched over a wire frame or onto a gauze mask held over nose and mouth (Fig. 13–2). There are no valves or delivery tubing; therefore resistance to respiration is minimal. Dead space is determined by the closeness of fit to the face or by the thickness of the gauze placed about the mask to prevent escape of the anesthetic. Measures taken to increase the concentration of anesthetic result simultaneously in an increase in dead space carbon dioxide and water vapor and a reduction in oxygen tension beneath the mask. If room air is breathed, a lower Pa_{O_2} results but is corrected by flowing 500 ml of oxygen/min beneath the mask; however, the higher the flow of oxygen, the lower the concentration of anesthetic.

An important aspect of this technique is the effect of mask temperature on vaporization of liquid anesthetics. As the anesthetic vaporizes, the temperature of the gauze falls, retarding further vaporization as well as induction of anesthesia. Condensation of water vapor on the gauze also interferes with vaporization of the anesthetic. The cooler the gauze, the more rapid the condensation of moisture in expired air, further increasing the dead space and leading to accumulation of carbon dioxide.

The open drop method is seldom used in modern practice, although some find it useful with halothane for brief anesthesia in children for eye examination or myringotomy.

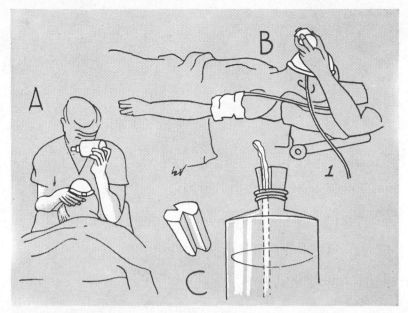

FIGURE 13–2. Technique of "open drop" anesthesia. *A*, Method of supporting the head with the arms; *B*, lateral view showing support of head and insufflation of oxygen *(1)* beneath the mask; *C*, cork cut and wick in place to drip the anesthetic.

AYRE'S T-PIECE

This device was introduced primarily for use during endotracheal anesthesia in infants and young children undergoing repair of harelip and cleft palate. The T-piece consists of a metal tube 1 cm in diameter into which gases and vapors are "injected" through a small inlet tube at a right angle to the main limb (Fig. 13–3). One end of the T-piece is connected to an endotracheal tube, the other is open to the atmosphere. Rubber tubing can be attached to the open end to constitute a reservoir for anesthetic gases, most of which would otherwise escape. If the capacity of the reservoir is equal to one third respiratory tidal volume, the total flow of gas into the system to prevent dilution of the inspired anesthetic mixture should be about twice the respiratory minute volume. This flow rate minimizes accumulation of carbon dioxide. Since reservoir bag and valves are absent, resistance to respiration is minimal.

The technique is often modified. Some use a Y-piece rather than the T-piece, substituting corrugated tubing for the reservoir and adding a reservoir bag or escape valve. The reservoir bag permits assisted respiration, thereby conferring greater

F = 2 × minute volume

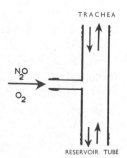

TRACHEA

N$_2$O

O$_2$

RESERVOIR TUBE

FIGURE 13–3. The Ayre T-piece. Nitrous oxide and oxygen supplemented with volatile anesthetic enter through the side tube. The tracheal end of the T-piece is connected to the endotracheal tube. The end marked "reservoir tube" is vented via a scavenging system. (From Ayre, P.: Br J Anaesth 28:520, 1956.)

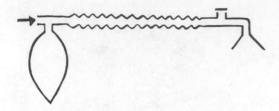

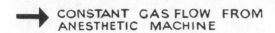

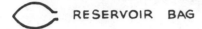

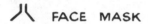

CONSTANT GAS FLOW FROM
ANESTHETIC MACHINE

RESERVOIR BAG

CORRUGATED TUBING

EXPIRATORY VALVE

FACE MASK

FIGURE 13–4. The Magill attachment. See text for description of operation of system.

versatility. The technique is appropriate for infants and small children if high gas flows are used, but again the drying effect on the respiratory mucosa and the potential toxic effects of waste anesthetics on operating room personnel must be considered. Both of these disadvantages can be overcome by humidifying and scavenging the exhaust gases. The original technique, however, remains simple and useful, particularly for children up to the age of four (see Chapter 25).

THE MAGILL ATTACHMENT

In this attachment the expiratory valve is close to the face mask or tracheal tube, separated from the reservoir bag by corrugated tubing (Fig. 13–4). Gas enters the system from the supply source at a constant flow rate. The expiratory valve opens when pressure in the system is slightly higher than that of the atmosphere. During the early phase of expiration, fresh gas flows directly into the bag while expired gas flows back into the corrugated tubing, forcing gas from the tubing into the bag. When the pressure in the bag equals the opening pressure of the expiratory valve, the valve opens and expired gas escapes. Fresh gas continues to flow into the corrugated tubing, thus eliminating, via the valve, expired gas that had previously entered at the onset of expiration.

With inspiration, gas is drawn from the system faster than it is supplied from the machine; therefore, additional gas must be drawn from the reservoir, decreasing its volume. The corresponding reduction of pressure in the system causes the expiratory valve to close. The bag empties slowly until the inspiratory flow rate falls below that of fresh gas. Mapleson (1954) has found that if the flow of fresh gas into the system is at least equal to the patient's respiratory minute volume, rebreathing will not occur. Mapleson's adaptations of this system offer a combination of the Ayre and Magill principles (see Fig. 25–3).

The Magill system is a relatively simple means of administering inhalation anesthetics with less dependence on the competency of valves than with the purely open technique and lower gas flows. The problems of loss of water vapor and heat and dissemination of anesthetic agents with possible toxic effects on personnel are readily correctable by use of humidified gases and scavenging systems (see Fig. 25–3).

SEMICLOSED SYSTEMS

In a semiclosed system, exhaled gas passes into the atmosphere or mingles with fresh gases and is rebreathed, but a chemical absorber is placed in the breathing circuit. Carbon dioxide accumulation is therefore less of a problem than in the semiopen system, and maintenance of an adequate oxygen supply is the dominant factor. With semiclosed systems, denitrogenation is accomplished more slowly and induction of anesthesia delayed. Total gas flow should at least equal respiratory minute volume if the proportion of oxygen in inspired gas is equal to that of atmospheric air as shown on the flowmeter. If a lower flow rate is selected, rebreathing increases and a larger proportion of the fresh gas must consist of oxygen.

Inhaled gases are humidified to a greater extent in such a system, and loss of heat and water vapor is less than with the techniques previously described. The reservoir bag permits assisted respiration — not only constituting a convenience but becoming a true "reservoir" and providing maximal flow rate at peak inspiration. Semiclosed systems are probably the most commonly used systems today.

CLOSED SYSTEMS

Complete rebreathing of expired gas takes place in a closed system with practically all of the carbon dioxide chemically absorbed. Oxygen is added in amounts sufficient to supply metabolic demand. In the once popular to-and-fro technique, the gases pass back and forth through a chemical absorber without interposition of valves, an efficient method of absorption because the gases pass through the absorber twice. However, because of the chemical reaction and low flow of fresh gas, accumulation of heat is greater than with any other system. Channeling of gas through the absorber may occur, with the possibility of accumulation of carbon dioxide. The possibility of inhalation of soda lime dust is another hazard. The canister is heavy and needs to be supported close to the patient's face. Few anesthetists use the system today because it is too clumsy. Its chief value lies in minimal resistance to breathing and ease of sterilization after use in anesthetizing a patient with communicable disease.

In the circle system with inspiratory and expiratory valves, gas flow is directed so that a single passage is made in one direction through the absorber. A closed system is achieved only when it is impervious to leaks, that is, when the expiratory valve is closed and the mask fit is tight. A total flow rate of over 500 ml/min suggests that the system is not truly closed. From the equipment standpoint this method is convenient (see Chapter 7) and conservation of heat and moisture is maximal. The cost of anesthetics is reduced, as they are confined to the system. Resistance to breathing is enhanced, however, because of turbulent flow through the valves, the absorber, the tubing, and the connectors.

With a constant flow rate and no need for escape valve adjustment, the closed system aids in determination of depth of anesthesia by transmitting changes in chest wall and lung compliance as respiration is assisted or controlled. With the advent of highly potent halogenated agents, closed systems, while economical, are potentially hazardous without constant monitoring of inspired anesthetic concentrations.

FLOW RATES IN ANESTHESIA SYSTEMS

During inhalation anesthesia several considerations dictate the rate of gas flow. The volume of gas delivered to the breathing system is considered to have one or more functions: achievement and maintenance of a specified alveolar concentration of anesthetic; compensation for losses from the breathing circuit resulting from variations in absorption and leakage; dilution or elimination of other gases in the breathing circuit and from the lungs; the use of additional gas as a vehicle for volatile anesthetics; and, finally, matters of practicality.

MAINTENANCE OF ALVEOLAR GAS CONCENTRATION

In a nonrebreathing system, a change in flowmeter setting alters the inspired gas concentration immediately. However, in a closed circle system, especially one of large internal volume, change in flow alters the inspired concentration only slowly. The speed of induction of anesthesia, therefore, relates in some measure to the characteristics of the anesthesia system used. A patient breathing halothane via a to-and-fro canister and a 2-L reservoir bag will lose consciousness rapidly. The same gas flows in a circle system with a large canister and 4-L bag might not result in anesthesia for several minutes.

LOSSES FROM THE BREATHING CIRCUIT

Flow rate of gases is set according to loss from the system, including rate of biodegradation of the anesthetic; absorption of gas by tissues; losses by diffusion through rubber and skin, through surgical incision, and into body cavities; and leakage from the system, including escape valves, poor connections, and undetected perforations in rubber goods. Absorption of halothane, enflurane, and methoxyflurane by rubber is significant and continues long after induction of anesthesia; the gas is then slowly released.

The metabolic demand for oxygen is high. An adult of 1.7 sq m body surface requires approximately 240 ml oxygen/min. Most general anesthetics decrease metabolic rate by 10 to 15 per cent, whereas lowered body temperature reduces metabolic rate and fever increases it. The metabolism of anesthetics is low when compared with the large volumes absorbed in body tissues, but up to 20 per cent may be metabolized (see Chapter 12).

Planned loss via escape valves or leakage as a result of ill-fitting connections and perforations in rubber must be compensated by higher gas delivery. In high flow techniques the effect of leaks is negligible, but in low flow systems the effect is considerable. Leaks should be discovered and corrected prior to induction of anesthesia.

DILUTION OR WASHOUT OF GAS

When nitrous oxide, a weak anesthetic effective only at high partial pressures, is given, a high initial flow rate is necessary to wash out residual lung nitrogen and replace same with the anesthetic mixture. At the conclusion of anesthesia, high flows of oxygen or nitrous oxide in oxygen may be used to eliminate a more soluble agent such as halothane or enflurane, thus hastening emergence. However, conversion to an open system or breathing room air is more likely to be effective in this regard.

VAPORIZATION OF VOLATILE ANESTHETICS

When volatile anesthetics are administered, the characteristics of both vaporizer and agent influence the selection of gas flows. Some vaporizers yield a stated concentration only at specified flow rates. The Fluotec vaporizer, for example, requires at least a 4-L flow to deliver the concentrations indicated on the dial. Divergence from the indicated concentration is greatest below 1 L and above 10 L per minute flow.

In a system delivering all of the oxygen required through the vaporizer, a potential danger exists if the anesthetist is forgetful and shunts the vaporizer out of the system. This was more often seen when methoxyflurane was in use, but the lessons learned then should not be forgotten. Oxygen is a vital carrier gas that should always be supplied via a flowmeter separate from that supplying the vaporizer. These are common problems when the vaporizer is located outside the circle system; if within the system, all inspired gases pass through the vaporizer. In this circumstance an inefficient vaporizer may produce a higher concentration of anesthetic than an efficient one.

PRACTICALITY

Simplicity of Calculations. With efficient vaporizers the concentration of anesthetic delivered is easily calculated; certain flow rates simplify the mathematics. For instance, at ambient temperature if total gas flow is 5 L per minute, comprising 1.5 L of oxygen and 3.5 L of nitrous oxide, approximately 1 per cent halothane will be delivered for each 100 ml of oxygen going through the Copper Kettle or Vernitrol vaporizer. Perhaps the best method is to have at hand a graphic representation of concentration of anesthetic delivered according to temperature, total gas flow, and gas flow through the vaporizer.

The Escape Valve. Another factor in choice of flow rate is the adjustment of the escape valve. It should be possible to adjust the valve during controlled or assisted respiration so that pressure on the breathing bag first inflates the lungs and then vents excess gas. Some valves are not easily adjusted; with these it may be more convenient to empty the bag periodically, at other times leaving the valve closed. Some find it difficult to judge adequacy of ventilation unless the escape valve is closed.

Dictates of the Operation. Circumstances during operation may require changes in gas flow. For example, during a thoracotomy in which a bronchus has been divided, high flows are necessary to compensate for leakage as suturing is done.

Limitations of Equipment. Some vaporizers impose limitations on flow for optimal vaporization and therefore cannot be relied on for accurate concentrations of anesthetics at all flow rates, as in the Fluotec device with low vaporizer flow. Rotameters are often more accurate in the upper two thirds of the scale than in the lower third. A Vernitrol vaporizer designed for ether offers a flowmeter range of flows up to 1300 ml/min; this flowmeter cannot be relied upon to deliver exactly 100 ml of oxygen per minute to vaporize halothane or enflurane.

Economy. For prolonged procedures, considerable saving in the cost of anesthetics is made possible by use of a semiclosed breathing circuit with low flows or a closed system. By definition, a semiclosed system is one in which fresh gas inflow is low to provide considerable rebreathing. Many anesthetists utilize high flows for the first 30 to 60 minutes and convert to low flows for the duration of a long operation.

Environmental Contamination. Appreciable quantities of anesthetics are detectable in the operating room environment, the concentration varying with distance from the anesthesia machine, total gas flow, concentration of volatile agents, patterns of room ventilation, and efficiency of scavenging systems.

REFERENCES

Ayre P: The T-piece technique. Br J Anaesth 28:520, 1956.
Bain JA, Spoerel WE: Prediction of arterial carbon dioxide tension during controlled ventilation with a modified Mapleson D system. Can Anaesth Soc J 22:34, 1975.

Eger EI II: Anesthesia Uptake and Action. Baltimore, Williams and Wilkins, 1975.

Fitton EP: A theoretical investigation of oxygen concentrations in gases inspired from various semi-closed anaesthetic systems. Br J Anaesth 30:269, 1958.

Lowe HJ, Ernst EA: The Quantitative Practice of Anesthesia: Use of the Closed Circuit. Baltimore, Williams and Wilkins, 1981.

Macintosh RR, Mushin WW, Epstein HG: Physics for the Anaesthetist. 3rd ed. Philadelphia, FA Davis. 1963.

Mapleson WW: The elimination of rebreathing in various semi-closed anaesthetic systems. Br J Anaesth 26:323, 1954.

Tayyab MA, Ambiavagar M, Chalon J: Water nebulization in non-rebreathing systems during anesthesia. Can Anaesth Soc J 20:728, 1973.

INTRAVENOUS ANESTHESIA AND TRACHEAL INTUBATION

Chapter 14

INTRAVENOUS ANESTHESIA

An early effort to produce insensibility by means of intravenous injection of opioids was made in 1665. Oré published the results of a trial of administration of chloral hydrate by vein in 1875. However, it was not until the introduction of the rapidly acting barbiturates in the 1930s that the intravenous method achieved popularity.

Induction of anesthesia by the intravenous administration of a rapidly acting barbiturate is not an unpleasant experience. A patient who has been anesthetized this way usually prefers it to all others. Thus it is difficult to avoid starting general anesthesia with an intravenous agent regardless of the anesthetic subsequently used for maintenance. Since the technique is simple, it appeals to individuals not qualified by experience or training to use it safely. It has been aptly said that thiopental is fatally easy to give.

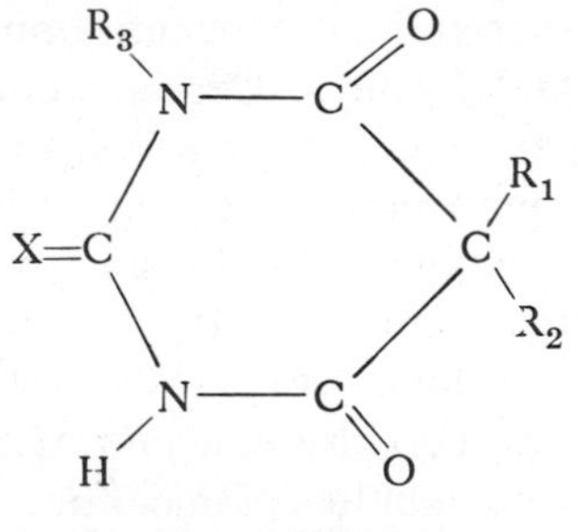

GENERAL FORMULA

	R_1	R_2	R_3	X
Thiopental (Pentothal)	Ethyl	1 methylbutyl	H	S
Thiamylal (Surital)	Allyl	1 methylbutyl	H	S
Methohexital (Brevital)	Allyl	1 methyl 2 pentynyl	CH_3	O

FIGURE 14–1. Chemical configuration of the barbiturates used intravenously for general anesthesia.

This chapter outlines the principles involved in the safe use of intravenous anesthetics. Barbiturates are the most popular intravenous induction agents, and the barbiturate most commonly used is thiopental. Thiamylal (Surital) is still another thiobarbiturate, whereas methohexital (Brevital) is the oxybarbiturate (Fig. 14–1) most commonly used. All are similar in action and will be discussed together. The chapter also describes the use of other anesthetics given by the intravenous route, including neuroleptics, ketamine, diazepam, opioids, and steroids.

BARBITURIC ACID DERIVATIVES

THEORETIC CONSIDERATIONS

Controllability

Barbiturate anesthesia differs from that produced by inhalation agents in that once the drug has been injected, there is little the anesthetist can do to facilitate removal. Dissipation of effects, as will be shown, depends on redistribution of the drug from brain to other tissues and, to a lesser extent, on biotransformation. With anesthetic vapors or gases, the partial pressure in blood can be altered at will by varying the concentration of agent in the inspired mixture. With overdosage of an inhalation agent, concentration can be diminished rapidly by ventilating the lungs with oxygen. Opioid injection can be countered by the use of antagonists. However, controllability with intravenous barbiturates is improved by the use of solutions varying from 0.2 to 2.5 per cent, the more dilute solutions given by continuous infusion and the higher concentrations injected intermittently. Theoretically, the lower the concentration or total quantity injected per unit time, the better the controllability of the level of anesthesia; but practically, the infusion is often forgotten during stressful times. As overdosage is therefore more likely to occur, we do not recommend routine continuous infusion of barbiturates.

Pharmacokinetics

The intravenous barbiturates are metabolized in liver and the metabolites excreted in urine. However, it is not biotransformation that terminates their action but redistribution in tissues. As an illustration we shall follow the course of a single injection of thiopental.

Initially, upon intravenous injection the drug is diluted in the central pool of blood in heart and lungs, passing then in high concentration to the organs of highest blood flow — brain, heart, liver, and kidneys. Cerebral concentration rises rapidly, peak concentration reached in approximately 50 seconds, and unconsciousness ensues. With recirculation, as equilibration with lean tissues begins, thiopental is removed from brain and the plasma concentration declines. Muscle, skin, bone, and, lastly, fat begin to take up thiopental, 15 to 30 minutes required for equilibration with the first three, whereas equilibration in fat takes several hours (Fig. 14–2).

Through redistribution, the cerebral concentration decreases sufficiently so that the patient awakens, often within minutes of injection, despite the fact that only a small amount of the drug has undergone biotransformation. Although the exact amount is controversial, the rate of this process is taken as 10 to 15 per cent per hour of the total dose injected.

If instead of a single injection multiple doses are given, more drug is stored in the body, and large total doses may lead to saturation of lean as well as fatty tissues. Under these conditions even small additional doses may be excessive, so that caution must be exercised. Recovery is slow, largely because of the slow release of drug from fat.

Considerable quantities of barbiturate are bound to plasma protein, particularly the

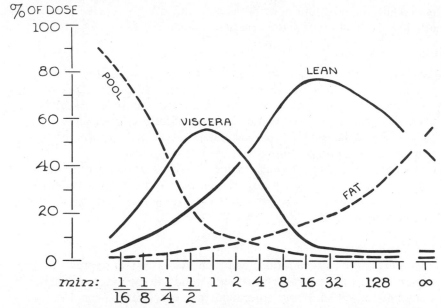

FIGURE 14–2. Distribution of thiopental in different body tissues and organs at various times after intravenous injection. (Reproduced with permission from Price HL, Linde HW, Price ML: Clin Pharmacol Ther 1:298, 1960.)

albumin moiety. Tissues come into equilibrium only with the unbound fraction, since the bound part is not readily available for diffusion. Equilibration between tissues and unbound portion is dependent, in part, upon the hydrogen ion concentration of blood. Acidosis reduces protein binding of the drug, tending to increase cell penetration; acidosis also increases the amount of undissociated drug present. For both reasons the acidosis resulting from carbon dioxide retention causes plasma thiopental levels to decline and anesthetic depth to increase. Respiratory alkalosis has a reverse action.

The rate at which barbiturates penetrate the central nervous system correlates with the lipid solubility of the un-ionized molecules — or the partition coefficient between lipid and aqueous phases. For example, the onset of hypnotic action following intravenous administration of pentobarbital is slower than that following comparable doses of thiopental. While thiopental is largely non-ionized at pH 7.4, it has a high partition coefficient (3.3). Pentobarbital, on the other hand, is ionized to a lesser extent and is much less protein bound, but it has a far lower partition coefficient (0.05); thus, penetration and hypnotic action are slow.

The thiobarbiturates undergo metabolic degradation by desulfuration and oxidation, principally in liver, with some biotransformation occurring in brain and kidney. Inactive metabolites are excreted via the kidneys except for methohexital, a significant amount of which is eliminated in feces. Biotransformation of the oxybarbiturates occurs only in liver. Narcosis with the latter, therefore, can be expected to last somewhat longer in patients with hepatic decompensation.

Acute tolerance to the thiobarbiturates can develop. A patient given 2 gm of thiopental in increments, following an initial dose of 500 mg, may regain consciousness with a blood level of 20 mg per 100 ml. Another patient given only 1 gm of barbiturate with an initial dose of 250 gm may regain consciousness with a blood level of about 10 mg per 100 ml. Time of awakening differs little between the two subjects. Viewed in practical terms, individuals given large initial doses of a thiobarbiturate will require larger increments to maintain anesthesia than those who receive smaller doses for induction. The mechanism of acute tolerance is unknown.

Alkalinity of Solutions

Solutions of thiopental, thiamylal, and methohexital are highly alkaline, the pH of 2.5 per cent solutions in distilled water being about 10.6. As a result, intravenous injection of the barbiturate may be followed by thrombophlebitis, nerve injury, or tissue necrosis, (in the event of extravasation), or intra-arterial injection can lead to arterial spasm and gangrene. If a thiobarbiturate is injected into the tubing of an intravenous infusion, these complications are less likely to occur.

The alkalinity was once though to lend "self-sterilizing" properties. Solutions were kept for weeks or until precipitation occurred. We know now that solutions of the barbiturates can support bacterial growth, so it is recommended that solutions unused within 24 hours be discarded.

Anesthetic Action

Intravenous barbiturates produce central nervous system depression ranging from mild sedation to coma. The totality of effect depends on the extent of excitability at the time of administration and any tolerance that may have been induced by prior exposure. The mode of action of barbiturates is believed to involve depression of short synaptic pathways in the central reticular core of the brain stem, sparing direct spino-lemnisco-thalamic pathways. For these reasons, barbiturates differ from inhalation anesthetics in their lesser ability to block afferent sensory impulses. An antianalgetic action has been demonstrated for the thiobarbiturates, but this is of doubtful clinical significance.

Recognition of these fundamental differences among the anesthetics is essential for the rational use of intravenous barbiturates. Healthy muscular individuals may require excessive doses for adequate anesthesia. Often the degree of anesthesia appears adequate, but with surgical stimulation movement or struggling occurs, responses indicative of poor afferent blockade. Minor pharyngeal stimulation may precipitate laryngospasm or cough, suggesting that thiopental sensitizes vagal nerve endings, leading to laryngospasm.

RESPIRATORY EFFECTS

The respiratory effects of thiobarbiturates are the result of direct depression of the medullary and pontine centers for respiratory control. Actions on pulmonary stretch receptors, afferent and efferent nerves concerned in respiration, and the neuromuscular junction are negligible. Immediately following injection, respiratory depression may be pronounced. Central stimulatory responses to carbon dioxide are depressed at all levels of anesthesia and are ultimately abolished as anesthesia deepens. Responses to peripheral chemoreceptor excitation persist longer but are also extinguished at profound depths of anesthesia. At ordinary levels of anesthesia, tidal volume is diminished and respiratory rate increased, and the thorax tends to assume the end-expiratory position.

CIRCULATORY EFFECTS

Barbiturates depress the activity of hypothalamic autonomic centers regulating the force of cardiac contraction. Myocardial contractility is reduced, whereas vascular tone is increased by direct action. Baroreceptor reflexes, conduction in autonomic nerves, and sympathetic ganglion transmission are little affected. The end result of these actions is that cardiac output is reduced whereas total peripheral resistance is increased. The barbiturates used for anesthesia do not sensitize the autonomic tissues of the heart to the arrhythmic effect of the catecholamines to any significant extent.

CENTRAL NERVOUS SYSTEM EFFECTS

Thipental reduces cerebral metabolism and oxygen consumption, suggesting that large doses protect against cerebral damage from hypoxia (Chapter 27). This reduction in metabolic activity leads to parallel reductions in cerebral blood flow. Because of the low flow (as much as one third in light anesthesia and up to one half in deep anesthesia) cerebral blood volume and CSF pressure diminish; thus use of the barbiturates is recommended in patients with increased intracranial pressure.

CLINICAL USE OF INTRAVENOUS BARBITURATES

Selection of Patients

Intravenous barbiturate anesthesia is not suitable for all patients. Caution is advised in those with bronchial asthma. Individuals with poor superficial veins may be unsuitable choices merely because of technical problems. Patients with masses encroaching upon the air passages may become hypoxic with loss of consciousness, muscle relaxation, and engorgement of cervical tissues unless a satisfactory airway is first established, as by tracheal intubation with the patient awake. Individuals with acute or chronic respiratory infections often react poorly to barbiturate anesthesia, developing chest wall spasm and cough. Patients with acute intermittent porphyria may undergo exacerbation of symptoms following barbiturate administration; a rapidly progressive fatal course has been described.

Barbiturate anesthesia is inadequate for many types of operations even when nitrous oxide is inhaled. For operations requiring muscle relaxation, a thiobarbiturate is used for induction, with analgesia provided by nitrous oxide and an analgetic, and relaxation achieved with a neuromuscular blocker.

Rapid induction of anesthesia for tracheal intubation is a popular technique; 3 to 6 mg of tubocurarine are given intravenously to prevent muscle fasciculations caused by succinylcholine while the patient is given 100 per cent oxygen to facilitate nitrogen washout. This is followed by 250 to 500 mg of barbiturate, administered simultaneously with, or followed by, a paralyzing dose of succinylcholine. However, the technique is inherently hazardous, as a high blood concentration of anesthetic is produced in a short time. If used in the poor risk patient with cardiovascular disease or upper intestinal tract obstruction, mortality may be high. Cough and bronchospasm may appear upon recovery of respiratory reflexes because of the irritant effect of the tracheal tube in an essentially unanesthetized patient. Furthermore, subsequent overdose with an inhalation anesthetic may result from attempts to quiet the patient.

Anesthetic Management

Anesthesia should not be induced with a barbiturate unless an anesthesia machine is at hand, with oxygen ready and the usual assortment of resuscitative equipment available. If opioids are administered for premedication, and they are an essential part of a balanced technique, the anesthetist can anticipate a greater degree of respiratory depression following injection of an intravenous barbiturate.

Although we prefer to inject the barbiturate into the tubing of an intravenous infusion, some patients have venous constriction upon arrival in the operating room. There is little excuse for exposing a patient to painful, multiple needle punctures in an effort to provide a seemingly pleasant induction of anesthesia. It is sensible to abandon the intravenous route and use an inhalation agent for induction.

Induction

A test dose of not more than 50 mg should be given at first. This can be done during preliminary oxygenation. Pain at the site of injection suggests extravasation of drug but more commonly is the result of venospasm caused by the high pH of the solution. Ordinarily, drowsiness occurs soon after initial injection. If loss of consciousness follows the initial dose, the amount of drug subsequently needed for anesthesia is likely to be relatively small. In general, incremental doses are preferred over single, large doses.

When the initial injection of barbiturate is to be followed by inhalation anesthesia, sufficient time should elapse to ensure unconsciousness. If too much barbiturate is given, the resulting respiratory depression will delay induction of inhalation anesthesia.

An intravenous barbiturate may be used as the sole anesthetic for brief surgical procedures such as closed reduction of a fracture or dislocation or incision and drainage of an abscess. When combined with nitrous oxide, longer operations not requiring relaxation can be accomplished. During maintenance, nitrous oxide can be given in equal volumes with oxygen or in a combination of as high as four parts to one of oxygen. A total gas flow of 6 to 8 L per minute is supplied for the first three to five minutes to denitrogenate the lungs and is subsequently reduced to 2 to 3 L per minute. If respiration is depressed by the initial injection of barbiturate, assistance is provided until tidal volume returns to normal levels.

Maintenance

The amount of barbiturate required depends on the physical condition of the patient, premedication given, and the nature and duration of operation. Persistent tachycardia, pupillary dilation, sweating, tachypnea, movement, and arterial hypertension are manifestations of pain perception and inadequate depth of anesthesia. Under such conditions, if a considerable quantity of barbiturate has already been given, the anesthetist may elect to change to a more potent inhalation anesthetic or to inject small doses of analgetic intravenously (morphine 1 to 2 mg, meperidine 10 to 25 mg, fentanyl 0.05 to 0.1 mg). Assisted or controlled respiration is necessary if the patient is given a neuromuscular blocker, combined with tracheal intubation to facilitate respiratory control.

Barbiturates and neuromuscular blockers have been given in combination from the same syringe. Because of chemical incompatibilities that result in precipitation, the choice of drugs is limited. Separate use of the agents allows for more accurate titration in relation to need.

COMPLICATIONS

Extravascular Injection

In the conscious patient this complication is suggested by pain at the injection site, but in the anesthetized patient detection is possible only by careful observation. If extravasation occurs, treatment consists of injection of 5 to 10 ml of 0.5 per cent lidocaine into the involved area to dilute and neutralize the barbiturate solution and to prevent vasospasm; otherwise neuritis or ulceration of the skin may result.

Intra-arterial Injection

This is most likely to occur with injection at the antecubital space but can take place at any site where artery and vein are in proximity or where an artery is superficial. Arteries, particularly the radial artery, often follow an anomalous course. Intra-arterial injection is detected by sudden onset of severe pain described as hot or scalding. The lesion seen after intra-arterial injection is a chemical endarteritis that destroys endothelial and subendothelial layers of the vessel. In severe cases the muscle layers may also be involved, with diffuse thrombosis. Injury takes place immediately, requiring only brief contact, the degree varying with concentration and amount of drug injected. The necrotizing effect is a property of the drug itself and is not related to alkalinity. Experimental work suggests that local release of norepinephrine is perhaps the cause of the arterial spasm. Other work proposes that gangrene results from precipitation of thiopental crystals with occlusion of capillaries on the venous side. The ultimate result is not likely to be disastrous unless concentrations greater than 2.5 per cent are used; to our knowledge, gangrene has not been reported following use of 2.5 per cent thiopental.

No single regimen has proved effective in treatment. However, any or all of the following measures may be tried. If possible, the needle should be left in place and 10 ml of 0.5 per cent lidocaine injected. Lidocaine dilutes and neutralizes the barbiturate solution. Local heparinization has been advised, and local injection of phentolamine, an alpha-adrenergic blocker, is theoretically justified. Stellate ganglion block or general anesthesia with halothane may be elected to promote vasodilation. If thrombosis occurs, amputation may ultimately be necessary. Some patients have recovered completely without treatment and others have developed gangrene in spite of therapy.

Cough and Laryngospasm

Together these constitute the most common complications of intravenous barbiturate anesthesia. One is not likely to forget the development of cough, chest wall and laryngeal spasm, anoxia, and cyanosis in a patient with bronchial asthma or chronic bronchitis. Pharyngeal secretions, early stimulation of the pharynx or trachea by airway insertion, movement of head or neck, or painful peripheral stimuli may also be precipitating events. Should cough or laryngospasm appear, treatment depends on the precipitating factor. If secretions are present, they are aspirated after more barbiturate has been injected to diminish reflexes. When an airway causes cough, it is removed and anesthesia deepened before replacement. Laryngospasm can usually be overcome by positive airway pressure and forward thrust of the mandible. Should spasm persist, intravenous injection of succinylcholine (50 mg in the adult) followed by ventilation with oxygen is indicated.

Vomiting

Vomiting is uncommon during barbiturate anesthesia unless the pharynx is stimulated or the patient has been allowed to emerge into the second stage or has a distended stomach.

POSTANESTHETIC COURSE

As a rule, recovery from barbiturate anesthesia is gradual and uneventful. Time of awakening depends on the total dose of drug given and the physical condition of the patient. Some individuals appear to awaken quickly, only to return to the anesthetized state when undisturbed. Others, believing themselves completely recovered, request to sit up or stand. An attendant should be present the first time a patient is allowed out of bed after anesthesia.

Patients recovering from barbiturate anesthesia occasionally show muscle fasciculation and rigidity, stertorous respiration, and slight cyanosis. This syndrome is possibly of neurologic origin but in most cases appears to be related to temporary derangement of body temperature control, more commonly seen when environmental temperature is low. Treatment consists of warming. If cyanosis causes concern, oxygen is given even though the cyanosis is more a manifestation of vasoconstriction than hypoxia.

NEUROLEPTANESTHESIA

The designation "neuroleptic" characterizes a drug that reduces motor activity, diminishes anxiety, and produces a state of indifference during which the individual can respond appropriately to command. These substances are also adrenolytic, antiemetic, and antifibrillatory; they block ganglionic transmission and are anticonvulsants as well.

First used in the 1950s, the "lytic cocktail" of Laborit and Huguenard consisted of meperidine, chlorpromazine, and promethazine. Administration resulted in a form of "neuroplegia," wherein there was major blockade of the autonomic nervous system and marked circulatory depression. When combined with physical cooling, a kind of artificial hibernation resulted. The lytic cocktail achieved transient popularity. It was succeeded a decade later by "neuroleptanesthesia," consisting of intravenous administration of one of the butyrophenones (similar to the phenothiazine group) and a powerful opioid, either in fixed combination or individually, together with inhalation of nitrous oxide. When the latter is omitted the resulting state is termed neuroleptanalgesia. One ml of the fixed combination named Innovar contains 2.5 mg droperidol (Inapsine) and 0.05 mg of fentanyl, the former a butyrophenone and the latter an opioid related to meperidine (Fig. 14–3).

PHARMACOLOGIC ACTIONS

Central Nervous System

Droperidol produces marked tranquilization and some amnesia, adding to the effect of other central nervous system depressants: barbiturates, analgetics, anesthetics, and other tranquilizers. Therefore, these compounds should be used in reduced amounts when combined with droperidol. Moderate antiemetic action may last as long as seven hours postinjection. The incidence of extrapyramidal effects consisting of akathisia, dystonia, or parkinsonlike responses is as low as 1 per cent in adults but up to 15 per cent in children. Such responses may be enhanced in the presence of pyridoxine (vitamin B_6) ingestion.

Fentanyl is an analgetic, 70 times more potent than morphine with a brief duration of action. Effects can be seen within four minutes of intravenous injection, with maximal intensity in 10 to 15 minutes and duration of analgesia from 45 to 60 minutes.

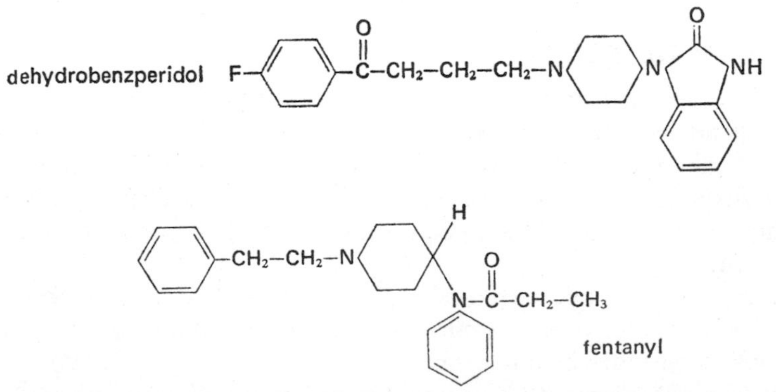

FIGURE 14–3.   Structural formulas of droperidol and fentanyl.

In the small doses used, fentanyl has little emetic effect in humans, the incidence being about 3 per cent. Miosis, bradycardia, bronchoconstriction, and biliary tract spasm occur.

Respiration

Droperidol exerts weak respiratory actions, causing a slight reduction in respiratory rate but a compensatory increase in tidal volume. Fentanyl reduces both tidal volume and respiratory rate, and as is the case with all opioids, respiratory depression occurs in equianalgetic doses. The carbon dioxide response curve is shifted to the right, the slope remaining essentially unchanged. The action of droperidol is not additive to that of fentanyl. It is well to remember that the respiratory depressant effect of the combination or of fentanyl alone outlasts that of analgesia, which is of relatively brief duration.

Cardiovascular System

Droperidol causes mild hypotension secondary to alpha-adrenergic blockade and peripheral vasodilation. The threshold to epinephrine-induced arrhythmias is raised by as much as 75 per cent in both dog and man. There is little evidence of myocardial depression. Fentanyl in average doses also produces mild hypotension and bradycardia, representing a parasympathomimetic stimulant effect that is blocked by atropine.

Musculoskeletal System

Droperidol has little or no action on this system in man. Fentanyl can produce skeletal muscle rigidity, particularly of the chest wall, when given in large doses or if given rapidly by vein. Neuromuscular transmission is unaffected, and the rigidity can be eliminated by a neuromuscular blocker or naloxone (Narcan).

CLINICAL USE

Although respiratory tract secretions are rarely a problem, a belladonna derivative is desirable because of the increased vagal tone induced by the combination of the sympatholytic action of droperidol and the parasympathomimetic stimulant properties of fentanyl. One to 2 ml of Innovar may be given intramuscularly for premedication if sedation is desired. Despite what may appear to be adequate sedation, about 10 per cent of patients complain of restlessness or vague feelings of dysphoria, a reaction often delayed as long as 60 to 90 minutes after administration.

For induction of anesthesia, a few anesthetists use a slow, intravenous infusion of Innovar, with the calculated dose added to 250 ml of 5 per cent dextrose in water, the amount titrated to the patient's reaction. In general, 1 ml of Innovar per 10 to 15 kg is given, the larger dose used in young, healthy individuals. Care must be taken not to give the induction dose too rapidly lest skeletal muscle rigidity result. To avoid this, many use droperidol and fentanyl separately, giving the droperidol for sedation and allowing for a slower, more controlled injection of opioid. In either event we recommend individualizing the dose to the patient's requirements. The induction dose is given over a period of five to six minutes. Gradually the patient becomes sleepy, with spontaneous eye closure; the patient may appear to be asleep but still responds to oral commands. As sedation increases respiratory effort decreases, and at times the patient may indeed forget to breathe. Oxygen by mask should be given as soon as tidal volume begins to diminish. Cardiovascular signs remain stable as long as the patient is not moved or tilted head up. When the response becomes markedly depressed, nitrous oxide and oxygen are added and consciousness is rapidly lost. We caution that the reported cases of cardiac arrest associated with the administration of Innovar have resulted from overdose and lack of recognition of the potential for respiratory and circulatory depression.

If muscle relaxation is needed, any of the neuromuscular blockers can be used. Owing to the long duration of action of droperidol (7 to 12 hours), droperidol or Innovar is rarely given after induction or used at all in ambulatory surgical units. Supplemental injections of fentanyl are given to counteract any of the following: tachycardia, increase in blood pressure, sweating, grimacing, or muscle movement. Early in the course of anesthesia a tracheal tube is poorly tolerated; this can be overcome by topical local anesthesia prior to intubation.

Anesthesia is terminated by discontinuing nitrous oxide and allowing the patient to breathe oxygen first, then room air. As a rule consciousness returns within a few minutes, although amnesia may persist for another 30 to 60 minutes.

POSTOPERATIVE COURSE

A patient who has been anesthetized with Innovar can easily be neglected in the recovery room or on the ward; uncomplaining, his condition alternates between being awake and asleep. The patient is easily aroused but not alert, and takes deep breaths or coughs on command. Analgetic requirements immediately postoperative are reduced. This results in part from droperidol sedation. Nausea (5 per cent) and vomiting (1 per cent) are uncommon. The chief postoperative complaints are confusion, inability to concentrate, and mental depression. The most annoying consequence is the development of extrapyramidal signs; the incidence is low and control is possible with 0.5 mg of atropine, 25 mg of diphenhydramine, 1 to 2 mg of benztropine, or 1 to 2 mg of physostigmine.

APPRAISAL

Neuroleptanesthesia is a safe, simple technique that has no demonstrable toxic effects on liver or kidneys. The cardiovascular system remains stable unless the patient is hypovolemic or change in position occurs. The method has proved useful in aged and poor risk patients. Tracheal intubation using topical anesthesia in the patient with a full stomach is facilitated by the injection of small amounts of Innovar or droperidol. Tranquilization produced by droperidol renders the patient cooperative and receptive to suggestion. The droperidol-fentanyl mixture without nitrous oxide can be used for diagnostic procedures, including bronchoscopy, pneumoencephalography, and carotid arteriography, as well as to provide sedation and analgesia for simple procedures such as burn dressings. As with any potent opioid or tranquilizer that produces marked depression and sedation (unconsciousness with overdosage), the patient must be observed continuously, and life support devices and drugs must be at hand.

Drugs other than droperidol and fentanyl have been used for neuroleptanesthesia. Chlorpromazine has proved to be an unsatisfactory substitute for droperidol in that inadequate sedation is produced. Diazepam, on the other hand, offers the advantages of avoiding extrapyramidal tract reactions and distinctly lessening the incidence of dysphoria. Substitutes for fentanyl include alphaprodine (Nisentil), meperidine, morphine, and a more potent derivative, sufentanil. Although muscle rigidity may accompany rapid intravenous administration of single doses of most opioids, the amount necessary to produce that occasionally seen after fentanyl is usually high.

DISSOCIATIVE ANESTHESIA

Anesthetic drugs with specific sites of action in the central nervous system have been sought as alternatives to the general anesthetics, which exert far-reaching effects

phencyclidine (CI-395) ketamine (CI-581)

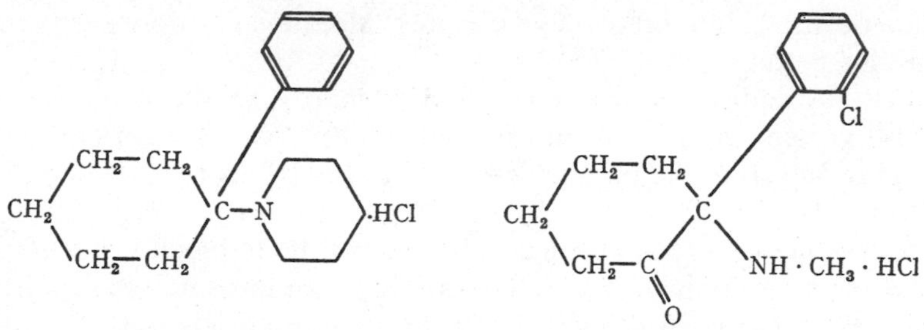

FIGURE 14–4. Structural formulas of phencyclidine and ketamine.

on the brain. The most successful of these to date has been ketamine (Ketalar) (Fig. 14–4), a substance permitting surgical operations on patients who appear to be awake in that movement may occur and the eyes remain open. So far as recollection or awareness is concerned, however, the individuals are anesthetized.

Ketamine is related to the hallucinogens, so that unpleasant dreams during awakening, not uncommonly extending into the postoperative period, constitute a drawback. Characteristics of ketamine anesthesia include profound analgesia, preservation of normal pharyngeal and laryngeal reflexes, normal to increased skeletal muscle tone, circulatory stimulation evidenced by hypertension and tachycardia, and an increase in CSF pressure. Some but certainly not all of these are desirable effects. The airway is usually easily maintained. Respirations tend to become rapid and shallow for a few minutes after injection but thereafter return to normal. Airway obstruction and severe respiratory depression can occur in all age groups but are most common in the adult, probably representing overdose. In patients with moderate to severe bronchospastic disease, a decrease in airway resistance has been demonstrated after ketamine injection. Changes are dose related, attributed by some to endogenous release of catecholamines. Similar changes are not seen in normal subjects.

Current thinking vis-à-vis the mechanism of action of the drug implicates interruption of cerebral association pathways, relative sparing of the reticular activating and limbic systems, and depression of the thalamo-neocortical system. The evidence for these assumptions is incomplete, however. The cardiovascular responses, which can be reduced by alpha-adrenergic or sympathetic ganglionic blockade, are thought to be secondary to inhibition of baroreceptor reflexes. It has been shown that myocardial oxygen consumption is increased with ketamine; thus its use in patients with severe coronary artery disease may be inadvisable.

CLINICAL MANAGEMENT

Premedication should include a belladonna drug to reduce salivary secretions. Many believe that an opioid lessens the total dose of ketamine required. Induction via the intravenous route is accomplished with 2 mg ketamine per kg injected over a 60-second period. Thirty to 40 seconds later the patient becomes unconscious and is usually ready for operation. Some patients show purposeless movements, nystagmus, eye opening, or vocalization. Blood pressure and pulse may rise as little as 10 or as much as 50 per cent. The airway is usually well maintained in children and young adults, but older patients may require airway correction, ranging from elevation of the mandible to placement of an oral airway. Complete airway obstruction is usually indicative of overdose. Maintenance of anesthesia is achieved by repeated injection of 30 to 50 per cent of the induction dose as often as every five to seven minutes. Induction may also be achieved via the intramuscular route. Three to 5 mg per kg are injected, with operation begun within three to five minutes. Maintenance doses are usually given intravenously for better control.

Indications for additional drug are based primarily on the response to surgical stimulation. Movement must be distinguished from that which occurs in response to a surgical stimulus and from the purposeless type normally seen in some patients given ketamine.

The drug produces profound analgesia but does little to block visceral pain; hence it is not useful for intra-abdominal or intrathoracic procedures unless supplemented by nitrous oxide or other inhalation agents. The increase in muscle tone that results from ketamine requires administration of a neuromuscular blocker when relaxation is needed. Increase in intraocular pressure seen after ketamine is probably the result of increased tone in the extraocular muscles.

POSTOPERATIVE COURSE

Time of recovery from ketamine depends on total dose given. An aggregate large dose with repeated injections for maintenance results in a prolonged awakening time. Recovery is frequently complicated by vivid dreams, and in 10 to 15 per cent of patients dreaming is accompanied by psychomotor activity of varying degree. Such emergence delirium can be terminated by the intravenous injection of thiopental 50 to 75 mg or diazepam 5 to 10 mg. In an effort to decrease emergence phenomena, many anesthetists substitute a tranquilizer for the last ketamine dose or resort to an opioid-tranquilizer combination; recovery is more tranquil but correspondingly prolonged. Skillful neglect, that is, allowing the patient to awaken undisturbed and unstimulated, also results in a more peaceful course.

INDICATIONS

Ketamine has proved useful in diagnostic procedures, especially in neuroradiology, as well as for superficial operations of short duration. The compound has found its chief use in the anesthetic management of children and young adults and is quite effective as an induction agent for general anesthesia in the poor risk patient and in hypovolemic states. It has also been proved useful in patients with asthma.

CONTRAINDICATIONS

Ketamine is contraindicated in patients with hypertension, prior cerebrovascular accident, psychiatric disorders, increased intracranial pressure, and upper respiratory infection, as well as in those who have demonstrated sensitivity to the drug and those undergoing intraocular surgery. Some of the problems seen with ketamine represent overdose; dosage should be based on lean body mass (1.9 mg/kg) rather than body weight. With this technique, circulatory changes are minimal and emergence delirium is reduced. Similar reductions in adverse effects have been achieved by combining ketamine with diazepam for induction of general anesthesia. Some believe strongly that the use of ketamine should be restricted to children and patients under 30 years of age.

Experience with the use of this drug has indeed shown that careful selection of dose and patient results in fewer complications and increases the effectiveness of the agent.

OTHER INTRAVENOUS AGENTS

DIAZEPAM

Diazepam (Fig. 14–5) is a tranquilizer of the benzodiazepine series, an anticonvulsant, a muscle relaxant, and an amnesic. The amnesic action is anterograde and

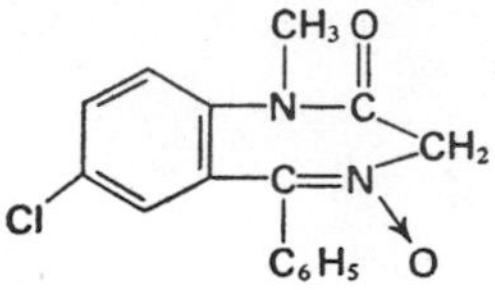

FIGURE 14-5.   Structural formula of diazepam.   diazepam

involves the input or "consolidation" process rather than retrieval of information. The drug causes slight respiratory depression — chiefly in reduction of tidal volume. Elevations in Pa_{CO_2} have been found, but patients are usually capable of adequate respiratory exchange.

Circulatory changes are minimal; the slight fall in blood pressure may be partly or wholly explained by simple sedation. There may also be some direct or reflex vasodilatory effect on the peripheral vessels.

Compared with thiopental for induction, diazepam causes less hypotension and bradycardia. If heart rate and mean aortic pressure are constant, diazepam significantly improves left ventricular function. The mechanism of this effect is unknown, but it may be the result of a decrease in coronary vascular resistance with a subsequent increase in coronary artery flow.

Diazepam is a highly effective anticonvulsant drug and is good for controlling muscle rigidity and spasm in patients with tetanus and cerebral palsy. This action seems to be at spinal reflex pathways, but a more peripheral action has also been implicated. The drug provides useful sedation if the trachea is to be intubated in the awake patient.

PROPANIDID

Eugenol is the chief constituent of clove oil and cinnamon leaf oil. Several of the eugenols possess anesthetic properties differing from those used in common practice.

Propanidid (Fig. 14-6) is the only eugenol currently used for anesthesia in European countries. Onset of action is comparable to thiopental or methohexital and may be accompanied by involuntary muscle movements. Recovery is rapid owing to enzymatic breakdown of the compound by plasma pseudocholinesterase. Profound and precipitous hypotension has followed overdose with propanidid. Hyperventilation is common and may relate to stimulation of the carotid chemoreceptors. The period of apnea that usually follows hyperventilation also appears to be dose related. Propanidid is not available in the United States.

STEROID ANESTHESIA

In 1927 Cashin and Moravek reported that large doses of cholesterol will produce general anesthesia, whereas Hans Selye some 30 years ago found that progesterone,

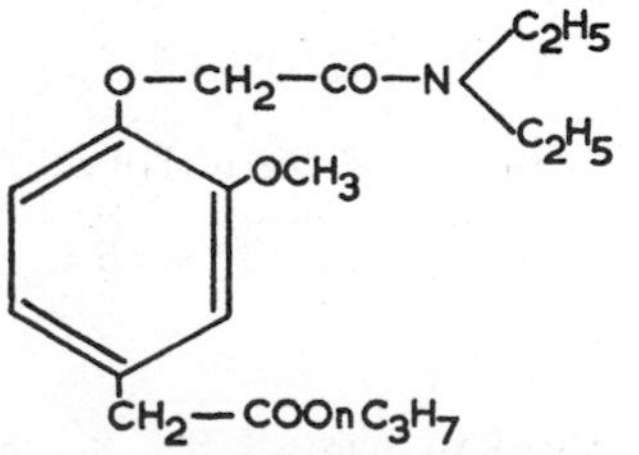

FIGURE 14-6.   Structural formula of propanidid.   propanidid

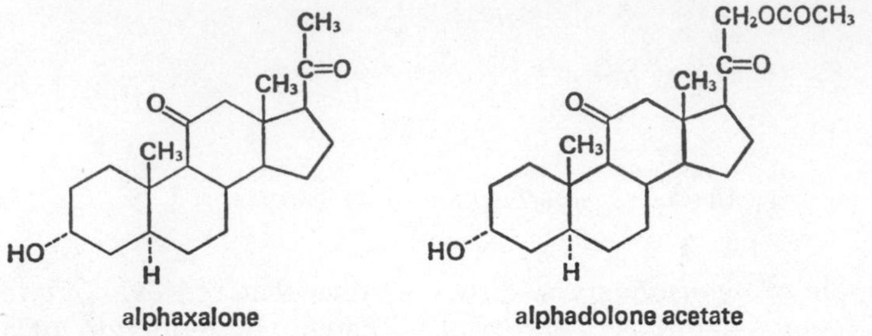

FIGURE 14–7. Structural formulas of the two steroids constituting Althesin.

desoxycorticosterone, and pregnanedione also induced general anesthesia. In 1955 hydroxydione (Viadril), a pregnanedione derivative described as endocrinologically inactive, was introduced as an anesthetic but achieved only modest success, in part because of local irritation upon intravenous injection. The newest derivative consists of a mixture of two pregnanediones (Fig. 14–7). With the mixture (Glaxo CT 1341 — Althesin), anesthesia is characterized by rapid induction, brief duration, and a rapid recovery. At present its prime role is as an alternative to the commonly used intravenous barbiturates, but the compound has not been approved for use in the United States.

The mechanism of action of commonly used general anesthetics is still speculative. It is not surprising that the same is true of the steroids, some of which produce convulsions. We mention this kind of compound primarily to indicate the wide spectrum of substances that can produce loss of consciousness and immobility in response to stimuli.

REFERENCES

Aldrete JA, Stanley TH: Trends in Intravenous Anesthesia. Miami, Symposia Specialists, 1980.
Dundee JW, Wyant GM: Intravenous Anaesthesia. Edinburgh and London, Churchill-Livingstone, 1974.

BARBITURATES

Brown SS, Lyons SM, Dundee JW: Intra-arterial barbiturates: A study of some factors leading to intravascular thrombosis. Br J Anaesth 40:13, 1968.
Skovsted P, Price ML, Price HL: The effects of short-acting barbiturates on arterial pressure, preganglionic sympathetic activity and barostatic reflexes. Anesthesiology 33:10, 1970.

KETAMINE

Ferrer-Allado T, Brechner VL, Dymond A., et al: Ketamine-induced electroconvulsive phenomena in the human limbic and thalamic regions. Anesthesiology 38:333, 1973.
Huber FC, Reves JG, Gutierrez J, Corssen G: Ketamine: Its effect on airway resistance in man. South Med J 65:1176, 1972.
Kothary SP, Zsigmond EK, Matuski A: Antagonism of the ketamine-induced rise in plasma free norepinephrine, blood pressure and pulse rate by intravenous diazepam. Clin Pharmacol Ther 17:238, 1975.
Lanning CF, Harmel MH: Ketamine anesthesia. Ann Rev Med 26:137, 1975.
Tweed WA, Minuck M, Mymin D: Circulatory responses to ketamine anesthesia. Anesthesiology 37:613, 1972.

STEROID ANESTHESIA

Carson IW: Group trial of althesin as an intravenous anesthetic. Postgrad Med J (Suppl 2) 48:108, 1972.
Tammisto T, Takki S, Tigerstedt I, Kauste A: A comparison of althesin and thiopentone in induction of anaesthesia. J Anaesth 45:179, 1973.

DIAZEPAM

Abel RM, Staroscik RN, Reis RL: Effects of diazepam (Valium) on left ventricular function and systemic vascular resistance. J Pharmacol Exp Ther 173:364, 1970.

Catchlove R, Kafer E: The effects of diazepam on the ventilatory response to carbon dioxide and on steady state gas exchange. Anesthesiology 34:9, 1971.

MORPHINE

Johnstone R, Jobes D, Kennell E, et al: Reversal of morphine anesthesia with naloxone. Anesthesiology 41:361, 1974.
Stanley TH, Webster LR: Anesthetic requirements and cardiovascular effects of fentanyl-oxygen and fentanyl-diazepam-oxygen anesthesia in man. Anesth Analg 57:411, 1978.
Wong K, Martin W, Hornbein T, et al: Cardiovascular effects of morphine sulfate with oxygen and nitrous oxide in man. Anesthesiology 38:542, 1973.

PROPANIDID

Conway CM, Ellis DB: Propanidid. Br J Anaesth 42:249, 1970.
Doenicke A: General pharmacology of propanidid. Acta Anaesth Scand (Suppl) 17:21, 1965.

Chapter 15

NEUROMUSCULAR BLOCKING AGENTS

There is more to anesthesia than simply rendering a patient unconscious and free from pain. To provide an optimal surgical field, an anesthetist must also control muscle tone. Since one of the major objectives in the use of neuromuscular blocking agents is suppression of muscle tone, a review of neuromuscular physiology is in order.

Skeletal muscle functions most effectively if the resting muscle is not limp, so that when a sudden response is required time is not wasted in taking up the slack. Since a voluntary muscle cell responds in an all-or-none fashion, all muscle cells cannot be partially activated to produce the background tone. Rather, the motor centers produce a continual random discharge such that only a small fraction of the cells contracts at any moment. It is this background activity that the anesthetist must control to provide convenient access for the surgeon during operation.

One way to suppress tone is to abolish it at its origin with deep anesthesia. However, this has the disadvantage of requiring high concentrations of agents that are far from innocuous. A second option is to block the signals as they traverse the vertebral canal, as is done with spinal and peridural anesthesia. The third approach, that discussed here, became available in 1942 with the introduction by Griffith and Johnson of neuromuscular blockers to clinical anesthesia. These agents, as exemplified by tubocurarine, interfere selectively with the transmission of signals from the motor nerve to the voluntary muscle cell. Their use leads to a division of labor such that the anesthetic need be used only to produce unconsciousness and analgesia and therefore can be administered at lower and safer concentrations. Skeletal muscle contraction can then be controlled separately with a neuromuscular blocker. To use these drugs properly, one must understand how they act.

NEUROMUSCULAR PHARMACOLOGY AND PHYSIOLOGY

To further understand the mechanisms of action of neuromuscular blockers, one must first appreciate the physiology of the nerve, the muscle, and the neuromuscular junction. This subject is far too extensive for the present discussion, so the reader should review the physiology as presented by Katz in *Nerve, Muscle and Synapse* and the pharmacology reviewed by Waud and Waud in *Muscle Relaxants*. In particular, the reader should be familiar with the following points before proceeding further.

1. The resting membrane of nerve or muscle is polarized with the inside negatively charged. This voltage difference, the "membrane potential," results from the presence

of a semipermeable membrane between solutions of different ionic concentrations on the inside and outside of the muscle cell.

2. Excitable membranes may be divided into two classes: those that are electrically excitable, that is, respond to the passage of an electric current outward through the cell membrane, and those that are chemically excitable, that is, respond to the presence of a chemical agent. Chemically excitable membranes are found at the end-plate region of striated muscle, whereas the remainder of muscle membrane and nerve membrane is electrically excitable.

3. The resting polarized state of an electrically excitable membrane can be altered by application of an electric current. If a positive charge is injected into the cell, the membrane potential rises toward zero and the membrane is said to be depolarized.

4. In an electrically excitable membrane, small depolarizations can be graded. However, as the stimulus increases, a degree of depolarization is reached ("threshold") that creates an all-or-none process ("action potential"). The nature of the underlying mechanism is such that not only is the internal negativity abolished but the membrane actually reverses polarity so that the inside of the cell becomes positive ("overshoot").

5. The electric charge associated with the passage of an impulse along a nerve or muscle is self-propagating. Movement of Na^+ across the membrane produces a flow of positive charges into the cell. Since charges cannot accumulate at one point, the positive current flows along the core of the nerve or muscle cell and then outward through an adjacent part of the membrane ("local action current"). This outward current is the electric stimulation needed to depolarize the adjacent membrane. Thus the process is propagated along the cell.

6. Electrically excitable membranes show "accommodation." Normally, the stimulus activating a nerve or muscle membrane is a pulse that results in a single action potential. If, however, the stimulus is a steady current, an action potential can be recorded only when the stimulus is first applied. Although the current continues to flow through the membrane, further activity in the membrane cannot be seen, even when a stronger stimulus is applied. In other words, the electrically excitable membrane becomes inexcitable in the presence of a steady depolarization.

7. Chemically excitable membranes are activated by compounds typically bearing positively charged quaternary nitrogen groups. When exposed to these compounds, the membrane potential shifts in a positive direction. However, in contrast to the electrically excitable membrane, the chemically excitable membrane does not reverse its potential but seeks a level at which the inside is still slightly negative. Also, the response of the chemically excitable membrane is continuously graded and not an all-or-none process.

8. Just as the electrically excitable membrane behaves differently when a prolonged stimulus is applied, so, too, does the chemically excitable membrane. Prolonged application of an agonist is associated with a decreased degree of depolarization ("desensitization"). Note, however, that the time scale is quite different. Accommodation can appear within the duration of a single action potential, that is, within milliseconds, whereas desensitization may take hours to develop.

Accommodation and desensitization appear to underlie the two types of neuromuscular blocks seen with depolarizing blockers.

9. Within the axon the combination of choline and acetate, catalyzed by choline acetylase, forms acetylcholine, which is stored in vesicles in the nerve terminals as a readily available source and a more slowly mobilized reserve supply. When a nerve action potential reaches the nerve ending, the electric charge releases calcium inside the nerve ending with the result that the stored transmitter is released into the synaptic cleft — the area between the nerve ending and end-plate region of muscle.

10. The released transmitter reacts with specialized sites ("receptors") on the end-plate region of muscle membrane, leading to depolarization of the end-plate ("end-plate potential").

11. Released acetylcholine is eliminated by both diffusion away from the end-plate region and enzymatic destruction by cholinesterase, which is located around the synaptic cleft.

A useful and convenient frame of reference when examining neuromuscular transmission is shown in Table 15–1. The table indicates the sites of action of various classes of agents that interfere with the whole signaling system. We shall focus here on the neuromuscular blockers proper, that is, those drugs reacting directly with the postsynaptic receptor for the transmitter. Muscle relaxation can result from interference at any of the steps along the motor pathway.

Neuromuscular blockers are divided into two groups: those that combine with the acetylcholine receptor and cause depolarization of the end-plate region — the depolarizing agents — and those that combine with the acetylcholine receptor to prevent depolarization — the competitive agents.

ACTION OF DEPOLARIZING AGENTS

This group includes succinylcholine and decamethonium (no longer used clinically). Depolarizing blockers exhibit two phases of action; each of these is discussed in turn.

PHASE I BLOCK

Depolarizing neuromuscular blockers exert the same action at the neuromuscular junction as acetylcholine, that is, they react with the receptors at the end-plate region of muscle and lead to depolarization of the chemically excitable membrane. Depolarization of the end-plate, in turn, leads to local action currents that spread to and depolarize the adjacent electrically excitable membrane, thus causing muscle contraction. Clinically, this is seen as fasciculation, an uncoordinated contraction of muscle, a phenomenon that may cause the patient to complain of stiff, sore muscles postoperatively. Because succinylcholine and decamethonium are not as rapidly eliminated as acetylcholine, depolarization of the end-plate region persists. Unlike a brief stimulus, continuous passage of local action currents leads to inexcitability in the electrically excitable muscle membrane adjacent to the end-plate. Neuromuscular block ensues. The block is not at the end-plate but rather in the area of the electrically excitable membrane around the end-plate.

PHASE II BLOCK

Zaimis first showed that with time, the neuromuscular block produced by decamethonium changes its characteristics. For example, a tetanus became less well sustained, and the block could be antagonized rather than aggravated by neostigmine. The depolarizing agents were said to have "changed their mode of action," to have a "dual mode of action," or to have passed into phase II block. Speculation as to the nature of this change has been considerable.

What is known about the changing action of depolarizing agents? As a starting point, remember that the action of depolarizing agents is to depolarize the end-plate. Muscle contraction, muscle block, or both are secondary effects resulting from the depolarization. If we focus on the depolarizing effects of these agents, we find that although stable drugs can produce a depolarization that is prolonged, the effect is not of infinite duration. This reduction of depolarization that occurs with prolonged exposure

TABLE 15–1. Sites of Action of Chemical Compounds that
Affect Neuromuscular Transmission

Physiologic Process	Blocking Agents
Initiation of signal in CNS	Volatile anesthetics
Nerve action potential	Volatile anesthetics Local anesthetics
Acetylcholine release	Hemicholinium Antibiotics Botulinum toxin
Acetylcholine-receptor combination	d-Tubocurarine Pancuronium Gallamine Metocurine
Depolarization of end-plate	Volatile anesthetics
Muscle action potential	Succinylcholine* Decamethonium* Local anesthetics Volatile anesthetics Tetrodotoxin
Muscle contraction	Calcium chelating agents

*The assignment of succinylcholine and decamethonium reflects the fact that, although both drugs act at the acetylcholine receptor, the actual block of neuromuscular transmission is the result of accommodation of the electrically excitable membrane around the end plate.

is called "desensitization," and the degree of reduced effect and the duration of exposure needed to bring it about vary among animal species and muscle groups.

Next, if we compare the relationship between depolarization and twitch response, we find that, with repeated exposure to a depolarizing drug, less and less depolarization is needed to cause complete block (Fig. 15–1) until finally, exposure to the drug causes complete block without any depolarization. Thus, with time, something other than depolarization must be responsible for the block. The actual cause is unknown. There is, however, no reason to consider phase II block to be competitive in nature.

In summary, we can only say that phase II block exists, it is associated with a reduced contribution of depolarization to the block, and it occurs in situations such as prolonged or repeated exposures that predispose to desensitization. There appears to be no close relationship between the degree of phase II block and indices that can be measured clinically such as tetanic fade or post-tetanic facilitation (see comments in connection with monitoring, page 175 et seq.).

ACTION OF COMPETITIVE AGENTS

This group includes tubocurarine, metocurine (Metubine), gallamine, and pancuronium. These drugs combine with acetylcholine receptors but do not activate them. However, their presence on the receptor prevents access of the transmitter. The larger the dose of blocking agent, the more receptors occluded and the fewer receptors available for reaction with the transmitter. Decreasing the receptors available to acetylcholine progressively reduces the height of the end-plate potential until it no longer reaches threshold for excitation of the adjacent electrically excitable muscle membrane; neuromuscular block ensues.

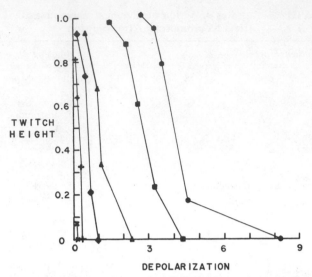

FIGURE 15-1. Changing mode of action of succinylcholine. Measurements from the dog tibialis anticus muscle. Ordinates: strength of muscle twitch in response to a single shock applied to the motor nerve (relative to control response). Abscissae: intensity of depolarization of end-plate region (millivolts, recorded with external electrodes). Single doses of succinylcholine 0.1 mg/kg were given at half-hourly intervals. During onset and offset of neuromuscular block a series of paired observations of twitch response and depolarization was made. For simplicity, only the recovery limbs are presented. The righthand curve (*full circles*) was obtained with the first injection. Note that about 8 mv of depolarization produced complete block. As the depolarization fell, the twitch gradually recovered. This is the typical picture of depolarization block. The remaining five curves were obtained following the second, fourth, sixth, eighth, and tenth injections. Note that with each succeeding dose, progressively less depolarization is associated with block, until at the last dose, complete block was associated with a barely measurable electrical effect, that is, something other than depolarization was producing the block. The shift from the first to the last curve illustrates the development of phase II block.

What fraction of the receptors must be blocked before neuromuscular transmission fails? On teleologic grounds one would expect that more acetylcholine receptors are available than are necessary barely to initiate an action potential in the muscle membrane; that is, there would be a margin of safety. Figure 15-2 shows the experimentally observed relation between the fraction of receptors blocked and the twitch response following motor nerve stimulation. One can see that until 75 to 80 per cent of the receptors are blocked, no interference with the twitch response can be measured and that transmission fails in all fibers when 90 to 95 per cent of the receptors are occluded. In other words, the more resistant fibers respond with less than one tenth of the receptor pool available, and all fibers function when only one fifth to one fourth of the receptors are free. As was expected, there is a large margin of safety in neuromuscular transmission.

Clinically, we may view the action of competitive antagonists as resembling an iceberg (Fig. 15-3). Because most of the receptors must be blocked before there is any decrease in twitch response, the first dose of an agent must be a relatively large one. The anesthetist works at the top 20 to 25 per cent of the iceberg, and it is only this small fraction of receptors that must be reblocked as the antagonist is eliminated. Subsequent doses, therefore, are smaller. The problems of surveying the bottom of the iceberg will be considered later.

The preceding description of the postsynaptic action of neuromuscular blocking agents is the classic view. Another opinion holds that these drugs exert some or most of their effect presynaptically, that is, at the nerve endings. It is possible, however, to explain the initiation of presynaptic effects by the action of a drug acting postsynapti-

FIGURE 15–2. Illustration of the margin of safety of neuromuscular transmission. Ordinates: fractional twitch height. Abscissae: fraction of receptors blocked by tubocurarine. Note that neuromuscular transmission is normal until about 80 per cent of the receptors have been blocked, whereas 90 per cent must be occluded before the most resistant fibers fail. (The reader will note a family resemblance of Figure 15–1 to Figures 15–2, 15–3, 15–5, and 15–6. This reflects the fact that response of a muscle to nerve stimulation represents the standard measure of neuromuscular transmission, whereas intensity of depolarization (Fig. 15–1) or receptor blockade (Figures 15–2, 15–5, 15–6) represent the direct effect of depolarizing and competitive agents, respectively.)

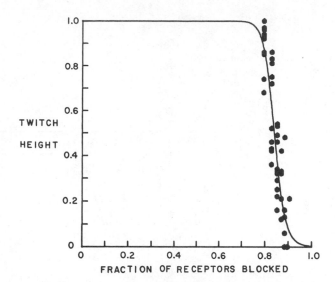

cally. Also, drugs such as tubocurarine display the kinetics compatible with competitive antagonism. The question might then be "Are the acetylcholine receptors presynaptic or postsynaptic?" Recently, it has become possible to separate the nerve endings from the end-plate region. By doing so, Kuffler has been able to show that acetylcholine receptors are situated primarily in the postsynaptic membrane of the end-plate region. Thus, presynaptic events are at most a side issue in the action of neuromuscular blocking agents.

EFFECTS ON OTHER ORGANS

Although neuromuscular blockers are reasonably specific in their action, some side effects deserve mention.

SUCCINYLCHOLINE

In addition to its effect at the neuromuscular junction, succinylcholine displays, to some extent, the actions of acetylcholine at other receptor sites. Thus, a patient may develop hypertension and tachycardia from stimulation of autonomic ganglia, or bradycardia, salivation, and increased bronchial secretions owing to a muscarinic action. These effects are more common on repeated intravenous injection and are seen most frequently in children. Incidents of cardiac arrest have been reported. The decreased heart rate following a second dose of succinylcholine may be attenuated by the prior administration of atropine, tubocurarine, or pancuronium. It has been suggested that the bradycardia results from a reflex response of the autonomic nervous system or from sensitization of the heart by the metabolic products of succinylcholine (succinylmonocholine or choline). Neither of these hypotheses has been verified.

Depolarizing agents can increase intraocular pressure, an effect usually attributed to contracture of the extraocular muscles. These muscles have many end-plate regions per muscle fiber. The distribution of chemically excitable muscle membrane all along the muscle fiber leads to a generalized depolarization of the muscle membrane by passive electrotonic spread. Contraction of these muscles can then occur without the presence of an action potential. Katz and Eakins have shown that in cats an increase in intraocular pressure occurs after the extraocular muscles have been severed, and they believe that contraction of the smooth muscles of the orbit is also involved. In any case,

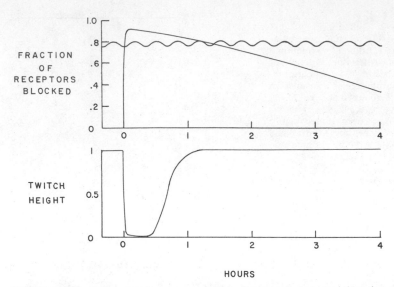

FIGURE 15–3. Diagrammatic representation of events during administration of a single dose of tubocurarine sufficient to produce maximal or near maximal relaxation at its peak effect. *Top:* Calculated fraction of receptors blocked as a function of time. As drug concentration rises in the muscle, receptors are quickly blocked; then, as the drug is slowly eliminated *(concentration* falls with a half-life of one hour), receptors gradually become free. *Bottom:* Corresponding twitch response calculated on the basis of results such as those in Figure 15–2, that is, when receptor occupancy reaches 75 to 80 per cent the twitch begins to fall, and by 90 per cent receptor occlusion, the twitch is essentially abolished. As receptors again become free the twitch response recovers and returns to normal when the receptor occupancy has fallen to 75 to 80 per cent. Note that the twitch response reflects only changes in receptor occlusion that occur above the 75 to 80 per cent level *(wavy line).* Thus monitoring the twitch allows one to examine only the tip of the iceberg, above this level.

since the duration of the increase in intraocular pressure is brief following a single dose of succinylcholine, there seems to be no contraindication to its use for tracheal intubation in patients with glaucoma. In patients with penetrating eye wounds, however, even a transient increase in intraocular pressure could lead to a loss of vitreous humor. Pretreatment with a small dose of competitive antagonist, tubocurarine, or acetazolamide has been proposed to prevent an increase in intraocular pressure from a subsequent dose of succinylcholine for tracheal intubation. Because the ability of these drugs to prevent such pressure increases is controversial and because their efficacy in traumatized eyes has not been established, the prudent anesthetist should avoid, whenever possible, the use of succinylcholine in patients with penetrating eye wounds.

It is generally believed that depolarizing agents, by causing fasciculation of abdominal muscles, can produce an increase in intragastric pressure sufficient to open the gastroesophageal sphincter. Miller and associates (1971) showed that the rise in pressure is proportional to the intensity of fasciculations. This phenomenon becomes important in patients who are in danger of aspirating gastric contents. The succinylcholine-induced increase in intragastric pressure may be diminished by prior administration of a small dose of a competitive agent (e.g., 3 mg tubocurarine).

A common complaint from patients who have received a depolarizing agent is muscle pain postoperatively. This occurs most frequently in young patients who undergo minor operations and early ambulation. Although occurrence of pain cannot be related to the degree of fasciculation observed, most investigators believe that uncoordinated muscle contraction is the cause. Suggested mechanisms of the pain include local damage to muscle fibers or muscle spindles, lactic acid production, and potassium flux. Fasciculation and the ensuing muscle pain can be eliminated by prior administration of a competitive agent.

TUBOCURARINE

The most common side effect of tubocurarine is a dose-related fall in arterial pressure. Although the cause of the hypotension is controversial, the two mechanisms most frequently suggested are ganglionic block and histamine release. Tubocurarine is an active ganglionic blocking agent. However, because its potency at the neuromuscular junction is greater than at the ganglia, there is some doubt that a clinical concentration of tubocurarine is sufficient to cause hypotension. Tubocurarine liberates histamine in man as well as in experimental animals. Furthermore, the extent of release correlates well with the magnitude of the fall in arterial pressure. In any case, if a patient is already hypotensive or if hypotension may become a problem, an anesthetist should consider using another blocking agent.

Histamine release has also been blamed for bronchospasm following administration of tubocurarine. Again, no direct proof has been shown. It is difficult, as well, to determine from clinical reports whether the bronchospasm in question is even the result of tubocurarine, as opposed to some other factor such as light anesthesia. The possibility of bronchospasm is not of major importance in the choice of blocking agent.

GALLAMINE

Gallamine causes tachycardia and an increase in arterial pressure. The increase in heart rate has been attributed to a tyramine-like action, i.e., a release of transmitter from sympathetic nerve endings in the heart. However, the concentration required is high. Clinical tachycardia may instead reflect a vagal blocking action demonstrable at therapeutic concentrations. Another neuromuscular blocking agent would be preferable in the presence of tachycardia and hypertension.

PANCURONIUM

Pancuronium also causes an increase in arterial pressure and heart rate, although both effects are less pronounced than those seen with gallamine. Pancuronium has been shown to exert a vagolytic action like that of gallamine.

METOCURINE

Metocurine shows minimal cardiovascular effects, although high doses may lower arterial pressure, presumably by releasing histamine.

UPTAKE, DISTRIBUTION, AND ELIMINATION

The uptake and distribution of the neuromuscular blockers are not remarkable; these drugs behave according to the general principles of pharmacokinetics. The easiest way to approach the matter is to consider first the simplest case and then superimpose any perturbations relevant to each specific agent. Decamethonium, which is not metabolized, is a good model. Thus one starts by picturing a charged compound, not metabolized and restricted to the extracellular space. Since the neuromuscular blockers are typically administered by rapid intravenous injection, their kinetics can be subdivided into two phases: redistribution and elimination.

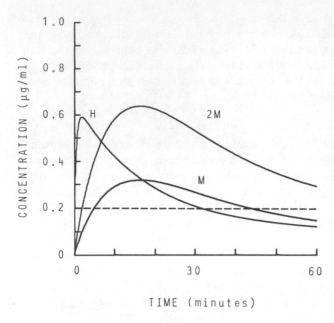

FIGURE 15-4. Calculated concentrations of pancuronium in muscle and heart following a single intravenous dose. Ordinates: concentration (μg/ml). Abscissae: time (minutes). Horizontal broken line represents concentration producing neuromuscular block. Curve labelled M is muscle concentration following a dose of 0.06 mg/kg. Curve labelled 2M is muscle concentration following double that dose. Curve labelled H is concentration in heart following 0.06 mg/kg. Note: a faster onset in muscle is possible with an increased dose but at the expense of prolonged duration of action; peak concentration in heart can be roughly twice that in muscle (and occurs considerably earlier).

REDISTRIBUTION

Immediately after injection, there is a high local concentration in venous blood flowing from the site of injection toward the heart. As this blood mixes with blood returning from other parts of the body, the drug is diluted. Passage through the lung distributes the drug through a still greater volume. Next the already somewhat attenuated bolus is swept out to the various tissues and the drug begins to be mixed throughout the entire extracellular space. During this period, the concentration in arterial flow to muscle exceeds the concentration in the extracellular space around the end-plate region of muscle, so the drug diffuses from muscle capillaries to the site of action.

The rate of equilibration of any drug with a tissue is governed by the ratio of flow to the volume perfused, i.e., by a perfusion rate constant that takes the dimensions of flow per unit volume. Anesthetists are accustomed to using drugs that exert their primary effect on the brain, where a volume of about 1.5 L is perfused with blood at a rate of 0.75 L/min to give a perfusion rate constant of 0.75/1.5 = 0.5/min. This means that the half-life for equilibration would be less than 1.5 minutes.* On the other hand, the primary action of neuromuscular blockers is in muscle where a volume of about 6 L is perfused by about 0.5 L each minute (note that in muscle we consider plasma flow, not blood flow, and extracellular fluid volume, not total tissue water, because our drugs of interest are quaternary compounds whose permanent charge restricts them to extracellular space). The calculated perfusion rate constant of 0.5/6 = 0.083/min corresponds to a half-life of 8.3 minutes. Onset of action would therefore be about six times slower than for a drug acting on the brain. Direct calculation (Fig. 15-4) shows that, following an intravenous injection, the peak concentration of a neuromuscular blocking agent would not be reached at the muscle end plate for 10 to 20 minutes, depending on the actual muscle blood flow.

---

*The rate constant and half-life of an exponential process (i.e., a process of the form $y = y_o e^{-kt}$) are related by the equation $t\frac{1}{2} = 0.693/k$. The derivation comes directly from the definition of $t\frac{1}{2}$ as that time at which y has fallen to half its previous value, i.e., to $y_o/2$. Thus, one can write either $y_o/2 = y_o e^{-kt1/2}$ or $\frac{1}{2} = e^{-kt1/2}$. Taking natural logs of both sides removes the exponential function, i.e., $\ln(\frac{1}{2}) = kt\frac{1}{2}$. Since the natural logarithm of $\frac{1}{2}$ is -0.639, $k = 0.693/t\frac{1}{2}$.

The only practical way to get a more rapid onset is to give a larger dose. Figure 15–4 illustrates this quantitatively. The horizontal line represents the tissue concentration that would have to be reached to achieve adequate paralysis. The lower curve (M) illustrates the time course of concentration that might be achieved with a dose that produces a block that wears off about 45 minutes after the dose is given. However, there is a delay of five minutes before onset of paralysis. The upper curve (2M) shows the time course following double the dose. (This curve is simply the first curve scaled up twofold.) Note that neuromuscular block comes on faster, at two minutes, but that the price paid is a longer total duration.

It is also important to note that, because of the larger perfusion rate constant of the heart (2/min for the extracellular compartment), any cardiac effects, such as tachycardia, would appear quickly and may be noticed before neuromuscular block is seen. Furthermore, the peak concentration achieved in the heart will be greater (see Fig. 15–4).

After three or four half-lives, i.e., about 30 minutes, muscle concentration will be close to that of the plasma. Thus, to picture the further course of the concentration at the end plate, we need only follow the plasma concentration. This brings us to the second phase of the distributional process.

ELIMINATION

The course of subsequent events can be deduced easily for the charged, unmetabolized drug. The major portal of exit is the kidney. Every minute, the glomeruli filter 120 ml of plasma, that is, 120 ml of extracellular fluid perfuse the renal tubules. Since all the drugs used as clinical neuromuscular blocking agents carry a permanent charge, they cannot diffuse back across the renal tubular membrane and hence are eliminated in the urine. Thus, the 12 L of extracellular space through which the drug is distributed are cleared of drug at a rate of 120 ml or 1 per cent per minute (i.e., the "elimination rate constant" is 0.01/min). This amounts to saying that the extracellular concentration will fall with a half-life of a little over an hour. (If the concentration fell linearly at the rate of 1 per cent per minute, then it would fall 50 per cent in 50 minutes and the half-life would be 50 minutes. However, as elimination proceeds, each 120 ml of glomerular filtrate contains progressively less drug, and the rate at which the concentration falls slows with time; that is, the concentration falls exponentially. The effect of this is to make the half-life longer than 50 minutes. As indicated earlier, the actual value works out to be 69.3 minutes.)

In summary then, the basic picture is a concentration at the site of action that rises for about ten minutes, levels off, and passes into an exponential decay with a half-life of a little over an hour. Variants can now be superimposed on this scheme.

BINDING TO PLASMA PROTEINS

At clinical concentrations, about half the tubocurarine in plasma is bound to plasma proteins. The effect of this is to make the plasma volume appear twice as big as it is, and thus the drug appears to be distributed through more than 12 L. The exponential elimination might be expected to be slowed slightly, but hardly enough to be perceptible clinically. The binding of metocurine (about 35 per cent), pancuronium (about 10 per cent), and gallamine is so low as to have a negligible effect on the kinetics.

METABOLISM

If the drug is metabolized, then the rate of elimination will be accelerated. Metabolism appears to be negligible with gallamine, tubocurarine, metocurine, and decamethonium. Pancuronium is deacetylated at either the 3 position, the 17 position, or both, to give metabolites, two of which show neuromuscular blocking activity. To further complicate the picture, the extent of any of the reactions involved is not known in humans. However, the metabolism does appear to contribute to the elimination of pancuronium, that is, its half-life appears to be on the short side of an hour. Succinylcholine is metabolized extremely rapidly to succinylmonocholine and choline (see further on).

BILIARY EXCRETION

Significant elimination of tubocurarine occurs through the bile. This feature may appear trivial until a patient with no renal function is considered. In such an individual, the half-life of tubocurarine will be greatly prolonged, but eventually the drug will be eliminated. On the other hand, the effect of gallamine or metocurine, which have no significant biliary excretion, can last so long that artificial dialysis may be required.

ULTRARAPID ONSET OF ACTION

A good example of very rapid onset of action is seen with succinylcholine, which has already been noted to undergo rapid metabolic destruction. This rapid elimination implies a brief duration of action, but the clinical significance relates not so much to rapid *offset* as to rapid *onset,* which facilitates rapid tracheal intubation and therefore minimizes the interval during which a patient is unconscious with an unprotected airway. This feature gives succinylcholine its prominent position in anesthesia. That rapid destruction should imply rapid onset of action may at first appear to represent a paradox. However, on reflection it may be seen that this trick has a biologic basis. Cholinesterase, which accelerates destruction of the transmitter, is placed at nerve endings to permit faster transmission of the signal. To get a rapid onset of action, one can give an overdose and get away with it if the drug is rapidly destroyed. Thus, in the usual clinical setting, when an intravenous bolus of succinylcholine is injected, an intentional overdose is given to achieve a rapid onset with the expectation of rapid curtailment of drug action by plasma cholinesterase.

This brings us to another peculiarity relevant to the pharmacokinetics of succinylcholine. Rarely, patients have an atypical pseudocholinesterase. In these individuals the overdose aspect is prominent since the drug effect is not abbreviated by rapid metabolism. Thus one ends up with "prolonged apnea" — a direct expression of overdose. The genetic aspects and diagnosis of this condition are discussed further on.

PLACENTAL TRANSFER

Although this can have little effect on duration of action in the mother, it might have important implications for the newborn's ability to breathe. However, neuromuscular blockers do not appear to cross the placenta in significant amounts.

FACTORS INFLUENCING ACTION OF NEUROMUSCULAR BLOCKERS

ABNORMAL PSEUDOCHOLINESTERASE ACTIVITY

Genetic

Under normal conditions, succinylcholine is metabolized by serum cholinesterase to succinylmonocholine and choline. Serum cholinesterase is determined genetically by allelic genes, four of which have been identified: the normal (N), the dibucaine-resistant (D), the fluoride-resistant (F), and the silent (S). These four genes can combine to form ten genotypes; of these, six (D–D, F–F, S–S, D–F, D–S, F–S) show a marked decrease in their ability to metabolize succinylcholine. An individual with such a genetic makeup will show a greatly prolonged effect from succinylcholine — the "overdose" mentioned previously. There is no danger to the patient as long as the condition is recognized and controlled ventilation instituted until the drug is eliminated.

Acquired

Liver Disease. Serum cholinesterase is synthesized in the liver. Foldes has shown that even moderate liver disease can reduce serum cholinesterase by 50 per cent and double the duration of action of succinylcholine.

Organophosphorous Compounds. Organophosphorous compounds such as echothiophate are irreversible cholinesterase inhibitors used as eye drops for the treatment of glaucoma. Systemic absorption has been shown to decrease cholinesterase activity significantly, and prolonged responses to succinylcholine have been reported.

SYSTEMIC DISEASES

Patients with myasthenia gravis are markedly sensitive to the actions of competitive agents. Depolarizing agents can be used but tend to reach phase II sooner than in normal individuals. The "myasthenic" syndrome associated with small-cell carcinoma of the lung (Lambert-Eaton syndrome) is also associated with increased sensitivity to both depolarizing and nondepolarizing agents. Although in theory one could handle the increased sensitivity to blocking agents by scaling down the dose, in practice the nature of myasthenia is such that a blocker is seldom necessary and if possible should be avoided.

Patients with myotonia congenita and myotonia dystrophica respond to depolarizing agents with muscle contracture rather than relaxation. The muscle spasm may be so intense that ventilation, either spontaneous or controlled, is impossible. The mechanism is not known.

Depolarizing neuromuscular blockers cause an increase in serum potassium of about 0.5 mEq per L in normal individuals. However, in patients with burns, massive trauma, tetanus, injury to the central nervous system, or lower motor neuron lesions, the serum potassium elevation is greatly exaggerated and may lead to cardiac arrest. It is not known whether this increased release of potassium associated with depolarization is caused by injury to the muscle membrane or is the result of an increase in the extent of chemically excitable membrane similar to that seen following chronic denervation. The period of greatest risk lasts from a few days to six months following the injury. The exaggerated potassium release may be diminished by prior administration of a competitive antagonist, but the effect is not predictable. It is therefore wiser to avoid depolarizing agents entirely in such patients.

Individuals susceptible to malignant hyperthermia (see Chapter 33) may respond to succinylcholine by developing generalized rigidity. The contraction is not reversed by competitive neuromuscular blocking agents.

Individuals with renal failure obviously should not be given drugs such as decamethonium or gallamine that are eliminated solely via the kidneys. Other agents such as tubocurarine and pancuronium may be used safely if it is remembered that the half-life will be prolonged.

ELECTROLYTES

Magnesium interferes with neuromuscular transmission by decreasing the release of acetylcholine. Because of a large margin of safety, acetylcholine output must be greatly decreased before a clinical response may be detected. During the treatment of eclampsia, enough magnesium sulfate may be given to cause muscle weakness directly. More often, however, magnesium levels will be low enough so that a noticeable effect will not appear until a neuromuscular blocker is administered. Then, the combination of low concentrations of magnesium and tubocurarine will summate the neuromuscular blocking properties of decreased acetylcholine output and those of fewer available acetylcholine receptors. Thus, patients receiving magnesium will require less tubo-curarine to produce visible neuromuscular block.

Calcium has both presynaptic and postsynaptic sites of action. The higher the plasma calcium level, the higher the concentration of blocking agent needed to produce neuromuscular block.

Potassium, like calcium, has both presynaptic and postsynaptic actions that, on the one hand, increase acetylcholine output and, on the other, decrease the effect of acetylcholine. The net effect is such that both acute and chronic hypokalemia lead to a decrease in the amount of tubocurarine needed to cause neuromuscular block.

Lithium has been reported to accentuate the action of both depolarizing and nondepolarizing blocking agents; the mechanism is not known.

ACID-BASE BALANCE

There is extensive literature concerning the effect of acid-base balance on the potency of neuromuscular blockers. Investigators differ in their opinions and in the design of their experiments. Also, it is not known whether differences in the extent of neuromuscular block are the result of pH changes *per se* or alterations caused by acid-base imbalance (e.g., changes in blood flow, serum electrolytes, or protein bind-ing).

TEMPERATURE

Lowering the temperature has been said to strengthen a depolarizing block and antagonize a competitive block. Recently the latter response has been questioned by investigators who have shown that tubocurarine-induced neuromuscular block is enhanced by hypothermia. Examination of the effect of temperature on the potency of tubocurarine and pancuronium *in vitro* suggests a possible explanation for the conflict-ing reports in the literature. Temperature changes produce minimal shift of the dose-response curve for either drug. However, both drugs produce steep dose-response curves. Thus, a change in temperature need shift a curve only slightly to generate a situation in which a single twitch response may be slightly blocked at 37°C yet markedly blocked at 25°C. Although this change will loom large if one happens to start at the right place, generally the effect of temperature on muscle sensitivity to neuromuscular blockers will be less than patient-to-patient variation.

Much more significant than these minor changes in sensitivity of the neuromuscu-lar apparatus will be the pharmacokinetic implications of cooling. Thus, slowing of metabolism and renal excretion could considerably prolong the effect of the drugs.

DRUG INTERACTIONS

It is obvious from Table 15–1 that the ability of a muscle to respond to nerve stimulation is a reflection of many events, and prevention of muscle contraction may result from drug action at any step along the way. A drug may act at one or more sites, or combinations of drugs may act at the same or different sites. In any event, the final neuromuscular response will be a summation of the individual drug effects. Since up to 80 per cent of the receptors may be blocked before any twitch depression is seen, it is easy to understand why many drugs, which, by themselves, are unlikely to cause noticeable neuromuscular block, can produce frank paralysis when combined with small doses of neuromuscular blockers. Magnesium has already been mentioned; further examples are given.

Antibiotics

Antibiotics, with the exception of penicillin G, cephradine, and cephaloridine, have been shown to cause neuromuscular block. The mechanism of action of these drugs is varied, as would be expected from the diversity of structure, and often controversial. Although the antibiotics by themselves produce block only in concentrations higher than those normally used clinically, the combined use of antibiotics and specific neuromuscular blocking agents produces synergistic effects. Such an interaction is seen most frequently when antibiotics are administered intraperitoneally or intravenously during operation. Careful monitoring of neuromuscular block is especially important in these situations because adequate reversal of the block may not be possible, and the patient's ventilation will need to be controlled until the neuromuscular effect has worn off. It is also important to realize that following the use of competitive antagonists the margin of safety of neuromuscular transmission is reduced for many hours, and administration of large doses of antibiotics in the immediate postoperative period may lead to a dangerous blocker/antibiotic block.

Local Anesthetics

Although local anesthetics can, by themselves, produce neuromuscular block, it is the interaction of local anesthetics with competitive antagonists that is important clinically. Synergism has been reported with all agents studied. In guinea pig isolated nerve-muscle preparations, only 1 per cent of the neuromuscular blocking concentration of lidocaine will cause profound twitch depression following administration of tubocurarine in a concentration that, by itself, will not show twitch depression. Similar concentrations of both drugs may be seen in patients in the recovery room, for example, if lidocaine is used to treat cardiac arrhythmias. It is important that surgeons and recovery room nurses as well as anesthetists be aware of the possibility of neuromuscular block in such situations.

Cardiovascular Drugs

Propranolol, quinidine, bretylium, trimethaphan, and nitroglycerine increase the effect of neuromuscular blocking agents and again are of particular interest to those dealing with patients in recovery rooms or intensive care units.

Inhalation Anesthetics

All the inhalation anesthetics augment the effects of neuromuscular blockers. As suggested by Table 15–1, the possible sites of action are numerous. In clinical concentrations, general anesthetics do not depress nerve conduction nor do they interfere with the acetylcholine-receptor combination. Some anesthetics, cyclopropane, for example, have an effect on the motor nerve terminals, but the importance of this on muscle relaxation is unknown. Volatile anesthetics increase the twitch response to both direct and indirect stimulation — if anything, an "antiblocker" effect. Inhalation anesthetics have their greatest effect at synapses. In this regard, their effect on spinal cord motor neurons and the neuromuscular junction appears to be similar.

At the neuromuscular junction the volatile anesthetics halothane, isoflurane, methoxyflurane, diethyl ether, fluroxene, and enflurane depress chemically induced depolarization of the end-plate region. Unlike neuromuscular blockers, which depress depolarization by combining with the acetylcholine receptor, the action of volatile anesthetics is on the muscle membrane distal to the receptor. The higher the anesthetic concentration, the greater the depression of depolarization. Only when depolarization is depressed by 50 per cent (1.5 to 5.0 MAC) does the indirectly stimulated twitch response begin to fall.

The effects of general anesthetics and competitive neuromuscular blockers on depolarization reinforce each other. Thus it is possible to use enflurane and tubocurarine, for example, in concentrations that by themselves have no effect on twitch response but that in combination cause complete neuromuscular block. Effectively, the

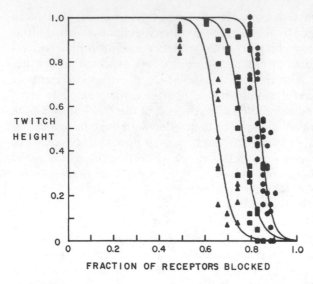

FIGURE 15–5. Effect of volatile anesthetics on the margin of safety of neuromuscular transmission. Plot as in Figure 15–2. Right-hand curve *(circles),* no anesthetic present. Middle curve *(squares),* halothane (0.75 per cent). Lefthand curve *(triangles),* enflurane (1.68 per cent).

action of inhalation anesthetics is to decrease the margin of safety of neuromuscular blockers (Fig. 15–5). The extent of such a decrease depends not only on the concentration of the anesthetic but on the anesthetic used. When the anesthetic concentrations are equal to MAC, tubocurarine requirement is decreased by about one third with halothane and by about two thirds with isoflurane or enflurane.

SUMMARY OF FACTORS AFFECTING BLOCKADE

The preceding list of factors influencing the action of neuromuscular blockers includes problems that vary widely in clinical significance. The effect of myasthenia gravis, for example, can be so marked that no additional relaxation is needed, whereas at the other end of the scale one encounters the temperature effect, which is still controversial even as to the direction of the shift. When the problem is clear-cut, the solution is obvious; for example, avoid depolarizing agents in situations in which exaggerated potassium release might be expected. On the other hand, the effects of acid-base balance, temperature, and electrolytes are of the same order of magnitude as random patient-to-patient variation and can be approached in the same way. Thus one should not give "cookbook doses" of blocking agents but rather titrate the drugs against the patient's response, as described further on.

CLINICAL USE OF NEUROMUSCULAR BLOCKERS

Patients show marked variation in their responses to both depolarizing and nondepolarizing blockers, regardless of whether the dose is calculated in mg per kg or mg per sq m of body surface. It is wise, therefore, to use a monitoring device such as a peripheral nerve stimulator (see further on) to determine the effect of the blocking agent used and to titrate the drug against the response of the patient. Katz showed that 7 per cent of patients who received 0.1 mg per kg tubocurarine showed complete depression of twitch response; therefore this dose is a good starting point. Comparable doses of gallamine and pancuronium would be 0.6 mg per kg and 0.02 mg per kg, respectively. Depending on the effect of this dose, the inhalation agent used, and the kind and duration of operation, an additional dose is given. Adequate relaxation for most operations is achieved when the twitch response at 0.1 Hz is depressed by 90 per cent.

Succinylcholine is most commonly used for tracheal intubation. Although 0.5 mg per kg is sufficient to cause complete neuromuscular block in most individuals, the duration of block is short. The extra time gained by using 1.0 mg per kg may be useful and is far safer than repeating the original dose (see earlier).

ASSESSMENT OF DEPTH OF NEUROMUSCULAR BLOCK

There are two situations in which one needs to know the level of neuromuscular block: (1) Is the patient relaxed enough for operation? (2) Has the patient recovered safely? Many indices have been used to answer one or the other of these questions. A brief list is useful.

The first group of indices involves direct measurements that, however, require specialized apparatus. The common feature is application of electric shocks to a motor nerve and observation or recording of the resultant muscular response. The simplest example is application of single shocks to the ulnar nerve every ten seconds, with monitoring of the resultant flexion of the fourth and fifth digits. (The electric activity of muscle also has been used as a measure of muscle response. However, it is hard to see any advantage over the simpler twitch response.) This particular index corresponds exactly to the physiologist's standard neuromuscular preparation. Thus the response can be interpreted directly in the framework of Figure 15–2. When the twitch is completely or almost completely abolished, the degree of relaxation is suitable for the operation. As a rule of thumb, the dose of a competitive antagonist required to produce such a twitch depression is twice the dose needed to depress the twitch response minimally. Thus, if, following administration of 9 mg tubocurarine, a slight depression of the twitch response is seen, 18 mg tubocurarine (total dose) will cause 90 per cent depression. It follows that the time taken for the twitch to recover from deep block to control levels will be the half-life of the drug. During recovery, when the simple twitch response has returned to normal, one can say that 20 per cent of the receptor pool is free. Fortunately, the diaphragm needs fewer receptors available to respond normally than do peripheral muscles. This is borne out clinically in that spontaneous respiration may be detected before an indirectly stimulated twitch response. However, a patient with 80 per cent receptor block may still be in a precarious position. Thus it is important to have a means of assessing when recovery has proceeded to a more adequate level. To this end, variants on the single shock have evolved. The simplest involves administration of a series of shocks at 30, 50, and 100 Hz. The rationale is that a tetanic response puts a greater demand on the neuromuscular synapse. As each successive stimulus arrives at the nerve ending, it depletes the local store of transmitter so that the amount of acetylcholine available for release by each succeeding stimulus falls. When the fraction of free receptors is also decreased, the tetanic response does not maintain its initial intensity; it fades. Thus the margin of safety is reduced for tetanic stimuli.

The higher the rate of stimulation, the greater the proportion of the receptor pool that must be free before a tetanic response does not fade. Unfortunately, the patient who has recovered to the level that could be examined with a tetanus is often conscious. Because production of a tetanic response can be painful, especially at the higher frequencies that yield the most information, tetanic stimulation has not proved practical clinically. An attempt to avoid this impasse led to the introduction of the "train-of-four" approach. In this test, the ulnar nerve is stimulated with four supramaximal stimuli 0.5 seconds apart, and the ratio of the fourth twitch to the first twitch is used to determine the degree of neuromuscular block. The procedure has two advantages: it is not painful, and the first response in the train provides a built-in control for the fourth response. This is a great convenience in the clinical situation in which factors such as patient movement can change the initial tension of muscle and hence the size of the twitch response. For practical purposes, the degree of block may be estimated by counting the number of twitches seen following the four stimulations. When only one twitch is present, there is greater than 90 per cent block. All four twitches appear when the single twitch is depressed by 75 per cent. Recovery from the block occurs when all four twitches in the train are the same height. At this time, about 25 per cent of the receptor pool is free. Thus, the train-of-four is a slightly more sensitive index of recovery than the simple twitch (Fig. 15–6).

A few comments are in order regarding determination of the nature of the block, a subject related to assessment of recovery. In this connection two phenomena may be mentioned: tetanic fade and post-tetanic facilitation (PTF). Tetanic fade has already been discussed. In the case of competitive block, the underlying mechanism is a progressive depletion of the transmitter stores. In PTF, the first twitches following a tetanus are larger than those immediately preceding it. The mechanism appears to reflect cumulation of calcium ions in the nerve terminal during the tetanus. However, this may not be the whole story or even the principal cause. The important point is that PTF itself, and in particular its relation to neuromuscular block, is not well understood and therefore does not provide a firm basis for interpretation of mechanisms. Unfortunately, PTF is often overinterpreted; this frequently applies as well to tetanic fade. But a few words of caution are in order. Typically, the indices are used to determine the nature of a neuromuscular block. Thus one encounters claims that a tetanus is sustained during depolarizing block, whereas it fades during phase II block. However, in well-controlled experimental situations, all possible combinations of fading and sustained tetani and phase I and phase II blocks may be demonstrated. Thus, the extent of fade should not be considered a reliable index of the nature of the block. The same caution applies to extent of PTF. It is also worth mentioning that the extent of PTF is not easily equated with depth of a competitive block.

The second group of indices of depth of block requires minimal or no specialized apparatus. Aside from the obvious maneuver of noticing whether there is sufficient relaxation for operation, the components of this group are directed toward assessing the extent of recovery rather than depth during operation. Examples may be listed in order of their appearance during recovery: (1) tidal volume (which is normal by the time the twitch response has reached control level), (2) vital capacity (which is 90 per cent of

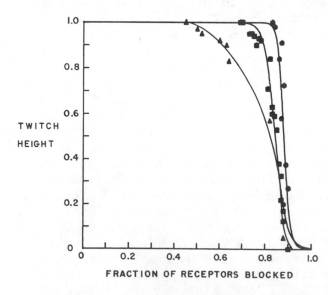

FIGURE 15–6. Comparison of twitch, train-of-four, and tetanus at 100 Hz as indices of receptor occlusion. Plot margin of safety as in Figure 15–2. Righthand curve *(circles)*, twitch responses. Middle curve *(rectangles)*, train-of-four. Lefthand curve *(triangles)*, 100 Hz tetanus. Note that more receptors must be available before train-of-four response returns to normal, but that 100 Hz tetanus requires about half of the receptor pool to be free before a normal response is obtained.

normal by the time a 50 Hz tetanus has recovered), (3) maximal inspiratory and expiratory force, and (4) head lift for five seconds. Note the relation of head lift to tetanic electric stimulation. Both allow one to probe more significant levels of recovery than can be monitored with a single twitch, but the head lift not only requires no apparatus but administers the tetanic stimulation painlessly. Eliciting a head lift does, however, require the patient's cooperation.

This brings us to another aspect of monitoring — the differential diagnosis of neuromuscular block from central mechanisms. For example, consider inadequate ventilation. Is the problem too much tubocurarine, too much morphine, or hypocarbia? A normal response to peripheral nerve stimulation and the ability to raise the head or take a deep breath on command rule out the first explanation.

REVERSAL OF NEUROMUSCULAR BLOCK

Competitive neuromuscular blockers can be antagonized by agents such as edrophonium (Tensilon), neostigmine, or pyridostigmine (Mestinon). These drugs appear to act by combining with cholinesterase, thus preventing the metabolism of acetylcholine, which is then available to compete more effectively with the antagonist for the receptor. Neostigmine also causes depolarization of the end plate by a direct action, but the significance of this action in the reversal of competitive antagonism is unknown.

The effect of acetylcholine is not only on the end plate of striated muscle but on structures innervated by the parasympathetic nervous system. Therefore, to prevent muscarinic responses such as bradycardia, bronchospasm, or salivation, atropine 0.5 to 1.5 mg must be injected before or simultaneously with the anticholinesterases.

Because of a short duration of action, edrophonium is not useful as an antagonist of competitive block. Both neostigmine and pyridostigmine are preferred. Pyridostigmine has a longer duration of action and a longer time to onset. The time from administration to maximum effect is 7 to 11 minutes with neostigmine and 12 to 15 minutes with pyridostigmine. The duration of action is 37 to 58 minutes with neostigmine and 51 to 83 minutes with pyridostigmine.

The dose of neostigmine or pyridostigmine necessary to antagonize a neuromuscular block is debatable. However, there is no basis for debate if the drug is titrated. When a peripheral monitor is used the dose may be titrated against the effect of nerve stimulation. For example, neostigmine can be given in increments of 0.5 mg until either satisfactory recovery is achieved or succeeding doses no longer cause improvement. Because of the large margin of safety of neuromuscular transmission, an additional increment of 0.5 mg neostigmine should be given after tetanus or head lift is sustained. Pyridostigmine is similarly used but with incremental doses of 2.5 mg.

It has been suggested that the effect of neostigmine might wear off faster than the competitive antagonist and lead to "recurarization." However, in the absence of gross prolongation of action of the neuromuscular block, as might be produced by anuria, a single course of neostigmine will suffice if the neuromuscular block is adequately reversed in the first place.

There is no reliable antagonist of depolarizing blockers. Anticholinesterases may either cause reversal of the block or increase it. Some authorities suggest that anticholinesterases increase phase I block and reverse phase II block. Since it is difficult at present to clinically differentiate phase I from phase II block, an appropriate clinical approach is hard to determine. Some authors suggest that a test of the short-acting edrophonium be used and if block is reversed, the longer-acting neostigmine can be given. In practice, the safest procedure is to control ventilation until spontaneous recovery occurs.

NEW NEUROMUSCULAR BLOCKERS

None of the neuromuscular blocking agents in general use is perfect. The only short-acting agent, succinylcholine, causes depolarization, with the associated fasciculation, potassium release, and phase II block. The competitive antagonists are not only long acting but also produce cardiovascular effects. It would be advantageous to have a competitive antagonist with a short duration of action and no secondary effects. Clinicians have studied many agents, only to discover that metabolism was less rapid, more histamine was released, or vagolytic action was more pronounced in human than in animal studies. The search goes on. At present, two agents are undergoing clinical investigation. Atracurium contains two tetrahydroisoquinolium structures reminiscent of tubocurarine with the nitrogen atoms connected by a bridge containing two ester bonds. A short half-life results from both ester hydrolysis and spontaneous dealkylation of the nitrogen atoms. Org NC45 is a monoquaternary analogue of pancuronium. The tertiary nitrogen appears to facilitate hydrolysis of the adjacent ester group. Note that in both cases the trend seems to be to depend more and more on an inherent chemical instability rather than an enzymatic mechanism (which can vary considerably among species and individuals) to eliminate the drug.

APPRAISAL

In summary, neuromuscular blockers are valuable, specific, and safe drugs when carefully used. Proper use requires a background knowledge of the pertinent physiology and pharmacology plus the patience to titrate the drug accordingly rather than to give standard doses.

REFERENCES

Ali HD, Wilson RS, Savarese JJ, et al: The effect of tubocurarine on indirectly elicited train of four muscle response and respiratory measurements in humans. Br J Anaesth 47:570, 1975.

Bowman WC, Norman J (eds): Symposium on ORG NC45. Br J Anaesth 52:Suppl 1, 1980.

Burns BD, Paton WDM: Depolarization of the motor end-plate by decamethonium and acetylcholine. J Physiol 115:41, 1951.

Farrell L, Dempsey MJ, Waud BE, Waud DR: Temperature and potency of d-tubocurarine and pancuronium in vitro. Anesth Analg 60:18, 1981.

Fogdall RP, Miller RD: Antagonism of d-tubocurarine and pancuronium-induced neuromuscular blockade by pyridostigmine in man. Anesthesiology 39:504, 1973.

Henschel O (ed): Malignant Hyperthermia: Current Concepts. New York, Appleton-Century-Crofts, 1977.

Katz B: Nerve, Muscle and Synapse. New York, McGraw-Hill, 1966.

Katz B: The Release of Neural Transmitter Substances. Springfield, Ill, Charles C Thomas, 1969.

Katz RL (ed): Muscle Relaxants. New York, American Elsevier Publishing Co, 1975.

Lee Son S, Waud BE: Potencies of neuromuscular blocking agents at the receptors of the atrial pacemaker and the motor end-plate of the guinea pig. Anesthesiology 47:34, 1977.

Miller RD: Antagonism of neuromuscular blockade. Anesthesiology 44:318, 1971.

Miller, RD, Van Nyhuis LS, Eger EI II, et al: Comparative time to peak effect and duration of action of neostigmine and pyridostigmine. Anesthesiology 41:27, 1974.

Miller RD, Way WL, Dolan WM, Stevens WC, Eger EI II: Comparative neuromuscular effects of pancuronium, gallamine, and succinylcholine during forane and halothane anesthesia in man. Anesthesiology 35:509, 1971.

Paton WDM, Waud DR: The margin of safety of neuromuscular transmission. J Physiol (Lond) 191:59, 1967.

Payne JP, Hughes R: Evaluation of atracurium in anaesthetized man. Br J Anaesth 53:45, 1981.

Waud BE: Decrease in dose requirement of d-tubocurarine by volatile anesthetics. Anesthesiology 51:298, 1979.

Waud BE: Interactions of muscle relaxants and other drugs. Refresher Courses in Anesthesiology 9:1981.

Waud BE, Waud DR: The relation between tetanic fade and receptor occlusion in the presence of competitive neuromuscular block. Anesthesiology 35:456, 1971.

Waud BE, Waud DR: The relation between the response to "train-of-four" stimulation and receptor occlusion during competitive neuromuscular block. Anesthesiology 37:413, 1972.

Waud BE, Waud DR: Comparison of the effects of general anesthetics on the end-plate of skeletal muscle. Anesthesiology 43:540, 1975.

Waud BE, Waud DR: Physiology and pharmacology of neuromuscular blocking agents. *In* Katz RL (ed): Muscle Relaxants. New York, American Elsevier Publishing Co, 1975, p. 1.

Waud DR, Waud BE: Depolarization block and phase II block at the neuromuscular junction. Anesthesiology 43:10, 1975.

Waud BE, Waud DR: Effects of volatile anesthetics on directly and indirectly stimulated skeletal muscle. Anesthesiology 50:103, 1979.

Waud BE, Waud DR: Interaction of calcium and potassium with neuromuscular blocking agents. Br J Anaesth 52:863, 1980.

Whittaker M: Plasma cholinesterase variants and the anaesthetist. Anaesthesia 35:174, 1980.

Chapter 16
INTUBATION OF THE TRACHEA

The advantages of intubation of the trachea are many: patency of the airway is reasonably assured, although not guaranteed; anatomic dead space is reduced by about half; control of respiration is facilitated; and secretions may be removed with relative ease from the tracheobronchial tree. Positive pressure can be applied to the airway without inflation of the stomach. The patient can be placed in any position for operation with less chance of compromising the airway, and the anesthetist can be situated at some distance from the patient's head and yet maintain control of respiration.

EQUIPMENT

LARYNGOSCOPE

Laryngoscopes are of three kinds: those with a straight blade, those with a curved blade, and the flexible fiberoptic instrument. Most laryngoscopes used by anesthetists have detachable blades that can be used interchangeably on a battery-containing handle, an arrangement both economic and convenient for cleaning the instrument. The novice can learn to intubate the trachea using any kind of laryngoscope, but initially, proficiency should be developed with one. For the difficult intubation, a flexible fiberoptic laryngoscope can be inserted into the lumen of a tracheal tube, permitting visualization of the larynx as the tube is threaded over it into the trachea. This technique is treated later in this chapter.

TRACHEAL TUBES

Tracheal tubes are usually manufactured from natural or synthetic rubber or plastic. A coiled wire or heavy nylon thread may be embedded in the wall to prevent collapse and an inflatable cuff incorporated. Natural rubber is more difficult to clean because its porosity permits absorption of bacteria-laden secretions, lubricants, and chemicals that may be used for cleaning. Although some plastic tubes stiffen with age and are thus more likely to produce trauma, others maintain their flexibility and are useful because transparency facilitates cleanliness and assurance of patency. Disposable tubes are the most convenient of all.

Tubes are chosen for durability, with thin walls and maximal internal diameters to assure minimal resistance to breathing, lack of compressibility, and ease of cleaning. All but those reinforced with the coiled wire may kink or undergo compression. Noncollapsible tubes are chosen in certain kinds of operation, such as for thoracic or cervical tumors compressing the trachea or in operations conducted in the sitting or face-down position when the head may be sharply flexed.

Endotracheal tubes are numbered according to outside diameter (Table 16–1). They are usually longer than necessary when received from the manufacturer and require shortening to lessen the possibility of bronchial intubation. The length of the tube is estimated for any patient by placing it alongside the face and neck, with the bifurcation of the trachea taken as the angle of Louis. Another method is to measure the distance from the cricoid cartilage to the tip of the xiphoid cartilage; this can be used as a rule of thumb for length of nasotracheal tubes; orotracheal tubes should be 2 cm shorter. Recommended lengths are given in Table 16–1.

Double lumen tubes are discussed in Chapter 26. A connector or slip joint is placed in the proximal end of the tube, fitting snugly and preferably distending the tube; otherwise it may be dislodged. Ideally, the connector should be situated at the level of the teeth; tubes that protrude from the mouth are subject to displacement into a bronchus or they may kink. The connector between adapter and breathing tubes of the anesthesia machine should be of large diameter, preferably curved, with smooth walls to minimize turbulence and resistance to gas flow (Fig. 16–1).

A *stylet* of malleable metal or plastic can be inserted to improve the curvature of an endotracheal tube. When placed within a tube the stylet is lubricated to aid in withdrawal; it should not protrude beyond the distal end. Some use a forceps to guide a flexible tube into the trachea rather than insert a stylet.

An *inflatable balloon or cuff* ensures a completely closed system, permitting easy control of respiration. When inflated, the cuff reduces the possibility but may not completely prevent passage of foreign material into the lungs. Cuffs may be of the high or low pressure kind, depending on the pressure used for inflation (see Chapter 37). Pressures higher than 200 torr have been measured at the interface between a high pressure cuff and tracheal mucosa; damage to the mucous membrane should be less with the low pressure kind (see Chapter 37). Modern endotracheal tubes have built-in cuffs, but if not, a cuff should be fixed to the endotracheal tube so that it cannot be displaced and occlude the distal end. Once in place, it is inflated with a measured amount of air, the extent of inflation tested by compressing the reservoir bag while simultaneously listening for escape of air at the mouth or nose. A small pilot balloon may be incorporated to indicate inflation of the cuff, and some cuffs are inflated through a self-sealing valve. A pharyngeal pack in conjunction with a cuffless tube is not recommended unless necessary, because of the added irritation.

Lubricants are used on cuffed tubes to facilitate passage through the glottis. Tap water or a water-soluble lubricant is adequate, although some believe that a topical anesthetic is useful. Nasotracheal tubes require more than the usual amount of lubrication. Suction catheters are likewise lubricated for easy passage through the endotracheal tube.

Figure 16–2 illustrates some essential pieces of endotracheal equipment.

TECHNIQUES OF TRACHEAL INTUBATION

GENERAL PRINCIPLES

Endotracheal tubes are packaged individually in clear plastic, marked as to size. A tube of appropriate diameter and length should be selected, though it is best to have several available because the appropriate size may be determined only after viewing the glottis. The tube is examined beforehand to assure patency and the cuff inflated to detect leakage of air. The laryngoscope bulb is tested and all equipment kept clean before use. Soiled equipment — masks, tubes, and airways — should be placed in a

TABLE 16–1. Dimensions of Endotracheal Tubes

		Endotracheal Tube Sizes (average in boldface)			Anatomic Distance		
		Diameters					
Age	Weight (lb)	French	Magill	Lengths (cm) Orotracheal	Teeth to Cords (cm)	Teeth to Carina (cm)	Sagittal Diam. Trachea (mm)
Newborn	to 8	10, 12, 14	0	**11**, 12	7–8	11–12	4
1–4 mo	8–10	12, 14, 16	1	11, 12			6
4–12 mo	10–20	14, **16**, 18	1, 1A	11, **12**	8.5	12–13	7
1–2 yr	20–25	16, **18**, 20	**1A**, 2	**12**, 13			7–8
2–3	25–30	18, **20**, 22	1A, **2**, 2A	13, 14	9	14	
3–4	30–35	20, 22, 24		**14**, 15		14.3	
4–5	35–40	22, **24**, 26	2, 3, 4	14, **15**, 16			8
5–6	40–45						
6–7	45–55		3, **4**, 5	**15**, 16, 17	9.5	15.5	8–9
7–8	55–60	24, **26**, 28					
8–9	60–65		4, **5**, 6	15, **16**, 17, 18			9
9–10	65–70	28, **30**	5, **6**, 7	16, **17**, 18, 19	9.5–10	15.5–17	
10–11	70–80				10–11	16.3–18.5	
11–12	80–90	30, 32, 34	6, 7, 8	17–24, **22.5**	11–15	17.5–25	9–11
12–16	90–140	34 (F)	7				11–15
Adults	130–200	36 (M)	8 (F)	23–26	12–15		
60–65		38	9 (M)	**24**		28–32	13–23
65 and over		40	10				

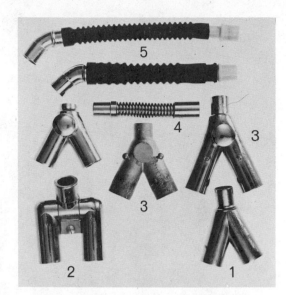

FIGURE 16–1. Types of endotracheal tube connectors. *1,* Y connector; *2,* Y connector with swivel neck; *3,* Y connectors with escape valve; *4,* flexible metal interconnector (rough, narrow interior walls predispose to turbulent air flow) not recommended unless respiration controlled; *5,* corrugated rubber interconnectors of two lengths and diameters, in which turbulence is of lesser importance because of a wide lumen.

separate container. Care and sterilization of endotracheal equipment are discussed in Chapter 8.

Before induction of anesthesia, certain observations are helpful in predicting the ease of tracheal intubation: relaxed submandibular tissues allow ready extension of the head, whereas inflexibility causes glottic exposure to be more difficult; a receding jaw causes difficulty in exposing the larynx via direct laryngoscopy; inability to open the mouth wide suggests ankylosis of the temporomandibular joint or trismus; patients with cervical arthritis often are unable to extend the head. The oral cavity is sometimes narrow and deep, with minimal space between the dental arches, so that the laryngoscope tends to block a good view of the glottis. A large tongue may be a hindrance, as is found in patients with cretinism, mongolism, or gargoylism.

The teeth are examined. Protruding upper incisors can be damaged by the laryngoscope and can predispose to difficulty in laryngeal exposure. Loose, chipped, capped, or diseased teeth should be identified preoperatively, a note made on the chart, and the patient advised of the risk of damage. If a tooth is found missing after intubation, it may be present in the mouth, pharynx, or nasopharynx. If it is not found, a chest x-ray is taken. Loose dental bridgework and partial plates are removed before intubation, and care is taken to avoid loss. Orthodontic appliances are removed if possible or protected against damage.

When the patient has healthy natural teeth with good supporting bone, careful manipulation of the laryngoscope, avoiding leverage against the teeth, will prevent damage. Teeth in jeopardy, even from minimal trauma, include those restored with fillings, crowns, or bridges. Alternatively, teeth with little supporting bone owing to periodontal disease may easily be loosened or dislodged, even with minimal force. Even in the absence of dental pathology, if difficult intubation is anticipated, a protective mouthguard should be available.

When dentition is poor, a dental consultation should be sought so that a custom-made Silastic mouthguard can be fabricated. Unfortunately, this practice is not always feasible in a busy hospital, so the anesthetist should be prepared to fabricate a simple dental splint in the operating room. A splint is constructed from a soft plastic mouth mold, as is used in dentistry for application of fluoride gels, or polyether rubber impression material. A plastic mold is closely fitted over the maxillary teeth; the mold is

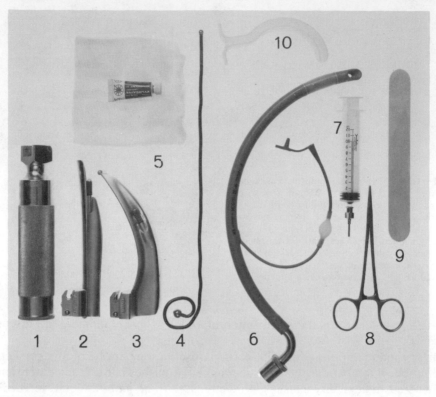

FIGURE 16–2. Equipment for tracheal intubation. *1*, Laryngoscope battery handle; *2*, straight blade; *3*, curved (Macintosh) blade; *4*, malleable copper stylet; *5*, sterile gauze with topical anesthetic lubricant; *6*, cuffed tube (uncut); *7*, syringe to inflate cuff; *8*, hemostat to hold cuff inflated; *9*, tongue blade for airway insertion; *10*, plastic oropharyngeal airway.

then filled with mixed impression material. Mold and rubber material are then placed over the teeth and held in position while the rubber sets. The mold is then removed.

A protective dental splint remains in place not only during intubation but throughout anesthesia and recovery. It is not unusual for a patient to bite with great force on an oral airway during recovery from anesthesia. When the patient is fully awake the splint is removed by gently sliding it away from the teeth.

The length and angulation of the epiglottis influence the ease of intubation. The relatively narrow and flexible epiglottis of the infant or child poses problems; in the adult the long, relaxed epiglottis, which falls back over the larynx when muscular relaxation is profound, can be difficult to control. Anatomic features of the upper airway are shown in Figure 16–3.

With this knowledge as background, skill in intubation is more quickly attained if a predetermined plan is followed.

Straight Blade Technique

1. The height of the operating table is adjusted so that the patient's face is approximately at the level of the standing anesthetist's xiphoid process. This allows for laryngeal suspension with the left arm flexed and the elbow held against the body at the level of the iliac crest.
2. The head, resting on a 4-inch firm pillow or pad, is brought into the "sniffing" position to bring the axis of trachea, pharynx, and mouth into line (Fig. 16–4).
3. The fingers of the right hand open the jaws widely, spreading the lips to prevent bruising them between laryngoscope and teeth.

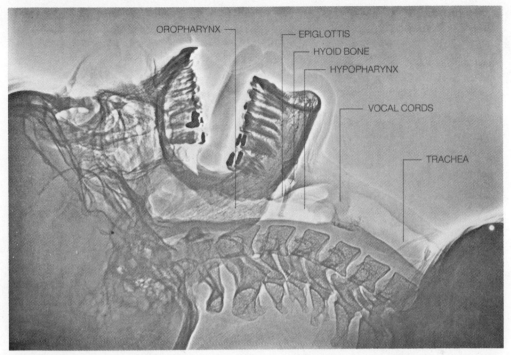

FIGURE 16–3. Xeroradiograph of a normal subject in "sniffing" position (flexion of neck and extension of head). The airway is straightest and greatest in size in this position. (From Applebaum EL, Bruce DL: Tracheal Intubation. Philadelphia, WB Saunders Co, 1976.)

4. A protective shield of lead or adhesive tape or a plastic mold placed over the upper incisors can prevent damage; gentleness and avoidance of pressure on teeth or gums are essential.
5. Held in the left hand, the moistened or lubricated laryngoscope blade is introduced at the right side of the mouth and advanced forward and centrally along the right side of the tongue. The epiglottis is seen at the base. The wrist is held rigid to avoid using the upper teeth as a fulcrum with the blade of the laryngoscope as a lever. The right hand is placed beneath the occiput to extend the head at the atlanto-occipital joint.
6. The blade is slipped just beneath the tip of the epiglottis, and exposure of the larynx is accomplished by an upward and forward lift at a 45-degree angle, elevating mandible and head. Exposure should not be obtained by leverage on the teeth. If the glottis is not easily exposed, depression of the thyroid cartilage may help; an extra pillow or pad beneath the head is also of value. Deep insertion of the laryngoscope blade results in elevation of the entire larynx and exposure of the esophagus rather than the glottis.
7. The endotracheal tube with cuff deflated, concavity directed laterally, is passed to the right of the tongue and laryngoscope through the glottis, 2 to 3 cm into the trachea in the adult or until the cuff just disappears beyond the vocal cords. Occasionally, intubation is accomplished only by a 90- to 180-degree rotation of the tube with return to the forward position in the trachea.

   Rarely, the glottis is not seen but intubation is possible if the arytenoid cartilages are visible. A curved stylet or a Magill forceps helps to direct the tube anteriorly. An olive-tipped urethral bougie inserted through the endotracheal tube, permitting the tip to pass into the barely visible glottis, may allow the tube to be "threaded" into the larynx.

Common causes of failure in tracheal intubation include inadequate muscle relaxation; insufficient depth of general anesthesia; poor position of the head; allowing the tongue to obscure the visual field; and lack of anatomic knowledge. On the other hand, hypoxia often occurs during intubation with the use of a neuromuscular blocker. The relaxation provided gives a false sense of security, and too long a time elapses before

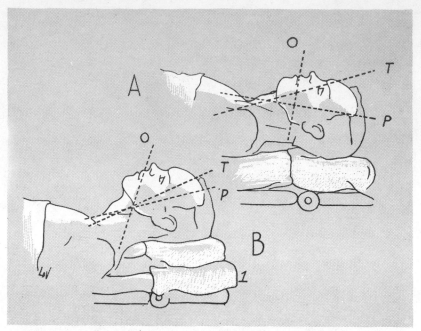

FIGURE 16–4. Position of the head for laryngoscopy and intubation of trachea. *A,* Ordinary position; *T,* axis of the trachea; *P,* axis of the pharynx; *O,* axis of the oral cavity. *B,* Modified position achieved with extra head rest. Flexion of cervical spine and extension at the atlanto-occipital joint bring the three axes more nearly into line.

respiration is resumed. Tracheal intubation is infrequently attempted today with general anesthesia alone.

Assuming that tracheal intubation is performed with a neuromuscular blocker, this should be preceded by several inflations of the lung to provide a reserve of oxygen. The instructor should place a limit of one minute for intubation, to be followed by another period of ventilation with oxygen. The interval can also be regulated if the anesthetist does not breathe during the intubation attempt; if the urge to breathe is felt, then the patient also needs ventilation.

Curved Blade Technique

Intubation with a curved blade involves the same maneuvers, but with a few modifications.

1. The blade is passed to the right of the tongue, then moved centrally, displacing the tongue to the left.
2. The epiglottis is not elevated; rather, the tip of the blade rests between the epiglottis and base of the tongue. Forward and upward lift of the laryngoscope stretches the hyo-epiglottic ligament, folding the epiglottis upward toward the blade and exposing the glottis. Failure to obtain good visualization is often caused by deep insertion of the blade, thereby fixing the epiglottis and preventing its movement. More often it is the failure to lift the blade at a 45-degree angle that causes difficulty.

The theoretic advantages of the curved blade relate to the sensory innervation of the laryngeal or undersurface of the epiglottis, derived from the superior laryngeal sensory branch of the vagus; stimulation by the straight blade is said to predispose to laryngospasm and cough. The pharyngeal surface is innervated by the glossopharyngeal nerve; stimulation of this surface by the curved blade is less likely to cause spasm. The curved blade allows more room for passage of the tracheal tube than a straight blade. Occasionally exposure of the glottis is not as good as that obtained with the straight blade, and a stylet may be required to ensure appropriate curvature of the tube. However, when the mouth cannot be opened wide, when the teeth protrude or are in poor condition, and in stout-necked individuals and those with a more cephalad larynx, the curved blade is more useful.

Orotracheal Intubation in the Conscious Patient

An anesthetist should be able to intubate the trachea with the patient awake when induction of general anesthesia is considered unsafe in the absence of an assured airway. Topical anesthesia is accomplished by means of a nebulizer, by application of cotton swabs to the pyriform fossae, or by transtracheal injection of a topical local anesthetic. Topical anesthesia is accomplished under direct vision with a laryngoscope or indirectly with reflected light and a laryngeal mirror. The structures are anesthetized in the following order: base of tongue, epiglottis, oropharynx, pyriform fossae, vocal cords, and finally, larynx and upper trachea by instillation through the glottis. A minimal amount of anesthesia is used to prevent untoward reactions, not more than 2 to 3 ml of 10 per cent cocaine, 1 per cent tetracaine, or 4 per cent lidocaine.

Orotracheal intubation with the patient awake is used to advantage in the following situations: in the presence of a full stomach when emergency operation is necessary; tumors of the neck or mediastinum displacing the trachea or larynx; tumor or inflammatory swelling encroaching upon the mouth or pharynx; malformation of the jaws; and intestinal obstruction when aspiration of vomitus during induction of anesthesia is a threat. In the latter instance, the cuff on the tracheal tube is inflated as soon as possible after intubation prior to induction of general anesthesia. During intubation, the head of the table is elevated to minimize regurgitation. Backward pressure on the cricoid cartilage helps to occlude the esophagus and to minimize regurgitation (the Sellick maneuver) (Chapter 33).

Blind Nasotracheal Intubation

Blind nasotracheal intubation is often the method of choice in oral and maxillofacial operations and is useful also in emergency situations when an airway is needed quickly, as in obese, stout-necked persons who easily become obstructed or patients with hypoglossal or cervical edema. Although indicated in a patient with trismus or a fractured jaw, nasal intubation is avoided in the patient with a fractured nose or nasal obstruction; it is also contraindicated in the presence of acute sinusitis and mastoiditis, since pathogenic bacteria may be carried into the trachea. Nasotracheal intubation may be done with the patient awake and well sedated or with general anesthesia and use of a neuromuscular blocker.

A nasotracheal tube should be soft and pliable so as not to injure the nasal mucous membrane or turbinates but of the proper consistency to resist compression and to maintain a reasonable curve. Tubes are stored to maintain the proper curvature and are well lubricated to minimize trauma. Prior topical application of cocaine or phenylephrine, 0.25 per cent, is useful in shrinking mucous membranes. A laryngoscope and Magill forceps are kept at hand in case intubation fails. Attempts at blind intubation are abandoned if not immediately successful, and the tube is inserted using direct vision and forceps.

When nasotracheal intubation is attempted, the occiput of the patient rests upon a firm pillow somewhat higher than with oral intubation, with the chin elevated. The tube is introduced with the concavity forward, hugging the floor of the nose. Advancement of the tube is slow and gentle, with rotation when resistance is encountered. Rough maneuvers, large-bore rigid tubes, poor lubrication, and use of force against an obstruction induce epistaxis. Guides to insertion are: observing the neck for bulging produced by the tip of the tube in the hypopharynx; increase or decrease in breath sounds if the patient is breathing; and resistance to passage of the tube. External, backward, or lateral movement of the larynx or rotation of the tube may be required.

Voluntary hyperpnea is helpful if the patient is awake, as is hyperpnea produced by hypercapnia if the patient is anesthetized but without neuromuscular block, providing maximal abduction of the cords during inspiration. Entry into the larynx is signified by loss of breath sounds if the patient is breathing and decrease in resistance, often accompanied by cough. Success is confirmed by connecting the tube to the rebreathing system and expanding the lungs. Commonly, blind nasotracheal intubation fails because the tube has poor curvature and the head is improperly positioned.

If a tracheal airway is required before induction of general anesthesia and this cannot be accomplished either by indirect or direct intubation under topical anesthesia, tracheostomy may be avoided by the use of fiberoptic laryngoscopy.

FIBEROPTIC LARYNGOSCOPY

The fiberoptic laryngoscope provides accuracy in tracheal intubation under the most difficult and unusual situations. It is also valuable for examination of the upper airway, verification of tracheal tube placement, assessment of laryngeal or tracheal damage, repositioning of endotracheal tubes in patients who are prone or with the head flexed, and changing an endotracheal tube with brief interruption of ventilation.

Principles of Fiberoptic Endoscopes

Glass fibers are flexible and efficient conductors of light and can be used for construction of fiberoptic endoscopes. Many glass fibers bound together at both ends make a flexible bundle useful for transmitting both light and images. To transport an optic image, the arrangement of fibers must be identical at both ends. When the ends are polished and objectives and oculars are placed on these ends, the fiberoptic laryngoscope or bronchoscope is completed. Such scopes are "frontal view," i.e., the lens is perpendicular to the longitudinal axis of the instrument.

Components of Fiberoptic Laryngoscopes

The flexible fiberoptic laryngoscope has three parts. (1) The control unit includes the tip deflection control knob, eyepiece, diopter adjustment ring, and working channel sleeve and plug (Fig. 16–5). (2) The flexible insertion cord consists of a coherent fiber bundle with a distal tip (objective) lens, and the illumination fibers and working channel for suction of secretions, instillation of medications, insufflation of oxygen or anesthetics, and passage of cytology brush and biopsy forceps. The semirigid nature of the insertion cord enables it to be rotated with the control unit of the instrument; this plus the ability to flex the tip of the insertion cord allows it to be maneuvered and advanced in any direction. (3) The light transmitting cord transmits light from an external source, usually supplied by an auxiliary source powered by A.C. current, although a snap-on battery handle is available.

In general, fiberoptic bronchoscopes are better made and offer superior resolution than laryngoscopes but are more expensive. Cleaning and sterilization of fiberscopes are time-consuming. Small amounts of secretion, blood, or fogging can cause failure. The available laryngoscopes are adequate for performing or teaching tracheal intubation but are not suitable for bronchoscopy. Smaller bronchoscopes are available for intubation in children (Table 16–2).

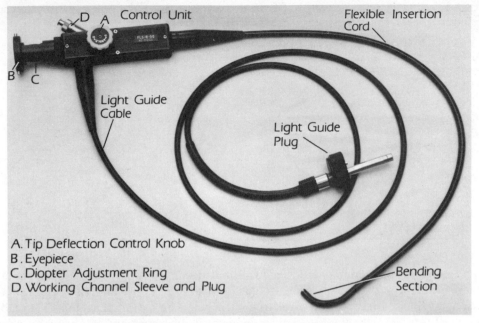

FIGURE 16–5.   Flexible fiberoptic laryngoscope.

Technique of Tracheal Intubation

The fiberoptic laryngoscope may be passed orally or nasally into the trachea to serve as a guide for the endotracheal tube. The operator constantly visualizes the anatomic relation of the airway, and intubation is easily accomplished and with little stress to the awake patient. Intubation is easier in the conscious patient, as tissue tone is maintained and the tongue and epiglottis do not relax to obscure the vocal cords. In an awake patient time required for intubation is unlimited, which is important in a teaching situation. The view differs from that seen with a rigid laryngoscope in that the pyriform sinuses appear more distal, as pathways to the glottis; the depth of vocal cords seems exaggerated and perhaps may not be seen until the false cords are passed; and the field of vision becomes limited as the fiberscope nears the structures. Secretions and blood may obscure the view. The following guidelines are useful when using this laryngoscope:

1. Be sure the light source is functioning properly.
2. Adjust the eyepiece by turning the diopter adjustment ring.
3. Inspect the eyepiece and distal objective lens for clarity.
4. Immerse the tip of the scope in warm water for a few minutes to prevent fogging.
5. Silicone or soapy water applied to the objective lens helps prevent fogging and adherence of secretions.
6. Lubricate the insertion tube, avoiding the objective lens.
7. Hold the scope in the right hand with the deflecting control knob between right thumb and forefinger (Fig. 16–6). The left hand is used to introduce and advance the fiberscope.

Nasal Approach

Sedation is provided according to need. Mucosal anesthesia is achieved with cocaine and anesthesia of larynx and trachea via translaryngeal injection of lidocaine. A well-lubricated, 8-mm nasotracheal tube is inserted through a nostril into the nasopharynx, the oropharynx is suctioned through the endotracheal tube, and the fiberscope is advanced into the oropharynx through the nasotracheal tube. The scope

TABLE 16–2. Characteristics of Two Fiberoptic Laryngoscopes and a Pediatric Bronchoscope

	Machida Flexible Intubation Scope Model FLS-6-50	American Optical Flexible Laryngoscope Model LS-7	Olympus Bronchofiberscope Model BF 3C4
Optical system			
Field of vision (degrees)	70	60	55
Depth of focus (mm)	5–50	5–30	3–50
Direction of observation	Forward	Forward	Forward
Angle deflection (degrees)			
Upward	120	120	160
Downward	120	120	60
Length (mm)			
Total	670	700	770
Insertion tube	500	500	595
Diameter (mm)			
Insertion tube	6.0	6.4	3.6
Working channel	2.0	2.0	1.2

glides along the posterior pharyngeal wall and usually past the tip of the epiglottis without difficulty. The vocal cords are easily visualized in the majority of cases, and the scope is passed through the cords to midtrachea. The nasotracheal tube is threaded over the scope into the trachea. Topical anesthesia of larynx and trachea may be enhanced by topical anesthesia spray through the working channel after exposure of the cords.

After gaining experience in awake patients, fiberoptic nasotracheal intubation can be attempted in anesthetized patients breathing spontaneously or after neuromuscular blockade. In the latter, upper displacement of the mandible by a second person results in easier exposure. In anesthetized and paralyzed patients, intubation time should not exceed 45 to 90 seconds, depending on the patient's condition.

Oral Approach

The oral approach is more difficult, especially in anesthetized patients, as the tip of the scope enters at an acute angle to the epiglottis and posterior pharyngeal wall, thus making it more difficult to expose the cords. In awake, sedated patients after topical anesthesia of the base of the tongue, pharynx, glottis, and trachea, a bite block or airway is used to prevent accidental biting on the scope, which can damage the instrument beyond repair. A Berman type II oral airway is effective for this purpose, as it also keeps the tongue from prolapsing posteriorly and blocking the view. An endotracheal tube is then placed inside the Berman airway, the tip of the tube flush with the end of the airway, which is then placed in the mouth. The scope is then passed through the endotracheal tube into the oropharynx for glottis exposure. Airway and endotracheal tube must be in the midline to avoid entering the pyriform sinus or the side of the mouth. A large relaxed epiglottis, the tip either close to or touching the pharyngeal wall, results in poor glottis exposure.

In an anesthetized, paralyzed patient in whom intubation attempts have failed, either oral or nasal fiberoptic intubation can be substituted. Bleeding and secretions may obscure the landmarks. The lungs should be oxygenated via face mask followed by suctioning and then fiberoptic laryngoscopy. If not successful, the patient is allowed to resume spontaneous breathing to provide better tissue tone. In addition, movement of the epiglottis and vocal cords assists in locating and identifying the glottis.

Pediatric Usage

The large diameter of the fiberoptic laryngoscope and most bronchoscopes prohibits the use of the previously described techniques in infants and small children.

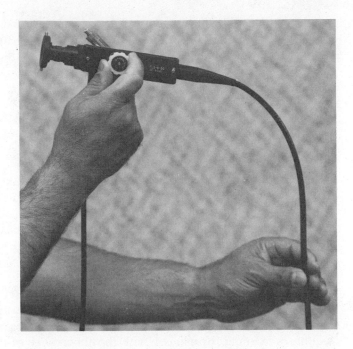

FIGURE 16–6. Flexible fiberoptic laryngoscope.

Stiles has described a method of using a fiberoptic pediatric bronchoscope and a cardiac catheter with a pliable guide wire for tracheal intubation in infants.

After general anesthesia is established, a fiberoptic bronchoscope is passed as far as the vocal cords, if possible through the cords, to the level of the cricoid cartilage. An assistant threads the cardiac catheter guide wire through the suction port of the scope; when the wire is seen at the tip, threading is continued until the wire meets resistance, which is assumed to be in the peripheral bronchial tree. The bronchoscope is then withdrawn, leaving the wire in the trachea. At this time the lungs may be ventilated, although if breathing spontaneously the cords may close, necessitating use of a neuromuscular blocker. A cardiac catheter is then passed over the guide wire into the trachea, and an endotracheal tube is slipped over the catheter into the trachea. The catheter and its guide wire are withdrawn as one, leaving the endotracheal tube in place.

Another approach is to insert a small fiberscope through one nostril, identifying the glottis, then pass a well-lubricated nasotracheal tube through the opposite nostril to the supraglottic area. With visualization of the nasotracheal tube through the scope it is then possible to manipulate the tube through the vocal cords into the trachea.

Miscellaneous Uses of the Fiberoptic Laryngoscope

Fiberoptic evaluation of upper airway obstruction in children permits differentiation of epiglottitis from subglottic edema and other less common causes of airway obstruction and can be utilized to intubate the trachea in the presence of epiglottitis.

The extent of laryngeal and tracheal injury following long-term tracheal intubation can be evaluated following extubation, photographs taken for the record and for follow-up comparison. In an intensive care unit the position of the tip of the endotracheal tube in relation to the carina can be verified with the fiberscope, excluding the need for a chest x-ray to detect endobronchial intubation.

To change an endotracheal tube expeditiously without losing control of the airway, the scope is passed through a fresh endotracheal tube nasally or orally placed and advanced alongside the already positioned endotracheal tube into the trachea until the carina is exposed. The used endotracheal tube is then withdrawn and the fresh endotracheal tube advanced over the scope into the trachea.

Cleaning and Sterilization

The control unit of the scope is cleansed with alcohol, the insertion cord cleansed with disinfectant solution such as 2 per cent glutaraldehyde, and the working channel flushed with the same solution. For cold sterilization only the insertion cord should be soaked in disinfectant solution, for 10 to 20 minutes.

A fully automatic portable washer for flexible endoscopes is available using foaming water and disinfectant to clean the interior channels and exterior insertion tube of endoscopes. Automatic processing minimizes handling of delicate scopes during washing and provides rapid uniform cleaning.

Ethylene oxide can be used for sterilization of the entire scope. The recommendations of the manufacturer should be followed to avoid damage to the instrument.

Appraisal

Complete familiarity with the fiberoptic laryngoscope and its use is essential for successful employment of the instrument. Such experience is gained in patients with normal airways under elective circumstances. Practice with a tracheobronchial model facilitates learning. Familiarity with the appearance of the airway as seen through the fiberscope and problems created by secretions may be gained by exposure of the epiglottis and vocal cords immediately postoperatively.

CARE AFTER TRACHEAL INTUBATION

The first steps after intubation include observation for chest movement while the lungs are inflated with oxygen and listening for breath sounds bilaterally high in the axillae to be sure that the trachea, not the esophagus or bronchus, has been intubated. A long tube may easily enter the right main stem bronchus, which comes off the trachea at a lesser angle than the left. Failure of the left side of the chest to move with ventilation or absence of breath sounds suggests bronchial intubation. Inflation of the cuff can be detected with the fingers straddling the trachea just above the manubrium; this suggests that bronchial intubation has not occurred. After orotracheal intubation, an oropharyngeal airway or soft bite block is placed between the teeth to prevent biting on the tube. The tube is secured with adhesive or umbilical tape tied around the neck. Suturing into place may be required for some maxillofacial operations. When there are excessive secretions, as in the face-down position, or when solutions used to prepare the operative field may loosen the adhesive, preparation of the skin with tincture of benzoin before application of the tape is helpful. Nasotracheal tubes should also be securely fixed with the connector at the level of the nares but not pressing on cartilage.

Cough after intubation frequently occurs when topical anesthesia is inadequate, in light planes of general anesthesia, and when the tube touches the carina. If cough is mild, transient hypertension and tachycardia result. In the more severe reaction, the spasm of thoracic muscles and bronchospasm may be difficult to overcome; ventilation may be impaired, resulting in hypoxia. If the tube is touching the carina, it should be withdrawn slightly. In more intractable cases, intravenous injection of a small dose of tubocurarine or pancuronium accompanied by controlled ventilation will relieve chest wall spasm.

After cuff inflation and fastening of the tube, the anesthetist should again be sure that bronchial intubation has not occurred. If so, the tube should be withdrawn until breath sounds are equally audible bilaterally. Sometimes there is increased resistance to respiration if the bevel of the tube lies against the tracheal wall.

When the patient's position on the operating table is changed, the position of the tube should again be verified. Flexion of the head or steep Trendelenburg position may cause the tube to enter the right main stem bronchus.

Occasionally the tracheal tube may be inserted into the esophagus. This is suggested by the absence of distinct breath sounds and progressive development of cyanosis. Listening over the stomach with a stethoscope should detect entry of air as the reservoir bag is compressed. If doubt exists, the tracheal tube should be removed immediately and ventilation carried out by means of a face mask. After tracheal intubation is accomplished, the stomach should be emptied of gas.

EXTUBATION

At the conclusion of anesthesia, extubation may result in unwanted sequelae. The tube should be removed to avoid laryngospasm and cough, either at a relatively deep plane of anesthesia or when the patient has reacted sufficiently to have reflex control. If a neuromuscular blocker has been used, extubation is delayed until spontaneous respiration has returned. Although it is essential to rid the trachea and pharynx of secretions prior to extubation, one should not persist to the point of causing continued cough and cyanosis. Secretions are aspirated from the upper airway, and the lubricated catheter is then passed through the tracheal tube, secretions aspirated, and the catheter withdrawn. Before and after aspiration, oxygen is administered; the cuff is deflated and the tube removed with the lungs inflated. A tube should not be removed with the aspirating catheter in place, for oxygen cannot be given; and if the catheter brushes against the vocal cords, bleeding or laryngospasm may occur. After removal of the tube, the patient is again given oxygen. Laryngospasm commonly follows but is less threatening if the lungs have been oxygenated prior to extubation.

A tracheal tube should not be removed in the presence of cyanosis, when respiratory exchange is inadequate or not controllable with mask and bag, or when the operation compromises the airway. In patients with intestinal obstruction, the tube is left in place as long as possible, and the stomach emptied via gastric tube before extubation. After maxillofacial operations resulting in a compromised airway, elective tracheostomy is performed before extubation. In the presence of inadequate respiratory exchange the tube is left in place and ventilation continued mechanically in the recovery room, an increasingly common practice in the anesthetic management of the critically ill and those who have been given a combination of opioid, nitrous oxide, and a neuromuscular blocker.

COMPLICATIONS

Tracheal intubation has become a commonplace technique often used for the convenience of the anesthetist rather than for the good of the patient. Some believe there are few complications, but we have seen many.

TRAUMA AT INTUBATION

Intubation may result in lacerated or bruised lips and tongue; chipped, loosened, or dislodged teeth; laceration of the pharynx; dislodged adenoid tissue, submucosal hemorrhage of the vocal cords; epistaxis; mediastinal and subcutaneous emphysema; and pneumothorax (see Chapter 33).

COMPLICATIONS DURING INTUBATION

Increased Resistance to Breathing.   Narrow tubes and adapters or acutely angulated connectors cause turbulent air flow, increasing the work of breathing and producing respiratory fatigue. Added resistance results in hypercapnia, hypoxia, hypertension, and tachycardia, predisposing to cardiac arrest.

Obstruction of the Tube.   This occurs as a result of collapse, kinking, foreign body, or secretions within the lumen; occlusion by biting; a dislodged cuff overriding the distal orifice; bevel of the tube against the tracheal wall; or imperfections in the tube causing flaplike valves.

Esophageal Intubation.   This is sometimes difficult to detect, a complication discovered by listening for breath sounds laterally over the chest and epigastrium. Failure to recognize esophageal intubation has resulted in cardiac arrest within minutes.

Bronchial Intubation.   This can be avoided by estimating the length of tube for each patient and by inserting the tube only 2 to 3 cm beyond the vocal cords. Bronchial obstruction may also result from an overinflated cuff.

Dislodgment.   Failure to fasten an endotracheal tube properly may cause displacement into pharynx or bronchus or dislodgment from nose and mouth.

Prolonged Cough and Chest Wall Spasm.   If these result from light anesthesia, the level of anesthesia is deepened. If chest wall spasm does not respond to positive pressure with oxygen within a reasonable time, a neuromuscular blocker is given to permit expansion of the lungs.

COMPLICATIONS FOLLOWING EXTUBATION

Laryngospasm.   Vocal cord spasm may follow extubation in lightly anesthetized patients; this is often alarming, particularly in infants and children, and is better prevented than treated. Treatment includes administration of oxygen under pressure with reservoir bag and mask, or injection of succinylcholine intravenously.

Tracheal Collapse.   Weakening of cartilaginous rings may be associated with large cervical tumors or goiter, and tracheal collapse may follow extubation.

Edema or Infection of Larynx or Trachea.   Improperly sterilized equipment, contaminated lubricants, insertion of an oversized tube, or an allergic response to the lubricant, rubber, or plastic may cause these reactions.

Hoarseness and Sore Throat.   Some degree of denudation of respiratory tract epithelium is inevitable upon intubation. Postoperatively, many patients experience sore throat and hoarseness, which invariably disappear within a day or two.

Ulceration of Tracheal Mucous Membrane.   This usually occurs on the anterior wall where the tip of the tube has abraded the epithelium.

Ulceration and Granuloma of Vocal Cords.   This complication is suspected when hoarseness persists for more than a few days. Contributing causes are trauma during intubation, tightly fitting tubes, protracted cough, undue movement of the head or tube, and allergic reaction to a lubricant. Most granulomas of the vocal cords seen by otolaryngologists are not attributable to anesthesia.

Aspiration of Gastrointestinal Contents.   This is commonly seen in the patient with intestinal obstruction extubated before protective reflexes return and may take place despite preventive measures in the aged and debilitated or in those with neurologic disease (see Chapter 33).

Vocal Cord Paralysis.   Unilateral cord paralysis may be seen after thyroidectomy. Bilateral paralysis can occur for other reasons, but we have seen this complication on several occasions after endotracheal anesthesia alone. Tubes sterilized with ethylene oxide may cause such paralysis despite presumed adequate airing, therefore it is probably a toxic effect.

This list of complications is impressive. We do not mean to dissuade anesthetists from intubation but rather to remind them of the consequences of a careless technique. Sequelae occur more commonly during the training period of the anesthetist, becoming less frequent as skill is achieved. Critical analysis of one's technique as well as that of others does much to increase the safety and comfort for the patient when intubation is performed.

REFERENCES

Applebaum EL, Bruce DL: Tracheal Intubation. Philadelphia, WB Saunders Co., 1976.

Bowes JD, Kelly DF, Peacock JH: Intubation trauma: Effect of short-term intubation on tracheal mucous membrane of the pig. Anaesthesia 28:603, 1973.

Gillespie NA: Endotracheal Anesthesia, 3rd ed, revised and edited by Bamforth BJ, Siebecker KL, Madison, University of Wisconsin Press, 1963.

Kaban LB: Dental and oral surgical problems in the preoperative patient. *In* Vandam LD (ed): To Make the Patient Ready for Anesthesia: Medical Care of the surgical patient. Menlo Park, Addison-Wesley, 1980.

Klainer AS, Turndorf H, Wu WH, et al: Surface alterations due to endotracheal intubation. Am J Med 58:674, 1975.

McGinnis GE, Shively JG, Patterson RL, et al: Engineering analysis of intratracheal tube cuffs. Anesth Analg 50:557, 1971.

Ovassapian A, Dykes MHM, Golmon ME: Fiberoptic nasotracheal intubation: A training program. Anesthesiology 53:S354, 1980.

Raj PP, Forestner J, Watson TD, et al: Technics for fiberoptic laryngoscopy in anesthesia. Anesth Analg 53:708, 1974.

Rosenbaum SH, Rosenbaum LM, Cole RP, Askanazi J, Hyman IA: Use of the flexible fiberoptic bronchoscope to change endotracheal tubes in critically ill patients. Anesthesiology 54:169, 1981.

Stanley TH, Kawamura R, Graves C: Effects of nitrous oxide on volume and pressure of endotracheal cuffs. Anesthesiology 41:256, 1974.

Stiles CM: A flexible fiberoptic bronchoscope for endotracheal intubation of infants. Anesth Analg 53:1017, 1974.

Vauthy PA, Reddy R: Acute upper airway obstruction in infants and children — evaluation by the fiberoptic bronchoscope. Ann Otol 89:417, 1980.

Chapter 17
EVALUATION OF THE RESPONSE TO ANESTHETICS: THE SIGNS AND STAGES

The need to evaluate a patient's response to anesthetics has existed from the very beginning. John Snow recognized certain signs as guidelines for the administration of ether or chloroform. As early as January of 1847, Plomley had described three stages of anesthesia; later Snow added a fourth. To facilitate teaching during World War I, Guedel codified a system that had been used clinically for ether administration for nearly 70 years. He clearly defined the four stages of anesthesia and described the respiratory changes, pupillary alterations, eye movements, and swallowing and vomiting responses that allow estimation of depth of ether anesthesia in any patient. In 1943, Gillespie added reflex responses; laryngeal and pharyngeal reactivity, lacrimation, and the respiratory response to surgical incision.

The Guedel system applied only to the unpremedicated patient allowed to breathe spontaneously during ether anesthesia, a situation that no longer exists in modern practice. Most patients receive either opioid or anticholinergic drugs as premedicants, and both alter the reliability of pupillary changes. The agents on which the system was based are now seldom used in the Western world. Halothane, enflurane, and isoflurane do not dilate the pupil but do cause a dose-related depression of blood pressure in the unstimulated patient. Respiratory tract secretions, lacrimation, and heightened airway reflex responses are usually absent. The variability among anesthetics is so great that no uniform system to evaluate depth of anesthesia is likely to evolve. Respiratory signs, the keystone of Guedel's system, are usually invalid in today's practice of controlled ventilation and use of neuromuscular blockers. Nevertheless, evaluation of the patient's physiologic response is an important guide to anesthetic dose requirements. Guedel's system will be described in brief, followed by a discussion of modifications of his approach required to assess the level of anesthesia in current practice.

GUEDEL'S SIGNS AND STAGES OF ETHER ANESTHESIA

A graphic presentation of the signs and stages of ether anesthesia is given in Figure 17–1 as taken from Gillespie's chart, which emphasizes reflex alterations. The converging lines indicate progressive loss of reflex activity as anesthesia deepens.

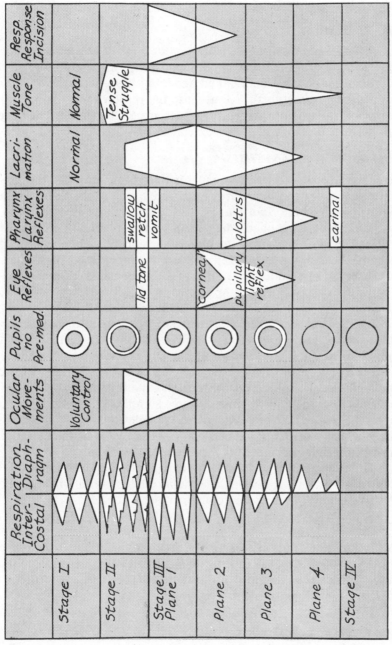

FIGURE 17–1. The signs and reflex reactions of the stages of anesthesia. (Reproduced with permission from Gillespie NA: Anesth Analg 22:275, 1943.)

STAGE 1 — AMNESIA AND ANALGESIA

Stage 1 is defined as lasting from the beginning of anesthesia to the loss of consciousness. Commonly called the stage of analgesia, sensation of pain is not absent and the pain threshold is apparently unchanged, but the patient's reaction to pain is altered. If warned, the patient will usually tolerate procedures that normally would not be accepted, e.g., minor operations or the pain of the second stage of labor.

STAGE II — DELIRIUM

Stage II, or the stage of delirium, lasts from the time of loss of consciousness to onset of a regular pattern of breathing and disappearance of the lid reflex. This is the state of unconsciousness with uninhibited reaction. Patients should not undergo stimulation of any kind during this stage because the response may be injurious. It is unwise to begin operation before the ensuing third stage has been reached because of the possibility of inducing movement or excitement.

STAGE III — SURGICAL ANESTHESIA

This stage lasts from the onset of a regular pattern of breathing to the cessation of respiration. Most surgical procedures are performed at one of the levels of this stage, which is arbitrarily divided into four planes.

Plane 1. This plane is reached when the lid reflex is abolished and respiration becomes regular. The eyes may oscillate and not infrequently are eccentrically fixed. The pupils become distinctly smaller when well into the first plane. The vomiting reflex in response to insertion of an oral airway is gradually abolished, as is the secretion of tears. The tendency for respiratory rate and depth to increase in response to skin incision decreases.

Plane 2. This plane lasts from the time the eyes cease to move and become concentrically fixed to the beginning of a decrease in intercostal muscle activity or thoracic respiration. Respirations remain regular but tidal volume is diminished, the rate tending to rise. The pupils begin to dilate. Reflex closing of the vocal cords or laryngospasm begins to disappear. Muscle tone lessens as anesthesia deepens.

Plane 3. Intercostal activity begins to decrease in this plane; the upper intercostals seem to become less active before the lower. Complete intercostal paralysis occurs in lower plane 3, whereas respiration is carried on solely by the diaphragm. It is unwise and unnecessary to maintain plane 3 for very long.

Plane 4. This plane extends from the time of paralysis of the intercostal muscles to cessation of spontaneous respiration. The pupils dilate and no longer react to light. There is little muscle tone, even in the robust person.

STAGE IV

Stage IV lasts from the time of cessation of respiration to failure of the circulation, where respiration fails first because of a high concentration of anesthetic in the central nervous system. This stage is premortem. Most reflexes are absent and the circulation is about to fail, a plane of anesthesia arrived at only in error.

CLINICAL ASSESSMENT OF ANESTHETIC REQUIREMENTS

Anesthetists currently use an approach different from that proposed by Guedel to evaluate the effects of anesthetics. His was a static system: ether at a given dose (although then unknown) produces a given effect. He neglected the patient as a responsive organism in whom graded stimuli produce graded responses. Anesthetics alter patient reactivity, allow input of multiple stimuli, yet limit the response. To evaluate the effect of an anesthetic, the anesthetist must consider both the stimulus and the response. Gillespie recognized this concept when he added response to surgical incision to Guedel's scheme. Today's anesthetists use a stimulus-response assessment to classify adequacy of anesthetic level; it is less well defined than Guedel's scheme but more operational.

STIMULUS-RESPONSE ASSESSMENT

Guedel's stages I and II are usually not seen during induction of anesthesia today because of the nearly routine use of intravenous induction techniques. Even during inhalation induction the two stages are not differentiated but are regarded together as presurgical anesthesia. Excitement may occur during this stage, and stimulation of the patient during induction must be avoided. Three signs generally identify surgical anesthesia: loss of lid reflex, muscle relaxation, and rhythmic respiration. If these have not occurred, then the patient is at a presurgical level and stimulation must be avoided.

Three levels of anesthetic depression are recognized with the stimulus-response assessment: presurgical anesthesia, surgical anesthesia, and overdose. Three planes of surgical anesthesia are accepted: too light, adequate, and too deep (Fig. 17–2). The thoughtful anesthetist follows a specific method in judging a patient's status: evaluation of afferent input to the nervous system; estimation of observable physiologic responses; and assessment of the interaction among patient, stimulus, and anesthetic and the level of surgical anesthesia.

Stimulus Assessment

This assessment is arbitrarily classified somewhere between strong and weak; strong stimulation resulting from a skin incision, anal or cervical dilation, periosteal stimulation, and the like; weak stimulation resulting from uterine curettage, retroperitoneal dissection, wound debridement, and the like. No appreciable stimulation occurs during surgical dissection of brain, muscle, and connective tissue; bowel or lung resection; and suturing. Inflammation usually enhances the intensity of the stimulus.

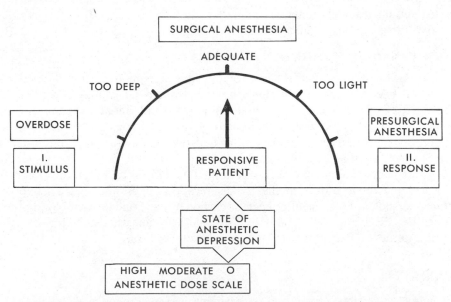

FIGURE 17–2. Schematic representation of evaluation of anesthetic requirements.

Careful surgical manipulation may diminish the stimulus, as does advancing age and diminishing physical status.

Response Evaluation

Woodbridge, recognizing the many subtle observations the anesthetist must make, cited four components of the anesthetic state: sensory, motor, mental, and reflex functions. Table 17–1 attempts to classify the intensity of responses that may be observed in reference to Woodbridge's components. Note that observations evaluating depression in any one component involve nearly all body systems, and a single response may relate to several components. For example, if a patient takes a deep breath, moves, and develops tachycardia and hypertension when an incision is made, it is obvious that sensory depression is inadequate. Whether motor depression is inadequate depends on the site of operation. The low intensity responses listed are undesirable in virtually every case, and most anesthetists avoid drug doses that result in such responses. Utilization of this system permits logical evaluation of specific drug effects in each of Woodbridge's components.

Depth of Anesthesia and Arterial Pressure.   Hypotension is the chief clinical sign of depth of anesthesia with halothane, with or without nitrous oxide. Hypercarbia, although not condoned, counteracts hypotension, and with time during administration of halothane the arterial pressure rises. Both effects probably are related to increased sympathetic nervous activity. Pain perception during light anesthesia causes arterial pressure to rise. Enflurane and isoflurane resemble halothane in their actions on blood pressure.

Evaluation of Anesthetic Requirement.   A comparison of strength of surgical stimulus and observation of intensity of response allows for evaluation of specific anesthetic requirements. If the response is excessive in a specific area, compensatory adjustments are needed. A higher concentration of inhalation anesthetic may be administered with recognition that this may increase depression in all areas; alternately, a specific drug, a neuromuscular blocker, may correct the defect. Observations are repeatedly made and adjustments instituted. Occasionally, the system is disturbed by design to test the resulting response; the anesthetist may increase or reduce the inhaled concentration of anesthetic to observe the effect. In fact, as anesthesia progresses, the anesthetist should gradually reduce the inhaled concentration and observe the effect to prevent overdose as body tissues become saturated.

ADDITIONAL OBSERVATIONS

A correlation of the clinical signs of anesthesia with the arterial level of the anesthetic has been attempted. Although the depth of anesthesia may correlate closely with the arterial concentration of anesthetic for any one individual, the same concentration of anesthesia in a population of individuals gives wide deviations in depth. For this reason and because arterial concentration of anesthetic is ascertained only after some delay, it is rarely used as a clinical guide to depth.

The electroencephalogram (EEG) has limited usefulness as a monitor of anesthetic depth. Each anesthetic differs in the EEG alterations it produces (see Chapter 12). Other factors, such as tensions of oxygen or carbon dioxide and level of blood pressure, can alter the EEG and thus the EEG response to anesthetics. Moreover, each anesthetic interacts differently with these modifying factors.

APPRAISAL

In many ways, this procedural assessment is a restatement of what the good clinician has always done. As powers of observation improve and experience increases,

TABLE 17–1. Evaluation of Response Intensity

Woodbridge Component	Sensory	Motor	Mental	Reflexes Circulatory	Reflexes Respiratory	Reflexes Gastrointestinal
High intensity response	Breath holding Deep breathing Stiff chest Phonation Laryngospasm Tachycardia Rise or fall in BP Movement with stimulus Pupillary dilation Sweating Coughing	Fine or gross movement Abdominal tightness Muscle potentials on ECG	Movement upon stimulation Delirium Uninhibited speech or actions	Bradycardia and hypotension or Tachycardia and hypertension Arrhythmias	Spasm: laryngeal bronchiolar chest wall Salivation	Nausea Retching Vomiting Swallowing
Acceptable response	Minimal response to painful stimuli followed by accommodation Stability of cardiovascular and respiratory systems	Quiet surgical field Relaxation of muscle	Amnesia Ataxia Sleep	Absence of troublesome cardiovascular, respiratory, and gastrointestinal reflexes		
Low intensity response	No response	Muscle flaccidity Inability to reestablish normal ventilatory function at end of anesthesia	Prolonged obtundation in pre- or postanesthetic period	Bradycardia Tachycardia Hypotension Arrhythmias Intolerance to position change	Respiratory arrest*	Intestinal atony Postoperative ileus

*In the absence of neuromuscular blockers or hypocarbia.

the beginner will find that a combination of signs provides a satisfactory guide to anesthetic depth. It is well known, for example, that reactivity to stimuli diminishes with age and is always less marked in the critically ill. The anesthetist must be alert and observant to prevent overdose.

General anesthesia usually appears to be deeper than it actually is. It is usually easier to lighten than to deepen anesthesia. Therefore, induction should be carried a little further than seems necessary for the incision, so that the difficulties associated with inadequate anesthesia are not encountered. A middle course must be steered between light and unnecessarily deep anesthesia.

REFERENCES

Artusio JF: Diethyl ether analgesia: A detailed description of the first stage of ether anesthesia in man. J. Pharmacol Exp Ther 3:343, 1954.

Clark DL, Hosick EC, Rosner BS: Neurophysiologic effects of different anesthetics in unconscious man. J Appl Physiol 31:884, 1971.

Cullen DJ, Eger EI II, Stevens EC, et al: Clinical signs of anesthesia. Anesthesiology 36:21, 1972.

Eger EI II: Anesthetic Uptake and Action. Baltimore, Williams & Wilkins Co, 1974.

Gillespie NA: The signs of anesthesia. Anesth Analg 22:275, 1943.

Guedel AE: Inhalation Anesthesia. 2nd ed, New York, The Macmillan Co, 1951, pp. 10–52.

Woodbridge PD: Changing concepts concerning depth of anesthesia. Anesthesiology 18:536, 1958.

REGIONAL ANESTHESIA

Chapter 18

LOCAL ANESTHETICS

The introduction of local anesthesia followed that of general anesthesia by about 40 years. Niemann, in 1860, first observed the numbing effect on the tongue of cocaine, an alkaloid obtained from the coca plant. In 1884, after Koller had produced topical anesthesia by instillation of cocaine into the conjunctival sac, the principle of local anesthesia gained quick acceptance. Perhaps this resulted from a dissatisfaction with the general anesthesia given at the time; furthermore, surgeons could now provide anesthesia for their own operations. The subsequent development of local anesthesia was assured by the synthesis of more reliable local anesthetics and the introduction of new techniques of regional anesthesia.

Local anesthesia is useful for the following reasons:

1. Simplicity: The costs are reasonable, the agents injectable, and the equipment required minimal. The need for postoperative care of the patient is lessened.

2. Most of the undesirable side effects of general anesthesia are avoided. A localized area of the body can be operated upon without loss of consciousness, hence the term ''regional'' anesthesia. Modern studies support the anoci-association theory of Crile, which held that impulses from the operative area could be stressful and could cause circulatory collapse. Regional anesthesia decreases the autonomic and endocrine response to stress through interference with afferent nerve conduction.

3. The methods are appropriate for ambulatory patients, for brief and superficial operations, and in situations in which recently ingested food poses the threat of regurgitation and aspiration during general anesthesia. If the patient's cooperation is needed, local anesthesia is a valuable technique.

Some of the reasons why regional anesthesia is not more widely used are as follows:

1. Lack of patient acceptance; patients choose to be unaware of the operation. This opposition results in part from an ineffectual approach to the patient and from anesthetists' lack of skill in the performance of nerve blocks.

2. The impracticality of anesthetizing some body areas. For example, the number of injections, the quantity of anesthetic required, and the time consumed in providing local anesthesia for a modified radical mastectomy would be prohibitive.

3. Insufficient duration of local anesthesia: the patient fears that the anesthesia will wear off prematurely. There are, however, agents and special techniques that prolong anesthesia considerably.

4. Rapid absorption of local anesthetics into the bloodstream with untoward, but

rarely fatal, reactions. Although the mechanisms and the means of prevention and treatment are understood, reactions may occur because of variations in human responsiveness. These reactions, however, should be minimal if precautions are taken.

THEORIES OF ACTION

Local anesthetics applied to the body surfaces and injected about nerves are used primarily to prevent pain during surgical procedures. They are also used in the treatment of pain associated with trauma or disease. A good way to explain their action is to relate anesthetic activity to the transmission of the nerve impulse.

Nerve fibers, like all cells, possess a lipoprotein membrane that separates the intracellular from the extracellular fluid. Concentration gradients between the intracellular fluid containing potassium, the major cation, and the extracellular fluid containing sodium are maintainted by an active metabolic process. Properties of this membrane are such that permeability to different ions alters with variations in transmembrane potential. In the resting state the membrane is relatively permeable to potassium but much less so to sodium, so that the concentration gradient for potassium is the major determinant of the membrane potential (-70 to -90 mv), with the exterior positive relative to the interior. As the nerve impulse spreads, partial depolarization triggers depolarization via a major increase in permeability to sodium (Fig. 18–1A). The membrane potential transiently approximates that predicted from the concentration gradient of sodium (the outside becomes negative relative to the inside), and depolarization is electrically conducted to adjacent areas of the membrane (Fig. 18–1B). This sequence of events occurs successively as the impulse spreads along the nerve. During the later phase of depolarization, the membrane again becomes less permeable to sodium, which is extruded by an active process, and the nerve returns to the resting state, ready within milliseconds to repeat the response.

Local anesthetics increase the threshold for electric excitation in the nerve; slow the propagation of the impulse, reduce the rate of rise of the action potential, and eventually block conduction. These compounds act on nerve fibers by interfering with the ability of the membrane to undergo the specific change in permeability to sodium as a response to partial depolarization. The membrane is said to be stabilized at resting potential.

There are two theories as to how a local anesthetic may interact with the membrane. First, binding of local anesthetic molecules to receptors at the cell

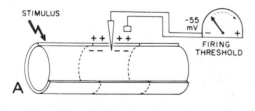

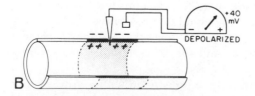

FIGURE 18–1. A, Upon stimulation, voltage across the membrane reaches -55 mv, the axon's firing threshold. B, Depolarization now complete, with the interior of the membrane 40 mv, positive in relation to the exterior. (Reproduced with permission from de Jong, RH: Physiology and Pharmacology of Local Anesthesia. Springfield, Ill., Charles C Thomas, 1970.)

membrane may increase stability and prevent the opening of channels or pores for passage of the electrolytes. The anesthetic may act internally or externally at the channel opening. A conformational change in proteins associated with lipids may lead to expansion of the membrane, hence the membrane expansion theory. A second explanation involves the binding of calcium, which is displaced from the membrane during impulse transmission, thereby allowing more ready access of sodium. Local anesthetics may increase the binding of calcium to the membrane. This is known as the surface charge theory.

In myelinated nerve, in which the speed of conduction is facilitated by saltatory conduction, local anesthetic action takes place at the nodes of Ranvier, where the neurilemma or sheath of Schwann is present but the myelin sheath is interrupted.

DIFFERENTIAL BLOCKADE

Passage of an impulse between electrodes placed on a peripheral nerve can be displayed on an oscilloscope, with delineation of a characteristic mixed action potential. As shown by studies on electric potentials in mixed nerves, fibers of different size conduct impulses at different speeds; conduction velocity is proportional to fiber diameter. On this basis fibers may be classified as belonging to an A, B, or C group. The A fibers, from 1 μ to 22 μ in diameter, carry afferent and efferent somatic impulses at rates up to 90 m per sec. Large fibers also have the lowest excitability threshold. The smallest fibers, those carrying impulses for superficial pain, temperature, and autonomic activity, conduct slowly, and these modalities are for the most part blocked early by local anesthetics; as a corollary, weak concentrations of local anesthetics interrupt conduction in small fibers first. No theory has yet been proposed that adequately explains why the small myelinated fibers are more susceptible to block than the large. The ability to block nerve fibers differentially has been useful in diagnosis and therapy, as, for example, in differential subarachnoid block when one wishes to determine whether pain is visceral or somatic in origin.

When a local anesthetic is deposited at the site of a peripheral nerve that carries both afferent sensory and efferent motor fibers, onset of anesthesia occurs first in those fibers that are peripherally located, i.e., in the mantle. Thus the pattern of onset of anesthesia does not follow that predicted for small and large fibers.

LOCAL ANESTHETIC DRUGS

More than a few reliable local anesthetics are available, but the anesthetist should understand the characteristics of a few drugs, employ those with the greatest advantages, and use only those that have passed the test of time. The attributes of an acceptable local anesthetic are complete reversibility of action, freedom from local irritation, high potency, effectiveness topically as well as regionally, minimal systemic toxicity, ready metabolism, stability during storage and sterilization, and a readily soluble synthetic molecule that permits chemical assay.

ESTER COMPOUNDS

Cocaine

Cocaine is still employed today in the form of hydrochloric acid salt, used in 4 to 10 per cent concentrations for topical anesthesia of the nose, pharynx, and tracheobronchial tree. No more than 200 mg should be applied at a time. The vasoconstrictive property of cocaine, unequaled by other local anesthetics, is useful in decreasing bleeding and in shrinking congested mucous membranes. Vasoconstriction occurs because cocaine prevents re-uptake of norepinephrine at nerve endings; thus epinephrine should not be added to cocaine solutions. Cocaine was abandoned in ophthalmology because it causes opacity of the cornea and retards corneal epithelial regeneration, as do other topical anesthetics. The high incidence of toxic reactions after injection of this drug, the liability to addiction, and the difficulty in preparing sterile solutions led to a search for a synthetic compound with better properties.

The clue to anesthetic activity lies in the structure of cocaine, an ester of benzoic acid, and the methylated base, ecgonine; the latter is related to tropine, the basic portion of the atropine molecule. Many local anesthetics subsequently synthesized have retained the ester structure and the chemical suffix "caine" in their nomenclature. The prototype of the esters consists of an aromatic lipophilic group, an intermediate group of several carbon atoms (ester linkage), and a hydrophilic group. The structure is as follows:

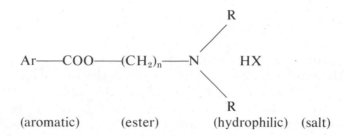

The basic part of the ester is usually a tertiary amino alcohol, which combines with acids to form soluble salts of weakly acidic reaction. The other portion of the ester is usually an aromatic acid with substituted radicals at various locations in the phenol ring. Most useful local anesthetics are secondary or tertiary amines, the compounds existing both as uncharged molecules (B) and as positively charged substituted ammonium cations (BH^+). The relative proportion of the two forms depends on the pH of the solution and the pK_a of the anesthetic according to the Henderson-Hasselbalch equation (see Chapter 4).

Local anesthetic solutions are marketed in the salt form and thus are more stable chemically and more water soluble than the free base. There is good evidence indicating that the salt form must be neutralized to the free base before the drug can penetrate nerve membranes. There is agreement that the tertiary amines penetrate the nerve membrane in the uncharged form and block the action potential from inside the membrane in charged form.

The ester compounds are hydrolyzed by esterases in plasma, of major importance in their metabolism when absorbed into the bloodstream. The amino group bears resemblance to the quaternary amine structure of neuromuscular blockers. Since the latter compete with acetylcholine at receptor sites, some of the adverse reactions of local anesthetics may result from interference with central or peripheral synaptic transmission.

Procaine

Einhorn in 1904 synthesized procaine, an ester of diethylaminoethanol and p-aminobenzoic acid. Procaine hydrochloride lacks topical activity but was once widely used because of minimal systemic toxicity, lack of local irritation, ease of sterilization, short duration of action, and low cost. The brevity of action and lack of a cumulative, toxic concentration in plasma result from the rapid hydrolysis by pseudocholinesterase.

Chloroprocaine

Halogen substitution in the aromatic portion of the procaine molecule yields substances that are rapidly hydrolyzed in plasma and therefore less toxic than the parent compound. Chloroprocaine hydrochloride (Nesacaine), like procaine, is not topically active but is more potent and has a shorter duration of action. It is probably the safest local anesthetic from the standpoint of systemic toxicity; hence it is advocated for use in continuous peridural anesthesia. Concentrations employed for anesthesia range from 0.5 to 2.0 per cent in doses not exceeding 1 gm. Concern has arisen over the development of sensory and motor deficits following use of chloroprocaine for epidural anesthesia when the subarachnoid space was inadvertently entered. Some would attribute this reaction to the highly acidic nature of the anesthetic solution.

Tetracaine

The third drug in the ester series is tetracaine hydrochloride (Pontocaine, Pantocaine, Amethocaine). The potency of this compound is higher and the duration of action longer than those of the other anesthetics mentioned, the systemic toxicity being correspondingly greater. The slow rate of hydrolysis in plasma explains in part the high incidence of reactions, but the low total dosage counteracts this disadvantage. Tetracaine is injected in 0.1 per cent concentration when the duration of anesthesia required is longer than several hours. It is the most commonly employed anesthetic for spinal anesthesia, usually combined with an equal volume of 10 per cent dextrose to increase the specific gravity and thereby control spread of the solution. As a topical anesthetic in the pharynx and tracheobronchial tree, tetracaine is employed in 1 to 2 per cent concentrations. In the conjunctival sac tetracaine retards corneal epithelial regeneration. The rapid rate of absorption from the respiratory tract mucosa accounts for the many adverse reactions reported; quantities greater than 100 mg should not be applied at one time.

AMIDES

The structure of the amide local anesthetics is essentially the same as that of the esters except for the amide linkage. As a consequence, these compounds are less readily metabolized and tend to accumulate in plasma, and the liability of adverse reactions is greater. On the other hand, some have significant antiarrhythmic effects on the heart.

Dibucaine

Dibucaine hydrochloride (Nupercaine, Percaine, Cinchocaine), a substituted amide, is a potent anesthetic with high systemic toxicity and long duration of action. However, because of the lesser concentration needed, there are fewer adverse reactions. Dibucaine is used infrequently for topical anesthesia of mucous membranes as an ointment in 0.2 per cent concentration; it was once popular for spinal anesthesia and is still available.

Lidocaine

Lidocaine hydrochloride (Xylocaine), an acetanilid derivative, has achieved widespread acceptance since its introduction by Löfgren in 1948. Its major advantages are rapid onset of anesthesia and freedom from local irritation. Potency and duration of action are moderately greater than those for procaine, and topical activity, although good, is not as effective as that of cocaine. Lidocaine lacks the vasoconstrictive property of cocaine and because of the amide structure is slowly detoxified in circulating plasma. Some of the drug is metabolized in liver microsomes and part is excreted unchanged in urine. For these reasons the drug is considered twice as toxic as procaine, and doses greater than 0.5 gm should not be used when the recommended 0.5 to 2.0 per cent concentrations are employed for injection. Concentrations of 4 per cent are employed for topical anesthesia; 80 mg seems to be a safe dose. Lidocaine is remarkably free from allergic reactions and therefore is a good substitute for the ester compounds when reactions to the latter have occurred.

Mepivacaine

Mepivacaine hydrochloride (Carbocaine) incorporates an amide radical linked to a saturated heterocyclic ring of the piperidine group. In comparison to lidocaine, mepivacaine acts equally quickly, but duration of anesthesia is approximately 20 per cent longer. For this reason the addition of epinephrine is not required for nerve block of ordinary duration. Concentrations suggested range from 1 to 4 per cent for injection and topical anesthesia, with the maximal dosage no higher than 500 mg. Adverse reactions are few, and studies on its metabolism are not extensive. Although tissue irritation is minimal, the drug has not been used in spinal anesthesia.

Bupivacaine

Bupivacaine hydrochloride (Marcaine) was synthesized in 1957 by Ekenstam and has been extensively used since. The compound, an anilide derivative, differs from mepivacaine in that a butyl group is substituted for the methyl. More potent and with a markedly longer action than lidocaine or mepivacaine, probably as a result of increased tissue protein binding, the drug is used in concentrations ranging from 0.25 to 0.75 per cent for the complete span of regional nerve blocks. Epinephrine in 1:200,000 concentration is added to the solution when indicated; the total amount of drug injected at a time should not exceed 200 to 500 mg, since its toxicity approximates that of tetracaine. With weaker concentrations, motor fiber block is inadequate, 0.75 per cent being necessary for that purpose in abdominal operations. Although onset of anesthesia may be somewhat slower than with lidocaine or mepivacaine, the duration is two to three times longer. Upon repeated injection the drug accumulates in the bloodstream, with arterial concentrations 20 to 40 per cent higher than the venous; the placental barrier is readily crossed. The drug has been only sparingly used for spinal and intravenous regional anesthesia.

Etidocaine

Etidocaine (Duranest), the most recently introduced of the local anesthetics, is an amide structurally similar to lidocaine but of greater potency and longer duration of action. Its properties in relation to the others are shown in Table 18–1; its general pharmacologic and toxicologic actions differ little from the group characteristics.

Table 18–1 lists the local anesthetics discussed in this chapter and their structure-activity relationships, whereas Table 18–2 lists some data of practical use in regional anesthesia.

LONG-ACTING LOCAL ANESTHESIA

In the treatment of postoperative and chronic, intractable pain, the need exists for a local anesthetic with a duration of action longer than six to eight hours. Hence bupivacaine and etidocaine have been useful additions to the existing armamentarium of local anesthetics. One must bear in mind that local anesthesia by definition is a reversible process. In this respect, the long-lasting effects of certain proprietary compounds do not represent true anesthesia; careful histologic examination after experimental injection of these compounds often reveals destruction of nerve fibers.

Solutions of local anesthetics in oil were once thought to act as repositories from which the anesthetic was gradually released, thereby extending its action. Prolongation of anesthesia has not been demonstrated by this means. In some instances the oily base remains at the site, causing abscess or granuloma formation. Proprietary long-acting anesthetic mixtures often contained benzyl alcohol, eugenol, bromosaligenin (Bromsalizol), salicyl alcohol (Saligenin), or phenol. These agents are not local anesthetics and are destructive to nerve fibers. One must be certain never to inject these solutions near the larger peripheral nerves or in the vicinity of the spinal cord, for the resulting neuritis may lead to pain more severe than that originally experienced or may cause transverse myelitis. However, in the treatment of the intractable pain of terminal malignancy or to relieve the muscle spasm of paraplegia, weak solutions of ethyl alcohol or phenol, 6 per cent, have been injected into the subarachnoid space. In these situations the resulting neurologic deficit is overbalanced by the therapeutic effect.

INTRAVENOUS USE OF LOCAL ANESTHETICS

Although high blood levels of local anesthetic are responsible for most adverse systemic effects, several of the local anesthetics have been given intravenously either as adjuncts to general anesthesia or in the treatment of a miscellaneous group of ailments. Procaine was once given not only to treat cardiac arrhythmias but as a continuous infusion in 0.1 per cent concentration to add to the effect of general anesthesia. Although central nervous system stimulation was not observed if the drug was given carefully, the frequent appearance of hypotension led to abandonment.

Intravenous injection of lidocaine has been advocated for the same reasons that led to the use of procaine. Lidocaine appears to depress laryngeal and tracheal reflexes, thereby permitting maintenance of pharyngeal and tracheal airways in light planes of general anesthesia. Patients thus treated are said to require less analgetics for pain and to vomit less postoperatively. Because of its antiarrhythmic properties, lidocaine is effective during cardiac surgery, in resuscitation after cardiac arrest, and for treatment of irritability in myocardial infarction.

TOPICAL ANESTHESIA

Topical anesthesia is often inexpertly done, thus the incidence of adverse reactions is high. Preliminary topical anesthesia of the respiratory passages is useful in eliminating pharyngeal and tracheal reflexes and cough when airways are inserted before induction or during light planes of general anesthesia. The drugs used for this purpose have been described, and the safe dosage limits are listed in Table 18–2. Preferably only one topical agent should be used for a procedure. Blood levels of local anesthetic during topical anesthesia may equal those obtained after intravenous injection, and primary myocardial depression is the probable cause of sudden collapse; therefore, preparation should be made for resuscitation should such a reaction occur.

Because topical anesthetization is an uncomfortable procedure, appropriate preanesthetic sedation should be provided and atropine given for the drying effect. Salivary secretions interfere with anesthesia by diluting the anesthetic and preventing sufficient contact with mucous membranes.

Anesthetic ointments should be water soluble and sterile. Ointments are often applied to airways before insertion but unless preceded by topical anesthesia they do not immediately prevent cough. At least one minute is required for onset of anesthesia with most topical drugs, the duration of anesthesia being no longer than 20 to 30 minutes. Either a water-soluble jelly or solution may be introduced into the pharynx. Once anesthesia of the pharynx has been obtained, a small amount of anesthetic can be

Table 18–1. Structure–Activity Relationships of Local Anesthetics

Agent	Chemical Configuration			Physico-Chemical Properties		Biological Properties		
	Aromatic Lipophilic	Intermediate Chain	Amine Hydrophilic	Partition Coefficient	% Protein Binding	Equi-Effective* Anesthetic Conc.	Approx. Anesthetic* Duration (min.)	Site of Metabolism
A. Esters								
PROCAINE	H_2N-⟨benzene⟩	$COOCH_2CH_2-$	$-N(C_2H_5)(C_2H_5)$	0.6†	5.8§	2	50	Plasma
TETRACAINE	$H_9C_4-N(H)-$⟨benzene⟩	$COOCH_2CH_2-$	$-N(CH_3)(CH_3)$	80†	75.6§	0.25	175	Plasma
B. Amides								
MEPIVACAINE	⟨dimethylphenyl⟩	NHCO	⟨N-CH₃ pyrrolidine⟩	0.8‡	77.5‖	1	100	Liver

BUPIVACAINE		27.5‡	95.6‖	0.25	175	Liver
LIDOCAINE		2.9‡	64.3‖	1	100	Liver
ETIDOCAINE		141‡	94‖	0.25	200	Liver

*Data derived from rat sciatic nerve blocking procedure
†Oleylalcohol/pH 7.2 buffer
‡n-Heptane/pH 7.4 buffer
§Nerve homogenate binding
‖Plasma protein binding—2 μg/ml
Reproduced with permission from Covino BG, Vassallo HG: Local Anesthetics. Mechanisms of Action and Clinical Use. New York, Grune & Stratton, 1976.

TABLE 18–2.   Suggested Uses, Concentrations, and
Maximal Dosage of the Local Anesthetics*

Drugs	Topical	Dose (mg)	Injection	Dose (mg)
Esters				
Cocaine hydrochloride	Respiratory tract 5–10% (4–2 ml)	200	Not employed	
Procaine hydrochloride Novocain Ethocaine	Ineffective		Infiltration 0.5% (200 ml) Peripheral nerves 1–2% (100–50 ml)	1000
Chloroprocaine hydro- chloride Nesacaine	Ineffective		Infiltration 0.5% (200 ml) Peripheral nerves 2% (50 ml)	1000
Tetracaine hydrochloride Pontocaine Pantocaine	Respiratory tract 1–2% (8–4 ml)	80	Infrequently used for infiltration and nerve injection, 0.1 to 0.25%	100
Amides				
Dibucaine hydrochloride Nupercaine Percaine Cinchocaine	Infrequently used 0.2% (15 ml)	30	Infrequently used	
Lidocaine hydrochloride Xylocaine lignocaine	Respiratory tract 2–4% (10–5 ml)	200	Infiltration 0.5% (100 ml) Peripheral nerves 1–2% (50–25 ml)	500
Mepivacaine hydrochloride Carbocaine	No data		Infiltration 0.5–1.0% (100–50 ml) Peripheral nerves 1–2%	500
Bupivacaine hydrochloride Marcaine	No data		Infiltration and periph- eral nerves 0.25–0.75%	500
Etidocaine hydrochloride Duranest	No data		Infiltration and periph- eral nerves 0.25–0.75%	500

*Use of local anesthetics for specialized techniques is not shown.

instilled into the trachea under direct vision. Spraying or atomization is commonly employed but is often ineptly done because the droplets vary so much in size. Large droplets from an ordinary spray cause cough and lead to overdose, whereas small droplets from a nebulizer traverse finer bronchioles and are rapidly absorbed, with toxic effects. The most efficient atomizers supply droplets ranging in size from 30 to 100 μ; these devices should incorporate a reservoir so that the quantity of drug used can be readily observed. Prepackaged syringes containing lidocaine for topical anesthesia are commercially available.

A safe concentration and volume of anesthetic (tetracaine 1 per cent or lidocaine 4 per cent, 2 ml total) can be injected into the trachea percutaneously through the cricothyroid membrane; the resulting cough helps to spread the anesthetic. At the same time, superior laryngeal nerve block can be done. This is done aseptically and is used only in situations where anatomic relations are clearly defined and there is no local disease. Vigorous cough is hazardous in certain types of valvular heart disease in which hypoxia and the Valsalva effect can lead to circulatory collapse.

ADVERSE EFFECTS OF LOCAL ANESTHETICS

Untoward reactions to local anesthetics are often erroneously ascribed to sensitivity or idiosyncrasy, whereas they can be explained on known pharmacologic grounds even though exceedingly small doses may have been responsible for the effects observed.

SYSTEMIC REACTIONS

Cause

The systemic reactions encountered involve the central nervous, respiratory, and cardiovascular systems. These reactions result from absorption via the bloodstream of toxic amounts of the drug into the CNS, causing convulsions, drowsiness, or unconsciousness. Whether a depressive or excitatory response occurs seems to depend on a balance of effect between inhibitory and excitatory centers in the brain. The excitatory response is enhanced by respiratory and metabolic acidosis. The depressant effect on the medullary centers may lead to apnea and vascular collapse. Local anesthetics depress the myocardium directly by a quinidinelike effect on conduction, contractility, and irritability. For this reason, procaine and lidocaine have been employed as antiarrhythmic agents. The hypotension resulting from the action on the myocardium is compounded by a peripheral vasodilatory action. Part of the depressive action may be countered by reactive sympathetic activity. Some or all of these effects occur rapidly in response to injection of much less than the expected toxic doses. The most feared outcome is simultaneous respiratory and cardiac arrest.

Because the circulating blood level of anesthetic is a prime factor in systemic reactions, the site of injection is of paramount importance. The intravenous route is most dangerous, but absorption from the pharyngeal, tracheal, and bronchial mucosa yields high blood concentrations almost as rapidly because of the vascularity of these areas, rapid absorption of anesthetic from the lungs, and direct circulation of the drug to the myocardium. Thus it is not surprising that most instances of sudden cardiovascular collapse involve topical anesthesia of the respiratory tract. Other hazardous injection sites include tissues about the head and neck and the paravertebral region; least dangerous are the subcutaneous areas of the trunk and limbs. Hyaluronidase, because of its spreading action, is sometimes added to local anesthetic solutions to increase the percentage of successful nerve blocks, but systemic reactions occur more frequently because of rapid absorption. Anesthetic solutions taken by mouth and swallowed result in few reactions, probably because of absorption into the portal venous system and rapid metabolism in liver.

A second factor in the causation of reactions is the rapidity of hydrolysis once an anesthetic reaches the circulation. The enzymes involved are cholinesterases formed in the liver. Hydrolysis of the ester compounds proceeds at varying rates, toxicity being related quantitatively to this factor alone. The generalization may be made, therefore, that the esters are less likely to be toxic than the amides.

Prevention

Total Amount of Anesthetic. The least possible amount of anesthetic should be used. Total amount of drug injected over a period of time is more significant than the initial concentration or volume. Thus it is essential to employ the minimal effective concentration and the smallest volume, bearing in mind that sensory nerve impulses are blocked by lesser concentrations.

Use of Epinephrine. The rate of absorption of anesthetic should be retarded in every way possible; this is accomplished by slow injection and repeated aspiration for blood, particularly in vascular areas, to avoid intravenous injection. The vasoconstrictive property of epinephrine slows absorption; additional benefits are prolongation of anesthesia and decreased bleeding. Near maximal prolongation of anesthesia and probably maximal protection are obtained with 1:200,000 concentrations of epinephrine, or 0.5 mg per 100 ml of solution. Even a 1:400,000 concentration is effective. Epinephrine should be measured with a syringe rather than added to the anesthetic solution according to the number of drops. Only minimal effective concentrations should be employed because epinephrine carries a toxicity of its own. Many so-called reactions to local anesthetics represent the pharmacologic effects of epinephrine: apprehension, tremor, pallor, sweating, tachycardia, and palpitation. Epinephrine is dangerous in the patient with myocardial disease or coronary arteriosclerosis because of the increased work of the heart resulting from the positive chronotropic and inotropic actions as well as arrhythmogenic properties. Local injection of anesthetic solutions containing epinephrine may result in gangrene when injected into closed spaces such as the finger. Little benefit derives from adding epinephrine to topical anesthetics; certainly it is an added hazard with cocaine.

Barbiturates and Diazepam.   Preanesthetic administration of a short-acting barbiturate, secobarbital, or pentobarbital in sedative doses, once believed to protect against the central stimulating properties of local anesthesics, provides little more than relief from apprehension. Narcotic rather than sedative doses of the barbiturate are necessary to prevent convulsions. Diazepam may be more effective in prevention and therapy. deJong has shown in the cat that the median convulsant dose of lidocaine (8.4 mg per kg) is approximately doubled by the prior use of 0.25 mg per kg diazepam, the equivalent of 15 mg in a 60-kg adult.

Treatment

Rapid intravenous injection of pentobarbital or thiopental has been the initial treatment of choice for incipient or fully developed convulsions, but the barbiturates may add to the circulatory and respiratory depression already present. Recently diazepam has been employed intravenously in 5 mg doses for the treatment of convulsions. The dangers of a convulsion derive from cerebral hypoxia, bodily injury, the possibility of the aspiration of vomitus, postictal depression, and respiratory and circulatory arrest attendant upon the hypoxia. Consequently, oxygen should be given by inhalation immediately and simultaneously with injection of the drug. It has been suggested that the short-acting neuromuscular blocker succinylcholine be used to stop convulsive movements. Although this may minimize oxygen demands secondary to muscle contractions, it does not prevent the cerebral hypoxia contingent upon cortical hyperactivity. We believe that the production of apnea by succinylcholine in inexperienced hands may lead to more problems in the way of pulmonary ventilation. Furthermore, succinylcholine is seldom available in the place where reactions are most likely to occur — the physician's office.

Circulatory depression as indicated by hypotension or a weak pulse should be treated with a vasopressor drug given intravenously or intramuscularly. Ephedrine or phenylephrine should be at hand. It matters little which vasopressor is given in an emergency so long as myocardial depression and peripheral vasodilation are reversed before cardiac standstill occurs. Cardiac arrest should be managed according to the plan suggested in Chapter 26.

ALLERGIC REACTIONS

True allergic reactions to the local anesthetics are infrequent. One might anticipate such reactions in the patient with a history of atopy. We have observed an anaphylactic reaction in a patient with multiple allergies who developed bronchospasm and cardiac standstill following topical application of cocaine for tonsillectomy. It has not been possible to predict allergic reactions reliably by either skin patch tests or conjunctival instillation. Dermatitis following repeated exposure to local anesthetics, particularly procaine, occurs not infrequently in professional personnel, and cross-sensitivity has been demonstrated; further use of local anesthetics calls for subsitution of a compound of a different chemical nature. Allergic reactions to the amide anesthetics are remarkably infrequent.

PRACTICAL SUGGESTIONS FOR THE USE OF LOCAL ANESTHETICS

A patient scheduled for nerve block should refrain from eating or should eat an easily digested meal not less than four hours before the procedure. Vomiting may occur as a psychogenic response or may accompany a systemic reaction to the local anesthetic. A sedative dose of one of the short-acting barbiturates or diazepam can be prescribed to allay apprehension. If ambulatory, the patient should be accompanied by a relative or friend and not be permitted to drive an automobile after a sedative has been given. Patients should be questioned for untoward reactions to the local anesthetics, and the physical condition as well as essential laboratory data should be known.

A patient should be recumbent at the time of injection and the skin prepared with an antiseptic that will not stain clothing or bed linen. Sterile, single dose ampules or vials of the drug are used. One calculates in advance the quantity of anesthetic to be injected, keeping well below the toxic dose. This is done by choosing the minimal effective concentration, understanding the anatomic course of nerves, and injecting at a point at which maximal effect is obtained with the least amount of solution. Use of epinephrine has already been discussed. A common mistake is not to wait long enough for the anesthetic to take effect or to inject only into the subcutaneous tissues, thereby missing intracutaneous nerve fibers. Injection should be unhurried, with frequent aspiration for blood and constant observation. Observation of the face may disclose muscle twitches that precede a more generalized reaction. Continuous conversation serves to reassure the patient and to allow detection of garrulousness, excitement, or loss of consciousness.

Upon completion of a procedure using a local anesthetic, particularly a complicated one, the patient should be observed for some time to detect delayed complications. If an untoward reaction to the anesthetic has occurred, the patient should be fully informed so that repetition is avoided. Lastly, a record must be kept of the procedure as a protection for both patient and physician.

REFERENCES

Covino BG, Vassallo HG: Local Anesthetics. Mechanisms of Action and Clinical Use. New York, Grune & Stratton, 1976.

deJong RH: Physiology and Pharmacology of Local Anesthesia. Springfield, Ill, Charles C Thomas, 1977.

deJong RH, Heavner JE: Diazepam prevents local anesthetic seizures. Anesthesiology 34:523, 1971.

Gissen AJ, Covino BG, Gregus J: Differential sensitivities of mammalian nerve fibers to local anesthetic agents. Anesthesiology 53:467, 1980.

Lee AG: A consumer's guide to models of local anesthetic action. Anesthesiology 51:64, 1979.

Munson EA, Wagman IH: Diazepam treatment of local anesthetic-induced seizures. Anesthesiology 37:523, 1972.

Symposium on local anaesthetics. Br J Anaesth 47·Suppl, 1975.

Chapter 19

SPINAL ANESTHESIA

Spinal anesthesia involves the injection of a local anesthetic into the subarachnoid space. Introduction of the method followed the invention of the hollow needle and syringe in the middle of the 19th century, the discovery by Koller of the local anesthetic properties of cocaine in 1884, and the initial performance of lumbar puncture by Quincke in 1891. Administration of the first spinal anesthesia has been attributed to Corning, who in 1885 attempted to anesthetize the lower half of the body of a patient by injecting cocaine into the region of the spinal column. The anesthesia, which reached completion after a lapse of about 20 minutes, possibly resulted from diffusion of cocaine into the peridural space. Three surgeons — Bier in Germany, Matas in America, and Tuffier in France — independently in 1898 and 1899, were among the first to administer spinal anesthesia in the true sense of the term.

ACTION AND FATE OF ANESTHETICS IN THE SUBARACHNOID SPACE

When a local anesthetic is injected into the subarachnoid space there is almost immediate onset of anesthesia. Spinal nerve roots, dorsal root ganglia, and the periphery of the cord to some extent are the loci of action. The main effects probably result from anesthetization of the anterior and posterior nerve roots. Because of the high initial concentration gradient and lipoid solubility of the local anesthetic, absorption takes place rapidly into nerve fibers. Fibers of smallest diameter are affected first, possibly because of more rapid diffusion through the myelin sheath, possibly because of the large surface area and the lesser distance in penetration. Disappearance of neural function occurs more or less in the following order: autonomic activity, superficial pain, temperature sensation, vibratory and position sense, motor power, and finally, touch.

As the anesthetic spreads from the lumbar region, more and more fibers are affected, with gradually decreasing concentration in the cerebrospinal fluid (CSF), until at the upper reaches conduction is interrupted only in autonomic fibers and those mediating pinprick. The concentration of procaine in CSF necessary for block of superficial sensation is approximately 0.2 mg per ml and for tetracaine, 0.02 mg per ml. A span of several dermatomes is present between complete motor block and the highest point of sensory or autonomic interruption. Thus, it is possible to produce abdominal muscle relaxation without paralyzing the upper intercostal muscles or diaphragm. On the other hand, mere sensory blockade does not guarantee sufficient muscle relaxation for performance of operation.

216

Anesthesia wanes as the anesthetic is absorbed into the systemic circulation from nerves and CSF via lymphatics and capillaries. Ultimately the anesthetic is metabolized in the liver and excreted in urine. For ester compounds, hydrolysis takes place in the circulation and liver; the concentration of esterases in CSF is negligible. Thus, duration of spinal anesthesia depends on the vascular and lymphatic supply of the spinal cord and the rapidity of absorption. Duration of anesthesia also relates to the amount of anesthetic injected. A small amount injected into the subarachnoid space and then permitted to spread widely results in incomplete anesthesia of short duration, whereas a larger quantity concentrated in one area produces more complete and longer-lasting effects.

PHYSIOLOGIC EFFECTS

Circulation. Appearance of marked degrees of arterial hypotension after administration of spinal anesthesia was an early concern and is still considered a relative disadvantage despite use of vasopressor drugs and intravenous fluids to support the pressure. The hypotension of spinal anesthesia results from interruption of sympathetic nerve impulses to systemic blood vessels and interruption of baroreceptor reflexes that control blood pressure. The higher the level of sympathetic block, the more consistent and profound is the fall in pressure and the less chance for compensatory vasoconstriction in unanesthetized areas of the body. Blood pressure tends to decline more if the initial level of pressure is high. Postural effects are marked as in any type of neurologic hypotension, and the lowering of pressure is further aggravated in the presence of hypovolemia.

Circulatory studies indicate that a decrease in total peripheral vascular resistance accounts for the drop in pressure in some individuals; in others, a decrease in cardiac output is found. The latter probably results from venous dilation and pooling of blood, with decreased venous return to the heart. Accessory factors include bradycardia resulting from block of accelerator impulses to the heart or decrease in endogenous release of norepinephrine from sympathetic nerve endings, thereby reducing myocardial contractility. Vasoconstriction in unanesthetized areas of the body may compensate partially for the hypotension. With total autonomic block, the reflex vasoconstrictive response to hypotension initiated from the baroreceptors is interrupted.

Respiration. Under ordinary circumstances, paralysis of intercostal muscles does not cause respiratory insufficiency if the cervical origin of the phrenic nerves is not reached by the anesthetic; diaphragmatic action alone should provide adequate ventilation. During abdominal operation, however, movement of the diaphragm may be limited by retractors or packs; thus, respiratory assistance with oxygen should be provided. When diaphragm and intercostal muscles both are paralyzed, this emergency is treated as is any other instance of respiratory failure. Patients often complain of difficulty in breathing during spinal anesthesia because of lack of perception of abdominal and thoracic movements.

Bowel and Urinary Tract. Because of sympathetic block, the effect of spinal anesthesia on the bowel is that of unopposed parasympathetic activity, the intestines being contracted and hyperactive, the sphincters relaxed. However, opioids oppose this action, and high doses of atropine tend to minimize vagal influence. Spillage of feces during intestinal anastomosis or defecation may occur, although uncommonly. The ureters show peristalsis with relaxation of the ureterovesical orifice; this may aid in removal or elimination of ureteral calculi. Renal blood flow tends to decrease unless the aterial blood pressure is maintained.

The usual adrenocortical response to stress is lacking during spinal anesthesia because of the block of afferent impulses from the operative field.

CHOICE OF SPINAL ANESTHESIA

In the majority of cases, spinal anesthesia is given for operations on the lower abdomen, inguinal regions, or lower extremities, although in some clinics it is used for upper abdominal operations as well. The conditions provided for intra-abdominal operation are unrivaled because of the excellent muscle relaxation, contracted bowel, quiet breathing, and relative decrease in bleeding owing to the hypotension usually present. Some of the conditions for which spinal anesthesia is the method of choice are as follows: in husky muscular patients; when food has recently been ingested; in cesarean section for prematurity; in the patient with alcoholism or barbiturate addiction; when a difficult airway problem exists; and in the presence of hepatic, renal, or metabolic disease. Spinal anesthesia should not be given without consideration for the patient's emotional and physical make-up and the needs of the surgeon. Among the contraindications are prior difficulty with spinal anesthesia, residual neurologic deficit, backache, the presence of neurologic disease, and concurrent use of anticoagulants. Other deterrents are the prospect of difficult lumbar puncture or the possibility of introducing infection. The patient's back is examined beforehand to anticipate these matters and to determine the best position for puncture. Lesser contraindications include very young patients, mental aberration, morbid fear of this kind of anesthesia, decreased blood volume, severe anemia, and a marked increase in intra-abdominal pressure.

Common reasons for dislike of spinal anesthesia are the patient's fear of being conscious during the operation, apprehension that anesthesia may wear off prematurely, and worry about complications such as headache or residual paralysis. It is unwise to force spinal anesthesia on an unwilling patient.

PREPARATION FOR ANESTHESIA

Premedication is given to allay apprehension and an opioid used to lessen the pain of lumbar puncture. A drying agent is not used unless supplementation with general anesthesia is planned, although some believe that atropine decreases nausea and vomiting and diminishes the parasympathetic effect of spinal anesthesia on the bowel. Before spinal anesthesia, the same preparations are made as for general anesthesia (see Chapter 5), including having an anesthesia machine readied for use.

EQUIPMENT

The local anesthetics should be reputable products. A variety of disposable spinal anesthesia trays containing all the materials necessary and sterilized in ethylene oxide is now commercially available (Fig. 19–1). When ampules of local anesthetic are wrapped separately, they are sterilized at 260°C and 12.25 kg pressure for 10 minutes in ethylene oxide. As a rule, drugs are not resterilized even though little deterioration takes place with autoclaving; this includes epinephrine, whose potency is not reduced by such treatment. Sterilization of ampules by immersion in antiseptic solutions is unacceptable because the antiseptic can penetrate a cracked ampule; detection of contamination is difficult, and neurologic damage has followed injection.

LUMBAR PUNCTURE AND INJECTION

TECHNIQUE

The lateral decubitus is the routine position for lumbar puncture; however, if difficulty is expected, puncture is often easier in the sitting position. A prone position is

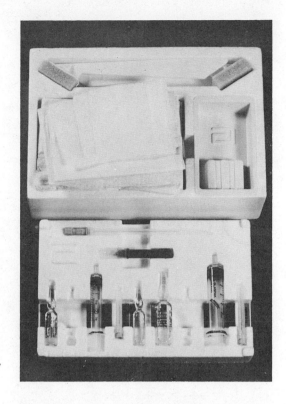

FIGURE 19–1.   Disposable spinal tray. (Courtesy of Abbott Laboratories.)

used when anesthesia in the lumbar and sacral dermatomes is induced with hypobaric solutions. If a hyperbaric solution is given, the side to be operated upon should be lowermost, and uppermost if a hypobaric technique is chosen. An assistant should flex the back, support the patient, and prevent exposure. At this time the skin of the back may be shaved. The anesthetist palpates the vertebral spines, selecting the appropriate interspace; an imaginary line between the iliac crests (Tuffier's line) intersects the spine at the third or fourth lumbar space, both below the level of the estimated termination of the spinal cord at the second lumbar space.

After washing the hands, the anesthetist dons sterile gloves and opens the spinal tray. Equipment is approached with a ''no touch'' technique; that is, the barrels of syringes and tips of needles are not handled. Ampules are identified, inspected for imperfections, and the questionable ones discarded.

The patient is forewarned before each maneuver. Lumbar puncture is done carefully to avoid injury to soft tissues, ligaments, or periosteum. Trauma is probably responsible for many complaints after spinal anesthesia including backache and sciatic radiation of pain. The skin is prepared with a colored antiseptic, avoiding contamination of needles and syringes. Beginning at the lumbar puncture site and working concentrically, the back is painted over a wide area. The sponge stick is set aside and the back covered with a sterile drape. The anesthetist is seated with the spine at eye level (Fig. 19–2) and the skin is not touched until dry. A skin wheal is raised, using the 25-gauge needle and small syringe with infiltration to the supraspinous ligament. The lumbar puncture needle is grasped in the manner in which a pencil is held, between thumb and forefinger. With stylet in place, the needle is advanced through the skin wheal perpendicularly to the plane of the back, but slightly cephalad. Tissues penetrated are the supraspinous and interspinous ligaments, the ligamentum flavum, and lastly the dura. After some experience one learns to distinguish these structures by a sense of touch. If bone is met, the needle is withdrawn subcutaneously and

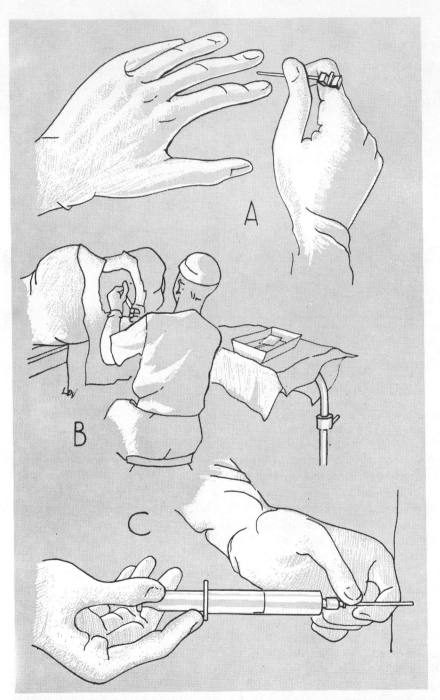

FIGURE 19–2. Details of spinal anesthesia technique. *A*, Insertion of lumbar puncture needle. Left hand fixes skin over chosen lumbar intervertebral space. *B*, Position for lumbar puncture. Anesthetist sits with eyes at level of lumbar spine. Spinal tray on separate table to right. *C*, Position of hands to aspirate and inject fluid.

redirected. Usual causes of failure include poor positioning of the patient, selection of the wrong interspace (too low), and failure to advance the needle in the midline. If the midline structures are calcified, the needle is directed toward the interlaminar space via a lateral approach. For the sacral or Taylor approach, a longer needle is inserted at the second sacral foramen and is directed medially and cephalad toward the midline of the lumbosacral space, a technique useful with the prone patient and also helpful in surmounting calcific or bony obstruction at higher sites.

Rotation of the needle places the bevel well within the subarachnoid space at an average depth of 6 cm from the surface. Blood-tinged CSF or lack of free flow contraindicates injection of the anesthetic; blood-tinged fluid that clears is not a contraindication. One should not inject the anesthetic in the presence of a paresthesia, as the needle tip may lie within or against a nerve root; permanent neurologic damage will follow intraneural injection. However, another interspace can be tried.

At this time a vasopressor drug may be injected into the lumbosacral muscle if a major fall in blood pressure is expected. Pressor drug and dose are matters of individual preference (see Chapter 32). The anesthetist then stands, and, with the needle supported to prevent dislodgment, the syringe is firmly attached to the needle hub. If CSF can be aspirated easily, the anesthetic is injected at a slow rate, avoiding mixing during injection. Syringe and needle are removed after final demonstration of a free flow of CSF.

FACTORS INFLUENCING SPINAL ANESTHESIA

The composition and volume of the solution injected into the subarachnoid space and the technique of injection are influenced by duration, intensity, and level of anesthesia desired; body height or length of the vertebral column; intra-abdominal pressure and obesity; and anticipated position of the patient during operation. One can combine the measures listed further on to influence duration, intensity, and level of block.

Duration of Action.   The average duration of anesthesia with the commonly used drugs is 60 minutes for procaine and lidocaine and 120 minutes for tetracaine. For operations of indeterminate duration, the continuous technique may be chosen. We are not yet ready to advocate the use of bupivacaine for spinal anesthesia.

The duration of the anesthetic action may be increased by addition of epinephrine to the anesthetic mixture, 0.5 mg being the optimal amount. An average increase in duration of approximately 30 to 100 per cent can be expected, depending on the concentration of epinephrine and the degree of dilution in CSF. Phenylephrine, usually 2 mg, also increases the duration but to a lesser extent. Extension of anesthesia is thought to result from prolonged exposure of nerve fibers to the anesthetic, possibly with more thorough penetration and fixation, and slower release of the anesthetic from CSF.

When epinephrine is given with tetracaine, the onset of anesthesia is slower; whether as a result of the vasoconstriction and slow penetration of nerve fibers or the change in the physical characteristics of the solution has not been determined. The slow onset often prompts the anesthetist to lower the head of the operating table in an effort to spread the block with a hyperbaric solution, but this usually leads to a level higher than that desired. Since a high level results, the anesthetist is tempted beforehand to reduce the total dose of anesthetic and this, in turn, leads to inadequate anesthesia. A disadvantage of long-acting anesthesia is that the patient is left with numbness and paralysis for a long time postoperatively.

Dosage.   The average anesthetic dose of tetracaine for individuals of varying height and for expected levels of sensory anesthesia is shown in Table 19–1 and Figure 19–3. We believe that height provides a better index than body surface area. Sacral levels permit performance of operations on the perineum; levels at the groin allow for operation on the legs and thighs; xiphoid levels permit lower abdominal procedures; and a sensory level to the nipples is necessary for upper abdominal operations. It must be remembered that the upper level of anesthesia as tested by pinprick is merely a sensory level and that motor nerves to muscle are only blocked several dermatomes below.

Specific Gravity of Solution. The specific gravity of CSF varies, depending on temperature and solute content (average 37°C, 1.005 ±0.003). By dissolving the local anesthetic in distilled water, a solution with a specific gravity less than that of CSF results (hypobaric); with CSF or 10 per cent dextrose as the diluent, a hyperbaric solution is obtained. Differences in specific gravity when combined with position, during and after injection, are used to influence the spread of anesthetic. If, for example, a hyperbaric solution is selected and the patient is seated during and after injection, a low block is obtained; injection of a hypobaric solution would result in a higher level of anesthesia. When a heavy solution is injected slowly into the subarachnoid space it remains more or less as a bolus acted upon by gravity. In none of these maneuvers is the anesthetic confined to the site, for the difference in specific gravity is equalized as the anesthetic solution spreads. However, the area exposed to the higher concentration remains anesthetized for a longer time. Dextrose solution mixed with tetracaine seems to shorten the time of onset and to prolong anesthesia as well as ensure uniform block, although some would claim these benefits for hypobaric anesthesia. Unilateral anesthesia is often attempted in an effort to diminish some of the undesirable physiologic effects of spinal anesthesia, but this is hardly successful unless the original position is maintained for about 40 minutes.

Because of the spinal curvatures (Fig. 19–4) a hyperbaric solution tends to reach the third to sixth thoracic segments if the patient lies supine with legs extended. The curves may be altered by flexing the thighs on the abdomen; the reduction in lumbar lordosis limits cephalad spread of a hyperbaric solution.

Intra-Abdominal Pressure. Increased intra-abdominal pressure dictates a reduction in volume and dose of local anesthetic used. Elevated pressures compress the vena cava and increase volume and pressure in the peridural plexus of veins, the resulting dilation encroaching upon the subarachnoid space, thereby lessening capacity. The solution, therefore, is injected into a lesser volume of CSF and spreads over a wider

TABLE 19–1. Dose of Tetracaine for Spinal Anesthesia*

	Height (cm)		
Operation	*152*	*167*	*184*
Upper abdomen	14†	16	18
Lower abdomen	12	14	16
Inguinal — bladder	10	12	14
Extremities	8	10	12
Rectal	4	6	8

*Tetracaine is injected as 0.5 per cent, in 5 per cent dextrose in water; for a 12 mg dose, mix 1.2 ml of 1 per cent tetracaine with 1.2 ml of 10 per cent dextrose in water. With procaine, the dose is 10 times that of tetracaine, injected as 5 per cent procaine in CSF. *These doses are approximate,* chosen to make memorization easy. Dose and body height are not the only factors influencing anesthetic level. Position before and after injection, volume and baricity of the solution, inclusion of vasoconstrictors, rate of injection, cough and straining, and pressure and volume of the CSF affect the level (see text).

†All doses are given in mg.

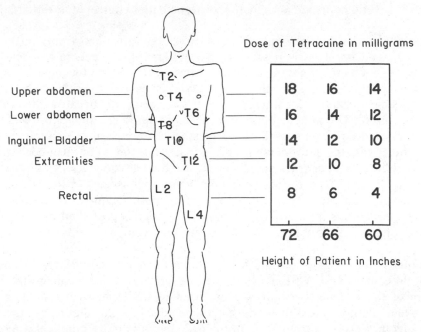

FIGURE 19-3. Approximate sensory levels of anesthesia required for the operative site indicated.

area. Pregnancy, ascites, large abdominal tumors, intestinal obstruction, and marked obesity are situations in which abdominal pressure may be elevated.

Position. Subsequent moving of the patient into position for operation is another factor in choice of anesthetic solution. Hypobaric solutions are of value for operations carried out in the lateral or prone position, since injection can be made with the operative site uppermost. If the Trendelenburg position is elected, as for a vaginal procedure, use of a hypobaric solution minimizes the likelihood of high block. If cholecystectomy is the procedure, a high, solid block is needed, and in our opinion a hyperbaric solution is best. Once spinal anesthesia is fully developed, a change in body position may be followed by hypotension (supine to lateral or prone position).

CONTINUOUS SPINAL ANESTHESIA

First described by Lemmon in 1940 and subsequently modified by Tuohy, this technique permits intermittent injection to provide anesthesia of unlimited duration. The method is chosen when the length of operation is indeterminate, when procedures

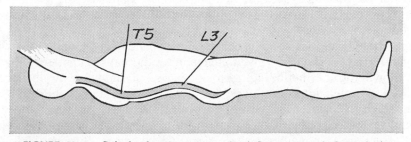

FIGURE 19-4. Spinal column curvatures that influence spread of anesthetic.

longer than several hours are anticipated, or when better control of anesthesia is essential.

After lumbar puncture with a Tuohy-Huber point needle, a previously marked plastic catheter with stylet is passed, the tip wedged in the needle tip. The stylet is withdrawn a centimeter or so, the catheter further advanced, and when it is certain that the catheter has passed the needle tip, the stylet is removed. Without the stylet it is hardly possible to pass the catheter beyond the needle tip because the warm CSF softens the plastic. The catheter is not inserted more than a centimeter or two because it may coil and interfere with spread of the anesthetic. Care is taken to avoid withdrawal of the catheter with the introducing needle in place, lest the tip be sheared: the catheter is advanced little by little as the needle is extracted while the markings on the catheter indicate the distance from the tip. A needle adapter is inserted in the free end of the catheter and the catheter fixed to the skin to prevent dislodgment. After aspiration of CSF, the anesthetic is injected. The anesthesia syringe is protected by a sterile towel and fixed to a small armboard to protect it and avoid accidental pressure on the plunger.

The most controllable solution for continuous spinal anesthesia consists of 3 to 5 per cent procaine in CSF. CSF is withdrawn and mixed with the local anesthetic before insertion of the catheter. Withdrawal of 10 ml of CSF causes a reduction in CSF pressure and dilation of vessels in the subarachnoid space; this diminishes the capacity and lessens the ease of introduction of the catheter. It is more practical, therefore, to use tetracaine 0.2 to 0.4 per cent in dextrose. Baricity of the solution also leads to better control of anesthesia. With either anesthetic, however, initial injection should be no more than 0.5 to 1.0 ml, as a larger volume may result in a high level of anesthesia. When continuation of analgesia or sympathetic blockade may be helpful, as follows vascular surgery, the catheter is left in place for several hours, with intermittent injection. It is probably unsafe to allow the catheter to remain in the subarachnoid space for a longer period.

With the increasing popularity of continuous peridural anesthesia, the continuous spinal technique is seldom used these days.

MANAGEMENT OF SPINAL ANESTHESIA

The time immediately following injection is critical. The initial position may be maintained for five to ten minutes if localization of anesthesia is desired, as in the sacral region or leg. During positioning for operation the patient is cautioned to relax, to permit passive turning. Straining or breath holding may raise the level of anesthesia to unwanted heights, and blood pressure may decline. For these reasons the anesthetist must devote full attention to the patient, alternately testing the level of anesthesia with pinprick and determining the blood pressure. Levels are tested and recorded over at least the first 10 to 15 minutes after injection. Motor power is tested by asking the patient to dorsiflex the feet (S1, S2), flex the toes (L4, L5), raise the knees (L2, L3) or tense the rectus muscles (T6 to T12) by lifting the head. Intercostal paralysis is detected by palpation in the intercostal spaces.

Onset of anesthesia is usually evident within one to two minutes of injection. Occasionally onset is delayed for five to ten minutes, perhaps because of slow diffusion or penetration of the anesthetic. Failure to obtain anesthesia, however, most commonly results from injection into the space between the dura and arachnoid. The term "rachi-resistance" was coined to describe spinal anesthetic failure, but even while admitting that in some individuals a slow onset of anesthesia occurs, we believe that technical errors are responsible in the majority of instances. Surgical incision should not be made unless it is certain that anesthesia is adequate. If anesthesia does not develop, the injection may be repeated if there is time, or general anesthesia may be substituted.

During spinal anesthesia the same careful observation is required as during general anesthesia. Respiratory insufficiency is not easily detected. If the slightest suspicion is aroused, however, oxygen is given by mask. High intercostal paralysis may be accompanied by a feeling of suffocation and signs of sensory and motor paralysis in the arms. If the phrenic nerve roots are blocked, accessory muscles of respiration may be called into action, although these too will be weakened. The patient is unable to speak for lack of ability to move air and may lose consciousness. Paralysis of respiration is treated with positive pressure oxygen via mask or endotracheal tube and is carried out until the high level of anesthesia recedes.

Arterial hypotension is considered to be present when significant lowering below preoperative values occurs or when systolic blood pressure declines below 80 torr. Hypotension is potentially more hazardous if coronary and cerebral insufficiency have been diagnosed preoperatively. Treatment consists of oxygen by mask, rapid administration of fluids, and intravenous injection of a pressor drug (see Chapter 32). Small doses are given intravenously to avoid excessive elevation of pressure, whereas a larger amount is given intramuscularly for sustained effect. If repeated injection of a pressor drug is necessary, continuous infusion is preferable to sustain the pressure. A pressor drug infusion may be started in the poor risk patient even before pressure falls.

The anesthetist should remain at the head of the table to encourage the patient, monitor vital signs, and supplement with general anesthesia when needed. Nausea and vomiting are not uncommon occurrences. Opioids used for premedication, cerebral ischemia, psychologic factors, or traction on viscera may be responsible for the gastrointestinal symptoms. Supplementation with general anesthesia is necessary when analgesia or muscle relaxation is inadequate, when nausea and vomiting are protracted, or when the patient chooses to be unconscious. As a rule, only a light plane of general anesthesia is needed. Circulatory depressant properties of most general anesthetics are magnified during spinal anesthesia because of lack of compensatory sympathetic activity.

COMPLICATIONS OF SPINAL ANESTHESIA

SEQUELAE OF LUMBAR PUNCTURE

Headache. The syndrome of decreased intracranial pressure, consisting primarily of headache but occasionally accompanied by difficulty in hearing and vision, is the most common complication of lumbar puncture. The opening in the dura made by the lumbar puncture may persist for days or weeks (Fig. 19–5). With escape of CSF, pressure falls. Headache is postural, appearing in the head-up position and suggesting that loss of CSF permits traction on intracranial pain-sensitive structures.

In a series of 9277 administrations of spinal anesthesia studied by the authors, the overall incidence of headache was 11 per cent. Headache occurred in highest frequency in patients in the third and fourth decades (Table 19–2). Frequency of headache was also higher in women, a result in part of inclusion of obstetric cases in the group, for headache followed vaginal delivery in 22 per cent of patients. Even if obstetric cases are not included, headache was still more frequent in women.

The incidence of headache diminished with decreasing diameter of needle used (Table 19–3); not only were there fewer headaches, but severity and duration were less. In this series of cases a 16-gauge needle was employed only for continuous spinal anesthesia. Technical difficulties were more common, and the incidence of headache and ocular complaints was high.

Treatment of headache consists of keeping the patient flat in bed, using analgetics,

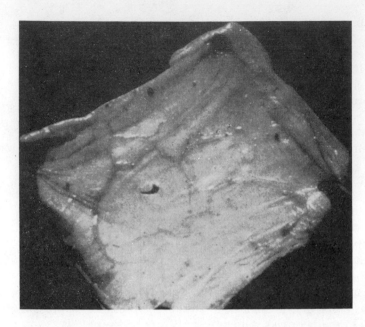

FIGURE 19–5. Puncture opening in dura, two days old. Diameter of needle 0.8 mm. Magnification 4×. (Reproduced with permission from Franksson C and Gordh T: Acta Chir Scand 94:443, 1946.)

or attempting to increase CSF pressure. Body hydration or application of a tight abdominal binder, thereby raising pressure in the peridural venous plexus, sometimes relieves the milder headache. The mechanism of relief of headache after peridural placement of fluid has not been established. When headache is protracted and severe, the symptoms may be completely relieved in a high percentage of cases by application of an autologous "blood patch." An epidural injection of 10 to 15 ml of blood serves to seal the dural fistula. However, back pain and signs of meningeal irritation have been noted in more than a few instances after this therapy.

Ocular and Auditory Complications.   Auditory complaints, noted in 0.4 per cent of 9277 anesthetized patients, consisted of buzzing, popping, clogging of the ears, humming, roaring, or loss of hearing altogether — with few exceptions associated with a postural headache. Auditory difficulties may relate to alterations in fluid pressure in the cochlea. Difficulty with vision occurred in 0.4 per cent of the patients; double vision, blurring, trouble in focusing, and spots before the eyes were the complaints. In all but eight of the 34 patients visual problems arose in association with postural headache. There were three cases of abducens or lateral rectus muscle paralysis, and the symptom of prolonged double vision in three others suggested that paralysis might

TABLE 19–2.   Relation of Age to Incidence of Spinal Headache

		Headache	
Age (yr)	Number of Anesthetics	No.	Per Cent
10–19	537	51	10
20–29	1994	321	16
30–39	1883	261	14
40–49	1759	192	11
50–59	1736	133	8
60–69	1094	45	4
70–79	297	7	2
80–89	27	1	3
Total	9277	1011	

TABLE 19–3. Relation of Gauge of Needle Used for Lumbar
Puncture and Incidence of Headache

Gauge	Number of Anesthetics	Headache	
		No.	Per Cent
16	839	151	18
19	154	16	10
20	2698	377	14
22	4952	430	9
24	634	37	6
Total	9277	1011	

also have been present. The six cases followed use of a 16-gauge needle for continuous spinal anesthesia. One theory holds that with brain displacement or traction, the abducens nerve with a long intracranial course is affected by stretch.

Traumatic Puncture or Infection.   Traumatic lumbar puncture without injection of the anesthetic has led to transient and permanent neurologic deficit. This usually occurs after repeated attempts, with production of paresthesias and recovery of blood or blood-tinged CSF. Epidural abscess and bacterial meningitis have followed lumbar puncture and spinal anesthesia. In the vast majority of instances, such complications must be ascribed to faulty technique.

SEQUELAE OF LOCAL ANESTHETIC INJECTION

The complication most feared is chronic, progressive adhesive arachnoiditis, which, we believe, is a nonspecific pathologic response to an intrathecal irritant. The ultimate effects of arachnoiditis relate to ischemia of the spinal cord. Transverse myelitis has also been described and perhaps is related to destruction of neural tissue by the injected substance or to intraspinal or intraneural injection. Either of these two processes may result in paralysis of the lower limbs and intestinal and bladder dysfunction as well as involvement of the spinal cord and roots at higher levels. Sensory changes alone may occur. In our study of spinal anesthesia there were no instances of adhesive arachnoiditis, cauda equina syndrome, or transverse myelitis. We believe that these good results relate to proper selection of the patient for this technique and its careful application.

Residual signs or symptoms of numbness following spinal anesthesia occurred in 0.8 per cent of the patients, in the majority restricted to the lumbar and sacral dermatomes. None of the patients had other neurologic signs, and most complaints disappeared within six months. Subjective complaints consisted of numbness, tingling, heaviness, or burning. Sensory deficit was not always found. These sequelae must relate to anesthetic injection.

Exacerbation of Pre-existing Neurologic Disease.   Although a cause-and-effect relation between spinal anesthesia and exacerbation of neurologic disease can rarely be proved, we believe that spinal anesthesia generally should not be given to patients with certain neurologic diseases. This reservation applies to congenital, active, or inactive disease. Exceptions to the rule are made only when a technique other than spinal anesthesia is potentially more hazardous or less safe in the hands of the administrator.

Detection of neurologic disease after spinal anesthesia calls for repeated postanesthetic visits, during which patients are questioned for difficulty in voiding, residual numbness, or paralysis. Any deviation from normal is investigated even at the expense of suggesting a relation to anesthesia. It is important to detect symptoms early, for we believe that progression of disease can be halted, perhaps by surgical exploration or in some cases by administration of corticosteroids. In many instances unrelated neurologic disease has been found.

In any instance of neurologic complaint, and this point cannot be emphasized enough, it is essential to seek other causes rather than to ascribe all to spinal anesthesia. The majority of serious neurologic symptoms appearing after spinal anesthesia, as administered today, can be attributed to coincident or previously unrecognized disease. Thorough neurologic examination must be performed, appropriate diagnostic methods used, and consultation sought.

APPRASIAL

It is not an easy matter to assess the role of spinal anesthesia in modern anesthetic practice. With the widespread use of balanced anesthesia techniques and the resurgence of interest in peridural anesthesia, one might expect decreased interest in the subarachnoid technique. Nevertheless, the manufacturers dispense millions of spinal sets annually. Because the method is more predictable in its results and the onset of anesthesia more rapid, these advantages still prevail in the choice over peridural anesthesia. General practitioners, surgeons, and obstetricians may find the method useful when an anesthetist is not available. However, headache after lumbar puncture remains a major problem, particularly in obstetrics, and neurologic sequelae are still reported.

REFERENCES

DiGiovanni AJ, Galbert MW, Wahle WM: Epidural injection of autologous blood for post lumbar-puncture headache. Anesth Analg 51:226, 1972.

Dripps RD, Vandam LD: Long-term follow-up of patients who received 10,098 spinal anesthetics: I. Failure to discover major neurological sequelae. JAMA 156:1486, 1954.

Ernst EA: *In vitro* changes of osmolality and density of spinal anesthetic solutions. Anesthesiology 29:104, 1968.

Giasi RM, D'Agostino E, Covino BG: Adsorption of lidocaine following subarachnoid and epidural administration. Anesth Analg 58:360, 1979.

Greene NM: Physiology of Spinal Anesthesia. 3rd ed, Baltimore, The Williams & Wilkins Co, 1981.

Lund PC: Principles and Practice of Spinal Anesthesia. Springfield, Ill, Charles C Thomas, 1971.

Phillips, OC, Ebner H, Nelson AT, et al: Neurological complications following spinal anesthesia with lidocaine. A prospective review of 10,440 cases. Anesthesiology 30:284, 1969.

Vandam LD, Dripps RD: Long-term follow-up of patients who received 10,098 spinal anesthetics: II. Incidence and analysis of minor sensory neurological defects. Surgery 38:463, 1955.

Vandam LD, Dripps RD: Exacerbation of pre-existing neurologic disease after spinal anesthesia. N Engl J Med 255:843, 1956.

Vandam LD, Dripps RD: Long-term follow-up of patients who received 10,098 spinal anesthetics: III. Syndrome of decreased intracranial pressure (headache and ocular and auditory difficulties). JAMA 161:586, 1956.

Vandam LD, Dripps RD: Long-term follow-up of patients who received 10,098 spinal anesthetics: IV. Neurological disease incident to traumatic lumbar puncture during spinal anesthesia. JAMA 172:1483, 1960.

Chapter *20*

PERIDURAL AND CAUDAL ANESTHESIA

We have presented the subject of spinal anesthesia first because we believe that the beginner should learn this technique before approaching peridural (epidural) anesthesia. In addition, the two methods are similar except for certain technical differences; that is, choice and application to the patient are almost the same, action and fate of the local anesthetics are similar, the physiologic consequences are almost identical, and management of anesthesia differs little. Throughout the discussion comparisons between the two methods will be made.

Peridural anesthesia results from injection of a local anesthetic into the space surrounding the dura mater, within the spinal canal. Note was made earlier that Corning in 1885 was possibly the first to do this, although it was done unsuspectingly. In 1901 Sicard and Cathelin independently introduced local anesthetics into the peridural space via the sacrococcygeal hiatus. Subsequently, sporadic attempts were made to approach the space at higher levels, but the method did not take hold until Pages in 1921 and Dogliotti in 1927 achieved anesthesia with greater consistency via a lumbar approach. Peridural anesthesia via the caudal route is used today for procedures performed in the sacral region — anorectal operations, vaginal procedures, and obstetric delivery. However, because of uncertainty in achieving the level of anesthesia via the caudal approach, the need for large volumes of local anesthetic solution, and a failure rate about 5 to 10 per cent, the lumbar approach to the peridural space is more commonly used for obstetrics. The latter has gained popularity because of a better understanding of technique and physiology and the availability of a wide spectrum of the amide group of local anesthetics.

ANATOMY

The anatomic features of the peridural space explain in part the action of the local anesthetics injected into it as well as the requirements for concentration and volume. In essence, the peridural space extends from the base of the skull to the coccyx. The spinal cord present within is enveloped by the meninges, the dura outermost, with the cord terminating at or just above the second lumbar vertebra and the subarachnoid space at the second sacral foramen. The outer limits of the space are formed by the ligamentum flavum and the periosteum lining the vertebral canal; traversing the space via the intervertebral and sacral foramina are the spinal nerves, enveloped by the dura to the point of exit at the foramina. Other structures within the peridural space are the peridural plexus of veins, loose areolar tissue, and fibrous connections between the dura and the spinal column, most prominent anteriorly and more extensive in the elderly.

The volume of the peridural space varies from region to region, depending on the configuration of the vertebral canal and the contents of the dural sac. The most prominent enlargements of the spinal cord are the lower cervical, the upper thoracic, the lumbar, and the upper sacral segments, corresponding to the brachial and lumbosacral plexuses, respectively. Areas of larger capacity in the peridural space are the caudal canal and the lumbar region. The peridural space varies in capacity, with alterations in volume of the dural sac owing to changes in position and to the volume of blood in the peridural plexus of veins, again influenced by position and intra-abdominal pressure.

NEGATIVE PRESSURE IN THE PERIDURAL SPACE

An important aspect of the peridural space is the negative pressure demonstrable upon initial entry with a needle, a useful sign. Although some claim this is an extension of the negative pressure developed within the thorax, negative pressure can also be demonstrated in the cadaver. Thus, it is thought that flexion and lengthening of the spine increased the volume of the relatively closed peridural space, creating a true vacuum. However, in the living subject the pressure in the thoracic region is subatmospheric, less negative in the lumbar region, and not demonstrable in the caudal canal. Probably the most likely explanation relates to the pressure in the peridural plexus of veins. Pressure in the space is negative as long as a body position favors a negative pressure in the veins. Perhaps also pertinent is the explanation that needle entry into the space "tents" the dura ahead of it, causing local expansion of the space with development of negative pressure; this is confirmed by a simultaneous rise in pressure within the subarachnoid space.

RESULTS OF PERIDURAL INJECTION

SITE OF ACTION OF THE LOCAL ANESTHETIC

The action of local anesthetics deposited within the peridural space is believed to occur in several ways. Perhaps the major action takes place at the nerve roots and dorsal root ganglia beyond the point of meningeal covering, the result of outward diffusion of anesthetic through the intervertebral foramina. On the other hand, the anesthetic is found in the subarachnoid space, access gained either by diffusion across the meninges or by retrograde diffusion through the intervertebral foramina via the perineural spaces and lymphatics. The periphery of the spinal cord is also affected so that block of ascending and descending pathways may be observed. At any time during peridural anesthesia a concentration of local anesthetic sufficient for sensory blockade is present in CSF.

SPREAD, ONSET, AND DURATION OF ANESTHESIA

The volume of fluid injected into the peridural space is the major influence in the spread of local anesthesia. Unlike spinal anesthesia, position and gravity influence distribution to a lesser extent, whereas the baricity of the anesthetic solution is of no importance. Spread is influenced more by the structures within the space and the changing volume of the space in the sitting or lateral position owing to the volume of the dural sac and venous plexus. Some believe rapidity of injection is another variable, for it may influence the escape of fluid through the intervertebral foramina and the extent of spread cephalad or caudad. Finally, concentration of the anesthetic solution determines the completeness of the block insofar as nerve fiber size and the number of fibers are concerned.

In summary, then, it is the mass of local anesthetic, concentration times volume, that determines the spread and solidity of the block. Differential block of nerve fibers can also be obtained by altering the concentration of the anesthetic. Latency and duration of anesthesia are affected by the aforementioned factors as well as by specific properties of the local anesthetic. Epinephrine slows vascular absorption and decreases peak concentrations of anesthetic in the bloodstream by approximately one half to one third. Termination of anesthesia depends on absorption of the anesthetic from the nerves and peridural space via vascular and lymphatic channels.

IMPORTANCE OF VASCULARITY

Because the peridural area is highly vascularized and the concentration and volume of anesthetic injected are relatively large, a significant incidence of systemic reactions to the local anesthetic may be expected as a result of absorption. For this reason, epinephrine is added to the anesthetic solution unless there is some contraindication to its use. Epinephrine increases duration of anesthesia; a concentration of 1:200,000 is usually employed. Under conditions of increased vascularity, as in pregnancy at term, the likelihood of absorption is increased.

PHYSIOLOGIC EFFECTS

Although the physiologic results of spinal and peridural anesthesia are almost the same, there is a difference in that absorption of the local anesthetic from the peridural space may give rise to systemic effects, a possibility already mentioned. Likewise, the systemic actions of epinephrine may be evident. Depending on the concentration of anesthetic employed, motor block may be less intense and slower to appear than in spinal anesthesia, whereas some sensory input may continue via large fibers.

Hypotension can follow peridural anesthesia for most if not all the reasons listed under spinal anesthesia. In comparisons of spinal and peridural anesthesia of equal extent, the hypotension encountered with the latter tends to be less profound. The concomitant use of epinephrine in peridural anesthesia does not prevent hypotension. Despite an increase in heart rate and stroke volume, peripheral resistance declines to a greater degree. In addition to the neurogenic effects on circulation, some of the changes noted may result from absorption of the local anesthetic into the bloodstream. It should also be emphasized that pressor drugs are rarely used prophylactically before peridural anesthesia.

TECHNICAL ASPECTS

EQUIPMENT

Basic equipment and principles of sterilization are the same as for the spinal technique. In peridural anesthesia the anesthetic should be added to the prepared tray in a single dose ampule rather than risk injection of a contaminated solution from a multiple dose vial. Additional equipment required is as follows:

1. For single dose anesthesia, a well-designed needle is required. The essentials are: a sizable hub that can be grasped firmly as the needle is advanced, a rigid shaft, and a short bevel point with rounded edges to minimize inadvertent dural puncture. We prefer a 19-gauge, thin-walled needle, about 9 cm in length.
2. For continuous anesthesia we use a 17- or 18 gauge, 7.6-cm, thin-walled Tuohy needle with a Huber point. In conjunction, a disposable vinyl plastic catheter is used, which

receives a 23-gauge Luer-Lok needle. The tubing is marked at 10, 11, and 15 cm, the leading edge beveled, and a fairly rigid stylet inserted. With a Teflon catheter, a stylet is not necessary.
3. A 10-ml Luer-Lok syringe for attachment to the catheter and serial injection.
4. An 18-gauge, short-bevel needle for puncturing the skin and ligaments to permit entry of the Tuohy needle.
5. A 10-ml, plain-tipped syringe is used for the "loss of resistance" test, whereas a 20-ml syringe may be used for initial injection.
All the equipment is commercially available in presterilized, packaged form.

AGENTS AND TECHNIQUE

Currently used local anesthetics, concentrations employed, approximate latency of onset, and duration of anesthesia are shown in Table 20–1. We employ 1.5 and 2.0 per cent lidocaine or mepivacaine and from 0.25 to 0.75 per cent bupivacaine. A few clinicians still employ dichloroprocaine for the continuous method to avoid cumulative concentrations in plasma, but others have abandoned the drug because of reports of neurotoxicity.

Single Dose Technique

The routine position of the patient is the lateral decubitus, with the anesthetist seated as for lumbar puncture. The spine need not be flexed as much as in spinal anesthesia, for some believe that inadvertent dural puncture is less likely with minimal flexion. The skin of the back is prepared and draped and the skin and deeper tissues then anesthetized. Entry is made at a spinal interspace corresponding as closely as possible to the dermatomes at the center of the area to be anesthetized. More uniform results can be expected from a standard midline insertion at L2 to L3.

Several techniques have been suggested to detect entry into the peridural space; the loss of resistance method is perhaps most commonly used. We prefer this when a smaller needle is employed for single injection. A syringe containing air, distilled water, or preferably saline is attached to the needle as it is advanced, maintaining steady gentle pressure on the plunger. After the ligamentum flavum has been pierced a sudden loss of resistance is experienced, fluid or air entering the peridural space and displacing the dura. If distilled water is used, pain may be experienced as it enters the space. When the hanging drop method of Gutierrez is selected, a drop of local anesthetic placed in the needle hub is sucked inward as negative pressure is encountered.

Once entry has been gained, aspiration is tried by rotating the needle in several quadrants to detect blood or CSF; if either is recovered the needle is removed and

TABLE 20–1. Action of Local Anesthetics in Single Dose Peridural Anesthesia*

Agent	Usual Conc. (%)	Volumes (ml)	Total Dose (mg)	Onset (min)	Duration (min)
Esters					
Chloroprocaine	1–3	15–30	150–900	–	30–45
Procaine	1–2	15–30	150–600	–	45–60
Tetracaine	0.25–0.5	15–30	37.5–150	–	180–360
Amides					
Lidocaine	1–2	15–30	150–500	15	60–180
Mepivacaine	1–2	15–30	150–500	15	60–180
Bupivacaine	0.25–0.75	15–30	37.5–225	16.5	180–360
Etidocaine	1–1.5	15–30	150–300	10.85	180–360

*Data compiled from reports in the literature.

inserted at another space to avoid intrathecal or intravascular injection. A trial injection of 3 ml of anesthetic is then made. Although not infallible, this measure should reveal subarachnoid puncture or intravenous injection, especially if epinephrine is used where the pulse rate will rise considerably; if not demonstrable, the anesthetizing dose of local anesthetic is injected. Usually 1.5 to 2.0 ml of anesthetic are required in the younger age group for each spinal segment anesthetized, with injection performed at a rate of 1 ml per second. A faster injection may produce paresthesias, a higher level of anesthesia, and a higher blood concentration; slow injection should result in more localized anesthesia. The anesthetic diffuses in both directions, usually more cephalad than caudad, particularly in the elderly. We do not recommend the use of thoracic peridural anesthesia by the beginner because of the greater hazards entailed.

Serial Technique

After performance of peridural puncture and injection of the test dose, the first anesthetizing dose may be injected. Then a catheter is passed through the needle, the tip wedged at the needle point. The wire stylet is then withdrawn a millimeter or two and the catheter further advanced; when it is certain that the catheter has passed the tip of the needle into the peridural space, the stylet is removed. Without the stylet, it is sometimes difficult to pass the catheter beyond the needle point. The catheter should be inserted into the peridural space not more than a centimeter or two because it may coil up and interfere with spread of the anesthetic or may traumatize nerves or blood vessels. Furthermore, paresthesias are almost uniform if the catheter is advanced further. Care is taken to avoid withdrawal of the catheter with the introducing needle still in place lest the tip of the catheter be sheared. An attempt is made to maintain the catheter in its initial position or to advance it slightly as the needle is extracted. The markings on the catheter indicating distance from the tip help in determining appropriate depth of insertion. A needle adapter is then inserted in the free end of the catheter and the catheter taped to the skin to prevent accidental withdrawal or kinking. Some may wish to inject the initial dose at this time. Subsequent injections of one half to one third of the initial dose are made every 45 to 60 minutes with agents of lesser duration. However, repeated injection may result in tolerance or tachyphylaxis, which may relate to local changes in hydrogen ion concentration. In the use of lidocaine, a slowly metabolized drug, the cumulative dose may reach toxic levels in plasma; as a rule, such concentrations are not attained during the course of an operation of average duration.

In using this technique precautions with regard to asepsis and avoidance of trauma must be assured. The anesthesia syringe is protected by a sterile cap.

MANAGEMENT AND SEQUELAE

Subsequent management of peridural anesthesia is the same as for spinal anesthesia, with attention paid to maintenance of normal circulation and respiration and supplementation with sedatives, opioids, or general anesthesia when called for. There has been no thorough study undertaken to detect development of neurologic sequelae after peridural anesthesia. However, isolated instances of neurologic complications have been reported. Major problems may be summarized as follows:

1. Inadvertent subarachnoid injection, with the resultant high spinal anesthesia requiring immediate treatment for respiratory paralysis and circulatory depression. Postural headache usually follows introduction of the large needle.

2. Systemic reactions to the local anesthetic in the form of convulsions, hypotension, and loss of consciousness — requiring special treatment. The systemic effects of

epinephrine are hazardous in the presence of arteriosclerotic heart disease, but the smaller total doses used in the elderly counteract this tendency. Furthermore, epinephrine intensifies the block.

3. Inability to obtain anesthesia or recovery of blood from the catheter dictates insertion at another level. Failure may be the result of catheter entry into a peridural vein. Onset of anesthesia may be absent or slow; the patient may manifest a circulatory reaction, and drowsiness or a convulsion may ensue.

CAUDAL ANESTHESIA

Although the first planned approach to the peridural space was made via the sacral canal and was subsequently called caudal anesthesia, the method was used largely in obstetrics, gaining popularity in the 1940s as a means of producing painless childbirth. Misapplication of the technique led to failures, complications, and a subsequent decline in popularity. However, the method is safe and useful, particularly for operations performed in the anal and sacral regions and for culdoscopy.

ANATOMY

The sacrum comprises the fused five sacral vertebrae. This triangular bone articulates with the lumbar spine above, the iliac bones laterally, and the coccyx below. The posterior midline crest represents the vertebral spines, whereas the sacral cornua below are remnants of the articular processes. Lack of fusion or absence of the laminae of the fifth or fourth vertebra gives rise to the sacral hiatus between the cornua. This area is covered posteriorly by the dense sacrococcygeal ligament formed from the supraspinous and interspinous ligaments as well as the ligamentum flavum. The posterior sacral foramina give passage to the posterior primary divisions of the sacral nerves. Osseous anomalies of the sacrum are frequent.

The sacral canal contains the following structures: the dural sac, which terminates at approximately the level of the second sacral foramen; the anterior and posterior divisions and dorsal root ganglia of the sacral nerves enveloped by the dura to their exits at the anterior and posterior foramina; a rich network of peridural veins; and some loose fat and areolar tissue. The capacity of the sacral canal varies according to body habitus and is more capacious in the female.

Because of the variable anatomy of the sacrum and the presence or absence of obesity and local contraindications, the sacrum should be examined during the preoperative visit to determine the feasibility of injection.

TECHNIQUE AND COMPLICATIONS

The patient lies in the prone position with the table flexed at the hips, the sacrum horizontal, and the heels turned outward to separate the buttocks and expose the hiatus. In the pregnant woman the left lateral decubitus position is elected. Important landmarks are the posterior superior iliac spines; the second sacral foramen, 1 cm below and medial to the spines; and the hiatus between the sacral cornua, about 4 cm above the tip of the coccyx (Fig. 20–1). The hiatus can be felt as a distinct depression.

The sacral area is thoroughly prepared with antiseptic and draped, a gauze sponge having first been placed between the buttocks to prevent leakage of irritating solutions onto the genitalia. Anesthetic infiltration of the skin and underlying ligaments is made with a hypodermic needle. A 20-gauge, 4-cm needle with stylet is used for injection; this is inserted almost perpendicular to the skin until a distinct feeling of penetration of the sacrococcygeal ligament is experienced. The needle is then advanced a centimeter or

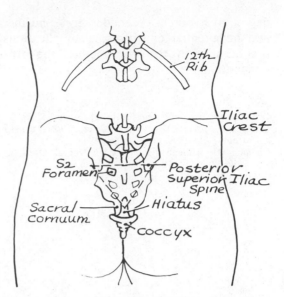

FIGURE 20–1. Landmarks for caudal anesthesia.

two somewhat parallel to the sacrum, with the bevel downward. The stylet is withdrawn and used to measure the distance inserted, certainly not as far as the S2 level. With a dry syringe, aspiration is gently done in four quadrants to detect the appearance of CSF or blood; recovery of either necessitates repositioning the needle. Five ml of air are then injected, with the fingers held over the site of the needle tip; a sensation of crepitus indicates that the needle lies on the dorsum of the sacrum, requiring re-insertion. If the needle is well positioned and there is no resistance to injection, an initial injection of 5 ml is made to be sure that subarachnoid entry has not occurred; the remainder of the anesthetic solution is then placed. Usually about 10 to 15 ml of 1.5 to 2.0 per cent lidocaine, mepivacaine, or procaine, with 1:200,000 epinephrine, are required for sacral anesthesia. Onset with lidocaine or mepivacaine is apparent in two to five minutes; with procaine, in five to ten minutes; complete anesthesia is obtained in about 15 minutes with any of the drugs. Because of the variation in capacity of the sacral canal as well as obstacles to diffusion of the drug, the resultant level of anesthesia may vary widely. Inadequate anesthesia can be corrected by repeat block or by transsacral injection, which is a paravertebral approach to the sacral canal. In 5 to 15 per cent of individuals the presence of ligamentous and osseous abnormalities precludes the attainment of satisfactory anesthesia.

Complications resulting from caudal anesthesia include systemic reactions to the local anesthetic and, in obstetrics, high levels of anesthesia with arterial hypotension and interference with the forces of labor. Injury to the fetal head has been reported when injection was made during the second stage of labor. Infection is a serious delayed complication.

APPRAISAL

Peridural anesthesia is a useful technique not only for surgical and obstetric procedures but in the diagnosis and treatment of pain and autonomic nervous system dysfunction, wherein prolonged neural blockade may be beneficial. The technical problems inherent in the method can be largely overcome through practice, but in every series reported there has been a higher failure rate than with spinal anesthesia. The chief reasons for selection of peridural rather than spinal anesthesia are the lesser degree of hypotension encountered and the avoidance of lumbar puncture headache and the potential for neurologic complications. If the beginner masters spinal anesthesia first because it is the easier method, the problems of peridural anesthesia will be better understood.

REFERENCES

Bromage PR: Epidural Anesthesia. Philadelphia, W. B. Saunders, 1978.

Cohen EN, Levine, DA, Colliss JE, et al: Role of pH in development of tachyphylaxis to local anesthetic agents. Anesthesiology 29:994, 1968.

Cousins MJ, Bridenbaugh PO (eds): Neural Blockade in Clinical Anesthesia and Management of Pain. Philadelphia, J. B. Lippincott, 1980.

Covino BG: Cardiovascular effects of spinal and epidural anesthesia. Reg Anesth 1:23, 1978.

Chapter *21*
REGIONAL NERVE BLOCKS

Although this is an introductory text, we believe it is important for the beginner in anesthesia to think at the outset in terms of regional anesthesia. Consequently, in this chapter we describe the techniques of nerve block most commonly employed for operation and in the treatment of pain and disease. There are other nerve blocks that anesthetists will wish to master as they gain experience. The descriptions given here are more or less in outline form, but with this as a background, proficiency ultimately will be attained with reading and experience. As with any form of anesthesia, the patient should be a suitable subject for the procedure, and the appropriate amount of sedative and opioid should be given for medication.

To perform nerve blocks, one should understand the anatomy of a typical spinal nerve (Fig. 21–1). Anterior and posterior nerve roots of a somatic nerve join at the intervertebral foramen to form the nerve trunk. In the immediate vicinity of the foramen the dorsal root ganglion is present, the spinal dura blends with the perineurium, and the anterior and posterior primary divisions of the nerve are formed. At this junction, the rami communicantes connect with the sympathetic chain, and a recurrent sympathetic branch enters the spinal canal. In general, the posterior primary divisions supply the skin and muscles posterior to the transverse processes of the vertebrae, together comprising the axial skeleton. The anterior divisions supply structures of the appendicular skeleton, anterior to the transverse processes, as well as the chest and abdomen. In the midline anteriorly the nerves overlap for a short distance, whereas any one area of skin receives a sensory contribution from at least three nerves, an overlapping of dermatomes. The approach to nerves for nerve block is dictated by the anatomy of the region involved, obviously differing for neck, thorax, and abdomen, and the extent of anesthesia sought. For the chest and abdomen, nerve blocks are usually done paravertebrally, whereas for the neck (to some extent) and the extremities, regional blocks involve the major somatic nerve plexuses and peripheral nerves.

PARAVERTEBRAL NERVE BLOCKS

CERVICAL PLEXUS BLOCK

The cervical plexus is formed from the anterior primary divisions of the first four cervical nerves. These nerves are interconnected, communicate with the last four cranial nerves, and receive gray rami communicantes from the cervical sympathetic chain. The most important contributions to the plexus are those to the ansa hypoglossi that supplies the infrahyoid muscles and to the roots of the phrenic nerve derived from

237

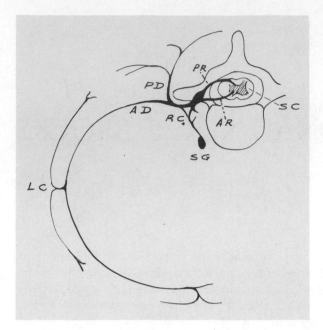

FIGURE 21–1. Diagram of a typical spinal nerve. *SC* = spinal cord; *PR* = posterior ramus; *AR* = anterior ramus; *AD* = anterior division; *PD* = posterior division; *RC* = rami communicantes; *SG* = sympathetic ganglion; *LC* = lateral cutaneous nerve.

the third, fourth, and fifth nerves. The first cervical nerve has no sensory component, but the others carry sensation from the head and neck via the superficial cervical plexus. The deep cervical plexus segmentally innervates those muscles that arise and insert on the corresponding cervical vertebrae and transverse processes.

The cervical plexus may be blocked from either a posterior or a lateral approach, the former more painful and offering less precise landmarks. For the lateral approach the patient's head is turned away to permit palpation of the transverse processes and to displace the sternomastoid muscle and carotid sheath anteriorly. After raising a skin wheal, injection of 10 to 20 ml of a 0.5 to 1.0 per cent solution of lidocaine or another anesthetic is made at the midpoint of the posterior border of the sternomastoid muscle; this should anesthetize the superficial cervical plexus, which carries sensation from head and neck (Fig. 21–2). The injection should "fan out" both superficial to and beneath the deep fascia, to reach all nerve filaments. Then the second, third, and fourth nerves are blocked at the anterior tubercles of the transverse processes. A landmark for the fourth transverse process lies just above the midpoint of the posterior border of the sternomastoid muscle, where the external jugular vein crosses the muscle. The upper border of the thyroid cartilage suggests the space between the third and fourth cervical vertebrae. After the transverse processes are identified, injection with 5 ml of 1.0 to 1.5 per cent lidocaine is made successively with the needle point against bone.

Possible complications of deep cervical nerve block include bleeding from the vertebral artery, subarachnoid or peridural injection, phrenic nerve paralysis, and laryngeal nerve block as indicated by hoarseness. It should not be a surprise if Horner's syndrome develops or if anesthesia spreads to involve the upper divisions of the brachial plexus. Actually, the cervical plexus is anesthetized when a large volume of local anesthetic is injected via the interscalene approach to the brachial plexus.

With superficial plexus block alone, operations can be performed between the jaw and the clavicle in the anterior and posterior cervical triangles. Deep cervical block provides relaxation of the strap muscles, but analgesia is not complete because afferent sympathetic fibers may remain unblocked. The surgeon should manipulate tissues gently and infiltrate with local anesthetic, if necessary, as the dissection proceeds.

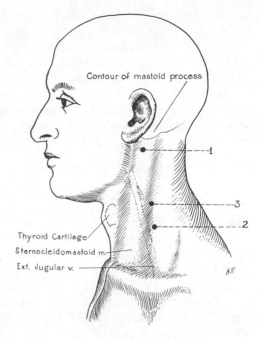

FIGURE 21–2. Landmarks for the cervical plexus; *1* is one fingerbreadth below the mastoid process, corresponding to *C2*; *3* is opposite the superior cornu of the thyroid cartilage corresponding to *C5*–also the midpoint of the posterior border of the sternocleidomastoid muscle where block of the superficial cervical plexus is done; *2* is at the level of Chassaignac's tubercle, or the sixth transverse process — also used as a landmark in stellate ganglion block and the interscalene approach to the brachial plexus. (Reproduced with permission from Labat GL: Regional Anesthesia. 2nd ed, Philadelphia, W B Saunders Co, 1928.)

Contour of mastoid process

Thyroid Cartilage

Sternocleidomastoid m.

Ext. Jugular v.

INTERCOSTAL BLOCK

The 12 thoracic nerves forming the intercostals present a peculiar anatomy of their own. In the intercostal space, vein, artery, and nerve relate to each other in that order from above downward. From the intervertebral foramen outward, the intercostal nerve lies between the external intercostal muscle and the internal intercostal membrane. Beyond the angle of the rib the nerve courses between the intercostal muscles, then forward, splitting the internal intercostal muscle so that the latter forms an internal and a medial muscle. At the costal cartilages the external intercostal muscle is no longer present. Thus, the nerves have varying relations, depending on the presence or absence of the intercostal muscles. The lower six intercostals pass posterior to the costal cartilages between the origins of the diaphragm and the transversus abdominis muscles to enter the abdominal wall; there they lie between the transversus abdominis and internal oblique muscles. A lateral cutaneous branch leaves the intercostal nerve anterior to the posterior axillary line and then splits into anterior and posterior divisions. Thus, the intercostal nerve must be blocked posterior to this point to obtain satisfactory superficial anesthesia of the abdominal wall. Furthermore, block of at least three somatic nerves is necessary for complete anesthesia at any site.

Intercostal nerve block provides satisfactory anesthesia of the abdominal wall, permitting relatively superficial intra-abdominal procedures such as liver biopsy, cholecystostomy, gastrostomy, or loop colostomy. In these instances the parietal peritoneum requires infiltration with anesthetic to avoid pain. More extensive intra-abdominal operations necessitate celiac and mesenteric plexus block to interrupt afferent visceral sympathetic impulses.

For unilateral intercostal block the patient is positioned with that side uppermost; for bilateral block the prone position, if tolerated by the patient, is more convenient. The ribs are identified with the injection made posterior to the posterior axillary line, using needles of the shortest possible length to avoid entering the pleura. We prefer to contact the rib above, perpendicularly, and to "walk off" the rib into the space below; the external intercostal fascia is sensed as the needle enters the space. A skin wheal is hardly necessary, and injection is made as the needle is advanced to the rib. No more than 3 to 4 ml of 0.5 to 1.0 per cent lidocaine are required for each space. As already noted, several nerves must be blocked above and below the proposed dermatomal site of abdominal incision. Thus, for the upper abdomen, thoracic nerves 5 through 11 should be injected. One should calculate in advance the total amount of local anesthetic needed to avoid injection of excessive amounts.

Multiple injection of the intercostal nerves is painful, requiring premedication with opioids if the condition of the patient allows this. Subsequently, operation is made more comfortable if 30 to 40 per cent nitrous oxide is given by mask.

PARAVERTEBRAL SOMATIC NERVE BLOCK

The landmark for any one of the spinal nerves is usually the corresponding vertebral spine; however, it not easy to identify the spines exactly. The most prominent is not always the seventh cervical, as stated (the vertebra prominens). The spines also vary in shape and slope, depending on segmental location. Thus, the cervicals are bifid and more or less perpendicular to the long axis; the thoracic spines are round at the tips, sloping downward acutely in the midthoracic region; and the lumbar spines are oblong at their tips and perpendicular to the long axis of the back.

For the dorsal approach to a somatic nerve, a point 4 cm from the midline is selected. The needle is guided perpendicularly onto the rib or transverse process. Then the needle is redirected inferiorly and inward at a 45-degree angle in both planes. If the needle is redirected upward after initial insertion, paresthesias are more frequent, and there is greater chance of subarachnoid injection through the intervertebral foramen. In the thoracic region the needle is advanced only 2 cm beyond the lower border of the rib or transverse process. Markers on the needle are helpful. The tip of the needle then lies between the external intercostal muscle and the internal intercostal membrane; deeper insertion carries the hazard of pleural entry. Five ml of 1 per cent lidocaine are sufficient to anesthetize not only the intercostal nerve but the sympathetic ganglion as well. In the lumbar region, depth of penetration to the transverse process is greater than in the thoracic region, and paravertebral injection, also at a greater depth, carries less hazard.

BLOCKS OF THE UPPER EXTREMITY

BRACHIAL PLEXUS

Soon after the introduction of local anesthesia in 1884, Halsted, a surgeon, injected cocaine under direct vision into the brachial plexus to perform radical mastectomy. After 1900 and with the synthesis of procaine, the plexus was anesthetized percutaneously — first via an axillary approach whereby the needle was advanced under and superior to the clavicle, then more or less directly via a supraclavicular insertion. Supraclavicular block remained the method of choice until Adriani resurrected axillary block, this time with perivascular injection about the axillary artery into the median, radial, and ulnar nerves. Finally, Winnie proposed the interscalene approach to the plexus, with insertion of the needle at the level of the sixth cervical transverse process. At present both the axillary and interscalene methods have supplanted the supraclavicular technique because of an appreciable incidence of pneumothorax with the latter procedure. The success of all these techniques rests upon a common anatomy.

Anatomy

Composed of the anterior divisions of the last four cervical and first thoracic nerves, the plexus can be envisioned as extending from the transverse processes to the apex of the axilla, where the terminal nerves are formed. All components are contained in a sheath of cervical fascia so that injection of a sufficient volume of anesthetic at any of the sites previously noted results in anesthetization of the plexus. The plexus itself is concentrated within a circumscribed area, just over the first rib, in relation to the cupula of the pleura between the anterior and middle scalene muscles. At this point the plexus is joined by the third portion of the subclavian artery, to form a neurovascular bundle continuing into the axilla. The prominent pulsation of the artery as it lies in the subclavian groove of the first rib can be used as a guide to the plexus in supraclavicular injection (Fig. 21–3). Landmarks such as the midpoint of the clavicle or the external jugular vein as it crosses the sternocleidomastoid muscle are also employed.

Finally, it should be noted that other nerves may be anesthetized as the large volumes needed for complete brachial block are injected: phrenic nerve with resulting diaphragmatic paralysis; inferior laryngeal nerve with vocal cord paralysis; the ascending nerves to the head in the paravertebral sympathetic chain causing Horner's syndrome; postganglionic autonomic fibers arising in the stellate ganglion; and the upper cervical nerves, which carry sensation from the back of the head, the anterior and posterior cervical triangles, and the cutaneous areas over the upper thorax and shoulder.

General Principles of Brachial Plexus Block

In all varieties of brachial plexus block the plexus should be approached with a clear concept of its location, the point of crossing the first rib; the relation to the pleural cupula immediately beneath; and a knowledge of other landmarks such as the scalenus muscles and the anterior tubercle of the sixth vertebral transverse cervical process. The anesthetist usually stands at the side of the recumbent patient, whose head may or may not be turned away, with the shoulder girdle drawn down or the arm abducted. The area is prepared and draped so that all landmarks are visible. Depending on the dexterity of the anesthetist, either hand may be employed for needle insertion. The needle should be the shortest possible length compatible with reaching the plexus; a 2- to 4-cm, 23-gauge needle is usually satisfactory.

Axillary Block of the Brachial Plexus

Because of the ease and accuracy of placement of the needle as well as a minimal incidence of complications, the axillary approach to the brachial plexus is the most

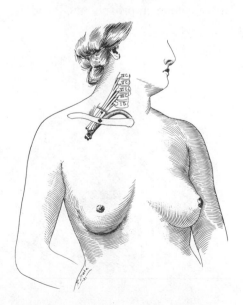

FIGURE 21–3. Landmarks for the supraclavicular block of the brachial plexus. (Reproduced with permission from Labat GL: Regional Anesthesia. 2nd ed, Philadelphia, W B Saunders Co, 1928.)

popular technique. Additional advantages are that the axillary block may be repeated if necesary during the course of a lengthy operation, and it is a technique easily applied to a child.

The skin of the axilla should be shaved and the arm abducted at 90 degrees, with the forearm flexed at a right angle and lying flat on a table (Fig. 21–4). The axillary artery is isolated and fixed between the index and middle fingers of one hand. A skin wheal is raised as high in the axilla as possible, usually 1 to 3 cm above the insertion of the pectoralis major muscle on the humerus. At this point the terminal nerves of the plexus have not yet begun to diverge from the artery. A 2- to 4-cm, 23-gauge, blunt-tipped needle is inserted at a 45-degree angle in the direction of the artery to enter the neurovascular sheath. A distinct impression of penetration of fascia may be experienced as well as production of paresthesias or perforation of the artery. The latter is of little moment when a small needle is used and immediately withdrawn. Pulsations transmitted to the needle are a good sign. Injection into the neurovascular sheath without repositioning the needle results in successful block. Volumes of local anesthetic in 1 to 1.5 per cent concentrations for lidocaine or carbocaine or 0.75 per cent concentration for bupivacaine (any agent with or without epinephrine) up to 50 ml may be required for complete anesthetization of the plexus. De Jong has described a technique for injection of the musculocutaneous nerve in the arm because this is frequently missed during axillary block. The intercostobrachial nerve is blocked merely by extending the initial skin wheal around the arm. This, however, does not prevent tourniquet pain.

Complications of axillary block are limited essentially to minimal extravasation of blood in a small percentage of cases. If properly performed, the solidity and extent of the nerve block are as good as in supraclavicular block, the anesthetic apparently diffusing upward to reach the supraclavicular branches of the plexus as demonstrated by injection of radiopaque solutions. When a large volume of local anesthetic is injected, the plasma concentrations approach the high levels achieved with caudal or paravertebral nerve blocks.

Interscalene Brachial Plexus Block

Winnie and Collins have described several perivascular techniques for block of the brachial plexus based on the concept that the plexus is enveloped in a fascial compartment extending from the cervical vertebrae to the distal axilla. In the interscalene approach, the head is lifted to accentuate the clavicular head of the

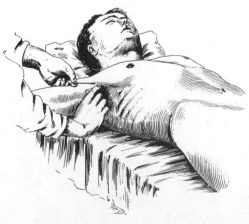

FIGURE 21–4. Perivascular axillary block of the brachial plexus. (Reproduced with permission from Labat GL: Regional Anesthesia. 2nd ed, Philadelphia, W B Saunders Co, 1928.)

sternomastoid muscle. Starting at the lateral border above the clavicle, the finger is rolled across the belly of the anterior scalene muscle to the groove between the anterior and middle scalenes. At the level of the sixth cervical transverse process or Chassaignac's tubercle, a 2.5- to 4-cm, 22-gauge needle is inserted into the groove perpendicular to the skin (thus slightly caudad, dorsal, and mesial). Penetration of fascia may be felt, a paresthesia elicited, or a transverse process touched. With the needle thus placed in the fascial compartment, 30 to 50 ml are injected into the space; volume is considered important for success. With large volumes both cervical and brachial plexuses are blocked. Although pneumothorax is avoided, Horner's syndrome and phrenic nerve palsy appear frequently, and inadvertent intravenous and subarachnoid injections have been reported.

Supraclavicular Block

A skin wheal is raised at a point 1 cm above the clavicle midway between the acromial tip and the sternoclavicular articulation, thus approximately at the lateral border of the first rib (see Fig. 21–3). To avoid puncturing the subclavian artery, the artery is depressed with the index finger of one hand while inserting the needle just above the fingertip. Direction of the needle is backward, inward, and downward. When paresthesias are elicited in the fingers, the anesthetic is injected slowly, usually 20 to 25 ml.

One of the important details of all these techniques is instruction of the patient in the accurate reporting of paresthesias, described as resembling "electric shock" or striking the "funny bone." Patient cooperation calls for just the right amount of sedation. If the rib is not reached at the expected depth, anywhere from 0.5 to 2.5 cm beneath the skin depending on the habitus of the patient, the needle is withdrawn to avoid entering the pleura and the direction altered. Once the rib is touched, the plexus has already been bypassed.

An intracutaneous and subcutaneous wheal is then made in bracelet fashion about the upper arm to interrupt sensory fibers of the second and third thoracic nerves carried in the intercostobrachial nerve. Although this is necessary for operations performed on the upper arm, it does not, as alleged, prevent tourniquet pain. This results from ischemia, the pain transmitted by autonomic fibers that travel perivascularly to enter the spinal cord through unblocked pathways.

The most serious complication of supraclavicular nerve block is development of tension pneumothorax, reported as occurring in 1 to 3 per cent of blocks. That pneumothorax develops gradually suggests slow escape of air from the lung rather than entrainment of air during injection. Phrenic nerve paralysis is found in approximately 25 per cent of patients. In a small number of patients persistent subjective paresthesias and sensory deficit have been noted. These are inherent in the technique, probably resulting from the deliberate elicitation of paresthesias and intraneural injection. It is thus apparent why the other techniques are favored in brachial plexus block.

NERVE BLOCK AT THE ELBOW

There is usually little need to block the radial, median, or ulnar nerve at the elbow because of the ease of performance of axillary block, but occasionally elbow block may be necessary. Block at the elbow does not prevent pain when a forearm tourniquet is used. The techniques of Labat described here are those commonly employed.

Median Nerve

Both median and radial nerves are approached at the arm where a crease is formed as the supinated forearm is held at a right angle; the forearm is then extended (Fig. 21–5). The tendon of the biceps is palpated, the pulsation of the brachial artery

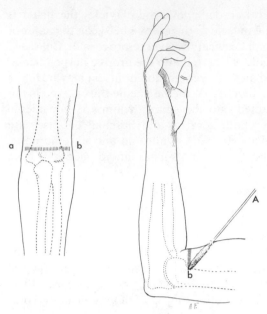

FIGURE 21–5. *A* is an applicator to show the level of injection of the median and radial nerves at the elbow. (Reproduced with permission from Labat GL: Regional Anesthesia. 2nd ed. Philadelphia, W B Saunders Co, 1928.)

identified, and a skin wheal raised just medial to the artery for block of the median nerve. This point is about midway between the medial condyle of the humerus and the medial border of the biceps. Occasionally the median nerve can be rolled beneath the finger. A 4-cm, 23-gauge needle is inserted perpendicular to the skin through deep fascia, where a paresthesia may be produced. From 2 to 3 ml of 2 per cent lidocaine are injected, or 5 ml are introduced fanwise in the absence of a paresthesia.

Radial Nerve

At the same level as for the median nerve, the needle is inserted 1 cm lateral to the biceps tendon through deep fascia, in a direction toward the operator's index finger as it is held against the posterior surface of the lateral condyle of the humerus. The intermuscular septum is thereby penetrated between the brachioradialis and brachialis muscles, about 10 cm above the lateral condyle, in the axis of the humerus. The needle is advanced to bone, where 10 ml of a 2 per cent lidocaine solution are injected fanwise over a distance of 6 to 7 cm. It should be recalled that once the radial nerve has supplied the muscles arising from the lateral condyle — the extensors, external rotators, and supinators — it is purely sensory to forearm and hand.

Ulnar Nerve

Block of the ulnar nerve at the elbow is easily performed because the nerve can be rolled beneath the finger as it lies in the groove between the medial condyle of the humerus and the olecranon process of the ulna. The patient is positioned to lie on the opposite side with the forearm extended, or supine with the forearm flexed and the arm held across the chest. Injection is made with a 2-cm, 25-gauge needle inserted from above downward into the groove, the nerve held immobile between two fingers. Paresthesias are easily produced, whereupon 1 to 2 ml of 2 per cent lidocaine are injected after slight withdrawal to avoid intraneural injection.

Block of the nerves at the elbow can be performed in rapid succession to produce anesthesia in the hand. For operations on the forearm, a bracelet injection of local anesthetic is made at the elbow to anesthetize the cutaneous nerves of the forearm.

NERVE BLOCK AT THE WRIST

Median Nerve

Satisfactory anesthesia for operation on the hand can be obtained by block of the nerves at the wrist. Block of the median nerve is made at a level corresponding to the tip of the styloid process of the ulna at a point between the tendons of the palmaris longus and flexor carpi radialis muscles (Fig. 21–6). The main part of the nerve lies beneath the volar fascia, either beneath or just to the radial side of the palmaris longus tendon. To identify the latter, the patient flexes the wrist against counterpressure with the fingers and thumb held straight. A 2-cm, 25-gauge needle is directed perpendicularly to a depth of 0.5 cm beneath deep fascia, and 1 to 2 ml of a 2 per cent solution of lidocaine are injected if a paresthesia is elicited; if not, an additional 2 ml are injected fanwise.

Ulnar Nerve

Ulnar nerve block at the wrist is performed at the same level as for the median nerve (see Fig. 21–6). With the hand supine and the tendon of the flexor carpi ulnaris held between the fingers, the needle is inserted perpendicularly, tangential to the tendon, beneath deep fascia where injection is made as for the median nerve. A good landmark is the ulnar artery, with injection beneath fascia just lateral to it, then both dorsally and subcutaneously to reach the smaller branches of the nerve. One to 2 ml of 2 per cent lidocaine are used.

Radial Nerve

At the wrist the radial nerve, now purely sensory, has diverged from the radial artery at the lower third of the forearm, turned dorsally, and pierced deep fascia to supply cutaneous branches to the wrist and the dorsum of the hand and the first,

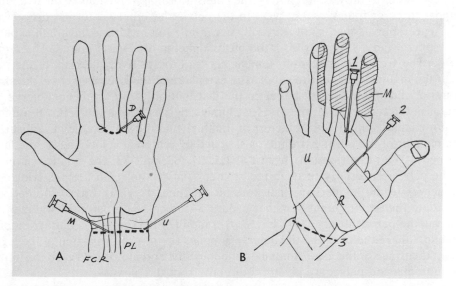

FIGURE 21–6. *A,* Palmar surface of the hand. Needles at *M* and *U* show points of injection for median and ulnar nerves, respectively. The dotted line is at the level of the styloid process of the ulna. Needle at *D* shows site of injection for field block of finger. *FCR* = flexor carpi radialis tendon; *PL* = palmaris longus tendon *B,* Dorsum of the hand showing cutaneous distribution of radial (*R*), ulnar (*U*), and median (*M*) nerves. Needles *1* and *2* indicate approaches to the interosseous spaces. The dotted line indicates bracelet injection for cutaneous nerves. (Reproduced with permission from Vandam LD: Anesthesia for hand surgery. *In* Flynn JE (ed): Hand Surgery. Baltimore, The Williams & Wilkins Co, 1966.)

second, and third fingers (Fig. 21–6). At the same level as for block of median and ulnar nerves, a subcutaneous and intracutaneous bracelet will anesthetize not only the radial branches but other cutaneous nerves of the forearm extending into the proximal part of the palm. Specifically, for radial nerve fibers, the radial artery is identified, the skin over it penetrated, and the needle then angled dorsally and parallel to skin, with injection subcutaneously for the length of the needle. Again, about 2 ml of a 2 per cent solution of lidocaine are used.

HAND AND DIGITAL BLOCK

Commonly employed nerve blocks of the hand are largely of the field and infiltrative variety. As a rule, it is best to inject via the dorsum of the hand rather than through the skin of the palm (Fig. 21–6). Injection should not be made into an infected area. In all instances it is important to avoid excessive distention of tissues and the use of epinephrine, which may compromise the circulation to the fingers.

The digits are anesthetized by cutaneous infiltration bilaterally at the base of the finger (see Fig. 21–6). Operations on the fifth finger involving palm and metacarpal bone can be performed with ulnar nerve block at the elbow or wrist. Extensive operations on the thumb require both median and ulnar nerve block as well as block of the radial and other cutaneous nerves. The other fingers and their respective metacarpals can be anesthetized by infiltration into the interosseous spaces. Injection is made from the dorsum, infiltrating the space down to the palm: about 5 ml of 1 per cent lidocaine are required. In interosseous injection, additional field block of the cutaneous nerves is necessary.

BLOCKS OF THE LOWER EXTREMITY

ANATOMY

The lower extremity is supplied by the anterior primary divisions of the five lumbar and upper three or four sacral nerves. In the pelvis these nerves form a deep-seated, widely spaced plexus that is not as readily accessible to block as is the brachial plexus. The peripheral nerves formed from the plexus emerge at several points. The femoral nerve derived from the upper four lumbar nerves crosses over the brim of the pelvis beneath the inguinal ligament to supply the extensors of the knee as well as the skin of the anterior thigh and part of the leg in the distribution of the saphenous nerve. The obturator nerve formed from the first four lumbar nerves leaves the pelvis through the obturator canal to supply the adductors of the thigh and the skin on the medial surface. The remainder of the lower extremity is supplied by the great sciatic nerve, the largest in the body. With contributions from L4, L5, S1, S2, and S3, the sciatic nerve exits from the pelvis posteriorly through the greater sciatic notch. On the posterior of the thigh, nerves to the hamstrings or flexors of the knee are given off; at the midpoint, division into the two terminal branches occurs — the common peroneal and the tibial. In general, the peroneal nerve (L4, L5, S1, S2) supplies all structures on the front of the leg and dorsum of the foot: the tibial nerve supplies the posterior portion of the leg and the plantar surface of the foot. A number of cutaneous and motor nerves to the muscles of the buttocks and pelvis are given off directly from the plexus.

FEMORAL NERVE BLOCK

The femoral nerve is blocked just below the inguinal ligament at the lateral border of the fossa ovalis. Three structures — femoral vein, artery, and nerve, medial to lateral — lie in the fossa. With a finger on the pulsating femoral artery, paresthesias of the femoral nerve are easily elicited, as it lies laterally. Five to ten ml of 1 per cent lidocaine are injected. Block of the nerve is not sufficient for operation on the anterior surface of the thigh unless combined with a lateral femoral cutaneous nerve block. The femoral nerve is sensory to the medial surface of the thigh by way of the intermediate and medial cutaneous nerves.

LATERAL FEMORAL CUTANEOUS NERVE BLOCK

The lateral femoral cutaneous nerve (L2, L3) is easily blocked just medial to the anterior superior spine of the ilium. Infiltration is performed fanwise to the iliac spine and beneath the inguinal ligament with 5 to 10 ml of 1 per cent lidocaine. This block alone is sometimes sufficient for superficial operation on the lateral surface of the thigh. Rarely, the nerve is involved in the syndrome of meralgia paresthetica (Roth), characterized by numbness and paresthesias in the distribution of the nerve, and injection may be made for relief.

OBTURATOR NERVE BLOCK

Block of the obturator nerve is so seldom performed and less easily done than the others that it is not described here.

SCIATIC NERVE BLOCK

Sciatic nerve block results in anesthesia on the back of the thigh and leg. With many other types of anesthesia available for the patient in a poor physical state, sciatic block is seldom used; however, as a means of relieving pain it is occasionally valuable. One hazard of sciatic block is intraneural injection; because the perineural sheath is dense, development of pressure may cause ischemia with resulting paralysis. Labat advises bisection of a line drawn between the posterior superior spine of the ilium and the posterior tip of the greater trochanter of the femur. The needle is introduced perpendicular to the skin 2 cm below, on a line drawn perpendicular to the first, where paresthesias are sought. Since the sciatic nerve is large, 10 to 20 ml of 2 per cent lidocaine are required. The sciatic nerve can also be blocked via an anterior approach, but the percentage of successful blocks with this method is much lower.

PERONEAL NERVE BLOCK

The peroneal nerve is easily blocked at the point where it encircles the fibula, just beneath the head. Some difficulty may be encountered in palpating the nerve, since it is flattened at this site. In this location the nerve is easily injured by pressure or stretch, thus accounting for postoperative foot drop. There is little need to block the nerve in the popliteal space.

TIBIAL NERVE BLOCK

If necessary, the tibial nerve can be blocked at the medial margin of the popliteal space just lateral to the tendons of the semimembranosus and semitendinosus muscles. As in sciatic block, 2 per cent concentrations of anesthetic should be employed.

ANKLE BLOCK

Anterior and posterior tibial nerves are both blocked at a level on the ankle corresponding to the uppermost ends of the malleoli of tibia and fibula (Fig. 21–7). The leg is positioned so that the knee is flexed, with the sole of the foot flat on the table. For anterior tibial nerve block the operator stands on the lateral side, introducing the needle between the prominent tendons of the tibialis anticus and extensor hallucis longus muscles. When the needle touches bone, it is withdrawn slightly and liberal infiltration made. For the posterior tibial nerve, the operator stands on the medial side and the

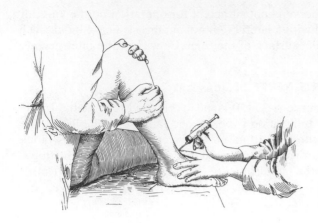

FIGURE 21–7. Approach to anterior tibial nerve block, same level as posterior tibial injection. (Reproduced with permission from Labat GL: Regional Anesthesia. 2nd ed. Philadelphia, W B Saunders Co, 1928.)

needle is inserted medial to the calcaneous tendon until bone is touched. Again, slight withdrawal and infiltration are done. Paresthesias are sought in both instances and are elicited relatively easily. Ankle block is completed with a superficial cutaneous bracelet infiltration and deep infiltration at the posterolateral compartment to block the sural nerve. Toe block is similar to that for the fingers.

SYMPATHETIC NERVE BLOCKS

STELLATE GANGLION BLOCK

Stellate ganglion block with interruption of sympathetic nervous impulses to the arm is beneficial in the treatment of peripheral vascular disease, sympathetic dystrophy, and perhaps as an adjunct to operation on the hand when vessel, nerve, or bone healing is in jeopardy. As noted earlier, brachial plexus and peripheral nerve block are also accompanied by sympathetic nerve anesthesia.

Anatomy

The sympathetic fibers that course through the ganglion supply blood vessels, sweat glands, and pilomotor fibers to the skin of the head, arm, and upper chest wall as well as the deeper blood vessels, pupils, salivary glands, heart, and lungs. Preganglionic fibers to the ganglion originate from the first through the eighth thoracic spinal segments and synapse either in the ganglion or in the upper cervical ganglia, thereafter accompanying blood vessels and nerves in a peripheral distribution. Deep pain sensation may be transmitted via perivascular autonomic fibers; these enter the cord via the posterior nerve roots and white rami communicantes, where the cell bodies are located in the dorsal sensory ganglia.

The stellate ganglion is usually composed of the conjoined ganglia of the inferior cervical and first thoracic sympathetic ganglia. It is a discrete, more or less encapsulated structure with its own blood supply, lying upon the seventh cervical vertebral transverse process and the neck of the first rib. Posteromedially situated is the longus colli muscle; posterolaterally, the scalenus muscles; and anteriorly, the cupula of the pleura. Adjacent structures include the carotid sheath, the first portion of the subclavian artery, the thyrocervical and vertebral arteries, the phrenic and recurrent laryngeal nerves, the esophagus, the vertebrae, and the spinal nerves.

Technique

Many approaches to stellate ganglion block have been described. These are classified according to point of entry in the neck and the relation to the sternocleidomastoid muscle — anterior, anterolateral, lateral, or posterior — paravertebral.

A safe technique is that described by de Sousa Pereira, utilizing the anterior tubercle of the sixth cervical transverse process (Chassaignac's, or the carotid tubercle — see Figure 21–2) as a landmark. With the patient semierect and the sternomastoid muscle and carotid sheath displaced medially, the tubercle may be felt just beneath the skin, easily reached with a short, small-gauge needle. Infiltration of 15 to 20 ml of 0.5 per cent lidocaine and downward diffusion produce effective block with little likelihood of major complications.

The simplest of all approaches in our experience is a median paratracheal injection made just beside the cricoid cartilage, corresponding to the level of the sixth cervical vertebra (Fig. 21–8). With the patient supine in a semierect position, the sternomastoid muscle is displaced laterally. A pillow placed beneath the shoulders so that the neck is hyperextended accentuates the anatomic landmarks. A 4-cm, 23-gauge uncapped needle is inserted perpendicular to the skin and tangential to the trachea until bone is met at a depth of from 2.5 to 4 cm. This may be either the sixth vertebral body or the base of the transverse process. The cervical sympathetic chain lies laterally at a distance no greater than 1.5 cm from the point of contact. After slight withdrawal of the needle to avoid injection into the longus colli muscle, 10 ml of 0.5 per cent lidocaine are injected slowly, with intermittent aspiration. At termination, the patient is tilted upright to facilitate downward diffusion to the ganglion.

The first sign of successful stellate ganglion block is usually ptosis of the eyelid on the blocked side, followed by miosis. Enophthalmos is an illusion seemingly produced by paralysis of the sympathetic component to the levator palpebrae superioris muscle. Scleral injection, warmth, and dryness of the face follow. These signs comprise Horner's syndrome, indicating interruption of the cervical sympathetic impulses to the head. To be certain of a satisfactory effect in arm and hand, warmth, anhidrosis, and vasodilation should be apparent.

Complications

As already noted, phrenic, recurrent laryngeal, or partial brachial nerve block may ensue. The patient should be warned beforehand of these occurrences, particularly of

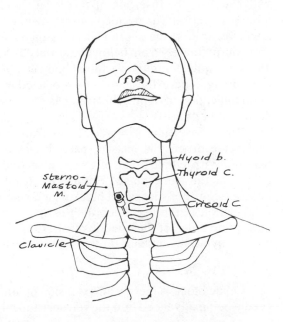

FIGURE 21–8. Median paratracheal injection of the stellate ganglion.

the ocular changes, the dryness of the face, nasal congestion, and possible hoarseness. Major complications resulting from stellate ganglion injection include pneumothorax, perforation of blood vessels, and subarachnoid injection. Block of the ganglion should not be attempted in the presence of a decreased clotting tendency or during use of anti-coagulants.

For sustained block, bupivacaine or etidocaine in 0.25 per cent concentration with epinephrine will produce block lasting up to 12 hours. Prolonged block with injection of 6 per cent phenol has been advocated to relieve chronic refractory pain, reputedly with little resultant neuritis. In this procedure, experience and placement of the needle under radiographic guidance are necessary to avoid complications.

PARAVERTEBRAL LUMBAR BLOCK

Apart from block of the stellate ganglion, paravertebral lumbar block is the most commonly performed sympathetic nerve block. The block is done as a diagnostic, prognostic, or therapeutic measure for vasospasm in the lower extremity or for sympathetic dystrophy.

Anatomy

The approach to the sympathetic chain is based on its presence on the anterolateral surface of the lumbar vertebral body in the retroperitoneal space, in close association with the celiac, semilunar, and mesenteric plexuses. Injection is made into the area of the first and second lumbar sympathetic ganglia — the lowermost portion of the thoracolumbar division of the autonomic nervous system, the site of maximal sympathetic outflow to the legs.

Technique

For unilateral block the patient may be positioned in the lateral decubitus position, but for bilateral block the prone position is more convenient. The trunk is bowed either by flexing the operating table or by placing a pillow beneath the abdomen to open the space between rib cage and iliac crests. Marked needles, 10 to 12 cm in length, 21- to 22-gauge, are required because of the depth of injection.

A line about 7 cm long is drawn from a vertebral spine to the point of intersection with the last rib. Insertion at this level should take the needle to the first or second lumbar vertebra. The needle is inserted either 4 or 7 cm from the midline at a 45-degree angle inward. At the shorter distance the transverse process of the lumbar vertebra is met approximately 5 cm below the surface. The needle is then redirected downward at a 45-degree angle until the vertebral body is touched from 7.5 to 10 cm below the surface; in so doing, a paresthesia may be produced in a lumbar nerve. After setting the marker as an indication of depth, the needle is progressively redirected until it slides just off the vertebral body.

When insertion is made 7 cm from the midline, contact with the vertebral transverse process is missed, paresthesias are less likely, and the procedure is less painful. With either point of entry, a second needle may be placed about 3 to 4 cm below, in the same plane. From 5 to 10 ml of 0.5 to 1 per cent lidocaine are then injected. Signs of successful block include increase in skin temperature, anhidrosis, and vasodilation in the leg. Recording of skin temperature or skin conductivity should be done as an index of therapeutic result. Complications are few: blood vessel perforation, arterial hypotension, and rarely, inadvertent subarachnoid block.

CELIAC BLOCK

Celiac block is merely an extension of lumbar paravertebral sympathetic block, the needle being advanced into the retroperitoneal space 1 to 2 cm beyond the anterolateral surface of the vertebral body. Care is taken to avoid penetration of the aorta on the left or the inferior vena cava on the right. Since the capacity of the retroperitoneal space is large and the celiac and mesenteric plexuses are diffuse, a large volume of anesthetic is required, from 30 to 40 ml of 0.5 per cent lidocaine.

Celiac block is usually performed for relief of abdominal pain in acute or chronic pancreatitis or carcinoma of the pancreas or in sympathetic imbalance involving the bowel such as acquired megacolon. Signs of a successful block include relief of pain and, sometimes, signs of sympathetic paralysis in the legs. Arterial hypotension is not infrequent because of widespread sympathetic blockade involving the splanchnic circulation and lower extremities. In situations in which prolonged block for a day or two might be beneficial, continuous lumbar peridural anesthesia is a more manageable technique.

INTRAVENOUS REGIONAL ANESTHESIA

Bier, in 1908, injected procaine intravenously between two tourniquets to produce anesthesia in the arm. After sporadic application, the method fell into disuse until reintroduced by Holmes in 1963. The method entails bloodless exsanguination of the extremity and subsequent injection of a measured quantity of local anesthetic, which is confined to the area by use of a pneumatic tourniquet above. Onset of anesthesia is prompt, probably relating to diffusion of the anesthetic to sensory nerve endings and, in part, to the pressure of the tourniquet on larger nerve fibers. Release of the tourniquet at the termination results in rapid disappearance of anesthesia but with the possibility of central nervous and cardiovascular symptoms relating to the entry of a bolus of local anesthetic into the systemic circulation. However, the concentration of local anesthetic reached in plasma is less than that following brachial plexus or caudal block. Three peak concentrations are observed, relating respectively to release of local anesthetic from the vascular space, the extravascular space, and the tissue compartments and neural elements. All precautions should be taken to detect and treat systemic reactions to the local anesthetic.

TECHNIQUE

For operations on the forearm or hand a double pneumatic tourniquet is applied just above the elbow, and for procedures on the foot the tourniquet is applied at the calf, with a web roll beneath to ease the pressure. Initially, the tourniquet is inflated just above venous pressure to permit venous puncture in a superficial vein adjacent to but not directly at the operative site. A scalp vein needle or a 22-gauge plastic catheter with plastic stylet is used and securely fixed in place, with a heparin lock attached. Tourniquet pressure is released, the arm or leg elevated above venous pressure for a minute or so, and an Esmarch bandage tightly applied beginning at the distal end and extending up to the tourniquet to provide maximal exsanguination and a bloodless operative field. First the distal tourniquet is inflated and then the proximal, after which the distal is released. Tourniquet pressure should reach at least 100 torr above arterial systolic pressure, about 250 torr for the arm and 350 for the leg. The extremity (presenting a cadaveric appearance) is then placed horizontally for injection of the local anesthetic. Any flushing of the skin should suggest loss of tourniquet pressure; injection is discontinued, and immediate steps are taken to treat a systemic local anesthetic reaction.

Usually 0.5 per cent lidocaine, 3 mg/k, or 0.2 per cent bupivacaine, 1.5 mg/k, is injected, with the ampule specifically marked for intravenous regional anesthesia. Obviously volume is important in filling the vascular and extravascular spaces, so that amounts up to 50 ml are commonly used.

In the ordinary course of events tourniquet pain is apt to develop after 45 minutes. Some believe that re-application of the Esmarch bandage after local anesthetic injection will force the anesthetic beneath the distal tourniquet, which is then inflated and is meant to avoid early onset of pain. Otherwise with onset of pain, the distal tourniquet is inflated and the proximal deflated. Pain is also mitigated by intravenous opioid administration or inhalation of subanesthetic concentrations of nitrous oxide.

Ordinarily, one would prefer to limit tourniquet inflation time to little more than an hour. At termination of operation, the part is wrapped and the tourniquet released, but never before 20 or 30 minutes. As noted previously, anesthesia wanes quickly. If the surgeon wishes to ascertain adequacy of hemostasis after tourniquet release, bupivacaine may be a better drug to use, as time will be allowed for wound closure; this is not so with lidocaine.

Intravenous regional anesthesia is employed largely for minor operations on the arm, less so on the foot or leg, and in either case when the procedure lasts less than an hour or so. Examples include incision and drainage; reduction of phalangeal or wrist fracture; excision of tumors or ganglia; removal of foreign bodies; repair of lacerations; and tendolysis and synovectomy. The time limitation is imposed by onset of tourniquet pain. Although toxic reactions to the local anesthetic are now rare, the anesthetist must be prepared to treat such occurrences by the recommended means (see Chapter 15).

APPRAISAL

There are distinct advantages in avoiding anesthesia if a regional technique will suffice. Regional methods, however, require much of the anesthetist, patient, and surgeon. Anesthetists must prepare their patients carefully through informative discussion and adequate premedication. A detailed knowledge of anatomy is required, as is a skilled, gentle technique. One must know the characteristics of the local anesthetic used, the potential for harm, and the treatment required should a toxic reaction develop. Finally, psychological support must be provided during the operation and appropriate supplemental drugs given when needed. The surgeon must be delicate in all manipulations and aware that the patient is awake. These admonitions are particularly important during intra-abdominal procedures. Some anesthetists and surgeons are unwilling to undertake these responsibilities, turning instead to general anesthesia as an easier but not necessarily better alternative.

REFERENCES

Adriani J: Labat's Regional Anesthesia. Philadelphia, W B Saunders Co, 1967.
Cousins MJ, Bridenbaugh PO (eds): Neural Blockade in Clinical Anesthesia and Management of Pain. Philadelphia, J B Lippincott, 1980.
Eriksson E (ed): Illustrated Handbook in Local Anesthesia. Philadelphia, W B Saunders, 1980.
Moore DC: Regional Block. Springfield, Charles C Thomas, 1975.
Ware RJ: Intravenous regional analgesia using bupivacaine. Anaesthesia 34:231, 1979.
Winnie AP, Collins VJ: The subclavian perivascular technique of brachial plexus anesthesia. Anesthesiology 25:353, 1964.

INTRAVENOUS SUPPORTIVE THERAPY

Chapter 22

INTRAVENOUS FLUIDS AND ACID-BASE BALANCE

The intravenous administration of drugs, electrolyte solutions, plasma, albumin, and blood components is an integral part of anesthetic management. In conjunction with principles of parenteral fluid therapy, this chapter is devoted to a discussion of the basic physiology of fluid, electrolyte, and acid-base balance. A subsequent chapter deals with blood transfusion and the technical aspects of intravenous administration.

THE BODY FLUID COMPARTMENTS

In practice the anesthetist is primarily concerned with monitoring the intravascular volume. Routine measurements such as blood pressure, pulse, central venous pressure (CVP), and ECG readings are all related to the adequacy or inadequacy of the circulating volume. The validity of these observations depends on an understanding of the relation between total body water and various subcompartments: the two major subcompartments — intracellular and extracellular — and the subdivisions of the latter, the intravascular and interstitial compartments, all are in equilibrium.

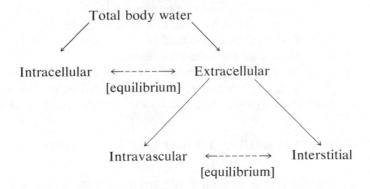

Total body water refers to the total amount of water in the body, expressed as a per cent of the total body weight. The lean body mass is defined as the functional tissues consisting of bone, essential fat, and all vital tissues. Studies have shown that approximately 70 per cent of the adult mammalian functional mass consists of water, but the human body contains a variable amount of fat, which has a much lower water content per gram than any other tissue. Therefore, a wide range of total body water exists among the sexes, with men having a higher content than women: 60 per cent mean for men (range 40 to 68) as compared with 50 per cent mean for women (range 30 to 53).

Measurement of body fluid volumes depends on the dilution principle. A known quantity of a measurable substance is injected intravenously into the fluid compartment, and the concentration is determined once the substance is in equilibrium.

$$\text{Fluid volume} = \frac{Q \text{ (known quantity of test substance)}}{\text{concentration}}$$

Estimation of total body water is made with substances that theoretically have equal distribution both inside and outside cells. Various substances, such as deuterium oxide (heavy water), urea, sulfanilamide, antipyrine, and creatinine have been used. Potential errors in measurement can be related to metabolism, protein binding, or inability of the substances to assume homogeneous distribution. The mean figures cited previously were obtained with deuterium oxide.

RELATION OF EXTRACELLULAR VOLUME TO BLOOD VOLUME

Extracellular fluid volume comprises approximately 20 per cent of ideal body weight or about one third of the total body water, and, as previously noted, consists of the intravascular or plasma volume and the interstitial fluid. The proportion of extracellular fluid present intravascularly is determined largely by the oncotic pressure of protein. Approximately one fifth of the extracellular fluid volume is plasma, whereas four fifths constitute interstitial fluid.

The body utilizes several mechanisms to maintain an appropriate balance between the size of the intravascular space and the intravascular volume to ensure adequate venous return to the heart. Homeostatic mechanisms include mobilization of protein via the lymphatics and vasoconstriction, primarily in capacitance vessels. Ultimately, changes in extracellular fluid are reflected by proportional changes in both interstitial volume and the plasma component of the intravascular space. Therefore, maintenance of a normal extracellular fluid volume is essential in the maintenance of blood volume.

Measurements of extracellular fluid compartments have been done with sucrose, inulin, or mannitol, all excluded from the cell interior. However, because these substances fail to enter all the extracellular fluid compartments uniformly, the measurements are not quite accurate. Plasma volume is determined by intravenous injection of a dye such as Evans blue or of radioactive iodinated human serum albumin (RIHSA). Whole blood volume is computed by adding the red blood cell volume as determined by injection of chromium-tagged cells. Average figures for the fluid compartments are given in Table 22–1.

RELATION OF EXTRACELLULAR TO INTRACELLULAR FLUID VOLUME

The distribution of water is not limited to any particular compartment, as it is a freely movable solvent for all the body solutes. Solute distribution, on the other hand,

TABLE 22–1.   Average Fluid Volumes

Measurement	Absolute Value		Relative Value (% Body Weight)	
	Male	Female	Male	Female
Weight (kg)	70	60	—	—
Hematocrit, large vessels (per cent)	44	40	—	—
Plasma volume (ml)	3150	2700	4.5	4.5
Red blood cell volume (ml)	2100	1500	3.0	2.5
Blood volume (ml)	5250	4200	7.5	7.0
Hematocrit, whole body (per cent)	40	36	—	—
Total body water (L)	42	30	60	50
Extracellular water (L)	16.4	14.2	23.4	23.7

has several limitations. The size of molecules, such as the plasma proteins, limits their movement from one compartment to another. Certain electrolytes, such as sodium, do not readily traverse cell membranes. The result is that water diffuses across the barriers to maintain osmotic equilibrium.

The concept of osmolarity is basic to understanding this solute-solvent relationship. One gm molecular weight (one mole) of a substance contains 6.023×10^{23} (Avogadro's number) molecules. One osmole is defined as one mole (Avogadro's number) of a nondissociating substance in 1 L of solution. The term milliosmol (mOsm) is defined as one thousandth of an osmole of the substance in solution. Osmolarity is equal to the number of osmoles per liter of solution, whereas osmolality is defined as the number of osmoles per 1000 gm of solvent. In dilute solutions such as exist in the human body, osmolality is approximately equal to osmolarity. Conventionally, these values are expressed in terms of mOsm, with the normal osmolarity of extracellular fluid equal to 285 to 295 mOsm/L.

The major extracellular cation is sodium; each cation is accompanied by an anion. Besides electrolytes, other osmotically active particles found in small amounts are urea and glucose. In patients with uremia or severe hyperglycemia, these molecules add significantly to the total osmolality. Other substances such as ethanol or mannitol can also increase the total osmolality. Both urea and ethanol readily cross cell membranes and therefore do not cause acute shifts in water between the extracellular and intracellular compartments. However, substances such as sodium, glucose, and mannitol do not readily cross cell membranes, therefore potentially causing loss of intracellular fluid. In clinical conditions such as heat stroke, water is selectively lost without solute. When this occurs, a hyperosmolar state exists, corresponding to a serum osmolality greater than 340 mOsm, a serum sodium greater than 160 mEq/L, or both. Some drugs, for example bicarbonate, given intravenously markedly raise osmolarity. A 50-ml ampule of sodium bicarbonate contains 50 mEq of $NaHCO_3$ (100 mOsm) per 50 ml or 2000 mOsm/L.

Excessive administration of salt-free water to a patient not on oral intake is associated with the hypo-osmolar state, corresponding to a serum osmolality less than 240 mOsm or a serum sodium less than 110 mEq/L. Rapidity of change of serum osmolality or serum sodium is another factor affecting a patient's tolerance to osmolar changes.

Administration of fluid containing 140 mEq of sodium expands extracellular volume without producing appreciable change in serum sodium concentration, as the solution is isotonic. Hypotonic salt solution increases the size of the extracellular space while decreasing serum sodium concentration. Clearly, serum sodium concentrations alone should not be used to estimate the size of extracellular fluid volume.

The volume of intracellular water is approximately twice that of extracellular water. Consequently, about two thirds of sodium-free water given a patient and not excreted in urine enters the intracellular compartment in response to osmotic equilibrium. Only one third of the water remains extracellularly, and in the absence of vasodilation or protein shift, only about one fifth of extracellular water is intravascular once osmotic equilibrium is established.

CHEMICAL STRUCTURE OF FLUID COMPARTMENTS

A diagram of the chemical composition of body fluid compartments expressed in mEq/L is shown in Figure 22–1. In the extracellular fluid compartment the important cations are sodium, 135 to 140 mEq, calcium, 4.5 to 5.5 mEq, and magnesium, 1.5 to 2.5 mEq. Changes in serum potassium levels induce cardiac effects such as arrhythmias long before any abnormalities cause fluid shifts secondary to osmotic effects. Similarly, changes in serum calcium and magnesium produce neurologic and cardiac signs before osmotic effects are observed. The clinical problems produced by the most common extracellular cation abnormalities and their treatment are summarized in Table 22–2).

The major extracellular anions are chloride, 100 to 106 mEq/L, and bicarbonate, 22 to 28 mEq/L. These anions are frequently referred to as exchangeable anions. When renal re-absorption of one anion is increased, renal excretion of the other is enhanced. A common example is the patient with chronic obstructive lung disease with carbon dioxide retention; values for bicarbonate between 35 and 40 are associated with those of chloride, between 85 and 95.

Recently, the importance of serum inorganic phosphorus has been recognized. An essential clinical effect of inadequate amounts of inorganic phosphorus can be traced to reduced adenosine triphosphate (ATP) and 2,3-diphosphoglycerate levels, both shifting the oxygen dissociation curve to the left, with diminished release of oxygen to the tissues (see Chapter 37). This kind of abnormality is found in the chronically ill patient in negative nitrogen balance through lack of oral intake and in some patients on a hyperalimentation regimen without inorganic phosphorus supplementation.

Normally the total sodium and potassium in mEq/L should not exceed the sum of chloride and bicarbonate by more than 15 mEq. Should a larger difference arise, increased amounts of other unmeasured anions, such as lactate, ketones, or salicylate, should be suspected. This phenomenon is defined as an anion gap:

$$Anion\ Gap\ [<15\ mEq]$$

$$[(mEq\ Na^+ + mEq\ K^+) - (mEq\ HCO_3^- + mEq\ Cl^-)]$$

The diagnosis and therapy of acid-base abnormalities are discussed later.

PHYSIOLOGIC CONTROL OF EXTRACELLULAR TONICITY AND VOLUME

The homeostatic systems for maintenance of extracellular tonicity are diagrammed in Figure 22–2. Sensors present in the posterior hypothalamus induce two compensatory responses when tonicity rises: thirst develops, increasing water intake; and more antidiuretic hormone (ADH) is produced and water resorbed from renal tubules. Restoration of normal tonicity occurs at the expense of increasing extracellular fluid

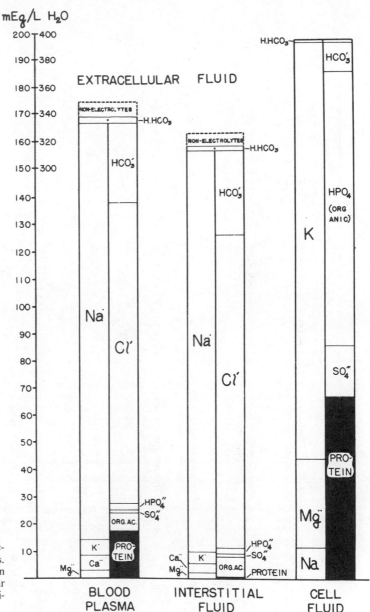

FIGURE 22–1. Chemical structure of the body compartments. (Reproduced with permission from Gamble JL; Extracellular Fluid. Cambridge, Harvard University Press, 1947.)

volume. The volume maintenance system then returns the extracellular fluid volume toward normal.

The mechanism for maintenance of extracellular fluid volume is shown in Figure 22–3, reacting to increased extracellular fluid volume by decreasing renin release from the renal juxtaglomerular apparatus. Renin cleaves a hepatic-produced plasma polypeptide to yield angiotensin II. A decreased level of angiotensin II leads to less release of aldosterone from the adrenal cortex, in turn resulting in less sodium resorption from the proximal renal tubules. Other poorly understood mechanisms reduce salt intake. Decreased sodium resorption and decreased sodium intake lower extracellular fluid tonicity. The decrease in tonicity causes shifts of water intracellularly, decreased thirst, and less ADH release, changes that return extracellular volume toward normal.

TABLE 22–2. Extracellular Cation Abnormalities and Their Treatment

	↑ K^+	↓ K^+	↓ Ca^{++}	↓ Mg^{++}
Major clinical problems	Cardiac arrhythmias: ultimately sinus arrest	Cardiac arrhythmias: ultimately ventricular fibrillation Muscle weakness or loss of reflexes	Inotropic cardiac failure Hyperreflexia and tetany	Hyperreflexia and tetany Psychiatric symptoms Increased arrhythmias with digitalis
Most common causes	Renal failure Acidosis Iatrogenic	Diuretic therapy; steroid therapy Treatment of acidosis; nasogastric suction Alkalosis Dehydration	Alkalosis Hypoparathyroidism Massive transfusion (rare)	Alcoholism Diuretic therapy Chronic renal disease GI losses
Laboratory values	>5 mEq/L	<3.5 mEq/L	<4.5 mEq/L <9 mg per 100 ml	<1.5 mEq/L <1.8 mg per 100 ml
ECG changes	Peaked T wave Loss of P wave Loss of peaked T wave Bradycardia Spread of QRS	ST depression T wave inversion U wave (may be a positive or negative wave)	Prolonged Q-T interval	No distinctive abnormalities
Acute therapy in 70-kg adult (life-threatening situations only)	100 mEq $NaHCO_3$ IV over 2 minutes 50 gm glucose, 20 U regular insulin IV	K^+ IV at 1 mEq per minute	$CaCl$ 250 mg IV every 5 minutes until symptoms reverse; if calcium gluconate is used, multiply dose by 3	$MgSO_4$ 5 gm per hour IM or IV

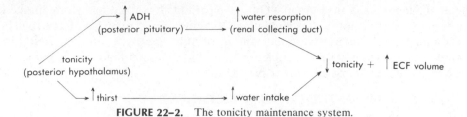

FIGURE 22–2.   The tonicity maintenance system.

Homeostatic mechanisms may be upset by many factors, the most important being restriction of oral intake; fluid and electrolyte deficits or excesses related to the primary disease; fluid and electrolyte deficits or iatrogenically produced excesses; inappropriate ADH secretion; and increased adrenocortical steroid secretion.

INTRAVENOUS FLUID THERAPY

ROUTINE PARENTERAL FLUID THERAPY IN ELECTIVE SURGICAL PROCEDURES

Most patients facing elective operation have oral intake withheld during the ten immediately preoperative hours, resulting in unreplaced solute and water loss. Water is lost from the body primarily via the kidneys, lungs, skin, and a small amount through the gastrointestinal tract. That portion lost from the lungs and skin constitutes the insensible loss, ranging from 800 to 1000 ml daily in the normal adult. In addition, a minimal obligatory 500 ml of urinary water are required for excretion of waste products. The optimal urine volume is expressed as 1 ml/kg of body weight per hour, approximately 1700 ml in a 70-kg adult. This potential water-conserving capability of the kidney provides a margin of safety, the chief means of adjustment when water must be conserved. The normal glomerular filtrate is approximately 180 L daily, equal to approximately 60 times the plasma volume. Obviously, most of this is re-absorbed in the renal tubules and returned to the circulation. Although renal function in adults can limit losses in the fluid-restricted patient, infants are less able to deal with unreplaced losses, in part owing to the increased ratio of surface area to weight. In adults not operated on until afternoon, an early clear liquid breakfast before oral intake is discontinued may be ordered or an intravenous infusion of a crystalloid solution may be given preoperatively.

In view of the loss of fluid preoperatively, it is logical to administer one third to one half of the estimated 24-hour fluid requirement parenterally during the course of a major operation in the adult. Thus, an average 70-kg adult would receive approximately 600 to 1000 ml of fluid during the course of a one- to two-hour operation. This presumes no significant fluid or blood loss. To minimize the hazard of excess free water administration, at least one third of the fluid should be a solute-containing solution, either as saline

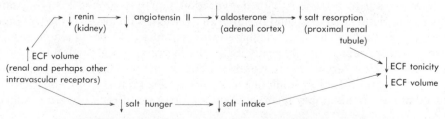

FIGURE 22–3.   The extracellular volume maintenance system.

or lactated Ringer's solution. As most of these patients have had no caloric intake over the preceding 10 to 12 hours, it is good practice to include 25 to 30 gm of dextrose in the fluid administered. Obviously modifications of this approach are required for the dehydrated or previously salt-restricted patient. Intravenous fluids are usually limited in healthy patients undergoing minor procedures.

FLUID THERAPY IN THE DEHYDRATED PATIENT

Patients with a history of vomiting, diarrhea, gastric suction, or intestinal fistulas may have suffered massive fluid losses from the gastrointestinal tract. In addition, those with peritonitis or bowel obstruction may lose large volumes of protein-rich fluid into the lumen of the gut or abdominal cavity. In the diabetic with hyperglycemia and acetonuria or in some kinds of renal failure, impressive deficits arise as a result of renal salt and water losses. Extensive burns result in massive losses of fluid, salt, and protein into the involved areas. Febrile patients or those exposed to tropical conditions can lose large amounts of fluid by sweating or through the respiratory tract. Finally, chronically ill or psychotic patients frequently fail to maintain adequate oral nourishment over prolonged periods.

The condition of this kind of chronically ill, malnourished patient falls into the category of the "depletion syndrome" because of several characteristics: depletion of essential substrates, amino acids, glycogen, fats, and caloric reserves necessary for vital system function; and a significant decrease in intracellular water with a corresponding slight increase in the extracellular component, occurring primarily in the interstitial compartment, with a concomitant fall in the intravascular compartment or plasma volume. These patients have a deficiency in total body potassium, phosphate, sodium, and serum proteins and a tendency toward a decreased serum osmolality. Frequently such patients appear stable until subjected to the stress of anesthesia and operation. Under these circumstances the circulation often rapidly decompensates and does not readily respond to treatment.

Useful signs in evaluating a patient with these problems include the state of consciousness and the degree of cardiovascular change in response to postural stress. Significant dehydration is generally accompanied by mental changes and obvious signs of hypovolemia. A fully conscious patient who can sit upright for at least a minute without a significant increase in pulse rate or fall in mean arterial pressure is unlikely to have more than a 10 per cent deficit in extracellular fluid volume. On the other hand, an obtunded patient with an obstructed or perforated small bowel causing peritonitis, with associated hypotension and tachycardia while lying supine, is obviously deficient in extracellular fluid volume. As morphine is a vasodilator of the capacitance vessels, intravenous injection of small doses may unmask a deficit in intravascular volume. Thus it is essential to restore extracellular fluid volume toward normal before operation to achieve adequate cardiovascular, cerebral, and renal function.

Other common signs of dehydration are furrowing of the tongue, dry oral mucosa, and loss of skin or tissue turgor. However, a dry oral mucosa is occasionally observed when a patient breathes through the mouth.

The approach to a patient with dehydration depends on the evolving physical findings and initial response to fluid therapy. In a patient with normal cerebral function, cardiovascular stability, and an adequate urine output, only documented losses and insensible loss are replaced. Alternatively, in the hypotensive, dehydrated patient, the extracellular space is repleted with isotonic saline or lactated Ringer's solution. It may be necessary to give 1 L of crystalloid every 15 minutes, up to 3 to 4 L, bearing in mind the nature of cardiopulmonary reserves. When more careful replacement is suggested, it is better to try a fluid challenge of 200 ml of crystalloid over a period of 10 minutes with observation of CVP or pulmonary wedge pressure. Fluids are continued until vital signs stabilize, urine output reaches 50 ml per hour, CVP rises excessively, or rales develop, as detected by auscultation. If signs of intravascular fluid overload appear before cardiovascular stability or adequate urine output occurs, fluid administration is slowed. Under these circumstances it is likely that the primary fault is inadequate myocardial function, and administration of a positive inotropic drug such as dopamine or isoproterenol should be considered, with simultaneous injection of the diuretic furosemide. Cardiovascular stability should be achieved before induction of anesthesia because vasodilation further compromises circulatory integrity. If circulatory stability cannot be reached before operation, minimal general or local anesthesia may be the only acceptable procedure.

For the reasons discussed, the serum sodium level cannot be used as an index of the amount of salt solution required. Misuse of the serum sodium level results in replacement errors both in magnitude and direction. A high hemoglobin or even a normal hemoglobin level in a chronically ill patient should heighten suspicion of severe dehydration. Modest decreases in hemoglobin or hematocrit indicate that the extracellular deficit has been effectively treated.

Some anesthetists and surgeons select blood or colloid over saline for treatment of dehydrated patients with peritonitis, bowel obstruction, or severe burns. Such patients can indeed suffer large internal losses of protien-rich fluid. Provided that insufficient amounts are administered, saline alone is almost always effective in restoring circulatory stability. However, an excess of saline may be required, involving the risks discussed later on. Hence, there is a reason to use colloid for at least part of the fluid replacement.

Some prefer a balanced salt solution to isotonic saline. The composition of the several available parenteral fluid solutions is given in Table 22–3. When using isotonic saline in large amounts, 30 mEq of bicarbonate are often added to each liter of solution administered. Provided that acid-base abnormalities are diagnosed by appropriate blood gas measurements and corrected with sodium bicarbonate, there is little proved advantage or disadvantage in using more expensive and complex salt solutions. Acid-base evaluation is mandatory in patients receiving massive replacement therapy regardless of solution chosen.

It is unwise to administer potassium routinely to the dehydrated patient without knowing the electrolyte status. The possibility of either hypokalemia or hyperkalemia exists, since severe dehydration can result in renal failure with resultant hyperkalemia. When hypokalemia is present, commercially balanced salt solutions usually fail to

TABLE 22–3. Comparison of Extracellular Fluid and Various Replacement Solutions

Solution	Na (mEq/L)	K	Cl (mEq/L)	Total Base	pH	Ca^{++} (mEq/L)	Mg^{++}	Calories per L
ECF	138	5	108	27	7.4	5	3	12
5% Dextrose/Water	0	0	0	0	4.5	0	0	200
Normal Saline	154	0	154	0	6.0	0	0	0
Lactated Ringer's	130	4	109	28	6.5	3	0	9
Normosol	140	5	98	50	7.4	0	3	24

supply sufficient potassium to correct the deficit. We add up to 40 mEq of potassium to replacement solutions given to the hypokalemic patient. Potassium should not be given more rapidly than 1 mEq/min/70 kg. Should the dose exceed 0.5 mEq/min/70 kg, the electrocardiogram must be monitored continuously and serum potassium measured before the start and at no less than two-hour intervals.

Ill-advised treatment frequently causes severe salt and water depletion. The effects of administering too little or too much water and certain solutes are shown in Table 22–4. Iatrogenic dehydration most often occurs in patients who are salt restricted and receiving diuretics for treatment of hypertension or congestive heart failure. Depletion may become evident only after the vasodilation that accompanies anesthesia, so it is preferable to establish CVP monitoring before induction of anesthesia. If both hypotension and a decrease in CVP follow induction, administration of isotonic saline or colloid is indicated. At times the intravascular volume needed to maintain cardiovascular stability during anesthesia proves to be too great after anesthesia. Nevertheless, anesthetists should realize that circulatory stability during the vasodilation of anesthesia may at times require administration of more volume than is best for the patient, once anesthesia is dissipated and remobilization of excess fluid occurs. Occasionally vigorous fluid restriction and diuresis are required after operation.

HAZARDS OF EXCESS FLUID AND ELECTROLYTE ADMINISTRATION

In addition to using parenteral fluids to treat dehydration, they may be given for other purposes: as a substitute for blood transfusion, to treat shock, and to protect the kidney during major operations. Before discussion of possible advantages of administering parenteral fluids to patients in excess of probable loss, we shall first examine the hazards.

WATER INTOXICATION

Release of ADH occurs in response to stress, general anesthesia, opioids, pain, blood loss, and positive pressure ventilation. Postoperatively, patients often develop elevated ADH levels despite normal or decreased extracellular fluid tonicity. When the extracellular fluid is already hypotonic, continued secretion of ADH is considered inappropriate. Unlike a patient whose tonicity maintenance system is intact, a patient with inappropriate ADH secretion fails to excrete excess free water. Administration of excess solute-free water to this patient results in dilutional hyponatremia, intracellular water shift with cell swelling, and cerebral symptoms ranging from mild lethargy and disorientation to delirium, coma, and convulsions. The condition can be worsened by administration of opioids in a misdirected effort to treat delirium. Symptoms of water intoxication usually begin on the first to third postoperative day, and if convulsions occur, the fatality rate is high. The syndrome is rarely seen in adults given less than 2 L of free water on any postoperative day, including water absorbed from irrigating solutions as during transurethral resection of the prostate. Water intoxication is more common in patients over 60 years of age. Serum sodium levels at the onset of symptoms are usually in the 118 to 131 mEq range, with 122 mEq an average value. Urine osmolality is higher than serum osmolality, with a typical value of 500 mOsm/L. Treatment includes fluid restriction to less than 1 L of isotonic saline per day with no free water intake. Oral intake of water by the uncooperative or confused patient must be prevented. Serum osmolality can be raised more quickly by the use of mannitol or other diuretics or by 2.5 per cent sodium chloride given intravenously. However, in the absence of serious symptoms, fluid restriction alone is effective. Symptoms may persist

TABLE 22–4. Effects of Administering Too Little or Too Much Water and Certain Solutes*

| Substance | Amount Administered | |
	Too Little	Too Much
Water	Serum solute and sodium concentration increased	Serum solute and sodium concentration decreased
	Highly concentrated urine	Very dilute urine
	Thirst	Polyuria
	Oliguria	Intracranial hypertension
	Fever	Headache, confusion, nausea, and vomiting
	Circulatory failure	Weakness
		Muscle twitching and cramps
		Convulsions
		Coma
Sodium	Extracellular fluid volume decreased	Extracellular fluid volume increased
	Hemoconcentration	Edema formation and congestive heart failure
	Lost tissue elasticity	Tendency to potassium deficiency
	Microcardia	
	Hypotension	
	Circulatory failure	
	Uremia	
Potassium	Apathy	Hyperpotassemia
	Lethargy	Electrocardiographic changes
	Muscle weakness	Muscle weakness
	Electrocardiographic changes	Cardiac arrest
	Ileus or diarrhea	
	Hypopotassemia	
	Metabolic alkalosis	
Phosphorus	Hypophosphatemia	Hyperphosphatemia
	Other effects	Hypocalcemia
		Tetany
Carbohydrate	Ketosis	Hyperglycemia
	Protoplasmic catabolism augmented	Glycosuria
	Tendency to greater water and electrolyte losses	Hepatic failure

*Reproduced with permission from Talbot NB, et al: N Engl J Med 252:856, 1955.

for days despite return of serum sodium levels to normal. Because of the hazard of water intoxication, administration of sodium-free water should be limited to replacement of demonstrated or probable losses, including those caused by overnight fluid restriction.

EXCESS SALT ADMINISTRATION

Just as ADH levels may be elevated postoperatively despite decreased extracellular tonicity, so, too, are adrenocorticoid levels raised despite increased extracellular fluid volume. As with ADH, elevations in circulating glucocorticoids and aldosterone are in part related to stress. However, part of the rise in aldosterone level may be a homeostatic response to a functional decrease in extracellular fluid volume when fluid is lost to sites from which it cannot be rapidly mobilized. Extracellular fluid in such locations comes more slowly into equilibrium with radioisotopic tracers used for measurement; that fluid which is sequestered presumably is not readily available for purposes of circulatory homeostasis. Many investigators have documented such functional losses of extracellular fluid following major operation or trauma. Moreover, the postoperative tendency toward renal salt conservation can be overcome by saline overloading, in contradistinction to postoperative renal free water conservation, which is not overcome by free water loading.

Nevertheless, large saline excesses are not without hazard. Previously healthy individuals given large amounts of isotonic salt solution (3000 ml or more) in the treatment of shock have developed fatal pulmonary edema. Smaller volumes may cause difficulty in pulmonary gas exchange even in the absence of overt edema. Pulmonary symptoms may not occur until several days postoperatively, with the mobilization of the sequestered (third space) fluid. Most patients tolerate excess saline better than excess free water; however, indiscriminate use of salt solution without demonstrable indication is poor practice.

INDICATIONS FOR ISOTONIC SALT SOLUTION OTHER THAN AS REPLACEMENT THERAPY

Several situations exist in which modest use of isotonic salt solution is justified in amounts exceeding probable losses. In a patient requiring intravascular volume replacement of less than 20 per cent of blood volume or for whom colloid or volume expander is not available, blood volume can be maintained with saline given in amounts two to three times the blood lost. Saline is substituted for much of the blood formerly used to prime heart-lung oxygenating devices (see Chapter 26). That kind of hemodilution has reduced the amount of hemolysis seen as a consequence of cardiopulmonary bypass and also conserves limited blood supplies.

A second use of salt solution is for rapid expansion of the intravascular volume prior to anesthetic techniques that result in vasodilation. Thus, rapid administration of 500 to 1000 ml prior to spinal anesthesia decreases the magnitude of hypotension and the need for vasopressors (see Chapter 19). Fluid necessary for overnight replacement therapy can be administered in this manner.

Finally, fluid administration beyond replacement of measured loss is commonly used to protect the kidneys. Studies suggest that an intraoperative diuresis of 50 ml per hour or more decreases the risk of postoperative renal failure, especially in patients with major trauma or those undergoing resection of an aortic aneurysm. Enhancement of urine output should initially be attempted in these patients by increased volume administration. However, excessive fluid may lead to pulmonary edema. In some cases, it is preferable to induce diuresis with mannitol or furosemide rather than via administration of excessively large fluid volumes. Exact figures on the limits of fluid administration above measured losses are not available; other factors to consider are the duration of operation; the operation per se, whether on abdomen, chest, or extremities; preoperative renal status; possible postoperative fluid losses; and myocardial reserves.

ACID-BASE BALANCE

An understanding of appropriate fluid and electrolyte therapy is not complete without an appreciation of basic acid-base balance. This subject is further considered in Chapter 37.

In simplified acid-base terminology, an acid is defined as a chemical substance that donates H^+ ions (proton donor) and a base as a substance that accepts H^+ ions (proton acceptor). In the body economy several different acids are found, such as hydrochloric acid in the stomach, lactic acid, organic acids, and carbonic acid, the end product of aerobic metabolism. Conversely, the several bases include ammonia and bicarbonate ion. A typical acid-base reaction occurring *in vivo* is:

$$H_2CO_3 \xrightleftharpoons{} H^+ + HCO_3^-$$
$$\text{Acid} \qquad\qquad \text{Base}$$

The acidity of a solution is determined by the concentration of H^+ ions, or more specifically, by H^+ ion activity. Acidosis implies an excess of H^+ ions in tissues, and acidemia is defined as blood H^+ ion concentration above normal. Conversely, alkalosis refers to a deficit of H^+ ions at the cellular level, whereas alkalemia is a less than normal blood H^+ ion concentration. Acidosis and alkalosis are clinical diagnoses, whereas acidemia and alkalemia are values obtained directly by analysis of arterial blood. Acidity is conveniently expressed by the symbol pH, which relates to H^+ activity, in dilute solutions approximated by free H^+ ion concentration.

Mathematically, pH is defined as the negative logarithm of the H^+ ion concentration. The pH scale is derived from the ionization constant of water, water representing the basic solvent. Water dissociates weakly into 1×10^{-7} H^+ ions and an equal number of OH^- (hydroxyl) ions. When the negative logarithm of this H^+ ion concentration is calculated, it is equal to a pH of 7.

$$pH = -\log_{10} [H^+]$$
$$= -\log_{10} 10^{-7}$$
$$pH = (-)(-7) = 7$$

At a pH of 7 it is apparent that the number of H^+ and OH^- ions is equal; therefore a chemically neutral solution exists. Blood normally has a pH slightly on the alkaline side of neutrality, with 4×10^{-8} mEq H^+ ion per liter. To convert an H^+ ion concentration of 4×10^{-8} mEq/L into pH, one takes the logarithm of 4, which equals 0.60, and adds to this the logarithm of 10^{-8}, which is -8.0. The resultant figure is -7.40. in pH terminology equaling $+7.40$.

Carbon dioxide and water constitute the major products of aerobic metabolism, and their combination into carbonic acid is unique in that it represents the only volatile acid produced by the organism. Elimination by the lungs of this potential source of H^+ ion via carbon dioxide and water enables the carbonic acid-bicarbonate system to be an effective physiologic buffering system. All other acids, both organic and inorganic, produced by metabolic processes are handled primarily by the kidney. It is essential that the body maintain a stable and narrow range of H^+ ion concentration for cellular enzymes to function properly. This is the reason for the existence of elaborate buffering systems. A buffer system is defined as a weak acid and its conjugate base or conversely as a weak base and its conjugate acid. A substance functioning in this manner is said to be amphoteric. Buffer systems are important in that they minimize changes in free H^+ ion concentration in spite of relatively large additions to or removal of H^+ ions from the system. Four major buffer systems function in the body: carbonic acid–bicarbonate system, reduced hemoglobin-oxyhemoglobin, serum proteins (carbamino compounds), and phosphates (major intracellular buffer).

Several expressions of the state of acid-base balance are in existence. One commonly employed is the Henderson-Hasselbalch equation, depicting the dependency of pH of blood on the bicarbonate-carbonic acid relation.

$$pH = pK + \log \frac{[HCO_3^-]}{[H_2CO_3]}$$

The relation between P_{CO_2}, dissolved CO_2, and H_2CO_3 permits manipulation of the H_2CO_3 term in the above equation. The chemical reaction, hydration of CO_2, is such that the concentration of dissolved CO_2 is approximately 1000 times greater than and proportional to H_2CO_3.

$$H_2CO_3 \propto \text{dissolved } CO_2 = (\text{solubility coef}) P_{CO_2}$$

Therefore in clinical practice the carbonic acid term is replaced by the solubility coefficient of dissolved carbon dioxide times the partial pressure of carbon dioxide (P_{CO_2}). The specific arterial blood gas measurements pH and P_{CO_2} provide a direct calculation of plasma bicarbonate.

$$pH = pK + \log \frac{(HCO_3^-)}{s \times P_{CO_2}}$$

$$where \; pK = 6.1$$

$$s = 0.03$$

Blood pH is dependent upon the ratio of bicarbonate to dissolved carbon dioxide, the normal being 20:1.

STATE OF ACIDOSIS OR ALKALOSIS

The normal pH range in arterial blood is between 7.35 and 7.45. Values below 7.35 represent acidemia, potentially harmful, whether of respiratory or metabolic origin, because cellular acidosis must be assumed until proved otherwise. More importantly, absence of acidemia does not unequivocally rule out cellular acidosis or at least localized tissue acidosis. At the cellular level, acidosis increases myocardial irritability, decreases myocardial contractility, and decreases responsiveness of the cardiovascular system to catecholamines, even though excess catecholamine secretion occurs as a response. Measurements of pH_a values alone are poor predictors of circulatory stability. For example, the heart of a young, vigorous, diabetic patient may withstand a pH_a value of 7.0 to 7.1, whereas an older patient with myocardial ischemia may be unable to tolerate a pH_a of 7.25. Also on clinical grounds a state of alkalemia (ph_a above 7.45), often considered innocuous, should not be viewed as such. Pa_{CO_2} normally ranges between 35 and 45 torr. Pa_{CO_2} levels above 45 represent hypercarbia or alveolar hypoventilation. On the other hand, Pa_{CO_2} levels below 35 represent hypocarbia or alveolar hyperventilation.

Clinical assessment of acid-base balance has been made easier by analysis of arterial blood gases. The interpretation is simple if the two directly measured variables, Pa_{CO_2} and PH_a, are used as the primary basis for interpretation (Table 22–5). Incorporating this information into the clinical picture and then using the information derived from blood gas measurements, such as bicarbonate and base deficit, the appropriate therapy is suggested. Once blood gas measurements have been obtained, the next step is to place them in the clinical context. For example, respiratory acidosis and metabolic acidosis may coexist. How can one decide whether the Pa_{CO_2} and pH_a abnormalities result entirely from the respiratory circumstances and if the pH_a change is appropriate to the change in Pa_{CO_2}. As a basic approximation for each increase of 10 torr in Pa_{CO_2} above 40, the corresponding pH_a decreases 0.05 units from a pH_a of 7.40. This oversimplification is sufficiently accurate for diagnosis and treatment of acute or combined acid-base disorders in the majority of situations. Table 22–6 lists approximate values of pH_a to be expected at different levels of Pa_{CO_2} assuming no metabolic component. An important assumption essential to initial determination that a blood gas sample has abnormal values is that the values represent deviations from normal, that is, Pa_{CO_2} equals 40 and pH_a equals 7.40. In patients with acute disease superimposed on a chronic ailment this assumption is frequently invalid, thus emphasizing the importance of obtaining blood gas data in patients with chronic cardiopulmonary disease preoperatively.

Acute Respiratory Acidosis

Acute respiratory acidosis can be corrected only by improving the alveolar ventilation, either spontaneously by the patient or mechanically. Intravenous adminis-

TABLE 22–5.   Blood Gas Analysis

	Pa_{CO_2}	pH_a
Normal respiratory state	35–45	7.45–7.35
Primary Pulmonary Dysfunction		
Acute respiratory acidosis	>45	<7.35
Chronic respiratory acidosis	>45	Norm. range
Acute respiratory alkalosis	<35	>7.45
Chronic respiratory alkalosis	<35	Norm. range
Primary Metabolic Dysfunction		
Uncompensated metabolic acidosis	Norm. range	<7.35
Partially compensated metabolic acidosis	<35	<7.35
Completely compensated metabolic acidosis	<35	Norm. range
Uncompensated metabolic alkalosis	Norm. range	>7.45
Partially compensated metabolic alkalosis	>45	>7.45
Completely compensated metabolic alkalosis	>45	Norm. range

tration of bicarbonate may result in transient improvement of pH_a at best and is to be avoided unless measures are taken simultaneously to ensure adequate alveolar ventilation.

Chronic Respiratory Acidosis

In chronic respiratory acidosis, the net fall in pH is minimized by renal compensation via re-absorption of bicarbonate. Thus, a patient in chronic CO_2 retention, a state of chronic respiratory acidosis, would be expected to have a pH only slightly lower than normal or at best a value in the low or normal range if one subscribes to the principle that the body usually does not overcompensate. Frequently, however, these patients show pH values slightly in the high normal range most easily explained on the basis of a superimposed metabolic alkalosis, since diuretic therapy may lead to hypokalemia and

TABLE 22–6.   Predicted pH at Different Pa_{CO_2} Levels in Absence of Metabolic Acid-Base Abnormality

Respiratory acidosis–Pa_{CO_2}, torr	Predicted pH (approximate)
100	7.1
80	7.2
60	7.3
Respiratory alkalosis–Pa_{CO_2}, torr	Predicted pH (approximate)
30	7.5
20	7.6
10	7.7

Note: Each change in Pa_{CO_2} of 10 torr when Pa_{CO_2} is greater than 40 torr produces a pH change of about 0.05 unit in the opposite direction.
Each change in Pa_{CO_2} of 10 torr when Pa_{CO_2} is less than 40 torr produces a pH change of about 0.10 unit in the opposite direction.

hypochloremia. Hypochloremia in moderately severe CO_2 retention should be expected as the kidneys augment excretion of chloride to enhance bicarbonate resorption. When these patients require mechanical ventilatory assistance, care should be taken to avoid normalizing Pa_{CO_2} too rapidly, as this will result in acute alkalosis, the hazards of which are discussed later.

Metabolic Acidosis

In metabolic acidosis, pH_a is less than normal in spite of a reduction in Pa_{CO_2}. If the blood is tonometered to a normal Pa_{CO_2} of 40 torr, further reduction in pH occurs. The resulting bicarbonate value is far less than expected from the pH-Pa_{CO_2} relation if the change is related solely to changes in Pa_{CO_2}. The discrepancy in bicarbonate values is referred to as base deficit, and the source of excess H^+ ions obviously resides in nonvolatile acids. The H^+ ions in turn combine with available bicarbonate and are eliminated through the lungs as CO_2 and H_2O. Approximate values for base deficit or excess when the $PaCO_2$ is kept constant at 40 torr are listed in Table 22–7.

The common causes of metabolic acidosis are diabetic ketoacidosis, lactic acidosis, renal failure, alcoholic ketoacidosis, and drug ingestion (salicylates and methanol).

When metabolic acidosis is present, the primary cause must be eliminated. However, in the interim, the cardiovascular system is supported with appropriate amounts of sodium bicarbonate intravenously, as follows:

1. Assume that the extracellular fluid volume is 20 per cent of ideal body weight and that bicarbonate is confined to the extracellular space.
2. The base deficit expressed in mEq is multiplied by the extracellular fluid volume: [(mEq/L) × (L)].
3. One half the calculated dose of sodium bicarbonate is given intravenously, and, after a short interval, arterial blood is analyzed for pH.

Several alternative methods are available to quantitate metabolic acidosis. Base excess or deficit can be calculated from a more exact nomogram or slide rule, available in most hospitals. Other methods include measurement of standard bicarbonate and CO_2 combining power.

Standard bicarbonate represents an estimate of blood bicarbonate concentration on the basis of titrating Pa_{CO_2} down to 40 torr. Standard bicarbonate is measured in an anaerobically drawn blood sample or equivalently corrected by a nomogram. Measurement is reported as bicarbonate level rather than deviation from normal.

CO_2 combining power differs from the standard bicarbonate primarily in that the sample is not handled anaerobically. Thus, blood drawn for CO_2 combining power is not reliable in providing data for Pa_{CO_2} or pH, especially in acutely ill patients. In addition, CO_2 combining power is usually reported in volumes per cent, which must then be converted to mEq/L.

TABLE 22–7.   Predicted pH_a at Different Levels of Acid or Base Excess When Pa_{CO_2} Is Kept Constant at 40 Torr

Acid excess, mEq/L (Reported as base deficit)	Predicted pH (approximate)
−21	7.1
−14	7.2
− 7	7.3
Base excess, mEq/L	**Predicted pH (approximate)**
+ 7	7.5
+14	7.6
+21	7.7

Note: For each 7 mEq of acid or base excess, pH changes about 0.10 unit in the appropriate direction. Acid excess is more commonly reported as base deficit or negative base excess; hence it is reported with a minus sign.

Respiratory Alkalosis

Respiratory alkalosis is most often secondary to hypoxemia and is also related to central nervous system disorders or iatrogenic-induced hyperventilation. If the primary cause is not corrected, the kidneys in time, should augment excretion of bicarbonate, resulting in a measured base deficit not to be confused with metabolic acidosis. In this situation, with Pa_{CO_2} below normal, the pH is on the high side of normal rather then below.

Metabolic Acidosis

Metabolic alkalosis correlates clinically with deficits of total body chloride, potassium, or a combination thereof. Reduced serum chloride values and hypochloremia are correlated well with reductions in total body chloride. However, a significant reduction in total body potassium is frequently present in spite of relatively normal serum potassium values. Blood gas values showing metabolic alkalosis should be considered as strong supportive evidence for inadequate body potassium stores irrespective of serum potassium values. Hypokalemia exerts several deleterious effects on the organism besides causing metabolic alkalosis; namely, increased myocardial irritability and generalized muscle weakness. To correct metabolic alkalosis it is important to supply not only potassium but chloride ion as well. This allows the kidneys to excrete the excess bicarbonate and to re-absorb chloride.

Additional adverse effects of metabolic alkalosis include deficient oxygen delivery to tissues owing to shift of the oxygen dissociation curve to the left and interference with central portion of respiration. These are discussed in Chapter 37.

Common causes of metabolic alkalosis include loss of gastric secretions in vomiting or nasogastric suction, diuretic therapy, chronic hypercarbia, inadequate dietary intake, chronic steroid administration, and excessive exogenous administration of bicarbonate as may occur in cardiac resuscitation.

APPRAISAL

The anesthetist is called upon to administer anesthesia to older patients who have considerable limitations of cardiopulmonary reserves for major operations, conditions that would have been unthinkable two decades ago. This challenge cannot be met by improved intraoperative anesthesia and operative technique alone. An appreciation is required of fluid, electrolyte, and acid-base physiology and a working knowledge of the various fluid therapy available for treatment. Assessment of these problems and institution of therapy are often required far in advance of operation for a successful outcome.

REFERENCES

Davenport HW: The ABC of Acid Base Chemistry. 6th ed. Chicago, University of Chicago Press, 1974.
Kassirer JP: Serious acid base disorders. N Engl J Med 291:773, 1974.
Loeb JN: The hyperosmolar state. N Engl J Med 290:1184, 1974.
Man SO, Carrol HJ: The anion gap. N Engl J Med 297:814, 1977.
Pitts RF: Physiology of the Kidney and Body Fluids. 3rd ed. Chicago, Year Book Medical Publishers, 1974.
Randall HT: Fluid, electrolyte, and acid-base balance. Surg Clin North Am 56:1019, 1976.
Sabatine S, Arruda JA, Kuntzman NA: Disorders of acid-base imbalance. Med Clin North Am 62:1223, 1978.
Schrier R: Symposium on water metabolism. Kidney Int 10:1, 1976.
Worthley LI: Symposium: Fluids and electrolytes. Anaesth Intensive Care 5:284, 1977.

Chapter 23

BLOOD COMPONENT THERAPY

Well-documented differences in blood volume exist between adult men and women and between adults and newborns and children, but the average percentages related to body weight are as follows:

Men	7.5 (75 ml/kg)
Women	6.5 (65 ml/kg)
Newborns	8.5 (85 ml/kg)

Muscularity and physical activity tend to increase blood volume, whereas obesity, inactivity, and chronic disease tend to decrease it.

When blood is lost, replacement with whole blood, its components, colloids, or crystalloids is necessary when: insufficient volume is present to fill the intravascular space, oxygen-carrying capacity per unit volume is inadequate to meet tissue oxygen needs at a reasonable cardiac output, or coagulation factors such as fibrinogen and platelets are insufficient to permit effective blood coagulation. The percentage of blood volume lost before these requirements can no longer be met differs among patients. Normal subjects suffer little functional impairment after a loss of 10 per cent in total blood volume, 20 per cent in oxygen-carrying capacity, or 40 per cent of coagulation factors. Losses twice these amounts may be compatible with survival but place extreme demands on the patient's reserves.

MAINTENANCE OF INTRAVASCULAR VOLUME

Cessation of blood loss is dependent upon protective local reactions at the bleeding site, vascular smooth muscle contraction in severed vessels secondary to both mechanical and reflex sympathetic stimulation, and formation of a fibrin clot, which depends on the integrity of clotting mechanisms.

An immediate compensation for loss of intravascular volume is a reduction in the size of the intravascular bed via vasoconstriction in the splanchnic system, the kidneys, and the venous capacitance vessels, the latter containing 60 to 70 per cent of the total blood volume. Vasoconstriction conceals the symptoms and signs of hypovolemia in healthy volunteers after an acute 20 per cent volume loss in the supine position or after a 10 per cent loss in the upright position. A good example of a 10 per cent blood loss is when a donor gives one unit of blood, approximately 400 ml, without the appearance of

270

tachycardia or postural hypotension. However, when losses exceed this amount or when anesthetics, drugs, or an adverse physiologic circumstance such as acidemia interferes with vasoconstriction, smaller blood losses may result in cardiovascular instability.

A second compensation for acute blood loss consists of transfer of interstitial fluid and extravascular protein to the intravascular space, thus replenishing plasma volume. Intravascular volume, following an acute blood loss of 10 per cent, is largely replaced by this mechanism in approximately 24 hours. The process is facilitated in the microcirculation by a lowered transcapillary pressure secondary to increased precapillary constriction and mobilization of interstitial fluid. At the same time lymph returned to the circulation, largely via the thoracic duct, is rich in plasma proteins.

Immediate treatment of blood loss maintains the intravascular volume and tissue perfusion without the need for activation of the normal homeostatic mechanisms. When the volume is not immediately replaced, little change in hemoglobin or hematocrit can be detected until interstitial fluid is mobilized. Since the process takes many hours, a change in hemoglobin concentration or hematocrit is a poor way to assess the magnitude of acute untreated blood loss. When volume expanders such as saline or dextran are used, the hematocrit decreases in proportion to replacement volume.

NONSANGUINEOUS VOLUME EXPANDERS

Albumin or plasma protein solutions are useful for limited expansion because they are more readily available than whole blood and do not transmit hepatitis or result in hemolytic transfusion reactions. When simple volume expansion, in the presence of adequate hemoglobin levels, is the sole therapeutic goal, these solutions are as effective as blood. Other oncotically active substances, such as high molecular weight dextran and hydroxyethyl starch (hetastarch), can also be used. On a logistic basis dextran, average molecular weight 70,000, is more readily available than albumin. The major deterrent to its use is an interference with clotting mechanisms when amounts in excess of 15 ml/kg are administered, approximately 1000 ml (2 units) in a 70-kg individual. Hetastarch (Hespan) is an artificial colloid with higher average molecular weights ranging between 60,000 and 450,000. To date, it has had limited use in the United States and has limitations similar to those of dextran.

Crystalloids such as 0.9 per cent sodium chloride and lactated Ringer's solution are widely used as volume expanders, both in emergencies and for definitive replacement. Compared with colloid, crystalloid solutions are more extensively distributed in the extravascular space, normally in a ratio of approximately 4:1. Therefore the amount of crystalloid required to maintain intravascular volume is three to four times larger than the amount of blood lost. As crystalloids are inexpensive and readily available, the need for larger amounts is not a disadvantage. However, in vulnerable patients the interstitial distribution also involves the pulmonary extravascular space, which can interfere with pulmonary gas exchange. This problem is magnified when there is altered alveolar-pulmonary capillary membrane function. The abnormally wide pores in the membrane facilitate movement of both crystalloids and colloids into the pulmonary interstitial space, leading to noncardiogenic pulmonary edema. Pulmonary complications are fewer when volume replacement is accomplished primarily with blood, followed by crystalloid and minimal use of colloid solutions.

Once large quantities of crystalloid are administered, the addition of albumin or other oncotically active substance to the circulation may cause increased mobilization of fluid into the intravascular space. This can lead to left heart failure in patients with limited cardiac reserves. Thus, colloid and crystalloid solutions should be used primarily as blood substitutes for replacement of modest blood loss, in an emergency for immediate re-expansion of blood volume, or in severe blood loss when blood is not immediately available. In clinical situations in which altered alveolar-capillary membrane function exists, volume replacement should be carefully titrated to minimize development of long-term pulmonary complications.

Large volumes of salt-free solutions such as 5 per cent dextrose in water are poor volume expanders, as they ultimately represent excess free water when the glucose is metabolized and pose the hazards of dilutional hyponatremia and water intoxication.

MAINTENANCE OF OXYGEN-CARRYING CAPACITY

Since most of the oxygen in arterial blood is carried by hemoglobin, a reduction in hemoglobin causes a decrease in arterial oxygen content. The amount of oxygen supplied to tissues depends on arterial oxygen content and cardiac output. If hemoglobin content is reduced, oxygen delivery to tissues must be maintained by a hyperdynamic circulation (see Chapter 37).

BLOOD REPLACEMENT THERAPY

Selective administration of blood components is preferable to routine use of whole blood, since most patients require only specific components (Table 23–1). This approach has been made possible by improvements in techniques of collection, processing, and storage of blood. Blood component therapy for the most part avoids the major adverse effects of whole blood adminstration, which include serum hepatitis, hemolytic reactions, and sensitization to minor erythrocyte antigens.

The once commonly used blood anticoagulant ACD, a mixture of citric acid, sodium citrate, and dextrose, has largely been replaced by CPD, a mixture of sodium citrate, citric acid, a phosphate buffer, and dextrose. CPD offers several advantages

TABLE 23–1. Blood Component Therapy

Blood Therapy Type	Indications
Whole blood (Type Specific)	Acute hemorrhage
Autologous	
Homologous	
Packed red blood cells	Severe chronic anemia
	Patient history—congestive heart failure
	Anemia in elderly debilitated patient
	Anemia in hepatic failure (cirrhosis)
	Anemia in renal failure (anuria, uremia)
Leukocyte-deficient red blood cells	Patient history—multiple transfusions
(washed RBCs)	Organ transplantation
Frozen red blood cells	Rare blood types
	Autotransfusion
	Organ transplantation
Platelet concentrates	Thrombocytopenic patient for:
	major surgery
	cancer (acute leukemia)
	postchemotherapy, radiation therapy
	Bleeding thrombocytopenic patient
	Intraoperative massive blood replacement
	with stored bank blood
Fresh frozen plasma	Intraoperative massive blood replacement
	with stored bank blood
	Specific coagulation factor deficiencies

over ACD in the decreased degradation of 2,3-diphosphoglycerate, a higher pH at equilibration, increased red blood cell survival, and lower potassium levels in storage.

Whole blood is best used only when blood loss is severe enough to cause hypovolemic shock. Under this circumstance there is a distinct advantage in the blood being as fresh as possible. In aging, the effectiveness of stored blood is diminished by reduced erythrocyte viability and a decreased oxygen availability secondary to changes in 2,3-diphosphoglycerate with left shift of the oxyhemoglobin dissociation curve, both significant in blood replacement.

Reactions to Blood Administration

Hemolytic Reactions.   Administration of incompatible blood leads to agglutination of the donor's red cells with resultant hemolysis. The signs and symptoms noted immediately or shortly after the start of transfusion may include any or all of the following: hives, chills, palpitation, fever, chest or flank pain, dyspnea, headache, and flushing of the skin. In severe reactions these symptoms may be accompanied by cardiovascular collapse, hemoglobinuria, and incoagulability of blood. Such reactions may be observed following transfusion of as little as 75 ml of incompatible blood. During general anesthesia the only signs of a hemolytic reaction may be hypotension, poor peripheral perfusion as evidenced by cyanosis, or diffuse bleeding at the operative site. A hemolytic transfusion reaction must be considered an emergency, varying directly with the amount of blood given. Therefore, the transfusion should be stopped immediately. Short of a fatality, the major long-term complication is development of anuria secondary to acute tubular necrosis (ATN). This lesion seems to result from renal cortical vasoconstriction induced by release of renin and formation of the potent vasoconstrictor angiotensin.

Treatment of circulatory collapse requires careful cardiovascular monitoring and, often, additional administration of fluids. At the earliest possible moment a urine specimen should be examined for the presence of free hemoglobin, which is often grossly apparent. There may be value in alkalinizing the urine, especially if done early to prevent precipitation of acid hematin in the tubules. Mannitol, 25 gm in 10 per cent solution, and furosemide, 40 mg, are administered intravenously to induce diuresis. Subsequently, if ATN develops, an anuric regimen is initiated to forestall overhydration and potassium intoxication, and consideration is given to either peritoneal or hemodialysis if a diuretic phase fails to appear or potassium intoxication is imminent.

The common cause of transfusion reactions owing to serologic incompatibility is misidentification of donor or recipient. Figures show that only 5 per cent of blood reactions result from serologic incompatibility detectable before transfusion. Because of the many minor blood groups one can never hope to give completely compatible blood, but major reactions are preventable by meticulous crossmatching and identification of donor and recipient.

The ordinary saline technique of crossmatching may fail to detect all antibodies capable of causing hemolysis. The end point of the normal crossmatch is agglutination of erythrocytes incompatible with the serum of a prospective recipient. However, recipient serum may contain incompatible antibodies that attach to the surface of donor cells, causing hemolysis *in vivo* without agglutination *in vitro*. These "incomplete" antibodies on the red cell surface can be detected by the Coombs test, which employs the serum of rabbits previously immunized against human globulin, causing agglutination of erythrocytes coated with the globulin.

Allergic Reactions.   These result from the transfer of allergens from donor to recipient and are manifested as pruritus, urticaria, asthma, angioneurotic edema, and, rarely, frank anaphylaxis. By and large these symptoms are not severe during general anesthesia, when antigen-antibody reactions and liberation of histamine seem to be depressed. Blood administration is not discontinued because of mild urticaria, but the rate of flow is slowed while appraisal is made; nor do we always give antihistamines for mild urticaria. For more severe manifestations, such as wheezing, an antihistamine such as diphenhydramine (Benadryl) is given, followed by epinephrine, aminophylline, and hydrocortisone if indicated. If an anaphylactic reaction occurs, aggressive therapy is instituted consisting of ventilatory support with oxygen, epinephrine 0.5 mg intramuscularly, aminophylline, hydrocortisone, blood volume expansion, and peripheral vasoconstrictors to support blood pressure.

Transmission of Disease

Hepatitis.   The disease most frequently transmitted by blood transfusion is type B viral hepatitis. It is not easy to determine the incidence of this complication because of nonicteric forms of the disease, but the incidence is lower when blood donor selection excludes high risk hepatitis carriers, drug addicts, and professional donors. The risk increases linearly with the number of units of blood transfused. The disease may also follow administration of plasma, pooled plasma, and some products of protein fractionation, and the incubation period may range from 14 to 60 days. A fatality rate of 12 per cent has been reported, but mortality is lower below the age of 40. According to recent reports, there is some hope of preventing or modifying the disease by the use of high titer immune globulins.

The discovery of a hepatitis-associated antigen, hepatitis type B surface antigen (HB_sAg), found in the blood of a high percentage of patients who develop serum hepatitis has proved helpful in studying the disease. Routine screening of blood donors for the presence of the antigen should reduce the incidence of serum hepatitis and is now mandatory in Red Cross blood banks and most hospital laboratories. However, screening does not detect a large percentage of carriers. Another approach that has reduced infection is limiting donors to volunteers rather than paid producers. It is important to know that infectious hepatitis can be transmitted by blood or blood products and that low levels of type B surface antigen capable of causing the disease may go undetected in blood.

Bacterial Contamination.   Patient reaction to massive bacterial contamination of bank blood is a rare complication, manifested by chills and hyperpyrexia and, in the severe case, cardiovascular collapse and death within a short time. The severe reactions apparently result from contamination of blood with gram-negative bacteria and their endotoxins. Vigorous treatment must be initiated with broad-spectrum antibiotics, myocardial inotropic agents, corticosteroids, and appropriate blood volume expansion. Careful bacteriologic control of bank blood, adequate refrigeration, and discarding blood containers that are opened and unused are the best preventive measures.

Similar reactions have occurred in patients receiving contaminated intravenous crystalloids or colloids. Therefore, all fluids to be infused must be routinely examined before use, and cloudy fluid or fluid in cracked bottles should be cultured and then discarded. Contaminated parenteral fluid supplies with low bacterial counts have gone undetected for long periods as the source of infections in recipients.

WHOLE BLOOD

Blood bank data from the mid 1970s onward reveal that approximately 30 to 35 per cent of blood administered is in the form of whole blood, with the remainder fractionated into component parts. A reasonable source of whole blood is autologous blood, i.e., blood taken from a patient and returned to that same patient. Replacement of blood loss by this technique avoids the problems of blood group incompatibility and immunogenicity and eradicates the possibility of serum hepatitis transmission. Three methods are available to facilitate blood replacement with this technique.

In elective operations, the technique of *preoperative collection and storage* can provide a patient with several units of his own blood. Over a period of several days prior to the procedure two or three units of blood can be withdrawn at timely intervals and stored up to 21 days; using frozen storage techniques the time limitations can be extended. Acute blood volume changes following withdrawal of a single unit are usually corrected within 12 to 24 hours. Furthermore, in healthy patients increased red blood cell production can re-establish stable hemoglobin levels following multiple unit withdrawals.

A second technique, thus far primarily used in open heart surgery entails immediate *preoperative collection and hemodilution.* The simultaneous collection of blood and augmentation of a patient's blood volume with crystalloid until the hematocrit is decreased to 30 per cent can provide up to three additional units of blood for subsequent transfusion. The reduction in oxygen-carrying capacity is not detrimental, and the decrease in blood viscosity may be beneficial in tissue perfusion.

The third technique, *auto transfusion* or *interoperative blood salvage,* has direct application in certain kinds of major trauma. The blood is aspirated from the operative field, and, with appropriate anticoagulation and filtration to remove debris it can be re-infused into the patient safely. This technique has its greatest application in the surgical care of chest, head, and extremity trauma since it avoids a problem of potential contamination in abdominal operations.

Homologous Blood. The administration of whole blood for rapid replenishment of circulating blood volume in severe hypovolemic shock probably remains the primary reason for its use. On the other hand, justification exists for use of whole blood in the transfusion of severely debilitated, chronically malnourished, or immuno-compromised patients. Under these circumstances, maximum benefit is obtained if the unit is administered almost immediately after collection.

PACKED RED BLOOD CELLS

Packed red blood cells are prepared by removing two thirds of the plasma and anticoagulant solution from a unit of whole blood by either centrifugation or undisturbed sedimentation, resulting in a hematocrit between 65 to 70 per cent. There are several advantages in using packed red blood cells as opposed to whole blood.

The most common indication for blood administration remains the restoration of oxygen-carrying capacity, a primary function of the red cells. A unit of packed cells has an oxygen-carrying capacity equal to that of a unit of whole blood with approximately one third the volume of plasma, thereby reducing the possibility of circulatory overload. This is of value in transfusions in patients with the potential for congestive heart failure, in the chronically anemic patient whose plasma volume is usually expanded, in the anuric patient, in those in chronic renal failure to reduce the acid and potassium load of a whole blood transfusion, and in the patient with severe hepatic dysfunction to minimize the ammonia and citrate load. Elderly debilitated patients with anemia, although hypovolemic, should be given packed cells because they are often unable to tolerate major increases in blood volume. With the development and use of extremely fine screen filters (40-micron pore size, in contrast to the traditional 170-micron filter) rapid, sustained infusion of multiple units of packed cells is occasionally a problem. This can be alleviated by use of a crystalloid solution, normal saline, as a priming volume.

LEUKOCYTE-DEFICIENT RED BLOOD CELLS

Often an allergic reaction to blood is caused by incompatible leukocytes. Leukocyte antibodies can be found in patients who have had multiple transfusions, in some multiparous women, and in those who have had tissue or organ transplantation. Lymphocytes and granulocytes also carry tissue antigens. The reaction is characterized by chills, fever, headache, nausea, and malaise. Prior sensitization of organ transplant recipients to incompatible antigens may jeopardize survival of the transplanted organ. Several methods are available to remove 70 to 90 per cent of the leukocytes normally found in blood, including centrifugation, nylon filtration, dextran sedimentation, red cells washed in saline, and reconstitution of frozen erythrocytes. Washing of red blood cells in saline requires that the cells be exposed to the environment, therefore the cell pack should be used within 24 hours to minimize bacterial contamination.

Reconstituted Frozen Red Blood Cells

Erythrocytes with an added cryoprotective agent such as glycerol can be frozen and stored for years, the freezing completely inhibiting cellular metabolism. Prior to transfusion the cells are thawed and the glycerol removed by washing, which removes the plasma and most of the nonerythrocytic formed elements such as leukocytes. The advantages of freezing include storage of red blood cells of rare type, accumulating blood for autotransfusion, stockpiling blood of various kinds without plasma proteins and few leukocytes, and building reserves in case routine blood bank supplies run low. A primary disadvantage is the higher cost of blood preparation.

MAINTENANCE OF COAGULATION FACTORS

Of the three independent problems resulting from blood loss, coagulation difficulties occur least frequently. Fortunately, only 10 to 20 per cent of labile coagulation factors are needed for effective coagulation. The labile coagulation factors (V and VIII) are found only in fresh blood or fresh frozen plasma — factor V or proaccelerin and factor VIII or antihemophilic globulin. Deficiencies of factor V or VIII result in prolonged clotting times. With meticulous technique (constant temperature block and predetermined tilt pattern), the one-tube clotting time is a useful and reproducible test, the normal clotting time being less than four minutes. Administration of 250 ml of fresh frozen plasma every time half the estimated blood volume is replaced should prevent bleeding owing to insufficient factor V or VIII.

Reduced platelet levels are another source of coagulopathy, not easily diagnosed and difficult to treat. Blood with insufficient platelets has an essentially normal clotting time, but the clot fails to retract normally. Viable platelets can be obtained only from fresh blood or from platelet concentrates. The normal platelet count ranges from 200,000 to 400,000 per mm^3 and can fall to 50,000 without impairment of the coagulation mechanism, provided that the platelets are functionally normal.

Patients with advanced liver disease and those receiving oral anticoagulants may develop hypoprothrombinemia. However, decreased levels of prothrombin are usually not a problem in replacement therapy, since adequate amounts of prothrombin are present in bank blood; the level must decrease below 40 per cent of normal before bleeding occurs. Hypoprothrombinemic patients usually have relatively normal clotting times but prolonged prothrombin times. If the problem is caused by oral anticoagulants and liver function is not impaired, intravenous vitamin K can correct the deficiency within four to six hours.

The third most common kind of intraoperative coagulopathy, increased fibrinolysis, occurs during massive transfusion with deficiency of labile clotting factors and thrombocytopenia. This is usually associated with intravenous release of thromboplastins, causing widespread inappropriate intravascular microclotting and depletion of clotting factors, especially fibrinogen and platelets. This entity, called consumption coagulopathy or disseminated intravascular coagulopathy (DIC), is observed after hemorrhage secondary to placenta previa, during prostatic and cardiopulmonary bypass surgery, and following hemolytic transfusion reactions and heat stroke or malignant hyperthermia. DIC is not easily diagnosed rapidly because the clot may not lyse at room temperature for many hours. With normal blood, lysis does not occur in 24 hours. In severe cases a poor quality clot forms or clotting does not take place at all. Specialized laboratory tests are available for diagnosis, but results may not be available for hours. The treatment of choice when diagnosis is certain is administration of heparin intravenously, a potentially dangerous therapy. Thus, hematologic consultation should be obtained whenever DIC is suspected. The use of antifibrinolytic agents such as ϵ-aminocaproic acid (EACA) is inappropriate and more dangerous than heparin.

PLATELET CONCENTRATES

Indications for platelet transfusion include patients scheduled for major operations in whom the platelet count is below 50,000 per mm^3 and patients with thrombocytopenia with pronounced bleeding. Usually thrombocytopenia in the nonsurgical patient is not severe enough to increase the risk of bleeding significantly until the platelet count falls below 10,000 mm^3. Cancer patients, acute leukemics or those who have had chemotherapy or radiation therapy often have moderate thrombocytopenia with platelet counts between 10,000 and 30,000 mm^3. When they are scheduled for operation, prophylactic treatment of the thrombocytopenia is necessary. Patients with thrombocytopenia secondary to increased platelet destruction derive minimal benefit from platelet transfusions because donor platelets are destroyed nearly as rapidly as the recipient's autologous platelets. Repeated platelet transfusion increases the risk of formation of antibodies to platelets, thus diminishing the response to subsequent platelet transfusions. Platelet concentrates should be given to the donor within a few hours of collection so that the platelets remain viable. Other sources of platelets include fresh whole blood, platelet-rich packed red blood cells, and platelet-rich plasma.

Platelet concentrates are prepared by plasmapheresis, a process by which whole blood is drawn into a special collecting system and plasma containing the platelets is separated from red cells by centrifugation. The remaining packed red blood cells can be re-infused into the donor or placed in the blood bank.

FRESH FROZEN PLASMA

To qualify as fresh, plasma must be separated from whole blood within four to six hours after collection, frozen and stored at -18 C. When frozen, it is used within two hours of thawing. Fresh frozen plasma contains all of the plasma clotting factors except platelets and the labile factors V and VIII, which disappear upon storage if unfrozen. Fresh frozen plasma is given only after proof of compatibility by typing and cross-matching. The prime indication for use is the treatment of major clotting factor deficiencies (V, XI, and XIII) and treatment of other specific clotting factor deficiencies (VII, VIII, IX, and X) when specific concentrates are unavailable. Fresh frozen plasma can be effectively used to treat the hemophiliac with factor VIII deficiency, but cryoprecipitated plasma is a preferred source, since factor VIII is thereby concentrated. Cryoprecipitate enriched with factor VIII is obtained by centrifugation at 4 C when fresh frozen plasma is thawed. The preparation is also indicated when multiple clotting factor deficiencies exist, as in severe liver disease and defibrination states, and during massive blood replacement with stored bank blood.

OVERLOAD OF THE CIRCULATION

In massive blood loss, whether replacement is with blood, colloid, or crystalloid, volume overload of the circulation can easily occur. It is possible to pass from a state of an inadequate blood volume to one of gross overload without receiving an unusually large volume. This occurs more readily in the elderly, in those with a history of congestive heart failure, and in debilitated patients. However, inadequate volume replacement with the consequent arterial hypotension can produce irreversible cardiac or cerebral damage before adequate perfusion is restored. The only approach is careful observation of all patients and use of the appropriate monitoring devices.

PRINCIPLES OF RAPID VOLUME REPLACEMENT

The need to give blood rapidly is modified by the state of the patient's cardiovascular system. The problem of what volume to give is simplified by determining the adequacy of venous return to the ventricles, hemodynamically referred to as assessing "preload function." Factors involved in preload function are the inotropic state of the myocardium and the relationship of intravascular space to intravascular volume.

Central venous pressure (CVP) is used to assess the return of blood to the right ventricle, and pulmonary wedge pressure (PWP, measured by a Swan-Ganz catheter) permits assessment of blood returned to the left ventricle (see Chapter 9). This discussion is confined to the use of these monitors as guides to rapid fluid replacement.

In many clinical situations the right and left ventricles have equal functional capabilities; therefore, measurement of CVP is an adequate estimate of overall myocardial function. CVP can be considered a reflection of myocardial pump function and the compliance characteristics or venous tone relative to volume in the capacitance vessels. The system can be assessed via sequential measurement called the "delta factor" or via a change in pressure from a previous baseline with intravenous administration of a finite volume of fluid. This is correlated with improvement observed in the systemic arterial circulation: increase in blood pressure, elevated urine output, and other evidence of improved peripheral circulation.

Several techniques permit a fluid challenge to monitor augmentation of intravascular volumes. Using the CVP monitor, one approach is a so-called 2 to 5 cm rule, which is as follows:

1. Give 50 to 200 ml of volume (usually crystalloid) over a ten-minute period; the exact amount depends on assessment of the patient's condition.

2. Observe the systemic circulation for improvement in blood pressure, peripheral circulation, and urinary output. Assess the pulmonary circulation by auscultation of the chest.

3. Evaluate changes in CVP. If the increase is less than 2 cm H_2O, administer more fluid. An increase of more than 5 cm H_2O suggests that continued volume expansion is unlikely to cause further improvement. If the increase is between 2 and 5 cm H_2O, wait ten minutes, then re-evaluate CVP and the clinical situation. If CVP returns to less than 2 cm H_2O increase, continue to give fluid. If CVP remains between 2 and 5 cm H_2O, give a smaller quantity of fluid and repeat the evaluation.

PWP is a more reliable guide to rapid fluid therapy in patients with a disparity between left and right ventricular function. An approach as outlined previously can be followed using a 3 to 7 torr rule. The probability of ventricular disparity is increased in patients with a history of recent myocardial infarction (especially if pulmonary edema was present), in septic shock, following massive trauma, and with chronic obstructive pulmonary disease with cor pulmonale. If pulmonary wedge pressure acutely rises 7 torr or more above normal baseline values, continued volume expansion should be re-evaluated, and therapy should be directed at improving left ventricular inotropic function.

Certain measures increase the safety of rapid blood transfusion: warming blood to body temperature and monitoring that temperature; continuous, direct monitoring of arterial blood pressure (systemic and pulmonary); measuring alveolar ventilation, arterial oxygenation, oxygen extraction, and acid-base balance; monitoring breath sounds via an esophageal stethoscope to detect pulmonary edema and evaluate heart sounds; and monitoring urine output, CVP, and PWP.

In spite of these measures, some patients may develop heart failure secondary to volume overload, often immediately postoperatively. This necessitates appropriate ventilatory support with oxygen and use of diuretic and positive inotropic drug therapy. In the awake patient, morphine given intravenously in repeated 1- to 5-mg doses is helpful, causing a decrease in venous tone and preload as well as providing sedation and analgesia.

The need for positive inotropic drugs and diuretics may be urgent. Furosemide, 10 to 40 mg intravenously, has immediate onset of action and a potent diuretic effect. Dopamine, with a positive inotropic effect increasing cardiac output and less potential for inducing tachycardia and arrhythmogenicity than isoproterenol, is the drug of choice following rapid transfusion resulting in a high PWP or CVP. At low doses (1 to 2 μg/kg/min), dilation of the renal vessels occurs with increased renal blood flow (see Chapter 32).

Calcium chloride or calcium gluconate is reserved for patients with hypocalcemia secondary to pre-existing disease or after massive blood transfusion in patients with myocardial dysfunction. Digitalis is not routinely recommended for acute myocardial failure during or immediately following anesthesia; however, if necessary, digoxin may be used. Other supportive measures for acute heart failure include utilization of PEEP (see Chapter 37) and phlebotomy.

INTRAVENOUS TECHNIQUE

APPARATUS

Disposable equipment, now universally used for intravenous fluid therapy, is both safer for the patient and economical. Occasionally, anesthesia for short procedures can be accomplished without an intravenous infusion but most operations require an intravenous route for blood, fluid replacement, or medication. Two categories of intravenous device are available: one is the so-called "butterfly needle," and the other is the plastic catheter. In the critically ill and in those given large volumes of fluid, the preferred device is a plastic catheter threaded well into a vein and stabilized externally.

The butterfly needle, available in various gauges, was devised for infusion into scalp veins of infants; it is also called a scalp vein needle. The needle is thin walled, with a plastic catheter extension terminating in a female adaptor for the infusion set. Plastic wings on the needle fold to form a grip for the fingers during insertion and are then flattened against the skin and taped in position. Although simple to use, the butterfly needle is not as reliable as a catheter threaded into a vein.

Two kinds of plastic catheter are available: the "intracath," introduced through a needle, and the "extracath," introduced over a needle. Once introduced into a vein the intracath is more flexible and more easily advanced, often deliberately into the central venous circulation. For routine peripheral use the extracath is preferred because it offers a larger bore for a given catheter size, causes less bleeding at the venipuncture site, and eliminates the possibility of catheter transection by the introducing needle. The latter usually results from improper technique.

The major disadvantages of the plastic catheter include high cost, an increased incidence of thrombophlebitis, and an increased potential for shearing and loss of the catheter to the circulation. Thrombophlebitis is usually of the aseptic variety, increasing with the duration of maintenance, and in part may be a consequence of rigid fixation in a small vein. Catheters are changed, or discontinued if possible, within 72 hours; the appearance of a sterile inflammation or thrombophlebitis is directly related to the time the catheter remains in situ. In the event of transection the fatality rate may be high if the loose catheter migrates to the lungs or heart; the catheter must be retrieved surgically during fluoroscopic localization.

When infusion of large amounts of fluid is anticipated, a minimum of two 16-gauge peripheral intravenous catheters should be placed exclusive of the one to measure CVP. The smallest catheter or needle permitting rapid blood administration is of 20 gauge, but this requires a high pressure head. A linear relation exists between hydrostatic pressure and laminar flow rate and a fourth power relation between the cross-sectional area of the catheter and flow; doubling the height of the infusion bottle doubles flow rate, whereas doubling the internal diameter of the catheter increases flow rate 16 times (Poiseuille's law). A unit of blood can be infused through a 14-gauge catheter in about five minutes using an elastic, cylindric in-line bulb with check valves or by applying external pressure via a hand-inflated air reservoir enveloping a plastic blood container. The once common method of introducing air under pressure into a blood container above the fluid level has been abdandoned because of the hazard of air embolism.

TECHNIQUE OF CATHETER INSERTION

The skin is routinely prepared for venipuncture with 70 to 90 per cent isopropyl alcohol. Mechanical cleansing is probably as important as the bactericidal action of the antiseptic, which is allowed to dry before venipuncture. Betadine solution may be preferred as an antiseptic. When using an 18-gauge or larger catheter, a skin wheal is made first with a 25-gauge needle, and 0.5 per cent lidocaine or procaine is given to minimize discomfort. The largest, straightest, and most visible vein that will remain accessible during operation is chosen for puncture. The veins on the dorsum of the hand are often excellent from the standpoint of size, visibility, and minimal chance of inadvertent arterial cannulation (Fig. 23–1), but it is sometimes difficult to maintain immobilization in the immediate postoperative period. Veins of the midforearm are more suitable for immobilization over long periods. Leg veins are avoided if possible because of the hazard of thrombosis. Spasm of veins can be overcome by dependent drainage, by application of moist heat, or by rubbing or tapping the puncture site. A tourniquet is applied as close as possible to the site without pinching the skin or pulling hair, best accomplished with a wide tourniquet; a blood pressure cuff inflated to 40 torr is also good.

The intravenous needle may be inserted attached to the adaptor of the infusion tubing or to a syringe, or it may be inserted independently. With anticipated easy venipuncture, the extracath may be directly introduced into the vein. Successful puncture is indicated by the appearance of blood in the proximal end of the needle. Some prefer to connect the intravenous tubing or a syringe for insertion of the needle. With the vein fixed proximally by the tourniquet and held distally by stretching the skin, the needle is inserted through the skin to one side of the vein and is advanced steadily and directly over the vein, with the bevel upward until penetration occurs. The needle is threaded into the vein with a slight rotary movement and the tourniquet removed before infusion is started. If an extracath is used, the entire unit is advanced into the

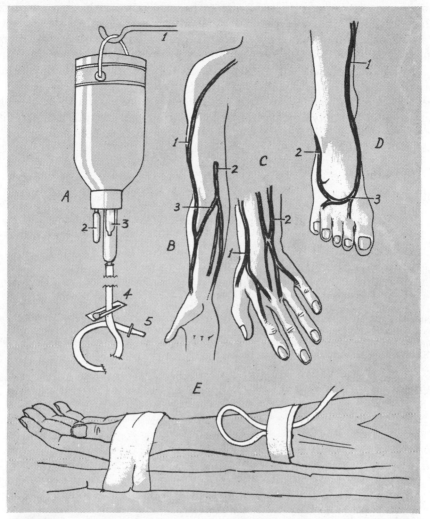

FIGURE 23–1. *A*, Components of intravenous apparatus: *1*, hook on pole of adjustable height; *2*, air inlet; *3*, drip bulb; *4*, pinch clamp for controlling flow of fluid; *5*, adapter for insertion into needle or catheter. *B*, Veins of arm: *1*, cephalic; *2*, basilic; *3*, antecubital. *C*, Veins of dorsum of hand: *1*, cephalic; *2*, basilic. *D*, Veins of dorsum of foot: *1*, great saphenous; *2*, small saphenous; *3*, dorsal venous arch. *E*, Fixation of intravenous needle and tubing to arm.

vein a few millimeters before sliding the catheter off the introducing needle. Catheters are not advanced past a venous valve lest a perforation occur. If a vein is torn or penetrated through and through, the needle should be removed, pressure applied, and the arm elevated above venous pressure to lessen hematoma formation.

The catheter is fixed with adhesive tape to maintain connection to the intravenous adaptor and to prevent accidental dislodgement; nonallergenic tape is used if there is sensitivity to adhesive tape. The wrist or elbow is held immobile on a padded board if the catheter site lies over those areas, and care is taken to avoid applying the tape to muscle or placing it circumferentially in such a way as to increase venous pressure (see Fig. 23–1). After insertion, the system is checked to make sure that infiltration has not occurred. Blood should flow back into the tubing if the container is lowered below heart level. The infusion site is re-examined for infiltration at intervals.

Some anxious, vasoconstricted patients benefit from having venipuncture done after inhalation anesthesia has produced vasodilation. When comfort alone is the issue, this is more pleasant for the patient than repeated and unsuccessful attempts at venipuncture. However, if vasoconstriction is the result of hypovolemia or if the patient has a full stomach, an intravenous route is mandatory before attempting anesthesia induction, even if a cutdown is necessary.

The following complications from intravenous therapy have been observed: localized cellulitis and lymphangitis, venous thrombosis or thrombophlebitis, air embolism, extravasation with tissue slough or neuritis, accidental injection of the wrong drug, and accidental intra-arterial infusion.

REFERENCES

Cullen DJ, Kunsmen J, Caldera D, et al: Comparative evaluation of new fine-screen filters. Anesthesiology 53:3, 1980.

Doenicke A, Grote B, Lorenz W: Blood and blood substitutes. Br J Anaesth 49:681, 1977.

Jesch F, Webber LM, Dalton JW, et al: Oxygen dissociation after transfusion of blood stored in ACD or CPD solution. J Thorac Cardiovasc Surg 70:35, 1975.

Lowe RS, Moss GS, Jilek J, et al: Crystalloid versus colloid in the etiology of pulmonary failure after trauma: A randomized trial in man. Surgery 81:676, 1977.

Mollison PL: Blood Transfusion in Clinical Medicine. 5th ed, Philadelphia, F. A. Davis Company, 1972.

Moss GS, Salletta JD: Traumatic shock in man. N Engl J Med 290:724, 1974.

Rice CL, Moss GS: Blood and blood substitutes: Current practice. Adv Surg 13:93, 1979.

Robertson HD, Polk HC: Blood transfusions in elective operations: Comparison of whole blood versus packed red cells. Ann Surg 181:778, 1975.

Rosenblum R: Physiologic basis for the therapeutic use of catecholamines. Am Heart J 87:527, 1974.

Slichter SJ: Controversies in platelet transfusion therapy. Ann Rev Med 31:509, 1980.

Umlas J: Washed, hyperpacked, frozen and shelf red blood cells. Transfusion 15:111, 1975.

Virgilis RW, Rice EL, Smith DE, et al: Colloid versus crystalloid resuscitation: Is one better? A randomized clinical trial. Surgery 85:129, 1979.

Part *E*
THE SPECIALTIES

Chapter 24
OBSTETRIC ANESTHESIA AND PERINATOLOGY

The first obstetric anesthetic comprised ether administered to a woman with a severely contracted pelvis by James Y. Simpson of Edinburgh in January 1847 during delivery of a dead baby by internal podalic version. Recognizing the effectiveness yet unpleasantness of ether, Simpson was determined to find a more suitable anesthetic. At the suggestion of David Waldie, chemist, Simpson later in that year successfully used chloroform, also effective in alleviating the pain of childbirth, for a more rapid and pleasant induction. Criticism arose at once, not only from physicians but from the clergy, who held that it was divinely ordained (Genesis 3:16) that women suffer in childbirth. Simpson answered his critics by pointing out that the Lord had anesthetized Adam when He created Eve from one of Adam's ribs (Genesis 2:21) and stated, "What God Himself did cannot be sinful." However, the morality of pain relief was not established until 1853 when John Snow gave chloroform analgesia to Queen Victoria during the birth of her eighth child, Prince Leopold. As the Queen was head of the Church of England, her action led to the moral acceptance of obstetric anesthesia.

While Simpson was using chloroform, Walter Channing, Professor of Midwifery and Jurisprudence at the Medical School in Cambridge (Harvard), used ether for obstetric anesthesia in April 1847. A year later Channing published a classic monograph entitled *A Treatise on Etherization in Childbirth* wherein he described use of ether, chloroform, and mixtures of ether, chloroform, and alcohol for anesthesia in 581 parturients.

GENERAL CONSIDERATIONS IN OBSTETRIC ANESTHESIA

Anesthetic care for mothers having vaginal delivery or cesarean section entails many considerations not pertinent to surgical patients. The anesthetist is required to provide anesthesia for two individuals simultaneously. Essentially all anesthetics given the parturient cross the placenta to affect the fetus — opioids, sedatives, tranquilizers, local and inhalation anesthetics, and, to some extent, neuromuscular blockers. These drugs should be given in minimal effective doses to avoid deleterious effects on the progress of labor, the intrauterine environment, and the condition of the neonate.

Unlike the usual surgical patient who comes prepared for anesthesia, the obstetric patient is rarely in optimal condition at the time. She must be suspected of having a full stomach, therefore being prone to aspiration of gastric contents, a leading cause of maternal anesthetic mortality. During labor, emergencies such as fetal distress, maternal hemorrhage, prolapsed cord, and uterine tetany demand immediate anesthesia if both mother and baby are to survive. Vaginal delivery requires the parturient to be awake and cooperative most of the time to assist the forces of labor. Common medical disorders, such as diabetes mellitus, heart disease, and endocrine imbalance are aggravated by pregnancy; others may be associated with the gravid state, such as preeclampsia/eclampsia and coagulation disorders occurring with abruptio placentae, intrauterine fetal death, and amniotic fluid embolism. For the most part the timing of delivery is not controlled; anesthesia must be readily available at all times. At delivery, the anesthetist must be prepared to assure care for both mother and newborn.

PHYSIOLOGIC CHANGES OF PREGNANCY AND ANESTHETIC IMPLICATIONS

RESPIRATORY CHANGES

Physiologic changes of pregnancy carry profound anesthetic implications. A generalized edema of the upper airway develops (thought to be a result of increased circulating levels of progesterone); thus airway obstruction is more likely to occur and the risk of trauma associated with airway insertion and laryngoscopy is increased. Edema of the larynx and vocal cords necessitates use of a smaller endotracheal tube, especially in teenage gravidas.

Changes in lung function during pregnancy are summarized in Figure 24–1. Although vital capacity is unchanged, total lung volume is decreased by approximately 5 per cent owing to elevation of the diaphragm. At term, alveolar ventilation is increased by approximately 40 per cent, primarily a result of an increase in tidal volume. These alterations cause a 15 per cent reduction in functional residual capacity, which enhances uptake of anesthetic gases. During labor without adequate pain relief, alveolar ventilation may approach three times normal, further increasing anesthetic uptake. Hyperventilation results in respiratory alkalosis, usually compensated by metabolic acidosis secondary to renal excretion of bicarbonate. At term, both basal metabolic rate and the quantity of oxygen required for physical exercise are increased by 15 per cent. These alterations, combined with a decrease in functional residual capacity, increase the likelihood of maternal hypoxia. Apprehension, increased oxygen consumption, and the demands of labor are associated with maternal metabolic and lactic acidosis. Effective analgesia during labor and delivery decreases maternal hyperventilation, oxygen consumption, and metabolic acidosis. The minimum alveolar concentration (MAC) of various inhalation anesthetics is decreased in pregnancy, postulated to be secondary to increased circulating levels of both progesterone and endorphins, thus subjecting the mother to possible overdose in inhalation anesthesia.

CIRCULATORY CHANGES

The total blood volume at term is increased by 30 per cent, an additional 1200 to 1500 ml. A larger increase in plasma volume occurs and results in a decreased hematocrit, thus explaining the relative anemia of pregnancy despite an increased red blood cell volume. With proper dietary intake, including vitamin and iron supplementation, hematocrit rarely falls below 35 per cent. About 800 ml of the increased blood volume is contained in the gravid uterus and is expressed into the peripheral circulation when the uterus contracts at delivery (Fig. 24–2). Simultaneously, vascular capacity is

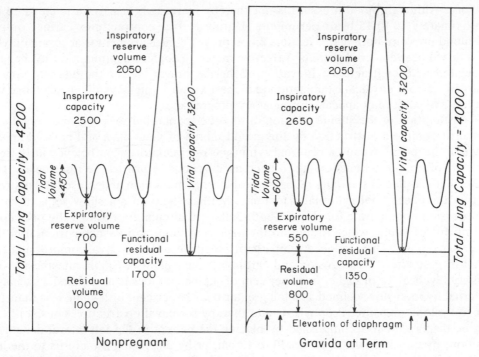

FIGURE 24–1. Comparison of pulmonary volumes and capacities in the normal gravida at term and nonpregnant woman. (Reprinted by permission from Bonica JJ: Principles and Practice of Obstetric Analgesia and Anesthesia. Philadelphia, FA Davis Co, 1967, p 24.)

decreased by an equal amount. This permits the healthy parturient to sustain a blood loss approaching 1500 ml without apparent difficulty. As the average blood loss in vaginal delivery and cesarean section seldom exceeds 500 and 1000 ml, respectively, transfusion with blood or colloid is rarely necessary.

Measured in the lateral decubitus position, maternal cardiac output is elevated to near maximum toward the end of the first trimester, remains elevated by about 35 per cent throughout pregnancy, and does not return to normal until two weeks post-

FIGURE 24–2. Cardiac output during pregnancy in the lateral and supine positions. In the lateral position, cardiac output reaches a near peak at the end of the first trimester and is maintained throughout pregnancy. (Reprinted by permission from Moir DD, Carty MJ: Obstetric Anaesthesia and Analgesia. Balliere Tindall, London, 1977, p 15. From data by Lees MN, Taylor SH, Scott DB, et al: A study of cardiac output at rest throughout pregnancy. J Obstet Gynaecol Br Commonw 74:319, 1967.)

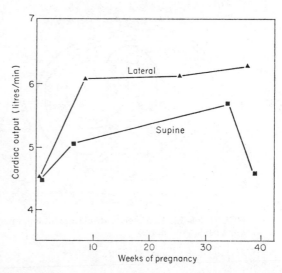

delivery. Although blood pressure is not thereby increased, heart rate is elevated by approximately 10 to 15 beats per minute. During uterine contractions, cardiac output and blood pressure both increase, thus blood pressure measurement is accurate only in the interval between contractions. Effective maternal analgesia minimizes the changes associated with contractions. Elevation of the diaphragm causes the heart to appear enlarged on both physical examination and chest x-ray. Benign systolic heart murmurs and left axis shift may appear as pregnancy progresses.

Assumption of the supine position during the second half of pregnancy results in partial to complete obstruction by the gravid uterus of vena cava and aorta. Maintenance of this position causes maternal symptoms of circulatory insufficiency in 10 to 15 per cent of gravid patients owing to decreased venous return to the right heart. The diminished cardiac output may reduce uteroplacental perfusion and cause fetal distress even in the absence of maternal symptoms. Mothers who do not show signs of caval compression compensate for this via both collateral circulation through the perivertebral plexus of veins, which drain into the azygos system, and vasoconstriction in the lower extremities. Drug-induced sympathetic blockade added to caval compression can result in precipitous hypotension and cardiovascular collapse. Spinal anesthesia with sensory levels at T8 or higher in 80 per cent of supine gravidas is associated with major maternal hypotension, defined as a fall greater than 30 per cent or a value less than 100 torr in systolic pressure. Prophylaxis and therapy for caval obstruction consist of left uterine displacement accomplished by placing the patient in the left lateral decubitus position, by elevating the right hip 10 to 12 cm, or by displacing the uterus to the left either manually or with a displacement device (Fig. 24–3). The gravid patient should not lie supine during the second half of pregnancy. During labor and delivery, left uterine displacement is assured until birth, a precaution especially relevant to utilization of general or major conduction anesthesia. Vena caval compression also results in dilation of perivertebral veins, so that accidental intravenous injection is more likely to occur during peridural block. Dilated veins decrease the volume of the peridural space and block the intravertebral foramina, possibly accounting for higher anesthetic levels obtained with peridural injection of local anesthetics. Dilation of peridural veins decreases the size of the subarachnoid space, perhaps explaining the 33 per cent decreased dosage requirement for subarachnoid block.

Compression of the aorta below the renal and common iliac arteries at the brim of

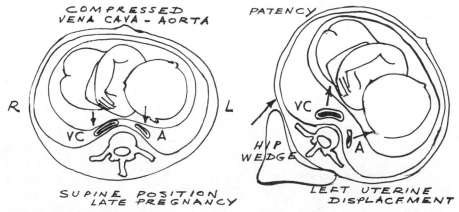

FIGURE 24–3.   Left uterine displacement employing a hip wedge: R = right; L = left; VC = vena cava; A = aorta.

the pelvis by the gravid uterus results in decreased uteroplacental perfusion and fetal compromise without maternal symptoms. Assumption of the left lateral decubitus position or left uterine displacement minimizes this effect.

GASTROINTESTINAL CHANGES

Both gastric acidity and secretion are increased during pregnancy. Gastric emptying time is prolonged by labor, apprehension, pain, and change in the position of the gastroduodenal junction effected by the gravid uterus. The gravid uterus also affects the gastroesophageal junction by producing a functional hiatal hernia with lesser competency and increased possibility of reflux. Likewise, the enlarged uterus and assumption of the lithotomy position for vaginal delivery elevate intragastric pressure. Together, these changes subject the sedated or unconscious gravid patient to a greater risk of pulmonary aspiration of gastric contents.

Many have suggested that the pathologic changes induced by pulmonary aspiration are eliminated by increasing the pH of gastric contents above 2.5 with antacids to avoid acid aspiration or Mendelson's syndrome. Antacids, particularly the insoluble suspensions of aluminum and magnesium salts, while increasing gastric pH, require up to 30 minutes for their action, do not lessen the possibility of aspiration, and have produced pulmonary lesions in animal models. The incidence of maternal mortality does not appear to have been reduced in women who have experienced aspiration despite use of antacids. Soluble solutions of antacids such as 0.3 m sodium citrate may be more effective as they offer more rapid neutralizing activity. The histamine blocker cimetidine (Tagamet) currently under study in gravid patients reliably increases gastric pH and decreases gastric volume when given either orally or intravenously. Unfortunately, 60 to 90 minutes are required to elevate gastric pH, and effects on uterine activity and the newborn are not known at present.

If pulmonary aspiration is to be prevented during regional anesthesia, competency of the protective laryngeal reflexes must also be maintained. If consciousness is lost or laryngeal reflexes compromised, the lungs must be protected by cricoid pressure followed by rapid tracheal intubation. The interval from last oral ingestion to induction of anesthesia is of little value in determining risk of pulmonary aspiration. Fasting women undergoing elective cesarean section are at nearly as great a risk as patients undergoing emergency section.

PAIN DURING LABOR AND DELIVERY

Parturition is associated with two distinct kinds of pain. One is visceral in origin, caused by uterine contractions plus dilation and effacement of the cervix, whereas the other is somatically induced through stretching of the vagina and perineum by the fetus during descent in the pelvis. The pain pathways involved in each instance are distinctly different, as shown in Figure 24–4. Although it is customary to refer to visceral pain as that of the first stage and somatic pain as that of the second stage, overlap of these two pain sources actually occurs.

As the uterus contracts, the presenting part of the fetus, usually the head, presses against the cervix and stretches it. The pain incited is ventrally referred to the lower abdomen between umbilicus and pubis and dorsally to the lower lumbar region. Early in labor this may be perceived as only a sense of pressure, but as contractions become stronger the pain becomes more intense and may be referred to hips and thighs. These sensations are mediated by small unmyelinated fibers passing from the cervix through the pelvic and hypogastric plexuses, enter the sympathetic chain at L3 to L5, and

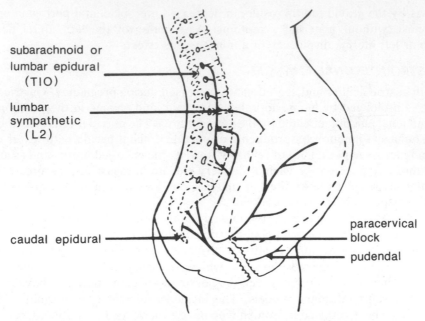

subarachnoid or
lumbar epidural
(TIO)

lumbar
sympathetic
(L2)

caudal epidural

paracervical
block

pudendal

FIGURE 24–4. Sensory pathways and sites of injection in obstetric regional anesthesia. Visceral pain from cervix and uterus is blocked by paracervical blocks, bilateral lumbar sympathetic blocks at T10 to L1. Somatic pain from perineum is blocked by pudendal nerve blocks, saddle (subarachnoid) block, or low caudal peridural block. All labor pain is abolished by a modified saddle (subarachnoid), lumbar peridural, or caudal peridural block extending from T10 to L5. (From Gutsche BB: Anesthesia and anesthesia for childbirth. *In* Reeder SJ, et al: Maternity Nursing, 14th ed. Philadelphia: JB Lippincott, 1980. Modified from Bonica JJ: Principles and Practice of Obstetric Analgesia and Anesthesia. Philadelphia, FA Davis, 1967, p. 492.)

finally reach the dorsal root ganglia and spinal cord via the white rami communicantes of T10 to T12, and possibly L1 as well. The majority of visceral pain is cervical in origin but may be partly the result of uterine ischemia.

Somatic or vaginal pain is perceived as the presenting part begins its descent through the vagina, usually at about 8 cm dilation of the cervix in the primigravida. Initially, this pain is perceived as a need to defecate, but with further descent the mother has an uncontrollable urge to bear down, thus activating accessory forces of labor. This helps not only to relieve discomfort, but is necessary to propel the fetus to the point where it can be delivered. The somatic pain component dominates the second stage and overshadows the visceral component as cervical dilation and effacement are completed. Somatic pain is conveyed primarily via the pudendal nerves in dorsal sacral nerve roots S2 to S4; additional components are conveyed through the ilioinguinal nerve, the genital branch of the genitofemoral and posterior femoral cutaneous nerves. Local anesthetic interruption of conduction not only abolishes somatic pain but eliminates the natural urge to bear down.

Pain during labor is experienced intermittently during contractions only when intrauterine pressure exceeds 30 torr; the degree of pain experienced varies greatly among parturients. Conditions surrounding conception, pregnancy, and delivery; the social background; and concepts of the birth process all influence a woman's behavior at delivery. Knowledge of the physiologic aspects of parturition, the presence of a supportive father, and attitudes of nurses and physicians can minimize the discomfort experienced. Encouragement, supportive conversation, and emphasis on the positive aspects and happy results of labor serve to decrease maternal anxiety, discomfort, and need for potent drugs.

RELIEF OF PAIN

The ideal form of analgesia for labor and delivery would meet the following requirements: satisfactory pain relief for mother, no significant interference with the progress of labor, little risk to either mother or fetus, and provision of satisfactory conditions for delivery and early interaction between mother and newborn, preferably in the delivery room. No one technique of analgesia or anesthesia provides all of these conditions. Often combinations of anesthetic techniques are required in a particular labor, which necessitate the availability of competent anesthesia personnel to modify or change techniques as circumstances dictate.

NONPHARMACOLOGIC METHODS OF ANALGESIA

Nonpharmacologic means of pain relief, including natural or prepared childbirth, hypnosis, and acupuncture, are advocated by many lay groups. However, there is little scientific evidence for their overall efficacy.

Natural or prepared childbirth encompasses a general philosophy of labor management based on the principle that prenatal education, encouragement of supportive persons (usually the father and labor floor personnel), and use of breathing and relaxation exercises will thereby abolish or minimize the need for pharmacologic intervention. This technique was first popularized by Grantly Dick-Read of the United Kingdom as the Read Method. Since then the psychophylaxis method of Lamaze and a modification devised by the Childbirth Education Association have become popular. These techniques provide satisfactory analgesia for some women, but for many pharmacologic pain relief is required as labor progresses.

Hypnosis has been sporadically used in childbirth. Formal hypnosis requires that the mother enter a trance, a state of focused attention and hypersuggestibility, which usually necessitates intensive training before parturition. The depth of trance obtainable in any individual varies from one that allows performance of surgical procedures to one that provides no analgesia, with most individuals falling between the two extremes. Acupuncture has not been extensively used for vaginal delivery. However, several studies have shown that some pain relief is provided, but it is usually incomplete, requiring pharmacologic supplementation.

ANALGESIA AND ANESTHESIA

Pharmacologic techniques of pain relief in parturition can be divided into four major categories: systemic medication for analgesia and sedation including opioids, tranquilizers, and dissociative drugs (e.g., ketamine); inhalation analgesia with subanesthetic concentrations of anesthetics; general anesthesia, which is rarely required for vaginal delivery; and regional or conduction techniques.

Ideally, every obstetric patient should be seen by an anesthetist prior to labor. Although logistics often make this impossible, arrangements to have an anesthetist speak to a group of mothers in a prenatal clinic and interview high risk patients individually are beneficial in allaying many of the apprehensions of obstetric patients. Upon arrival at the labor floor, the parturient can again be visited and her condition evaluated; plans for anesthesia can then be rationally discussed and informed consent obtained.

All patients receiving pharmacologic pain relief require continuous monitoring of vital signs throughout labor, in the delivery room, and during postpartum recovery. Trained labor floor nurses in constant attendance can perform this function most of the time, provided that an anesthetist is immediately available. During delivery, the presence of an anesthetist is required at all times for mothers receiving analgesia or anesthesia, as for any surgical patient. Postpartum visits are essential to document development or absence of anesthetic complications on the patient's chart. In general, patients in labor, particularly those receiving analgetics, require a reliable intravenous infusion through a 16- or 18-gauge catheter. This allows for hydration and nutrition, rapid infusion of blood if required, rapid induction of anesthesia, and treatment of complications should they arise.

SYSTEMIC MEDICATIONS

Drugs are often given parenterally to control pain and anxiety in the first stage, frequently providing sufficient analgesia throughout delivery in uncomplicated labors not requiring episiotomy. Although in the past these drugs were given intramuscularly, they are now often given intravenously in smaller doses but at more frequent intervals, as absorption and onset of action are more predictable. The opioids, which diminish awareness and the reaction to pain, comprise the mainstay of systemic medications. As equal analgesic doses of opioids cause the same degree of depression, choice of opioid is dictated by duration of action. The shorter-acting opioids, fentanyl among them, have largely replaced morphine in obstetrics. Although meperidine remains the most widely used opioid, attention has turned to the agonist-antagonists such as butorphanol and nalbuphine. The usual intravenous dose of meperidine is 0.5 to 0.75 mg/kg, repeated at half the initial dose every two to three hours. Even modest doses are associated with changes in neonatal neurobehavior, fortunately persisting only a day or two and not appreciably affecting neonatal feeding, weight gain, or development. Significant opioid depression is safely antagonized with naloxone.

Tranquilizers, including the antihistamines, phenothiazines, benzodiazepines, and occasionally a butyrophenone, are commonly included with the initial opioid dose to allay anxiety and for the antiemetic effect of some of them. Duration of action is generally long, often in excess of eight hours; when used alone in the presence of pain they may cause delirium and excitement. Furthermore, they rapidly cross the placenta to affect neonatal behavior, and there are no specific or reliable antagonists.

Barbiturates, widely used in the past, are rarely indicated as they offer no analgesia and antagonize analgesia otherwise obtained. They traverse the placenta rapidly and may cause neonatal depression. Scopolamine, usually combined with morphine or meperidine, was once widely used to produce "twilight sleep" during labor. When scopolamine was given alone or in combination with barbiturates, amnesia, excitement, and delirium were common; these are not desired by most women in labor today. The effects of scopolamine are readily antagonized by intravenous physostigmine.

Ketamine, a dissociative anesthetic, is a potent analgetic against somatic pain. Small intravenous doses of 0.25 mg/kg yield profound analgesia and amnesia lasting from two to five minutes. In these small doses, consciousness remains, and hallucinations and bad dreams are uncommon. Rapid analgesia can be provided for spontaneous or forceps vaginal delivery; incremental doses of 0.25 mg/kg not exceeding 1 mg/kg total may be given. Larger doses may result in maternal unconsciousness with loss of protective airway reflexes. Ketamine rapidly crosses the placenta, and total doses exceeding 1 mg/kg have been associated with newborn respiratory depression and muscle rigidity as well as heightened uterine contractility.

INHALATION ANALGESIA

A useful form of analgesia for vaginal delivery entails inhalation of subanesthetic concentrations of volatile or gaseous anesthetics. John Snow first described the technique in administering chloroform. Advantages include rapid onset of maternal analgesia; maintenance of protective airway reflexes; absence of significant maternal and neonatal depression regardless of duration of analgesia; frequent production of maternal amnesia; little effect on uterine activity or the urge to bear down; and rapid maternal recovery. However, the advantages of inhalation analgesia are derived only when the mother remains awake and responsive to command. Although intermittent administration of the more soluble anesthetics is effective, the maximum advantages are obtained with nitrous oxide inhaled continously in concentrations from 30 to 50 per cent in oxygen. Limitations of the technique include limited analgesia without progression to general anesthesia; possible delirium and excitement, indicating entrance into the second stage; and the need for constant trained supervision to avoid too deep an anesthetic level and unconsciousness. Continuous administration of 30 to 50 per cent nitrous oxide in high flows is usually effective for the latter part of labor, delivery, and postpartum examination. Forceps delivery is possible with inhalation analgesia if supplemented with small doses of ketamine and local infiltration or pudendal block. Intermittent methoxyflurane and trichloroethylene inhalation have also been successfully self-administered during the contractions of the latter part of the first stage.

GENERAL ANESTHESIA

General anesthesia for routine vaginal delivery is rarely indicated for the following reasons: prevention of maternal bearing down, thus allowing induction only when the fetus is deliverable; neonatal depression, which is directly related to depth and duration of anesthesia; predisposition to pulmonary aspiration; and prevention of maternal experience of the birth process and early maternal-neonatal interaction. Indications for use in vaginal delivery include control of a mother who becomes unmanageable on the delivery table; rapid delivery of a fetus in distress; and depression of uterine activity as in a tetanic uterine contraction or when intrauterine manipulation is required. Small doses of ketamine may obviate the need for general anesthesia in the uncontrollable mother or may permit rapid vaginal delivery. Intrauterine manipulation is rarely indicated in modern obstetrics except to perform version extraction of a second twin or manual removal of a placenta. The halogenated hydrocarbons, in concentrations of two MAC or greater, rapidly depress uterine activity. Today, the commonly used inhalation anesthetics for this purpose are halothane, enflurane, or isoflurane. Following attainment of uterine depression, the concentration is lowered, approaching two thirds MAC, if uterine atony and postpartum hemorrhage are to be avoided.

REGIONAL ANESTHESIA

Pain associated with labor and delivery is readily controlled with regional analgesia. The advantages are as follows: an awake, cooperative mother who can bear down; minimal neonatal depression; and minimal risk of pulmonary aspiration. Six basic techniques of regional analgesia are suitable for labor and delivery: paracervical block, bilateral lumbar sympathetic block at L2, local infiltration of the perineum, bilateral pudendal nerve block, subarachnoid sacral block (saddle), and peridural block, which includes both the lumbar and caudal approach.

Paracervical Block.   This block eliminates the visceral pain of cervical dilation and uterine contractions by interrupting conduction in afferent pain fibers as they exit from cervix and para-uterine plexus. The block is easily done by infiltrating just lateral to the cervix at 3 and 9 o'clock with dilute solutions of local anesthetic without epinephrine, 10 to 12 ml of 1 per cent 2-chloroprocaine or 0.5 per cent lidocaine. Somatic pain is not obtunded nor is the urge to bear down; in the absence of a local anesthetic reaction there are no ill effects on the mother. Unfortunately, the method has been shown to produce fetal bradycardia, fetal acidosis, and, rarely, fetal death in utero, particularly when epinephrine or larger doses of more concentrated anesthetic solutions were used. These complications have markedly curtailed the use of paracervical block for delivery of a viable fetus. To be avoided when the fetus is at high risk, the method is safe for delivery of a nonviable fetus, for therapeutic abortion, for postpartum curettage, or for repair of cervical lacerations.

Bilateral Paravertebral Lumbar Sympathetic Block at L2. This block interrupts visceral pain pathways as they traverse the sympathetic chain but provides no perineal analgesia. Although associated with maternal hypotension, fetal bradycardia is not an outcome. Sympathetic denervation of the uterus leaves parasympathic innervation intact, which may lead to increased frequency and duration of uterine contractions. As the technique is complicated, performance is usually relegated to an anesthesiologist. Each injection requires about 10 ml of a dilute local anesthetic solution, 1 per cent lidocaine or 0.25 per cent bupivacaine, best given for early, uncomfortable labor or if there is concern about the ability of the patient to bear down in the second stage. At the time these blocks are done, a lumbar epidural catheter can be inserted to provide perineal analgesia as labor progresses.

Bilateral Pudendal Nerve Block. This block yields anesthesia surrounding the introitus and anus; either a transvaginal or transcutaneous approach is employed, usually with the mother already in stirrups on the delivery table. Most of the somatic pain associated with vaginal and perineal stretching is eliminated. As overlapping innervation of the perineum is present, the urge to bear down is not completely abolished. Alone, the block provides complete analgesia for episiotomy and repair and is usually sufficient for low forceps delivery; supplementation with inhalation analgesia is required for midforceps application. Extensive perineal lacerations are more expeditiously repaired with pudendal block than with local infiltration. Each block requires 8 to 10 ml of 1 per cent lidocaine or an equivalent anesthetic with a latency of approximately five minutes. Properly performed, the method is not associated with maternal or fetal disadvantages and does not impede the progress of labor.

Subarachnoid Injection. This can produce either a true sacral block (L5 to S5) or a modified saddle block with analgesia extending from S5 to T10. It is usually performed with the subject sitting, using a hyperbaric solution of tetracaine, dibucaine, or lidocaine. For true saddle block, lumbar puncture is performed at L4 to L5 or L5 to S1, injecting 2 to 4 mg tetracaine or 20 to 30 mg lidocaine, with the sitting position maintained for two to three minutes. Adequate conditions are provided for forceps application and episiotomy without abolishing uterine pain. Modified saddle block is accomplished at L3 to L4 or higher by injecting 4 to 6 mg tetracaine or 35 to 50 mg lidocaine, with the sitting position maintained for 30 seconds. Not only does this block yield profound perineal analgesia, but the sensory level to T10 results in freedom from all pain, thus allowing cervical and uterine manipulation. Addition of 0.2 to 0.3 mg of epinephrine or 0.5 to 1.0 mg phenylephrine prolongs tetracaine analgesia to three hours or more. Onset of analgesia is rapid, permitting injection just before delivery; thus this block is an excellent choice when analgesia is required for emergency vaginal delivery.

The major adverse effects associated with saddle block include maternal hypotension, loss of the maternal bearing down reflex, possibility of a high sensory level, and development of lumbar puncture headache. Severe hypotension may develop within a minute following injection and is best prevented by preliminary rapid intravenous infusion of 500 to 1000 ml of a non-dextrose balanced salt solution plus continuous left uterine displacement when the patient is supine. Treatment is essentially the same plus intravenous administration of 10 to 15 mg of a vasoactive drug such as ephedrine or mephentermine. Potent vasoconstrictors, such as norepinephrine, methoxamine, and phenylephrine, while restoring maternal blood pressure, further compromise uterine blood flow and are to be avoided. As subarachnoid block abolishes the bearing down reflex and relaxes perineal muscles, the second stage may be prolonged and may be associated with an increased incidence of occiput posterior presentation. These complications can be minimized by delaying anesthesia until the occiput rotates anteriorly and the presenting part is on the perineum. Moreover, even though the patient loses the urge to bear down, she can be coached to do so with uterine contractions and the occiput can easily be rotated manually or with forceps; alternatively, the occiput can be delivered in the posterior position over a large mediolateral episiotomy. High sensory levels are avoided by using the correct dose of anesthetic, avoiding injection during contraction and preventing straining during positioning. Gravid patients develop the highest incidence of severe postlumbar puncture headache, best prevented by a single dural puncture with a 26-gauge needle. Adequate postpartum hydration of at least 3000 ml per day and application of a tight abdominal binder when the patient is ambulatory may provide additional prophylaxis.

Continuous Lumbar Epidural Analgesia. This form of analgesia has gained popularity over the past two decades in permitting completely pain-free labor and delivery with little or no depression of the newborn. The technique can be used for a trial of labor and the level easily extended to T4 if cesarean section becomes necessary. Initiated on onset of active painful labor, at 5 to 6 cm cervical dilation in the primigravida or 4 to 5 cm in the multipara, complete pain relief for labor and vaginal delivery is attained. With a catheter inserted at L2 to L3 or L3 to L4, from 6 to 10 ml of a dilute local anesthetic solution (0.25 per cent bupivacaine, 1 per cent lidocaine, or 2 per cent chloroprocaine) produce sensory block to T10, which interrupts visceral pain conduction from cervix and uterus. With descent of the presenting part and placement of the patient in a semisitting position plus injection of larger doses of anesthetic, the somatic pain of vaginal stretching is alleviated. Just prior to delivery with the patient sitting, a 10- to 12-ml dose of a more concentrated local anesthetic solution, such as 0.5 per cent bupivacaine, 1.5 per cent lidocaine, or 3 per cent 2-chloroprocaine, allows completely pain-free delivery including episiotomy and repair.

Lumbar epidural block as described is a major undertaking, requiring frequent monitoring of maternal vital signs, fetal heart rate, and uterine contractions. As the mother loses the sensation of uterine contraction, continuous monitoring of contractions is essential if labor is induced or enhanced with oxytocin. Hypotension with epidural block is slower in onset but can be just as severe as in subarachnoid block. Similarly, epidural anesthesia can abolish the urge to bear down, thereby resulting in an increased incidence of occiput posterior presentations. This problem can be minimized by using less concentrated local anesthetic solutions to avoid relaxation of the perineal sling and not initiating complete motor block until the presenting part is deliverable. As with saddle block, the mother can be coached to bear down with contractions.

Continuous Caudal Epidural Block. Once popular in obstetrics, this block has been largely replaced by continuous lumbar epidural block as the latter is more reliable, easier to perform, requires considerably less local anesthetic, can be performed in a less contaminated area, and can be reliably extended to allow for cesarean section. To obtain a T10 sensory level, caudal block requires approximately 20 ml of a dilute local anesthetic solution. The approach is useful for patients in whom lumbar epidural is not easily done or when delivery is imminent, as onset of perineal analgesia is more rapid with the caudal approach. A single injection of local anesthetic is made through a needle or catheter but is delayed until rectal examination confirms that needle or catheter has not entered the rectum or fetal cranium. In some institutions, a double catheter technique is employed, the lumbar catheter used for the first stage and the caudal catheter used for delivery.

ANESTHESIA FOR CESAREAN SECTION

The incidence of cesarean delivery has increased over the past decade from less than 10 per cent to over 15 per cent of all deliveries because of associated lowered neonatal mortality and morbidity as compared with difficult vaginal delivery or intrauterine manipulation plus minimally increased maternal morbidity. Section may be performed as either an elective primary or a repeated procedure in which either general or regional anesthesia is acceptable, although the latter is often preferred because of lesser associated neonatal neurobehavioral depression and decreased risk of pulmonary aspiration. Alternatively, section may be urgently indicated when a patient having had a previous section goes into labor, when labor does not progress, or when evidence appears of a deteriorating intrautine environment, albeit without overt signs of fetal distress. Again, either general or regional anesthesia is acceptable. True emergency section is indicated for overt fetal distress, prolapsed umbilical cord, or maternal hemorrhage for which general anesthesia is usually elected because of rapidity of induction. In the absence of maternal hypovolemia and with an epidural catheter in place, adequate analgesia can be obtained quickly if 17 to 20 ml of a rapidly acting local analgetic, such as 3 per cent chloroprocaine or 2 per cent lidocaine, is employed. Section must not be delayed to await administration or onset of spinal or epidural block.

Anesthetic techniques for section fall into three categories: local infiltration, regional anesthesia with spinal or epidural block, and general anesthesia. Local infiltration is rarely indicated today except in the absence of competent anesthesia care as it is time consuming, requires large amounts of local anesthetic, does not produce complete analgesia, and, following delivery, may require heavy maternal sedation or general anesthesia induced under unfavorable conditions.

Subarachnoid or epidural block to a T4 sensory level provides ideal conditions for section, although pain resulting from peritoneal traction or uterine exteriorization is not always obtunded. Subarachnoid block with hyperbaric tetracaine 7 to 10 mg or lidocaine 65 to 80 mg usually provides a T4 level. Severe maternal hypotension follows high subarachnoid block unless preceded by volume expansion with at least one liter of balanced salt solution and left uterine displacement. Many recommend that ephedrine, either 50 mg intramuscularly ten minutes before the block or 10 to 25 mg intravenously immediately following subarachnoid injection, be given to prevent the fall in pressure. If hypotension nevertheless develops, left uterine displacement, volume expansion, and intravenous ephedrine in 10- to 15-mg doses are continued.

Because of slower onset of hypotension and little threat of lumbar puncture headache, lumbar epidural analgesia has largely replaced subarachnoid block for section. Onset of analgesia requires 10 to 15 minutes depending on the local anesthetic chosen, but this need not delay skin preparation, draping, and initial skin incision. From 18 to 22 ml of 0.5 to 0.75 per cent bupivacaine, 1.5 to 2.0 per cent lidocaine, or 3.0 per cent chloroprocaine usually produce an adequate sensory level. With the continuous technique, two thirds to three quarters of the initial dose are given as supplementary doses at the first evidence of receding block. Hypotension, although slower in onset, can be severe and is treated by methods already described. If good maternal physiologic conditions prevail, the induction-to-delivery interval is not important in affecting the condition of the newborn, but a uterine incision–delivery interval exceeding three minutes may be associated with neonatal depression.

' General endotracheal anesthesia is indicated in the emergency, when the mother chooses or requires this technique, or when regional anesthesia is contraindicated, as in maternal hypovolemia, infection at or near the site of spinal or epidural injection, septicemia, neurologic abnormality, or coagulation defect. Although it is not within the scope of this chapter to detail general anesthetic management, several aspects require emphasis.

Parturients are always considered at risk for pulmonary aspiration and require tracheal intubation with a cuffed tube. Oral antacids given during labor do not exclude the need for intubation, which is usually accomplished in rapid sequence with cricoid pressure maintained following preoxygenation. Neonatal depression is directly related to induction-delivery and uterine incision–delivery intervals. Nothing is gained by delayed delivery to allow drugs to be dispersed in fetal tissues. Only a minimal plane of general anesthesia is required to provide analgesia and amnesia until delivery, induction requiring only thiopental 3 to 4 mg/kg or ketamine 0.75 to 1.0 mg/kg not exceeding 250 mg or 75 mg, respectively, including subsequent doses. Both depolarizing and nondepolarizing neuromuscular blockers cross the placenta. Full, blocking doses of nondepolarizers may cross the placenta in amounts sufficient to cause neonatal motor weakness. An inspired oxygen concentration of at least 60 per cent in nitrous oxide is provided until delivery, with maternal awareness prevented by addition of 0.5 per cent halothane, 0.75 to 1.0 per cent enflurane, or 0.1 to 0.2 per cent methoxyflurane. Left uterine displacement is maintained until delivery.

OBSTETRIC DRUGS AFFECTING MANAGEMENT OF ANESTHESIA

Anesthetic management can be markedly affected by drugs routinely administered in obstetrics, among them oxytocins and other substances influencing uterine activity. The synthetic oxytocins Pitocin and Syntocinon do not contain the vasopressin formerly found in biologic preparations. These drugs are used both to induce or augment labor and to strengthen postpartum uterine contraction. Dilute solutions exert no cardiovascular effects, but bolus injections may be associated with transient vasodilation, hypotension, tachycardia, augmented cardiac output, and occasional S-T wave changes in the ECG suggesting myocardial ischemia. These effects are largely avoided by rapid infusion of one liter of balanced salt solution containing 20 to 30 units of oxytocin until uterine contraction is adequate. Synthetic oxytocins do not cause hypertension or cardiac arrhythmias other than sinus tachycardia and hence are not contraindicated if vasopressors are concurrently given. A continuous oxytocin infusion exceeding 15 mU/min exerts an antidiuretic action, which may lead to subsequent water intoxication. A low sodium and low serum osmolality coupled with high urine osmolality and oliguria forewarn of this possibility.

Ergot derivatives, used only to contract the uterus postpartum, are associated with hypertension, nausea, vomiting, and agitation when given intravenously. Given in association with a vasoconstrictor drug, normal doses (0.2 mg) have resulted in severe maternal hypertension with the potential for cerebral hemorrhage. Thus the ergot compounds should be given cautiously in small fractional doses (0.5 mg = 0.25 ml) with blood pressure recorded frequently. Although similar events can occur after intramuscular injection, these are usually less severe even following doses of 0.2 mg.

The beta-2 adrenergics isoxsuprine (Vasodilan) and ritodrine (Yutopar) are being used to inhibit uterine activity and onset of premature labor. Adverse effects include maternal and fetal tachycardia, hypotension, increased cardiac output, and postpartum uterine atony. Prolonged use of these drugs to slow labor has resulted in congestive heart failure, particularly when given in conjunction with rapid hydration, magnesium for treatment of preeclampsia, or adrenal steroids to induce maturation of the premature fetal lung, and their use has been associated with maternal hypokalemia.

Preeclampsia/eclampsia is commonly treated with magnesium, which competes with calcium at the neuromuscular junction so that overdose may result in muscle weakness, respiratory embarrassment, and, rarely, cardiac arrest. The effects of magnesium are additive both to nondepolarizing and depolarizing neuromuscular blockers, particularly the former. Continued respiratory support may be required following delivery. At the time of induction and tracheal intubation, a full dose of succinylcholine (1.5 mg/kg) should be used to assure adequate relaxation, with subsequent doses given in small amounts and not until evidence of recovery from a previous dose is observed. Nondepolarizing blockers are best avoided in patients receiving magnesium. Calcium, while partially antagonizing the actions of magnesium at the neuromuscular junction, is potentially hazardous, as it also antagonizes the anticonvulsant properties of the latter ion. Patients receiving both neuromuscular blockers and magnesium require careful assessment of respiratory function at conclusion of operation.

FETAL MONITORING

Until the late 1960s, evaluation of the fetus *in utero* consisted primarily of intermittent auscultation of fetal heart rate and manual palpation of uterine contractions, crude indices that resulted in the birth of many a depressed neonate. Now, fetal monitoring before and during labor has permitted expeditious delivery of the newborn before development of acidosis and hypoxia with their associated neurologic, respiratory, and cardiovascular morbidity and mortality. Fetal monitoring during labor has taken two forms, biophysical and biochemical.

Biophysical monitoring, commonly used in high risk pregnancies, involves continuous determination of fetal heart rate related to uterine contractions. Fetal heart rate is counted either directly from the fetal ECG obtained via an electrode placed on the presenting part or indirectly via ultrasound utilizing the Doppler principle with a device placed on the maternal abdomen. Signals fed into a cardiotachometer are converted to a continuous, heart-rate tracing. Although direct measurement of heart rate is more accurate, is not affected by changing position, and allows accurate determination of fetal beat-to-beat variability, the method is not applicable until the membranes have ruptured and the cervix has dilated. Calibration of uterine contractions is likewise obtained directly via a catheter inserted into the uterine cavity, usually transcervically or indirectly via a tacodynamometer, a pressure-recording device placed on the abdomen. The latter technique measures onset and duration of contractions but does not allow quantitation of intrauterine pressure as in the invasive technique. A continuous, simultaneous tracing of heart rate and uterine contractions is recorded on hot stylus paper (Fig. 24–5). A stable fetal heart rate of 120 to 160 beats per minute is considered normal. In the mature fetus irregularity or beat-to-beat variability of 6 to 16 beats per minute occurs, a manifestation of a mature, fetal autonomic nervous system and normal heart. Absence of irregularity or a flat line tracing is ominous and may indicate fetal acidosis in the absence of other causes, such as prematurity or the use of certain drugs including local anesthetics, opioids, tranquilizers, anticholinergics, and magnesium.

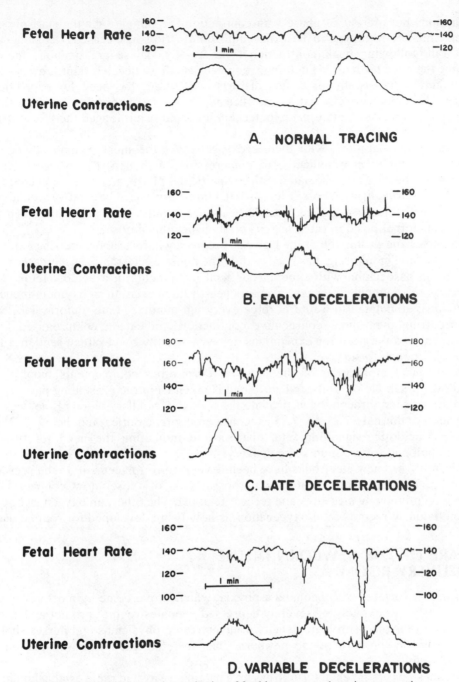

FIGURE 24-5. Bioelectronic monitoring of fetal heart rate and uterine contractions.

Decelerations of fetal heart rate and their relation to uterine contractions are important diagnostically; three basic types have been described: early uniform, late uniform, and variable. Early uniform decelerations are mirror images of uterine contractions. They begin and end with the contraction, the lowest rate corresponding to peak contraction (Fig. 24–5*B*) and are caused by compression of the fetal head but are unrelated to fetal acidosis or distress. Late uniform declerations resemble early decelerations but are out of phase with contraction, beginning after the start of contraction and not returning to base line until contraction has ceased, revealing the lowest rate following peak contraction (Fig. 24–5C). These are ominous indices signalling the need for fetal pH determination because these decelerations are associated with fetal acidosis, hypoxia, and distress and, often, the need for expeditious delivery. Uteroplacental circulatory insufficiency is another possibility resulting from aortocaval compression, maternal hypotension, or rapid or prolonged uterine contractions.

Variable decelerations with increased vagal tone, the most common kind, are thought to result from umbilical cord compression. Although usually seen during contractions, they are not associated with any particular phase, are irregular in contour, and are seen during many labors (Fig. 24–5D). Unless prolonged beyond 30 seconds or associated with bradycardia less than 70 beats per minute, they are usually benign. Changing maternal position often lessens or abolishes this pattern.

Prognosis and evaluation of the high risk pregnancy before labor, utilizing external noninvasive fetal monitoring, has been useful. The nonstress test utilizes increased fetal heart rate in association with spontaneous fetal movements in a healthy fetus. The contraction or oxytocin stress test monitors heart rate in relation to oxytocin-induced contractions, stimulated to a rate of three every ten minutes. Late uniform decelerations occurring over three consecutive contractions indicate a compromised fetal environment and the need for expeditious delivery, usually by cesarean section if the fetus is old enough to survive.

Biochemical monitoring of the fetus *in utero* often complements biophysical monitoring. A sample of fetal capillary blood is taken from the presenting part via an endoscope inserted through the vagina into the cervix. A capillary blood pH above 7.25 is considered normal, 7.21 to 7.25 is considered preacidotic, and below 7.21 is considered acidotic, signalling fetal distress and indicating the need for further determination and, often, immediate delivery.

Recently, two new electrodes have been developed for placement on the presenting part of the fetus for monitoring purposes. One of these, now commercially available, continuously measures and records fetal pH. The other, an oxygen electrode that continuously records fetal oxygenation, is now being developed for routine use.

CARE OF THE NEWBORN IN THE DELIVERY ROOM

Birth is associated with neonatal asphyxia, which is overcome by most newborns spontaneously. Moderately or severely depressed neonates require prompt and effective therapy to avoid neurologic deficits. Delivery room physicians and nurses should be competent in the care of the newborn, thus fostering their rapid adaptation to extrauterine life.

Certain steps are taken at birth to assure a patent airway and rapid establishment of ventilation and oxygenation. From birth until the upper airway is cleared, the newborn's head is maintained below the level of the torso, initially in the lateral decubitus position with the head in the sniffing position. Mouth and posterior pharynx are quickly cleared of secretions by gentle suction either with a mouth-operated device or a soft, rubber bulb aspirator. Nasal suction and aspiration of gastric contents often associated with bradycardia and further depression are delayed until adequate respiration, circulation, and reflex activity are present. With the airway assured, normal respiration usually appears. Gentle slapping on the soles of the feet encourages breathing, crying, and lung expansion; more vigorous forms of stimulation are traumatic. Should the neonate remain dusky or cyanotic despite normal respiration, oxygen in high concentration is given via a tight-fitting face mask until color improves. Gentle assistance of breathing should prove helpful.

Immediate evaluation of a newborn is still best accomplished by means of the Apgar score assessed at one and five minutes (Table 24–1). The one-minute score is indicative of the degree of depression at birth; a score of 7 to 10 indicates minimal or no depression, 3 to 6 moderate depression, and 0 to 2 severe depression requiring need for resuscitation. The five-minute Apgar score indicates severity of depression, effectiveness of resuscitation, and prognosis for future development. By subtracting points rather than adding, scoring can be completed in ten seconds, thus creating minimal delay in resorting to resuscitation, which is not to be delayed until the one-minute score is ascertained. If the neonate does not respond to initial routine treatment or if the one-minute score is less than 7, resuscitation is begun as in the adult, enumerated by the ABCDs of cardiopulmonary resuscitation (see Chapter 35).

Neonates remaining apneic with gasping or inadequate respirations following airway establishment require positive pressure ventilation. With the head in a sniffing position and an oral airway inserted, mouth-to-mouth ventilation is used initially but is changed as soon as possible to ventilation with mask and breathing bag and oxygen concentrations in excess of 50 per cent at 25 to 40 breaths per minute. Auscultation is done to assess adequacy of ventilation. Although pressures up to 60 cm H_2O are required initially to expand the neonatal lung, lesser pressures frequently initiate gasping followed by a normal breathing pattern. If the lungs cannot be expanded or if fetal heart rate remains below 100 beats/min beyond 30 seconds, tracheal intubation is done, followed by positive pressure breathing with oxygen. Unless pulmonary aspiration of meconium is suspected or heart sounds are absent, bag and mask ventilation should be done prior to intubation. Ventilation is continued until respirations become regular with effective respiratory exchange.

Meconium expelled by the fetus may be aspirated *in utero,* but more frequently aspiration occurs just after birth, causing mechanical obstruction to respiration and the possibility of chemical pneumonitis. Without immediate therapy in the delivery room, meconium aspiration is associated with a high incidence of neonatal morbidity and mortality. Babies delivered through a meconium environment in the vertex presentation should have the oral and nasal pharynx suctioned thoroughly by the obstetrician before delivery of the shoulders to prevent aspiration of meconium during the first

TABLE 24–1.   The Apgar Score*

Sign	0	1	2
Heart rate	Absent	Below 100 beats per minute	Over 100 beats per minute
Respiratory effort	Absent	Irregular, slow, gasping	Regular, rhythmic
Muscle tone	Limp	Some flexion of extremities	Active motion
Reflex response to stimulation	None	Grimace	Vigorous cry
Color	Pale, completely cyanotic	Body pink, extremities blue	Completely pink

*The Apgar method of scoring the condition of the newborn is done at exactly one and five minutes after complete delivery. The five objective signs are evaluated and each given a score of 0, 1, or 2. A score of 7 to 10 indicates minimal depression, 3 to 6 moderate depression, and 0 to 2 severe depression.

gasps. If, at birth, the neonate does not breathe at once or if signs of respiratory obstruction are evident, tracheal intubation is immediately done and meconium aspirated by applying negative pressure via mouth to endotracheal tube. Tracheal suction may be required several times before ventilation is adequate. A neonate born through meconium and breathing immediately is first oxygenated, then laryngoscopy is done to determine the presence of material below the cords. If meconium is found, laryngoscopy with repeated tracheal suction preceded by oxygenation is necessary. Aspiration of meconium dictates that the baby be placed in an intensive care environment to receive humidified oxygen and chest physiotherapy and care by a pediatrician.

Rarely does the newborn heart rate fail to accelerate over 100 beats/min with establishment of ventilation and oxygenation. Should cardiac arrest or heart rate of less than 100 be present after establishment of ventilation, closed chest cardiac compression at 120/min is initiated, with ventilation interspersed following every fifth compression. The sternum is compressed 1.5 to 2 cm at its midpoint against a firm resistance such as the resuscitator's other hand. Either two fingers of one hand or the thumbs of both hands can be used effectively as shown in Figure 24–6A and B. Elevation of the lower extremities may improve venous return. Cardiac compression is continued until a heart rate above 100/min is maintained. Definitive therapy based on umbilical arterial blood

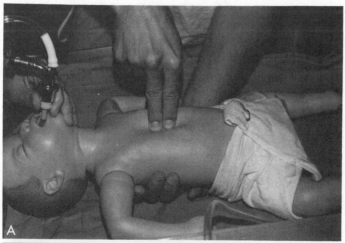

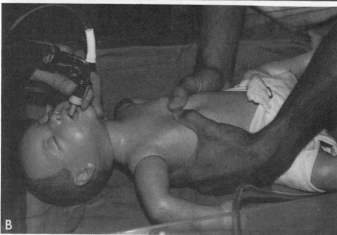

FIGURE 24–6. Two methods of closed chest cardiac compression of the neonate. *A.* The two-finger technique using the index and middle fingers of one hand. The other hand of the resuscitator is placed under the upper back to serve as a hard surface. *B.* The two-thumb technique, in which the remainder of the fingers are interlocked behind the upper back. Note that the pressure is applied on the upper sternum just above the midline. Also note the continued ventilation of the neonate via an endotracheal tube.

analyses consists of the following: correction of base deficit, correction of volume deficit, specific drug therapy, and establishment of a definitive diagnosis. Severely depressed neonates inevitably exhibit specific marked metabolic acidosis, requiring correction before the transition to neonatal circulation occurs. An Apgar score of 2 or less at two minutes or 5 or less at five minutes is presumptive evidence of metabolic acidosis requiring partial correction, which is best accomplished by 2 mEq/kg of sodium bicarbonate solution (7.5 or 8.4 per cent) diluted with an equal volume of 5 per cent dextrose injected into the umbilical vein over a two-minute period and repeated in three to five minutes if there is no improvement. Additional bicarbonate is not given without first ascertaining serum electrolyte values and acid-base status. Bicarbonate administration results in an increase in $PaCO_2$, which calls for adequate ventilation. Hyperosmolar bicarbonate solutions have been implicated in the development of intracerebral hemorrhage in the premature neonate. The dosages recommended here present little risk, especially when compared with the hazards of hypoxia and acidosis.

A poor response to therapy suggests an intravascular fluid deficit requiring correction with 10 ml/kg of 5 per cent albumin, packed red blood cells, or whole blood, the choice aided by a hemoglobin or hematocrit determination. Failure of heart rate to respond to these measures is ominous, thus warranting the use of cardiac stimulants such as epinephrine (0.25 to 0.5 ml of a 1:10,000 solution), calcium gluconate (1 to 2 ml of a 10 per cent concentration), or both, given through an umbilical venous line and *not* by direct cardiac injection. If respiratory depression is thought to be secondary to opioids given the mother, naloxone, 10 μg/kg, is given intravenously or intramuscularly. As the antagonism lasts only about an hour, observation for signs of recurrent depression is required. Absence of a response to naloxone suggests other causes for the depression.

The neonate is an obligate homotherm; cooling augments utilization of limited energy reserves and raises oxygen demand. The newborn loses heat rapidly by radiation, evaporation, and convection because of the large surface area in relation to body mass and the inability to shiver. To prevent heat loss the body should be immediately dried and the infant placed fully exposed under a suitable radiant warmer protected from drafts. When transported or viewed by the parents, the neonate should be wrapped in a warm dry blanket or kept in a warmed isolette.

Moderately or severely depressed neonates require pediatric consultation and, when possible, placement in an intensive care environment. These babies frequently develop apneic spells, respiratory distress, convulsions, hypothermia, and inability to accept oral feedings. They may require carefully monitored oxygen supplementation and ventilatory support to maintain normal blood gas values; care should be taken to avoid the problem of hyperoxia associated with retrolental fibroplasia and pulmonary oxygen toxicity. In addition, normal temperature maintenance, fluid balance, caloric intake, and other drug therapy require expert attention. With prompt resuscitation and continued neonatal care, prognosis for survival and normal development is excellent.

APPRAISAL

Anesthetic management of the parturient is demanding and very different from that of a surgical patient. Conditions surrounding labor and delivery are hardly controllable. The physiologic changes of pregnancy, which require comprehension by the anesthetist, predispose the mother to development of hypoxia, anesthetic overdose, cardiovascular derangements, and the possibility of pulmonary aspiration. These changes characterize the healthy, uncomplicated parturient as a high anesthetic risk. Anesthetic requirements for both vaginal delivery and cesarean section demand special consideration in choice and administration of various anesthetic techniques for the optimal outcome. Drugs commonly prescribed during parturition can interact adversely with anesthetics. Consideration must be given not only to avoid anesthetic related depression but to the care of the newborn. Established routines of anesthesia are rarely applicable to the parturient. Expertly administered anesthesia not only lessens the dangers of childbirth but is highly rewarding to the anesthetist's self esteem.

To help women through childbirth is to share in a mystery and a miracle. . . . It is also to touch life at a key point . . . there the opportunity is taken to grow in understanding and in love. There is more to having a baby than simply pushing an occiput-anterior out into the world. Birth is also implicitly an assent to life. Those who help women in childbirth have the privilege of sharing that act of assent.

S. KITZINGER

REFERENCES

Abouleish E: Pain Control in Obstetrics. Philadelphia, J B Lippincott Co, 1977.

Bonica JJ: Principles and Practice of Obstetric Analgesia and Anesthesia. Philadelphia, F A Davis, vol 1, 1967, and vol 2, 1969.

Carson BS, Losey RW, Bowes WA Jr, et al: Combined obstetrical and pediatric management of meconium staining. Pediatr Res 10:459, 1976.

Datta S, Alper MH: Anesthesia for cesarean section. Anesthesiology 53:142, 1980.

Gibbs CP, Schwartz DJ, Wynne JW, et al: Antacid pulmonary aspiration in the dog. Anesthesiology 51:380, 1979.

Gregory GA: Resuscitation of the newborn. Anesthesiology 43:225, 1975.

Hodgkinson R, Marx GF, Kim SS, et al: Neonatal neurobehavioral tests following vaginal delivery under ketamine, thiopental and epidural anesthesia. Anesth Analg 56:548, 1977.

Kouppila A, Koskinen M, Poulkka J, et al: Decreased intravillous and unchanged myometrial blood flow in supine recumbency. Obstet Gynecol 55:203, 1980.

Marx GF, Bassell GM: Obstetric Analgesia and Anesthesia. New York, Excerpta Medica, 1980.

Marx GF, Husain FJ, Shiau HF: Brachial and femoral blood pressures during the prenatal period. Am J Obstet Gynecol 136:11, 1980.

Moir DD: Maternal mortality and anaesthesia. Editorial. Br J Anaesth 52:1, 1980.

Ralston DH, Shnider SM: The fetal and neonatal effects of regional anesthesia in obstetrics. Anesthesiology 48:34, 1978.

Ralston DH, Shnider SM, deLorimier AA: Effects of equipotent ephedrine, metaraminol, mephentermine and methoxyamine on uterine blood flow in the pregnant ewe. Anesthesiology 40:354, 1974.

Scanlon JW: Effects of local anesthetics administered to parturient women on the neurological and behavioral performance of newborn children. Bull NY Acad Med 52:231, 1976.

Shnider SM, Levinson G: Anesthesia for Obstetrics. Baltimore, Williams and Wilkins, 1979.

Chapter 25
PEDIATRIC ANESTHESIA

The appropriate approach to anesthetizing the pediatric patient involves understanding the many differences between adult and child. In addition to smaller equipment, the anesthetist must be familiar with the varying anatomic, physiologic, pharmacologic, and psychologic considerations for the several age groups within the pediatric range. The premature newborn is as different from the one year old as the one year old is from an adult.

GENERAL CONSIDERATIONS

ANATOMY

Newborns usually are obligate nose breathers; the combination of small nares, relatively large tongue, small mandible, abundant lymphoid tissue, and short neck increases the susceptibility to airway obstruction. Pressure over the soft tissue of the neck while holding a mask over the face can easily obstruct the airway. The vocal cords lie more cephalad (C4 versus C6 in the adult), and the epiglottis — long, narrow, and U shaped — extends at a 45-degree angle to the cords. The narrowest part of the trachea is at the cricoid cartilage instead of at the vocal cords as in adults. Because of the small diameter at this point, edema owing to either mechanical irritation or infection can result in significant airway narrowing.

The ribs and sternum in the newborn or infant are cartilaginous and flexible, horizontally placed to form a cylindrically shaped thorax. Because of the rib placement and the relatively underdeveloped intercostal muscles, newborns are primarily diaphragmatic breathers, thus susceptible to ventilatory embarrassment by anything that would impede the diaphragm such as gastric distention following improper bag and mask ventilation or bowel obstruction. The ribs and sternum are especially pliable in the premature newborn, and the rib cage may actually collapse during the negative pressures of inspiration, leading to inadequate ventilation.

PHYSIOLOGY

Respiratory System

At birth, the functional residual capacity (FRC) is established within the first few breaths. The newborn's total volume (V_T), dead space (V_D), and other volumes are proportional to adult values (Table 25–1). However, the alveoli are incompletely developed both in number (10 per cent of adult alveoli) and structure (cuboidal epithelium). The newborn compensates for decreased alveolar surface area (one third

303

TABLE 25–1. Respiratory Data in the Adult and Neonate*

	Adult	Neonate
Alveolar Ventilation		
V_A (ml/kg/min)	60	100–150
V_T (ml/kg)	7	6
V_D (ml/kg)	2.2	2.2
D_D/V_T	0.3	0.3
f (min)	20	40
Lung Volumes		
FRC (ml/kg)	34	30
RV (ml/kg)	17	20
FRC/TLC	0.40	0.48
RV/TLC	0.20	0.33
Respiratory Mechanics		
Total respiratory compliance	20	1
Specific respiratory compliance (compliance/L lung volume)	1	1
Total flow resistance	1	12
Specific resistance	1	1
Acid-Base Status		
Pa_{CO_2} (torr)	38–40	32–35
Plasma HCO_3 (mEq/L)	24–28	17–22
pH	7.38	7.38
Alveolar-Arterial Oxygen Differences (AaD_{O_2})		
Pa_{O_2} (torr)	80–100	60–80
AaD_{O_2} (torr)	10 (105—95)	25 (105—80)

*From Nelson NM: Neonatal pulmonary function. Pediatr Clin North Am 13:769, 1966.

that of an adult) and increased metabolic rate (twice that of the adult) by increasing respiratory rate to yield proportionate minute volumes twice those of the adult over the first year of life. Although total respiratory compliance is lower and total flow resistance is much higher in the newborn than the adult, specific compliance and resistance values (corrected for lung volume) are equivalent, indicating that, in healthy patients, similar airway pressures should be used for ventilation of children and adults.

Control of ventilation differs in the newborn and adult. Although both respond in parallel fashion to changes in P_{CO_2}, the newborn under a week of age responds to a fall in P_{O_2} by hyperventilation followed by hypoventilation. This response is exaggerated in the presence of hypothermia. Newborn blood gases reveal signs of asphyxia immediately after birth but stabilize within an hour, whereas a mild hypocapnia (Pa_{CO_2} 32 to 35) and base deficit (−4 to −8) are seen in the first one to two years of life (see Table 25–1). Pa_{O_2} spans a lower range than normally seen in adults (60 to 80 versus 80 to 100 torr), probably on the basis of ductus arteriosus shunting and closing volumes close to and sometimes imposing on V_T. Premature infants and infants small for gestational age show similar values but over a larger range.

The idiopathic respiratory distress syndrome (IRDS) is seen mainly in prematures, with maternal diabetes, toxemia, hemorrhage, and prenatal asphyxia increasing the incidence. Insufficient surfactant levels lead to failure of development and maintenance of FRC, with consequent atelectasis, hypoxemia, and, lastly, ventilatory failure. Tachypnea, grunting respiration, and chest retraction appear soon after birth and are treated with cautious oxygen therapy, fluid restriction, CPAP, and, if necessary, mechanical ventilation. Patients who recover from the acute syndrome may continue to have apneic spells; they require enriched oxygen and may reveal abnormal pulmonary function throughout infancy.

TABLE 25–2. Cardiovascular Data in the Adult and Neonate

	Adult	Neonate
Stoke volume (ml)	70–80	4–5
Heart rate (min)	70	120
Cardiac output (ml/min)	4000–6000	500–600
Metabolic rate (cal/kg/hr)	1	2

Cardiovascular System

As the lungs are successfully expanded, a diminution in pulmonary vascular resistance and a large increase in pulmonary blood flow occur. The augmented return of blood to the left atrium leads to closure of the flaplike valve at the foramen ovale, and the rise in Pa_{O_2} results in functional closure of the ductus arteriosus, although significant bidirectional shunts may persist for at least 24 hours in the normal child. However, hypoxemia and acidosis can reverse these changes by increasing pulmonary vascular resistance and maintaining an open ductus, thus encouraging right to left shunting of deoxygenated blood, with worsening of hypoxemia, acidosis, and, ultimately, hypotension. As closure of the ductus is modulated by prostaglandins, prostaglandin inhibitors such as indomethacin are now given with some success in an attempt to close a persistent ductus. If this fails, surgical ligation may be required.

The newborn heart reveals biventricular hypertrophy, noncompliant ventricles with a fixed stroke volume proportionate to that of an adult (1 to 2 ml/kg), and a heart rate of 120 to 160/min (Table 25–2). These result in a cardiac index about twice that of an adult to compensate for the heightened metabolic rate of the newborn. It should be emphasized that cardiac output is dependent on rate with a fixed stroke volume and that bradycardia, whether the result of hypoxemia, hypovolemia, acidosis, or pharmacologic depression, must be quickly corrected.

The blood pressure of a newborn rises from 60/40 torr at birth to 80/50 torr at one week of age. These values rise to about 90/60 torr at six months, 100/70 torr at 6 years, and 120/70 torr at 15 years (Table 25–3).

Blood volume in the newborn is approximately 85 ml/kg, decreasing to 80 ml/kg at six weeks, 75 ml/kg at six months, 70 ml/kg at two years, and 60 to 65 ml/kg at adolescence (Table 25–4). The figures are approximate, as various studies have quoted the newborn blood volume as anywhere from 65 to 129 ml/kg.

Hemoglobin concentration at birth is 16 to 18 gm per cent, 70 to 80 per cent in the form of Hgb F. As Hgb F is replaced by adult Hgb A, total hemoglobin falls to 10 to 11 per cent at three months and then rises to 12 to 14 gm per cent by one year. Significant anemia (13.0 in the newborn, 9.5 at three months, and 10.0 over six months) compromises the oxygen-carrying capacity of the blood and, therefore, the margin of safety in a child. On the other hand, polycythemia (Hct > 65) in the newborn causes

TABLE 25–3. Blood Pressure and Pulse

Age	Approximate Systolic BP (torr)	Approximate Pulse Rate/(min)
2 hr	60	120–160
5 days	80	120–160
6 mo	90	110–130
6 yr	100	100
10 yr	110	90
15 yr	120	80

TABLE 25–4.　Estimated Blood Volume

Age	ml/kg
Newborn	85
Infant	80
Child	75
Adult	65

increased viscosity with attendant risks of sluggish capillary flow and infarction of brain, heart, kidney, or gut. This should be corrected by cautious hemodilution before elective operations. The sickle hemoglobin (Hgb S) concentration increases at the same rate as Hgb A after birth, therefore, a slide prep may not detect its presence until four months of age. However, sickle preps should be done on patients under four months, as major sickling may occur early, even *in utero*.

Fluid Balance and Metabolism

The newborn kidney matures rapidly so that it become "adult" in function one month after birth; nonetheless, before one month of age and especially before four to five days, kidney function reveals an obligate salt loss, slow clearance of fluid overload, and inability to conserve fluids. Thus, the newborn under five days of age is intolerant of both dehydration and fluid overload. Premature and full-term newborns need low maintenance fluid requirements for about the first five days, increasing over the first

TABLE 25–5.　Maintenance Fluids in Pediatric Patients
and Normal Urine Output

Electrolytes	Daily Dose (mEq/kg)
Na	3
K	2
Cl	2

Body Weight and Age	24-Hour Fluid Requirement
Premature and full-term newborn less than 5 days of age	50–70 ml/kg
Premature and full-term newborn over 5 days of age (5 days to 1 month of age)	150 ml/kg
3–10 kg (over 1 month of age)	100 ml/kg
10–20 kg	1000 ml plus 50 ml/kg over 10 kg
20 kg to adult	1500 ml plus 20 ml/kg over 20 kg

Normal Urine Output	
Age	ml/kg/hr
1 to 4 days	0.3–0.7
4 to 7 days	1.0–2.7
Over 7 days	3
Over 2 years	2
5 years to adult	1
Insensible loss	28

month. Serum electrolyte values and daily fluid requirements are equivalent to those of the adult (Table 25–5).

The distribution of water in the various body compartments differs in the premature, normal newborn, child, and adult (Fig. 25–1). The extracellular fluid compartment is largest in the premature and normal newborn, as is total body water volume. As water turnover is related to metabolic rate, the newborn is especially susceptible to dehydration on the basis of lesser intracellular fluid compartment reserves, high water turnover owing to high metabolic rate, and renal immaturity.

At birth, the newborn requires considerable energy to maintain pulmonary ventilation, cardiac output, muscular activity, and temperature regulation. Glycogen and fat stores are mobilized but are subject to rapid depletion, resulting in hypoglycemia. Prematurity, cold stress, and muscle activity compound the need for adequate caloric intake. Thus, sufficient glucose intake to maintain stores and avoidance of long periods without glucose are cornerstones of fluid replacement in newborns.

Temperature Regulation

The relatively large surface area, lack of subcutaneous fat, poor vasomotor control, and lack of ability to shiver make the newborn extremely sensitive to heat loss. The newborn responds to a cool environment with an increase in metabolism, derived from the highly vascular adipose tissue located between the scapulae, about the kidneys, and behind the sternum (brown fat). Norepinephrine is released by the sympathetic system in response to cold to activate hydrolysis of triglycerides and further oxidation of free fatty acids. This nonshivering thermogenesis produces heat but at the expense of considerable increase in oxygen consumption and organic acid production. When the ambient temperature falls below 33° C, oxygen consumption in the newborn begins to rise. To avoid added oxygen demand and acidosis, the patient is maintained in a neutral thermal environment through the use of incubators, infrared heating, blankets, and elevated operating room temperature. The smaller, premature newborn requires a higher environmental temperature to minimize oxygen consumption, in the range of 35° C for a 1000-gm neonate, decreasing with time so that 32° C becomes optimal after five weeks.

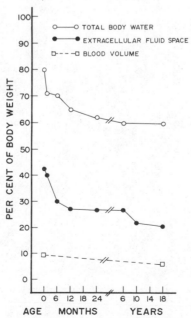

FIGURE 25–1. Body water and blood volume in the pediatric age group.

PHARMACOLOGY

GUIDELINES FOR DRUG USAGE

The actions, metabolism, and excretion of drugs vary with the age of the patient. Uptake of inhalation agents is more rapid in the newborn and infant because of increased minute ventilation. The bioavailability of drugs injected intramuscularly is capricious in the newborn. Distribution of pharmacologic substances is affected by several components that likewise affect uptake: a greater volume of both extracellular and total body water, lesser protein binding, smaller fat stores, and greater distribution of cardiac output to vessel-rich tissues as compared with the adult. Metabolism of anesthetic drugs in the newborn has not been well studied, but elimination of drugs metabolized by the liver, such as diazepam and some of the barbiturates, is significantly prolonged in the newborn. Diminished renal excretory capacity and lower plasma pseudocholinesterase levels may also contribute to decreased metabolism and elimination of drugs.

Newborns, especially under 12 hours of age, are sensitive to CNS depressant drugs but then develop an increased requirement for anesthetics. Patients under six months of age reveal a generalized, nondiscriminative response to pain that requires an anesthetic concentration about one third higher than in older children or adults, so that halothane MAC in newborns is 1.02 per cent and in adults 0.78 per cent. The increased requirement diminishes with age, with a slight rise during adolescence.

Several hereditary defects may cause abnormal responses to anesthetics that may be first discovered in childhood. Abnormal responses to succinylcholine (pseudocholinesterase deficiency, the myotonias), thiopental (porphyria), or anesthetic agents (malignant hyperthermia) may be the first signs of an underlying defect.

PEDIATRIC ANESTHETIC EQUIPMENT

APPARATUS

Standard anesthesia machines can be used for patients of all ages. Modern flowmeters accurate below 1 L/min flow are essential for the low flow rates utilized in

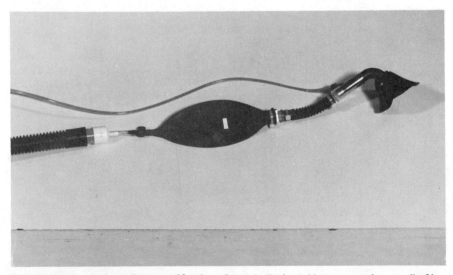

FIGURE 25–2.   Jackson-Rees modification of Ayre's T-piece. Note connection at tail of bag for anesthetic exhaust.

small children. The ability to entrain air into fresh gas flow is also necessary, and an oxygen analyzer to measure $F_{I_{O_2}}$ accurately is useful to ensure adequate oxygen concentration.

Circuits for the pediatric patient are designed with the following features in mind; minimal dead space, minimal resistance to flow, adequate humidification, simplicity, and light weight. The most commonly used circuit in neonates is the Jackson-Rees adaptation of Ayre's T-piece (Fig. 25–2). This is a valveless system that prevents rebreathing by having an adequate reservoir (tubing and bag) and a fresh gas flow of two and one half times minute ventilation. The system is lightweight and easily handled but requires scavenging because of high gas flows.

A variety of nonrebreathing circuits incorporate a nonrebreathing valve, such as the Sierra (Fig. 25–3B) or Stephen-Slater valve. These offer the advantages of easy gas scavenging and fresh gas requirements equal to minute ventilation; but the disadvantages of occasional valve sticking or incompetence and resistance to flow make them impractical for use with infants or small children.

The Bain circuit (Fig. 25–3A), a coaxial modification of the Mapleson D circuit, has become increasingly popular in pediatrics. This is a simple, lightweight, and low resistance apparatus, but it must be carefully inspected to ensure that the internal fresh gas line has not been disconnected at the entry, resulting in a large dead space. Recommendations for fresh gas flows vary widely among users but average about 100 to 150 ml/kg/min.

Circle systems work well for children above 30 kg, but high flow resistance can

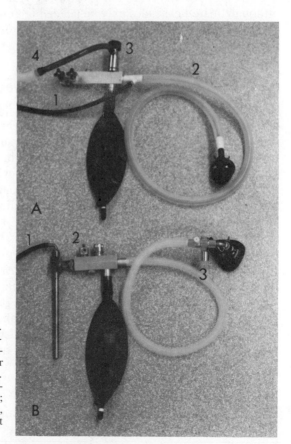

FIGURE 25–3. Two commonly used circuits. *A.* The Bain circuit, modification of the Mapleson D. *1,* Fresh gas flow from a cascade humidifier; *2,* combination fresh gas line and reservoir tubing; *3,* pop-off valve; *4,* exhaust tubing. *B.* The Sierra nonrebreathing valve in a Magill circuit. *1,* Fresh gas flow from a cascade humidifier; *2,* a Georgia valve for venting of excess flow; *3,* nonrebreathing valve with side port for exhaust tubing.

TABLE 25–6.   Endotracheal Tube Sizes for Pediatric Anesthesia

Age	Approximate French Size	Approximate Internal Diameter (mm)	Length (cm)
Newborn			
(under 2.3 kg)	11–12	2.5	10
(2.3 to 3 kg)	13–14	3.0	11
Infant			
to 6 mo	15–16	3.5	11
5 to 12 mo	17–18	4.0	12
12 to 20 mo	19–20	4.5	13
18 mo to 3 yr	21–22	5.0	14
3 to 4 yr	23–24	5.5	16
5 to 6 yr	25–26	6.0	18
6 to 7 yr	27–28	6.5	18
8 to 9 yr	29–30	7.0	20
10 to 11 yr	31–32	7.5	22
12 to 13 yr	31–32	7.5	23
14 yr	33–34	8.0	24

pose problems in smaller children. Although specially designed pediatric circle systems are available, simpler circuits seem preferable.

Humidification of gases is necessary in pediatric patients, not only to prevent drying of the respiratory mucosa and secretions but to prevent heat loss through vaporization of water in the respiratory tract. Nonheated cascades usually suffice, although heated cascades may be needed in newborns and infants to maintain adequate core temperatures. Hyperthermia and water overload pose dangers with heated humidifiers, thus the patient must be constantly monitored to avoid the consequences.

AIRWAYS AND ENDOTRACHEAL EQUIPMENT

Maintenance of the airway in children requires an appreciation of both qualitative and quantitative age differences. Masks for the pediatric patient, such as the Rendell-Baker-Soucek type, are designed for minimal dead space and mold closely to the relatively flat faces of infants and young children. Masks for the older child offer cushioned rims to maintain an airtight fit. Oropharyngeal airways must be of sufficient size to carry forward the relatively large tongue of the infant but not too large to obstruct the airway itself. Tracheal intubation in the newborn and infant is best accomplished with a straight blade because of the cephalad larynx and large tongue. A #0 Miller or other straight blade is best for the premature, whereas a #1 is adequate for a normal neonate. A curved blade can be used in older children. Use of the sniffing position is especially important in the newborn and infant; hyperextension of the head results in difficult visualization of the more cephalad placed larynx.

Clear, thin-walled endotracheal tubes are preferred and are cuffed when the child is over eight years of age (Table 25–6). A small leak should be allowed when positive pressure (30 cm H_2O) is applied to the airway to avoid mechanical trauma and subsequent subglottic edema. Armored latex tubes are useful when extreme flexion of the neck is necessary for operation, but they are easily dislodged. The Cole tube was designed to improve gas flow characteristics, but it is rigid, dislodges easily, and may produce glottic injury, thus making it less desirable than other tubes (Fig. 25–4). Several sizes of endotracheal tube should be at hand prior to attempted intubation, thus permitting a choice if one fits too tightly or too loosely (Fig. 25–5).

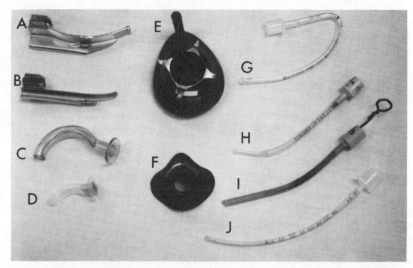

FIGURE 25–4. Pediatric endotracheal equipment. *A*, #2 Macintosh curved blade; *B*, #1 Miller straight blade; *C*, *D*, oral airways; *E*, child's anatomic mask; *F*, Rendell-Baker-Soucek mask; *G*, reverse angle endotracheal (RAE) tube; *H*, Cole tube; *I*, reinforced latex tube with stylet; *J*, plastic thin-walled tube.

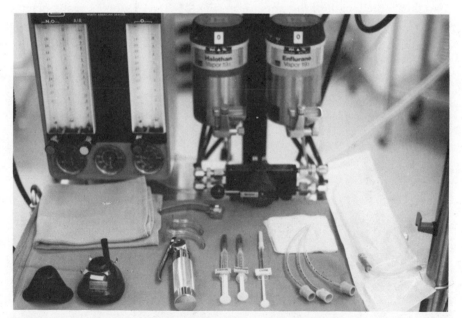

FIGURE 25–5. Basic equipment for pediatric anesthesia: appropriate sized masks, blades, airways, and endotracheal tubes. A suction catheter, atropine, and succinylcholine should be at hand for every case. Note that compressed air is available on the machine. (Not shown: oxygen analyzer distal to vaporizers.)

MONITORING

The basic principles of monitoring are the same in pediatric and adult populations, but differences in physiology and anatomy require modification of methodology.

Temperature should be monitored in all anesthetized pediatric patients and devices to maintain body temperature employed. Susceptibility to temperature change due to environmental factors, intravenous fluids, prepping solutions, bladder or bowel irrigation, and anesthetics demands that monitoring be continuous. Likewise, the possibility of development of malignant hyperthermia is a strong argument for continuous temperature monitoring (see Chapter 33). Temperature probes in the esophagus or rectum or at the tympanic membrane supply good approximations of core temperature, whereas axillary probes and temperature-sensitive papers are less reliable (see Chapter 9). A thermometer may be incorporated into a servo-control system with a warming mattress to maintain temperature, or it can be used as a guide to maintain temperature with heating lights (Fig. 25–6), warmed intravenous fluids, warmed inhaled gases, irrigation fluids, and elevated ambient temperature. Wrapping the patient and exposed viscera in cellophane or similar materials helps maintain thermal equilibrium.

A precordial stethoscope allows continuous monitoring of heart rate, sounds, and rhythm as well as breath sounds; because of the range of usefulness, this should be the first monitor applied and the last to be removed. The esophageal stethoscope is a useful alternate device.

Electrocardiographic monitoring is standard in pediatric anesthesia and is invaluable for detection and diagnosis of arrhythmias. As the baroreceptor reflexes are not fully developed in the newborn, changes in heart rate and blood pressure do not correlate well.

Blood pressure measurements require proper technique. Cuff width should be one half to two thirds the length of the upper arm (Fig. 25–7). A Doppler probe placed over the radial or brachial artery improves accuracy, especially at low pressures. Intra-

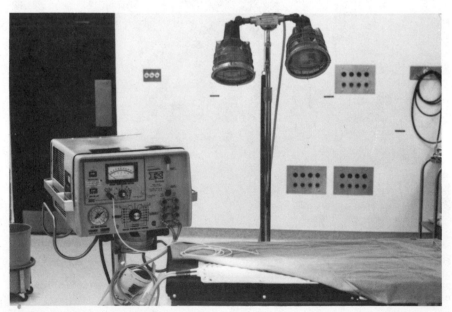

FIGURE 25–6. Two important methods of maintaining temperature intraoperatively: heating lights, and a servo-controlled water blanket.

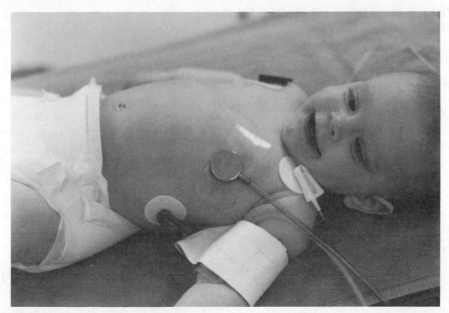

FIGURE 25-7. Basic monitoring devices for all pediatric cases — precordial stethoscope, ECG, and BP cuff.

arterial monitoring is useful when continuous pressure readings are needed and repeated arterial blood sampling is required. Central venous monitoring criteria for the child are the same as for the adult, although readings do not seem as reliable in the child.

Because of the danger of unrecognized hypoglycemia and, alternatively, hyperglycemia, intraoperative assessment of blood glucose levels is useful during major operations involving the newborn, especially the premature. Either venous sampling or capillary Dextrostix samples from a well-perfused limb are adequate.

Two newer monitors now used in pediatric anesthesia are pulmonary artery catheterization and transcutaneous P_{O_2} determinations. The pulmonary artery thermodilution catheter (Swan-Ganz), available in sizes as small as 5 French, permits measurement of pulmonary artery and wedge pressures and cardiac output (see Chapter 9). Although use of these catheters is not widespread, they will likely prove helpful in some major operations and in the critically ill pediatric patient. The transcutaneous P_{O_2} monitor was developed for use in the neonate and has proved useful in the neonatal ICU. Readings from currently available instruments appear to be unreliable in the presence of nitrous oxide, halothane, and poor perfusion states. Work in progress to perfect these monitors could conceivably provide an important addition to monitoring in infants and children.

The principal monitor in pediatric anesthesia is the anesthetist. Constant observation of the patient's color, chest expansion, the surgical field, and trends recorded on the anesthetic record offers essential information. Manual compression of the reservoir bag reveals changes in pulmonary compliance, whereas tactile contact with the patient can provide data relating to perfusion, temperature, and muscle tone. Similar vigilance is important in any anesthetized patient but even more so in the pediatric patient because of the rapidity with which changes occur.

PREOPERATIVE EVALUATION AND PREPARATION

The preoperative visit allows the physician not only to evaluate the patient but to prepare the parents and child psychologically for anesthesia and operation. Most often, children fear leaving their parents, but they also may have serious concerns about the pain of venipuncture, being awake during operation, mutilation, and death. Children from about one to five years of age are vulnerable to long-term psychic damage from this intrusion so that preoperative discussion with the child and parents reduces anxiety in both. Preoperative sedation may be especially useful in this age group, but no drug can compete with a friendly and reassuring preoperative visit. Photographs of the operating room, puppet shows, and personal handling of anesthetic equipment, particularly the mask, have been successful in preparation. One of the most helpful stratagems preoperatively and at anesthesia induction is to talk in a quiet and reassuring manner about matters familiar to the child.

The preoperative history centers on previous operations and anesthetics; underlying medical diseases and therapies; family history, especially of difficulty with operations and anesthesia; and acute physical problems such as an upper respiratory infection. A concurrent upper respiratory infection is reason for cancellation of elective operation because of the risk of airway obstruction from secretions, laryngospasm, laryngeal edema, bacteremia, and an otherwise stormy anesthetic course. Often it is difficult to distinguish between allergic rhinitis and infection, but a history of recent onset and the presence of purulent secretions and fever indicate an infective process.

Increasing numbers of pediatric procedures are being done on an outpatient basis, with the advantages of less exposure to infectious disease, less separation anxiety, and decreased costs. However, oral intake must be severely restricted, and a general description of expectations must be given to the family by the surgeon or anesthetist before admission. It is useful to emphasize during the preoperative visit that the family should feel free to contact the anesthesia department postoperatively if unexpected sequelae or questions arise.

Physical examination should, at minimum, estimate general status, the presence of significant congenital anomalies, and the cardiopulmonary situation. The state of hydration is evaluated by examining mucosal membranes, skin turgor, fontanelles, orbits, pulse, and temperature and capillary refill in the extremities (Table 25–7). Hematocrit, urine output and specific gravity, and weight changes aid in quantifying deficits. Significant dehydration should be corrected before inducing anesthesia. The fluid deficit can be estimated from per cent dehydration; 10 ml/kg/per cent dehydration is required. Half this amount should be given over six to eight hours, the remainder given over the next 16 hours. If the patient shows signs of cardiovascular decompensation, an initial bolus of 10 ml/kg of plasma or blood should be given, the remainder being lactated Ringer's or other balanced salt solution. As sodium, potassium, or water

TABLE 25–7.   Estimated State of Hydration in the Infant

Indication	Per cent Dehydration (Weight Loss)
Poor tissue turgor	5
Pale skin color	5
Sunken fontanelle	10
Dry mucosa	10
Oliguria	10
Sunken, soft eyes	15–20
Hypotensive	15–20
Anuria	15–20

deficits may exist, depending on the cause of dehydration, electrolyte and acid-base determinations should be ascertained and closely monitored. If metabolic acidosis is present, bicarbonate is given according to the formula mEq bicarbonate = base deficit × 0.3 × weight in kg, with half the dose given initially. Metabolic alkalosis, as seen with pyloric stenosis, usually requires potassium replacement as well.

Assessment of the cardiovascular system involves signs of perfusion, the presence of murmurs or arrhythmias, pulses, and signs of heart failure. Patients with congenital cyanotic heart disease, murmurs of undetermined origin, or heart failure require a cardiology consultation before proceeding. Lungs are evaluated by listening to breath sounds, examining for sternal or intercostal retractions, and reading the chest x-ray. However, chest x-rays need not be done unless there is reason to suspect disease. If the patient is in respiratory failure, preoperative tracheal intubation and ventilation may be needed for stabilization before operation.

Minimal laboratory work in pediatric cases consists of a hematocrit and urinalysis. In blacks, a sickle prep should also be done. Other tests, such as electrolyte determinations, are ordered as indicated.

The newborn and, especially, the premature are uniquely susceptible to hypoglycemia, hypothermia, hypocalcemia, hyperbilirubinemia, bleeding due to both vitamin K deficiency and disseminated intravascular coagulation, sepsis, periods of apnea, and IRDS. These conditions can complicate both the preoperative and intraoperative course.

Preoperative feeding is balanced between the need for an empty stomach and the fluid and glucose requirements of the child. Younger patients should be first on the surgical schedule, and, if delayed, intravenous fluids should be started on the ward. Clear liquids (water, apple juice, Pedialyte — but not milk) are given from midnight until four hours preoperatively in children under six months and six hours preoperatively in children under five years of age. Over five years, nothing by mouth is allowed after midnight. Patients with fever, diabetes, and other similar problems may require schedule modification.

Preoperative medication in pediatric anesthesia is a subject of controversy and personal beliefs. Atropine is given to attenuate the active cardiac vagal reflex and to reduce secretions and is preferred to scopolamine. Atropine is given intramuscularly (.03 mg/kg up to 0.6 mg) preoperatively or intravenously at induction (.03 mg/kg up to 0.4 mg). If repeated doses of succinylcholine are given intraoperatively, repeat doses of atropine are essential to prevent bradycardia. Atropine is omitted in patients with fever. Glycopyrrolate offers a reasonable alternative to atropine, with the advantage of decreasing gastric acidity but the disadvantage of increased cost (Table 25–8).

Preoperative sedation may be provided for patients older than one year and varies according to the needs of the patient and the anesthetist's preference; the goal is to provide calm but not depression. Opioids (morphine, pentazocine intramuscularly), barbiturates (pentobarbital intramuscularly or by mouth or rectum), and diazepam by mouth have all been used successfully. Children over seven years may not require premedication if they have undergone wise preoperative preparation. The two essential points about premedication are that it be tailored to the patient and given 45 to 60 minutes prior to induction to ensure effectiveness.

ANESTHETIC MANAGEMENT

INDUCTION

The safety of the patient is always the first consideration in anesthesia, so that a full stomach, an abnormal airway, hypovolemia, or respiratory failure requires special

TABLE 25–8. Drugs Useful in Pediatric Anesthesia

Drug	Dose	Remarks
Premedicants		
Atropine	0.03 mg/kg IV or IM up to 0.6 mg	
Diazepam	0.2–0.5 mg/kg PO	
Droperidol	0.1 mg/kg IM or IV	
Hydroxyzine	2–3 mg/kg PO	Give 45–60 min before procedure
Morphine	0.05–0.15 mg/kg IM	
Pentazocine	1–1.2 mg/kg IM	
Pentobarbital	2–3 mg/kg PO, PR, or IM	
Induction agents		
Ketamine	1–2 mg/kg IV; 5–10 mg/kg IM	
Thiopental	2–5 mg/kg IV; 20–25 mg/kg PR	2.5 per cent solution
Methohexital	2 mg/kg IV; 15–20 mg/kg PR	10 per cent solution
Maintenance agents		
Fentanyl	1–4 mcg/kg/hr	
Meperidine	1–1.5 mg/kg	Premedication dose
	0.5–1 mg/kg/kr	Maintenance dose
Morphine	0.05–0.2 mg/kg/hr	
Neuromuscular blockers		
Succinylcholine	2 mg/kg IV; 3–4 mg/kg IM	Newborn and infant dose
	1 mg/kg IV; 2 mg/kg IM	Child dose
D-tubocurarine	0.125–0.25 mg/kg IV initially, then ¼ initial dose for maintenance	Newborn and infant dose
	0.5 mg/kg IV initially, then ¼ initial dose for maintenance	Child dose
Pancuronium	0.05–0.1 mg/kg IV initially, then ¼ initial dose for maintenance	Newborn and infant dose
	0.1 mg/kg IV initially, then ¼ initial dose for maintenance	Child dose
Metocurine	0.25 mg/kg initially, then ¼ initial dose for maintenance	
Reversal Agents		
Neostigmine	0.07 mg/kg IV with atropine	Given slowly
	0.02 mg/kg IV	
Naloxone	0.005 mg/kg IM or IV	IM dose often given after IV dose to give longer lasting reversal
Resuscitation Drugs		
NaHCO$_3$	2 mEq/kg IV, then guided by blood gases	
Calcium chloride	20 mg/kg IV *slowly*	10 per cent solution
Epinephrine	0.1 ml/kg IV	1:10,000 solution
Lidocaine	1 mg (0.1 ml)/kg IV	1 per cent solution
Atropine	0.1–0.6 mg IV	
Other drugs		
Digoxin	Premature—0.04 mg/kg PO	Oral, digitalizing dose
	Newborn—0.05 mg/kg PO	Oral, digitalizing dose
	Over 2 years—0.04 mg/kg PO	2/3 oral dose if IV, ½ of which is given initially, then ¼ dose q 6–12 h
		Maintenance dose: 1/8 digitalizing dose q 12 h
Racemic epinephrine	0.25–0.5 ml in 5 ml saline	By aerosol or IPPB as needed for croup
Dexamethasone	4 mg IV	Under 2 years old
	8 mg IV	Over 2 years old
Furosemide	0.25–0.5 mg/kg IV	

attention. For elective procedures in healthy children, the ease and calm of induction are directly related to the anesthetist's ability to establish rapport with the patient, thereby gaining confidence and attention. A quiet operating room, a reassuring and soft voice, and gentle stroking or other physical cuddling aid in facilitating induction.

Inhalation induction is commonly used for elective procedures in children, halothane usually preferred over enflurane or isoflurane because the odor is better tolerated. To allay the fear of suffocation or restraint, the mask is often gradually applied from the chin upward, starting with high flows of nitrous oxide and oxygen (70/30) and gradually adding halothane in 0.5 per cent increments. As consciousness is lost, the mask is placed securely on the face and induction completed. Rapid increases in inspired concentration of volatile agents result in irritation of the respiratory tract and eyes, thereby causing coughing, breath holding, and laryngospasm in addition to frightening the still conscious patient.

Intravenous induction with thiopental or methohexital using a small, sharp needle or scalp vein cannula (27 gauge) is rapid and relatively painless but requires skill in venipuncture that the anesthetist who occasionally works with children may not possess. We do not recommend intravenous induction in patients in whom there is a question of upper airway obstruction.

Ketamine is a useful induction agent because it can be given intravenously (1 to 2 mg/kg) or intramuscularly (5 to 10 mg/kg) while maintaining cardiac output, blood pressure, and usually, airway and ventilation. The drug is especially useful in the burned or hypovolemic patient, those with cyanotic congenital heart disease, and the combative subject. However, the disadvantages include prolonged recovery with occasional emergence delirium, little visceral pain relief, increased cerebral blood flow, and occasional increases in upper airway reflex reactivity with development of laryngospasm. Emergence delirium can often be prevented or controlled with diazepam, either as premedication or given intravenously prior to emergence.

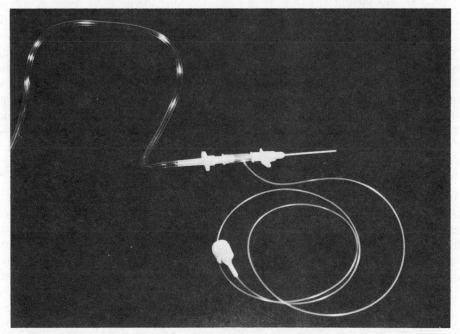

FIGURE 25–8. Intravenous side channel volume less than 0.1 ml for administration of drugs to neonate.

Rectal methohexital or thiopental (25 mg/kg) can be used for heavy premedication or as an induction technique in some children and offers the advantages of painlessly inducing sleep in the presence of parents. The rectal route is not recommended in children with anorectal disorders, a full stomach, or hypovolemia or for children of school age and older because of the psychic trauma possibly induced by rectal manipulation. However, this technique has proved useful for radiologic examinations and other short, often repeated operations. Once administered, the anesthetist must remain in constant attendance, prepared for any emergency.

Airway obstruction occurs readily during induction and usually responds to forward lift of the mandible while ensuring that the fingers do not compress the soft tissue of the neck; when necessary, an oral airway is inserted at the right time. Indications for tracheal intubation include a full stomach; thoracic, abdominal, and cranial procedures; the prone or sitting position; the use of neuromuscular blockers; and all surgical procedures in neonates. Intubation may be done with the newborn awake, especially when the airway is at risk, as in tracheoesophageal fistula. In older children, intubation is usually accomplished during deep inhalation anesthesia or with the aid of a neuromuscular blocker.

Intravenous fluids are given to all patients except brief elective cases. Vascular access for both fluids and drugs is usually maintained via plastic catheters, as they can be secured better than scalp vein needles (Fig. 25–8). Venous cutdowns may be needed to ensure access.

MAINTENANCE

All of the commonly used anesthetics can be used for maintenance of anesthesia, with halothane and nitrous oxide most common. Worth noting is that "halothane hepatitis" is practically nonexistent in the pre-adolescent population for reasons unknown. Ketamine, the opioids, and the other volatile agents are used in situations similar to those in the adult population. The critically ill newborn tolerates anesthesia poorly. To ensure the patient's safety in this situation, adequate ventilation, oxygenation, and cardiac support have priority. Fentanyl has been especially useful in these patients because of minimal cardiovascular effects.

Requirements for succinylcholine appear to be greater in the newborn (2 mg/kg intravenously or 4 mg/kg intramuscularly) than in the older child or adult (1 mg/kg intravenously or 2 mg/kg intramuscularly). On the other hand, debate exists over the requirements for nondepolarizing agents. Traditional teaching holds that neonates and infants present a myasthenic syndrome and require less tubocurarine or pancuronium than the older child or adult; recent data tend to refute this concept. Apparently, wide individual variations exist in response to nondepolarizers in the newborn and infant, so the best course is to use small doses and titrate the drug to clinical effect with neuromuscular monitoring as a guide.

Maintenance of adequate oxygen tension is always a concern. In the newborn adequate oxygenation must be maintained without exposing the infant to the hazards of oxygen toxicity. Retrolental fibroplasia, with neovascularization of the retina, appears often but does not always correlate with elevated inspired oxygen tensions. Pathology appears only when the retina is under development so that neonates and especially prematures under thirty-four weeks gestation are at risk. Current recommendations vary from source to source, but maintenance of Pa_{O_2} between 50 and 70 torr in the normal newborn and between 40 and 60 torr in the premature is usually advised. In healthy patients undergoing nonthoracic procedures, the Fi_{O_2} is kept below 0.4 per cent, adding air to the inspired mixture as needed. In cyanotic heart disease, during thoracic operations, and in the presence of pneumonia or IRDS, a higher Fi_{O_2} may be needed to maintain adequate blood oxygen tensions. The only certain method of ensuring adequate blood gas tension is measurement. The exact length of time in relation to an elevated Pa_{O_2} and the development of vascular damage is unknown.

Intraoperative fluid therapy depends on three variables: the preoperative deficit, maintenance requirements perioperatively, and blood and intraoperative third space losses. As already noted, preoperative deficits should be corrected prior to operation. Maintenance fluids comprise 5 per cent dextrose in 0.25 per cent normal saline except in the child under one week of age, in whom dextrose is increased to 10 per cent because of the hypoglycemic tendency. However, 5 per cent dextrose in lactated Ringer's solution is often infused in the patient over six weeks of age to cover maintenance and other losses. Blood loss is estimated on the basis of weighed sponges, calibrated suction traps, visual estimation of blood loss in the field and on the drapes, and the patient's vital signs and urine output. Assuming that the hematocrit is normal, losses below 10 per cent of total blood volume are replaced with two to three times the volume of lactated Ringer's solution or another balanced salt solution. Above 20 per cent blood loss, replacement is begun; although whole blood is desirable, it is often unavailable, and blood component therapy is resorted to. When massive transfusion is needed, blood is warmed to prevent onset of hypothermia, especially in small children. Metabolic acidosis in these situations usually results from poor perfusion and is not corrected when perfusion is restored. Bicarbonate therapy is guided by blood gas determinations, not empirical formulas. Albumin and fresh frozen plasma are given to replace protein-rich losses (visceral surgery or burns), coagulation protein defects

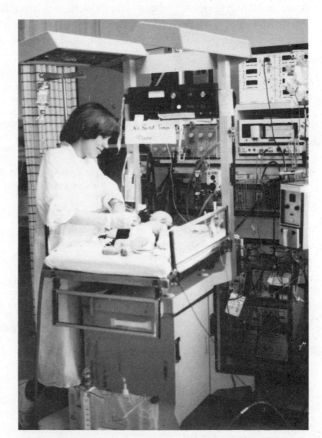

FIGURE 25–9. A bed with servo-controlled overhead warmers that allows easy access to the patient. This bed can be used in the operating room.

(congenital and due to transfusion), and volume deficits when whole blood is unavailable and when oxygen-carrying capacity of hemoglobin is not a major consideration.

EMERGENCE AND POSTOPERATIVE CARE

Oropharynx and stomach should be suctioned of secretions at the end of operation and all monitors left in place until the patient is fully awake and extubated. Safe emergence hinges on complete reversal of neuromuscular blockage; elimination of volatile anesthetics; and provision for normothermia, a normal acid-base status, and decent cardiopulmonary reserve. The acidotic, cold child does not respond with adequate ventilation or cardiac output.

The airway is probably the most common source of concern on emergence and immediately postoperatively. Extubation should be accomplished only in the fully awake newborn, in the critically ill, in the presence of a full stomach or compromised airway, or when there is residual anesthetic depression. Extubation may result in laryngospasm, usually corrected by positive airway pressure or requiring re-intubation. In all patients 100 per cent oxygen is given before extubation. Upper airway obstruction is usually relieved by forward displacement of the mandible.

Children are transported and maintained in the recovery room in the lateral decubitus position, thus allowing the tongue to fall from the pharynx. Oxygen is administered until consciousness is regained. Stridor sometimes develops after tracheal extubation, usually resolving if the patient breathes a heated mist; nebulized racemic epinephrine or intravenous dexamethasone may be needed.

The time in the recovery room is hazardous for the child, who must be constantly observed by well-trained staff. Aspiration, airway obstruction, hypothermia, hypotension, and emergence delirium (after ketamine) are all real possibilities to be anticipated. The newborn is best housed in an incubator or beneath heating lights to prevent hypothermia and subsequent increase in oxygen requirements (Fig. 25–9).

REFERENCES

Bennett EJ: Fluids for Anesthesia and Surgery in the Newborn and Infant. Springfield, IL, Charles C Thomas, 1975.

Earley A, Fayers P, Ng S, et al: Blood pressure in the first 6 weeks of life. Arch Dis Child 55:755, 1980.

Eckenhoff J: Some anatomic considerations of the infant larynx influencing endotracheal anesthesia. Anesthesiology 12:401, 1951.

Edmonds JF, Barker GA, Conn AW: Current concepts in cardiovascular monitoring in children. Crit Care Med 8:548, 1980.

Goudsouzian NG: Maturation of neuromuscular transmission in the infant. Br J Anaesth 52:205, 1980.

Klaus MH,Fanaroff AA: Care of the High Risk Neonate. 2nd ed, Philadelphia, WB Saunders Co, 1979.

Korsch BM: The child and the operating room. Anesthesiology 43:251, 1975.

Levin RM: Pediatric Anesthesia Handbook. 2nd ed. Garden City, NY, Medical Examination Publishing Co, 1980.

Liu LMP, Goudsouzian NG, Liu PL: Rectal methohexital premedication in children, a dose-comparison study. Anesthesiology 53:343, 1980.

Maze A, Bloch E: Stridor in pediatric patients. Anesthesiology 50:132, 1979.

Merritt JC, Sprague DH, et al: Retrolental fibroplasia: a multifactorial disease. Anesth Analg 60:109, 1981.

Seleny FL: Respiratory failure: Part II — The child. Curr Probl Anesth Crit Care Med 1978.

Smith RM: Anesthesia for Infants and Children. 4th ed. St. Louis, CV Mosby, 1980.

Steward DJ, Creighton RE: General anesthesia for minor surgery in healthy children. Curr Probl Anesth Crit Care Med 1977.

Wilkinson AR, Phibbs RH, Gregory GA: Continuous measurement of oxygen saturation in sick newborn infants. J Pediatr 93:1016, 1978.

Wolfer JA, Visintainer MA: Prehospital psychological preparation for tonsillectomy patients: Effects on children's and parents' adjustment. Pediatrics 64:646, 1979.

Chapter 26

CARDIOPULMONARY ANESTHESIA

For nearly a century after the introduction of anesthesia, operations within the thorax were rarely attempted because surgeons could not cope with the cardiorespiratory disturbances caused by pneumothorax. In the early 1900s pneumothorax was shown to shunt blood through the nonaerated lung; to solve this problem Sauerbruch, the authoritative surgeon of the era, used a negative pressure operating chamber that maintained lung inflation while the patient breathed spontaneously, head outside the chamber. This was done even though Matas had already demonstrated that intermittent positive pressure ventilation via endotracheal tube and a simple bellows device could maintain lung inflation. Sauerbruch's method prevailed; when the thorax was opened, the lung collapsed and paradoxical respiration occurred. During inspiration (Fig. 26–1*A*), dead space gas from the partially collapsed lung on the operated side was sucked into the inflated lung; on expiration (Fig. 26–1*B*), gas from the inflated lung re-entered the partially collapsed lung. A pendulum-like movement of air caused paradoxical shift of the mediastinum toward the intact hemithorax during inspiration and away from it on expiration. Respiratory and circulatory failures were common, and the mortality of thoracic procedures was prohibitive.

Rhythmic positive pressure endotracheal respiration was not universally accepted until the 1940s; the introduction of neuromuscular blockers abolished spontaneous respiratory movement, and cuffed endotracheal tubes allowed a tight seal of the trachea, setting the stage for modern thoracic anesthesia. However, the concept of adequate alveolar ventilation first had to be understood before thoracic anesthesia could develop.

Once the effects of pneumothorax were solved, operations on thoracic organs and vessels became common; pneumonectomy (1935) was followed by ligation of a patent ductus arteriosus (1938), repair of aortic coarctation (1943), and subclavian–pulmonary artery anastomosis for palliative treatment of tetralogy of Fallot (1944). Missile fragments from the chambers of a beating heart were removed during World War II, and in 1948, Bailey performed the first closed mitral valvulotomy for relief of mitral stenosis. In 1950, total body hypothermia extended the time of permissible brain and organ ischemia, allowing direct repair of intracardiac lesions. And in 1953, when heparin, protamine, and techniques of cardiac catheterization and extracorporeal oxygenation of blood became available, surgical correction of congenital heart defects and prosthetic replacement of diseased valves were permitted. Direct current defibrillators, external pacemakers, and demand implantable pacemakers allowed control of

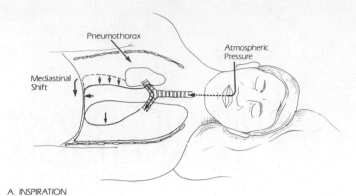

A. INSPIRATION

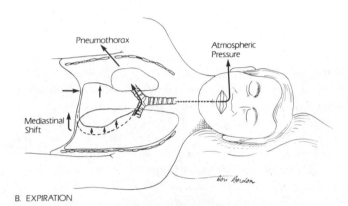

B. EXPIRATION

FIGURE 26-1. Pneumothorax. *A.* Effects of spontaneous inspiration. Note collapsed right lung and shift of heart and mediastinum to the left. *B.* Effects of thoracotomy and spontaneous expiration. Note slight expansion of right lung and movement of exhaled gases to right lung.

cardiac rate and rhythm. Angiography provided preoperative visualization of heart defects, and the discovery that contrast media could be safely injected into coronary arteries introduced the present era of coronary artery revascularization. Mechanical circulatory assist devices, diagnostic nuclear radiology for the assessment of reversibility of damage to the myocardium, surgical therapy of cardiac arrhythmias, and cardiac transplantation now challenge the field. We shall first consider concepts of anesthesia for pulmonary surgery, then for operations on the heart.

PULMONARY SURGERY

Since the early days of thoracic surgery, a dramatic change has occurred in diseases of the lung that present for operation. Tuberculous and wet bronchiectatic lungs are now rarities, whereas carcinoma of the lung and mediastinal lesions comprise the majority of lesions in thoracic operations today.

LUNG RESECTIONS AND PNEUMONECTOMY

Careful assessment and management of pulmonary and cardiac disease are essential prior to anesthesia for thoracic operations. Preoperative chest x-rays permit comparison with postoperative status. Preoperative pulmonary function tests and blood gas analyses are required on all patients for pneumonectomy and resections. The simplest measure of ventilatory adequacy is the FEV_1 (see Chapter 37); if FEV_1 is less than 35 to 40 per cent of predicted values, operability is questionable if large segments of lung would be removed. Complications of pulmonary operations include atrial fibrillation, retained secretions, air leak, atelectasis, emphysema, and hemorrhage — complications that are rare in nonpulmonary thoracic surgical procedures. Age of the patient, the extent of resection (pneumonectomy, lobectomy, segmental resection), and underlying lung and cardiac disease are factors that significantly affect morbidity and mortality.

Monitoring

Constant observation of the surgical field by the anesthetist is *pro forma*. Electrocardiogram, blood pressure, and body temperature must be monitored. Radial artery catheterization allows frequent assessment of blood gases and continuous observation of blood pressure. An esophageal stethoscope facilitates detection of pulmonary edema, airway secretions, and development of pneumothorax in the dependent hemithorax. Central venous pressure monitoring aids in assessing adequacy of volume replacement. Use of a Swan-Ganz catheter (see Chapter 9) is reserved for patients with left ventricular dysfunction or coronary artery disease.

Conduct of Anesthesia

We prefer controlled ventilation with a halogenated inhalation anesthetic and 50 per cent nitrous oxide and oxygen (some opt for oxygen without nitrous oxide), although intravenous opioids, nitrous oxide, and neuromuscular blockers are also satisfactory. The procedure is to induce anesthesia with thiopental, intubate the trachea with the aid of succinylcholine, and maintain anesthesia with halothane or ethrane, nitrous oxide, oxygen, and a nondepolarizing neuromuscular blocker. Although not essential when inhalation agents are used, neuromuscular blockers prevent coughing during dissection and manipulation about the hilum. The patient is usually placed in the lateral decubitus position, taking care to prevent stretching of the brachial plexus, with an axillary pad to permit better ventilation of the dependent lung.

At the end of operation, the anesthetist helps to extrude air from the pleural space by hyperinflation of the lung. After pneumonectomy, intrapleural pressure is adjusted by aspirating air to slightly below atmospheric pressure. Excessive negative pressure may cause hypotension by shifting the mediastinum and compromising cardiac output. The trachea may be extubated when adequate spontaneous respiration and reflexes have returned and secretions have been aspirated. If the patient's condition is precarious or if spontaneous respiration is inadequate, the endotracheal tube is left in place and mechanical ventilation begun postoperatively.

Oxygen should be given continuously via endotracheal tube or face mask and respirations assisted by using an Ambu bag during transport of the patient to recovery room or intensive care unit. If mechanical ventilation is elected postoperatively, some prefer to transport the patient directly to an intensive care unit. The patient should not be transported if emergence delirium, restlessness, or hypoxia is evident (see Chapter 36). In the critically ill, cardiovascular monitoring should be continued via intra-arterial monitor and ECG during transit to the recovery area.

In the recovery room the patient assumes the most comfortable position, provided that the position is changed frequently. A semierect position is favored, but varying the position to the horizontal with the thoracotomy side uppermost following segmental resection assists in drainage of secretions, facilitating expansion of residual lung. Postpneumonectomy, however, the intact lung is uppermost to drain secretions. The elderly or those with major cardiopulmonary disease may not tolerate the supine or lateral position; the key to the best positioning is frequent change.

PRINCIPLES OF CHEST DRAINAGE

Alveoli incised during segmental resection or lobectomy leak air to the pleural space until sealed. Prompt evacuation of air and fluid from the thoracic cavity via catheters connected to a water sealed system prevents atelectasis and encapsulation of the lung by scar tissue, further permitting accurate estimation of postoperative blood loss. The drainage tubes act as one-way valves, extruding air during expiration when intrapleural pressure overcomes the valve resistance, but preventing aspiration of air and fluid into the chest. The original three-bottle system (Fig. 26–2B) provided water seal and collecting bottles and another bottle for regulating intensity of suction and intrapleural pressure according to the depth of the tube beneath water level. Today, sterile disposable plastic units (Fig. 26–2A) permit both underwater seal and suction. A collection chamber collects drainage from the chest. The second chamber, a water seal chamber, is filled with sterile saline to a 2-cm level, and the third functions as a U-tube manometer. A positive pressure relief valve closes during suction and opens when air is expelled, preventing harmful intrathoracic pressures. The third chamber can be filled with saline to a level equal to the amount of suction desired, its port connected to a suction source. A water seal is maintained by keeping the unit upright at floor level to prevent aspiration of air and fluid into the chest. Recently, a chest drainage system has been developed to overcome the deficiencies of a water seal system; one-way positive-seal silicone rubber valves replace the water seal and positive pressure relief valve, eliminating the water and the need for a vertical position. After segmental resections, pleural air leaks may exceed 20 L/min at 30 torr negative pressure. Development of subcutaneous emphysema after thoracotomy suggests inadequate suction in the presence of an air leak.

One chest tube is positioned posteriorly to drain the pleural gutter; a second tube is required for air leak, its tip at the apex of the thorax. Following pneumonectomy, tubes

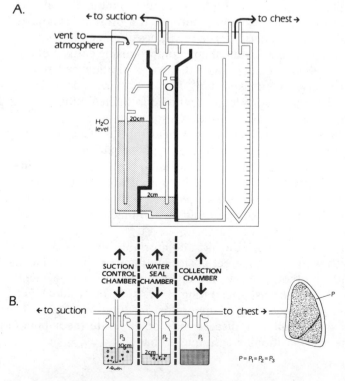

FIGURE 26–2. Chest drainage systems. *A,* Disposable plastic drainage unit. Note division of collection chamber into three continuous units. Suction can be adjusted according to the water level in suction control chamber. *B.* Three-bottle system for underwater seal suction. Note that pressure above water level in all bottles is equal to the intrapleural pressure minus 10 cm H_2O.

are not placed in the pleural space. After mediastinotomy if the pleural space has not been entered, the mediastinum is often drained because air and blood cannot be effectively evacuated via lung expansion alone. Chest tubes must not kink and should never be clamped. Even with minimal air leak, a sudden rise in intrathoracic pressure, as with coughing, may increase the air leak and cause tension pneumothorax if air cannot escape.

ENDOBRONCHIAL ANESTHESIA AND ONE LUNG ANESTHESIA

One lung anesthesia was once popular for patients operated on in the lateral decubitus position to prevent spillover of blood, pus, or excessive bronchial secretions from diseased lung into the nonoperated lung. Originally, single lumen endobronchial tubes incorporated one bronchial cuff and the anesthetist gave one lung anesthesia throughout the operation. Additional tracheal cuffs permitted ventilation of both lungs simultaneously or independently. The bronchial blocker, a two-channel catheter, one to inflate a blocking balloon and the other for suction, also achieved popularity, but it was difficult to position and did not provide an airtight seal. The Fogarty catheter, designed for embolectomy, can be used as a bronchial blocker. Although many anesthetists have not used the catheter, pulmonary hemorrhage is not a rarity, so that techniques for managing this potential catastrophe should be known.

The Carlens double lumen tube (Fig. 26–3*A*) isolates the lungs and permits individual ventilation depending on the surgical need. However, the small lumen increases resistance to gas flow, making passage of suction catheters difficult, and the carinal hook may cause laryngeal or tracheal damage. The Robert Shaw double lumen tube (Fig. 26–3*B*), with its larger lumen, is more popular and easier to insert.

Double lumen tubes are indicated in anesthetic management of bronchopleural fistulas, tension cysts of the lung, lung abscess, and pulmonary hemorrhage but need not be used routinely in thoracic operations. If one lung anesthesia is elected, at least 50 per cent oxygen (preferably 100 per cent) must be inhaled, and arterial blood gas monitoring is mandatory. Patients with poor respiratory function and low cardiac output are ill suited for one lung anesthesia.

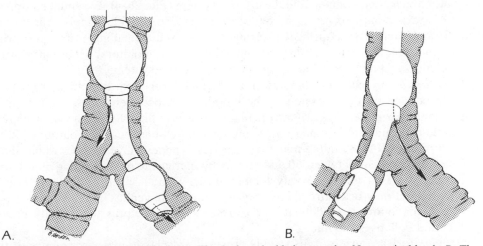

A.   B.

FIGURE 26–3. One lung anesthesia. *A.* The Carlens double lumen tube. Note carinal hook. *B.* The Robert Shaw double lumen tube. Note orifice of right endobronchial tube, which must be positioned at the lumen of the right upper lobe bronchus.

CARDIAC SURGERY

Anesthesia for cardiac surgical procedures differs little from that for other thoracic operations. Halothane was successful for open heart surgery because of its nonflammability, rapidity of induction and recovery, minimal side effects, and moderately good muscle relaxation; sympatho-adrenal depression rendered blood vessels more pliable. However, halothane is a myocardial depressant and predisposes to ventricular arrhythmias; nevertheless use of the agent in low concentrations (0.5 to 1.0 per cent) led to favorable results.

In the early 1970s Lowenstein popularized the use of large doses (0.5 to 3.0 mg/kg) of morphine for cardiac operations, doses large enough to depress respiratory drive and increase tolerance to endotracheal tubes during mechanical ventilation intra- and postoperatively yet not depressing cardiac output in patients with normal hearts or aortic valvular disease. As experience with morphine increased, problems developed: awareness during anesthesia, hypotension after induction, and hypertension during cardiopulmonary bypass. Some anesthetists substituted fentanyl for morphine; large doses (50 to 70 mcg/kg) produced complete anesthesia with less depression of blood pressure, peripheral vascular resistance, cardiac output, or heart rate. Although popular in many centers, fentanyl has disadvantages: it does not prevent hypertension; chest wall rigidity is common (see Chapter 14); bradycardia resulting in hypotension occurs; and the drug is costly.

The inhalation agent isoflurane may prove useful. Compared with halothane, it is less depressant to atrial and atrioventricular conduction and baroreceptor reflex control and does not sensitize the heart to the action of catecholamines. Although a myocardial depressant at light and moderate anesthetic levels, minimal change in myocardial contractility occurs; cardiac output remains stable, with a salutary decrease in peripheral vascular resistance. Compatibility with clinical doses of epinephrine, excellent muscle relaxation, and a stable cardiac output are characteristics that make isoflurane superior to halothane for cardiac operations. The propensity to tachycardia may be a disadvantage in patients with aortic or mitral stenosis.

CARDIOPULMONARY BYPASS

Over 150,000 bypass procedures are performed in 500 centers annually in the U.S. In this procedure, vena caval blood bypasses the heart, is drained by gravity into an oxygenator and is then pumped into the arterial system (Fig. 26–4). Essential equipment is as follows: a pump, oxygenator, oxygen and carbon dioxide supply, cardiotomy reservoir and suction system, heat exchanger, and circuit of tubing with appropriate priming solutions and filters. Pressure and temperature monitors, a coronary artery perfusion unit, and an anesthetic vaporizer complete the system.

The *roller pump* has been standard since the inception of cardiopulmonary bypass. Flow is produced by compression of the bloodstream between tubing, roller, and a curved metal back plate, thus driving the blood mass into the patient's aorta. This form of continuous, nonpulsatile blood flow should provide a basal cardiac output of 2.2 to 2.5 L/min/m² or 50 to 80 ml/kg/min at temperature ranges of 30 to 34C. Mean blood pressure is maintained between 60 and 80 torr by increasing or decreasing blood flow; less flow is required at lower body temperatures. Venous return is usually gravity implemented but may be controlled by a roller pump in the venous line; if venous return is low, a roller pump is inadequate, as excessive negative pressure usually creates bubbling and collapses the line.

Oxygenators are made of disposable presterilized plastic material and are of two kinds: the bubble and membrane varieties. Bubble oxygenators are the most popular;

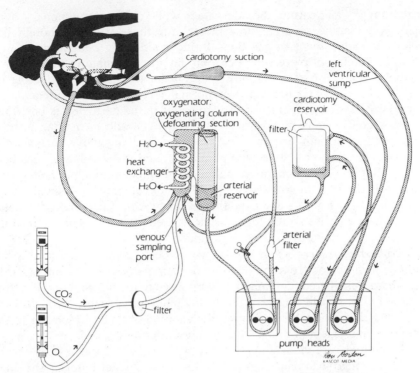

FIGURE 26–4. Cardiopulmonary bypass. Note the following: 1. gravity drainage from venae cavae to oxygenator; 2. heat exchanger with entrance and exit ports for water; 3. separate sources for oxygen and carbon dioxide; 4. left ventricular sump for decompression of left ventricle via right superior pulmonary vein with return of blood to oxygenator via cardiotomy reservoir; and 5. arterial filter bypass in the event of filter obstruction.

many models are available and all have three components: oxygenating column, a defoaming section, and an arterial reservoir.

Gas exchange occurs in the oxygenating column. Premixed oxygen and carbon dioxide filter directly into venous blood through perforations in a diffusing plate, microbubbles forming a large blood gas interface. Carbon dioxide and excess oxygen are eliminated through ports at the top of the chamber.

Gas bubbles are removed in the defoaming section, blood flowing over a large surface area provided by stainless steel wool mesh or polyurethane foam covered with an antifoaming agent. In some oxygenators, gas exchange also occurs here.

Defoamed blood is collected in the arterial reservoir. At standard perfusion flow rates the column of blood provides a 20- to 40-second blood reserve, forestalling accidental pumping of air into the patient should venous return be compromised by obstruction. Although today's bubble oxygenators are improved over earlier models, traumatized blood, platelet aggregates, denatured plasma proteins, and biochemical changes in blood remain problems, especially after prolonged bypass.

Membrane oxygenators have no blood gas interface. Thin, nonporous silicone or microporous Teflon or polypropylene sheets separate the oxygen mass from the blood film. The shim, an inflatable bag, exerts pressure on the membrane assembly, thus facilitating oxygen and carbon dioxide exchange. The postpump platelet count is higher and trauma to blood is less, but no convincing evidence suggests that these expensive, complex oxygenators are more advantageous.

Normal oxygen and carbon dioxide values while on cardiopulmonary bypass are maintained by adjusting separate flow meters for these gases, although fixed gas mixtures obviate adjustment of gas flow during rapid body cooling and rewarming. Although the solubility of oxygen and carbon dioxide are enhanced during hypothermia, metabolic rate decreases and low Pa_{CO_2} values can result, affecting cerebral perfusion. Pa_{CO_2} should be maintained at normal levels to ensure adequate regional blood flow regardless of temperature. Adequacy of tissue perfusion is best monitored by analyzing mixed venous blood for $P\bar{v}CO_2$ and $P\bar{v}O_2$ and measuring urine output. Pulmonary ventilation with helium, nitrous oxide, and oxygen with one of several techniques (mechanical ventilation, static inflation, and static collapse) has been used during bypass to prevent postoperative pulmonary complications, but no technique has proved superior to static lung collapse. With the development of small, disposable, bloodless priming oxygenators and expeditious surgery, the incidence of structural and functional alveolar changes after bypass has decreased markedly, and the postperfusion lung syndrome ("pump lung") is now uncommon.

The *cardiotomy reservoir and suction system* collects and recirculates blood. A roller pump collects blood from the heart cavity and pericardial sac into a cardiotomy reservoir, where it is filtered, defoamed, and returned to the oxygenator. The volume of blood returned may exceed that reverted to the pump oxygenator through the venous return line. The cardiotomy reservoir permits addition of fluid of blood to the system. This suction system is a major cause of hemolysis during bypass.

Heat exchangers are incorporated into oxygenators to control body temperature by heating or cooling blood as it circulates. Hot or cold water entering the unit at one end, with blood entering at the other, provides an efficient countercurrent flow system.

Arterial tubing of thromboresistant polyvinyl chloride returns blood from the oxygenator through a pumphead to aortic perfusion cannulas in the ascending aorta. The venous line returns blood from caval cannulas or a single atrial cannula to the oxygenator by gravity drainage, which is improved by elevating the patient above the oxygenator. The venous line should be inspected during bypass, as an air lock can develop and impede venous return. Filters in the oxygen delivery line and in the arterial line proximal to the aortic inlet and distal to the arterial pumphead function as traps for cellular debris, fat globules, fiber and silicone particulates.

A vent passed through the right superior pulmonary vein and the mitral valve decompresses the left ventricle, thus facilitating drainage of coronary sinus blood. The blood is either drained by gravity or sucked from the ventricle by a roller pump.

Many variations of cardiopulmonary bypass systems prevail, but bypass circuits should be simple and connections kept to a minimum.

An autologous blood recovery system has become an integral part of equipment used in cardiac surgery. This unit collects, washes, and spins blood drawn from the operative field prior to, during, and after cardiopulmonary bypass, thus providing packed cells that can be returned to the patient to alleviate the necessity for donor transfusion.

CONDUCT OF ANESTHESIA

Preoperative Preparation

Thorough preoperative evaluation of carotid and cerebrovascular disease may prevent neurologic sequelae, complications that have a higher incidence after cardiopulmonary bypass than after other operations. Preoperative medications must be reviewed and the effects of their withdrawal or continuation evaluated. The antiplatelet aggregation action of acetylsalicylic acid, for example, may prolong bleeding time and may result in unusual blood loss during and following operation. Quinidine may trigger an immunogenic thrombocytopenia by enhancing attachment of drug antibody complexes to platelets (see Chapter 4).

Monitoring

The Electrocardiogram. Patients scheduled for cardiac operations require extensive monitoring of the following: the ECG; intra-arterial and central venous or pulmonary artery pressures; body temperature; arterial blood gases; and, in some circumstances, serum electrolytes. We monitor a variety of ECG leads: standard limb leads (I, II, and III), unipolar augmented limb leads (AVR, AVL, and AVF), and a precordial lead (V_5); the last named aids in diagnosing ischemic injury in the zone of the left coronary artery, and lead II provides information related to the right coronary artery. Lead II is best for diagnosing arrhythmias. The ST segment is a monitor of myocardial ischemia. Although not a significant correlate of myocardial oxygen consumption ($M\dot{V}O_2$), a rise in pulmonary capillary wedge pressure or pulmonary artery diastolic pressure suggests an increase in ventricular wall stress and often precedes ECG evidence of ischemia. However crude, diastolic blood pressure, hematocrit, and oxygen saturation are the only clinical guides to myocardial oxygen supply, and rate pressure product (RPP) (the product of systolic blood pressure and heart rate) is a clinical correlate of $M\dot{V}O_2$.

Blood Pressure. A radial artery is usually cannulated for continuous monitoring of intra-arterial blood pressure. During operation for thoracic aneurysm when the distal aorta is to be cross-clamped, dorsalis pedis arterial pressure should also be observed for information relative to perfusion of kidneys and spinal cord. A Swan-Ganz catheter permits recording of pulmonary artery and pulmonary capillary wedge pressures (PCWP); this is especially valuable in patients with left ventricular dysfunction, since correlation between CVP and PCWP is poor in this situation. A combination of CVP for monitoring right heart pressure and an esophageal stethoscope to indirectly monitor left atrial pressure (rales or heart sounds [S_3]) may be used in patients with good left ventricular function and in those with tricuspid valve disease, atrial septal defects, or other congenital lesions.

Other Devices. These include esophageal, rectal, and myocardial cerebrovascular temperature recorders and bifrontal electroencephalographic monitors, useful in patients with cerebrovascular disease or those having combined carotid and cardiac operations. Arterial and venous blood gases, serum potassium, and urine volume measurements provide essential data on physiologic homeostasis. Cardiac output may be calculated intraoperatively by the thermodilution method including derived indices of peripheral vascular resistance.

Anesthetic Adjuvants

The immediate availability of a direct current defibrillator and a wide range of active drugs encourage a safe induction of anesthesia (Table 26–1).

Cardioplegia (induction of electromechanical cardiac arrest) in combination with profound cooling (cold cardioplegia) at 10°C is the accepted technique for myocardial protection during operation, resulting in significantly reduced perioperative myocardial damage as compared with noncardioplegic methods. Potassium, the most commonly used cardioplegic, 15 to 30 mmol/L at 4°C, is injected at the aortic root, blocking the initial phase of myocardial depolarization and resulting in cessation of electrical and mechanical activity. Hypothermia reduces oxygen consumption of the heart during ischemic aortic cross-clamping and allows tissue energy stores to support cellular

TABLE 26–1. Cardiovascular Drugs Used During Anesthesia for Cardiac Surgery

Drug	Indication	Preparation	IV Dosage	Remarks
Sodium bicarbonate 8.4 per cent	Acidosis Cardiac arrest	50-ml ampule (1 mEq 1 ml)	1 mEq/kg or 1 to 2 ampules	Repeat according to blood gas analysis
Atropine	Bradycardia Hypotension	0.4 to 0.6 mg	0.4 to 0.6 mg	Rule out anoxia
Lidocaine 2 per cent	Ventricular ectopic beats	5-ml ampule	1 mg/kg bolus	
Lidocaine	Persistent ventricular tachycardia	2 gm/250 ml D_5W	1 to 4 mg/min	Continuous infusion
Propranolol	Tachycardia Ventricular arrhythmia	1-mg ampule	0.2 to 1.0 mg	Use with caution in small doses
Phenylephrine	Hypotension at on- set of bypass	10 mg/250 ml D_5W	50- to 500-mcg bolus	Rarely needed
Methoxamine	Hypotension at onset of bypass	20 mg/ml	2- to 4-mg bolus	Rarely needed
Calcium chloride	Asystole	1 gm/10 ml	500-mg to 1-gm bolus	Slowly
Dopamine	Low cardiac output	200 mg/250 ml D_5W *	100 to 400 mcg/ min	Most commonly used cardiotonic
Dobutamine	Low cardiac output	250 mg/250 ml D_5W	125 to 500 mcg/ min	
Isoproterenol	Low cardiac output Pulmonary hypertension	1 mg/250 ml D_5W	0.5 to 0.2 mcg/min	Increases $M\dot{V}_{O_2}$
Epinephrine	Low cardiac output Cardiac arrest	2 mg/250 ml D_5W	1 to 4 mcg/min	Increases $M\dot{V}_{O_2}$
Nitroglycerin	Angina Hypertension	15 mg/250 ml D_5W	25 to 300 mcg/ min	Reduces preload
Sodium nitro- prusside	Hypertension	50 mg/250 ml D_5W	12 to 50 mcg/min	Reduces afterload
Verapamil	Rapid atrial filtration or flutter	5-mg ampule	0.075 mg/kg	Reduces rate

function and transmembrane gradients of sodium, potassium, calcium, and magnesium.

At 37°C, normally contracting heart muscle consumes 8 to 10 ml O_2/100 gm tissue/min. Myocardial temperature and resting wall tension determine energy demands in an electromechanically quiet heart. Whereas the fibrillating heart at 22°C consumes approximately 2 ml O_2/100 gm tissue/min, the electromechanically quiet heart consumes only 0.3 ml O_2/100 gm tissue/min. Although both crystalloids and whole blood are popular as carrier solutions for potassium cardioplegia, we favor the use of blood with its higher oxygen content; lower levels of lactate in coronary sinus blood and a higher incidence of spontaneous contraction during cardiac reperfusion attest to better myocardial oxygenation during ischemic arrest.

Prior to cannulation of the great vessels, the administration of heparin (3 to 5 mg/kg) through the CVP line ensures adequate anticoagulation for bypass. With measurement of activated clotting time (ACT) every 30 minutes, the anesthetist can maintain the ACT level above 400 seconds by giving additional heparin when necessary. After the pump run, reversal of heparin with protamine re-establishes clotting.

During induction of anesthesia, modifications of anesthetic technique may be necessary, and pharmacologic intervention with a vasodilator, especially nitroglycerin, may be required before institution of bypass to maintain heart rate, systolic arterial pressure, and pulmonary diastolic pressure below levels that could precipitate angina or ECG evidence of ischemia preoperatively. Vasodilators are useful in decreasing the overall operative risk of coronary bypass grafting, whereas a need for vasopressors is rare. By reducing preload, diminishing ventricular wall tension, and dilating collateral vessels, nitroglycerin improves concomitant ischemic ECG changes more often than does nitroprusside, but the latter dilates arterial resistance vessels and is more effective in reducing afterload.

A low output syndrome after cardiac surgery is best treated by improving preload via volume loading. If normal arterial and pulmonary artery diastolic pressures cannot be maintained, reduction in afterload (elevated systemic vascular resistance) with nitroprusside may decrease left ventricular filling pressure and improve output. If pulmonary artery diastolic pressure cannot be maintained at 15 to 18 torr without lowering arterial blood pressure below 100 torr, nitroprusside dosage should be reduced and dopamine or dobutamine given to support pressure. If these methods fail to produce the desired results, mechanical augmentation of the circulation with intra-aortic balloon pumping is indicated. Available data indicate that the calcium antagonists verapamil and nifedipine, which block the influx of calcium in cardiac and smooth muscle, may be of value in preserving the myocardium during coronary bypass; verapamil effectively and promptly controls the rapid ventricular response in atrial fibrillation and flutter.

Anesthetics

Thiopental, diazepam, or opioids are effective in inducing anesthesia. Rapid injection of large doses of thiopental is contraindicated in patients with poor ventricular function or fixed cardiac output. Small doses of thiopental may be used by an experienced anesthetist, but we believe that diazepam, which causes little or no cardiac depression, is safer.

Evidence for the superiority of one anesthetic or combination of agents over another for management of patients for open heart operations is unconvincing, despite the precise pharmacologic recipes recommended. We favor halothane, especially for coronary artery bypass operations. Experimental evidence suggests that halothane favorably influences the relation between myocardial oxygen supply and demand when coronary blood flow is limited. The diminished adrenergic response to operation and less frequent appearance of ST segment depression in lead V_5 suggest myocardial ischemia is less common compared with patients anesthetized with opioid.

Choice of anesthetic technique is a matter of judgment based on the skill of the anesthetist and familiarity with agents and their effect on a patient's disease and response to operation. With extensive monitoring, judicious use of vasodilators, and strict attention to the RPP (its limitations realized), both opioids and halothane are safe in patients with good ventricular function; opioids may offer greater advantage in patients with major ventricular dysfunction.

APPRAISAL

Anesthetists have responded to the rapid progress in cardiac surgery and have played active roles in improving intraoperative and postoperative care and the consequent diminishing mortality. Modifications in anesthetic management will undoubtedly occur in the future to improve current mortality figures. A continuing challenge to anesthetists lies in the decade ahead in anesthesia for cardiothoracic surgery.

REFERENCES

Fiser WP, Friday CD, Read RC: Changes in arterial oxygenation and pulmonary shunt during thoracotomy with endobronchial anesthesia. J Thorac Cardiovasc Surg 83:523, 1982.

Hoar PF, Stone JG, Faltas AN, et al: Hemodynamic and adrenergic responses to anesthesia and operation for myocardial revascularization. J Thorac Cardiovasc Surg 80:242, 1980.

Kaplan JA: Cardiac Anesthesia. New York, Grune & Stratton, 1979.

Kirklin JW, Conti VR, Blackstone EH: Prevention of myocardial damage during cardiac operations. N Engl J Med 301:135, 1979.

Lowenstein E, Hallowell P, Levin FH, et al: Cardiovascular responses to large doses of intravenous morphine in man. N Engl J Med 281:1389, 1969.

Mangano DT: Monitoring pulmonary arterial pressure in coronary artery disease. Anesthesiology 53:364, 1980.

Waller JL, Hug CC Jr, Nagle DM, Craver JM: Hemodynamic changes during fentanyl-oxygen anesthesia for aortocoronary bypass operation. Anesthesiology 55:212, 1981.

Wilkinson PL, Hamilton WK, Moyers JR, Graham B, Ports TA, Ullyot DJ, Chatterjee K: Halothane and morphine–nitrous oxide anesthesia in patients undergoing coronary artery bypass operation. J Thorac Cardiovasc Surg 82:372, 1981.

Chapter 27
NEUROSURGICAL ANESTHESIA

Safe anesthetic management of neurosurgical patients requires a detailed knowledge of the cerebral circulation, its physiologic and pharmacologic controls, and intracranial pressure (ICP) and the dynamics of its changes. The cerebral metabolic rate for oxygen ($CMRO_2$) and its alteration by drugs and disease represent additional important considerations in neuroanesthesia.

THE INTRACRANIAL COMPARTMENTS

The cranium is relatively noncompliant and consists of three compartments: brain tissue, which represents 80 to 85 per cent (1000 to 1200 gm) of intracranial contents; cerebrospinal fluid (CSF), which comprises 8 to 12 per cent (120 to 150 ml); and blood in the intracranial vessels, which constitutes 3 to 7 per cent (75 to 100 ml).

Total intracranial volume in an adult approaches 1200 to 1500 ml. Alterations in volume of any one intracranial compartment must, of necessity, produce change in the other two. Both the vascular and CSF compartments act as a common extracranial space, allowing for shift of blood and CSF out of the cranium to compensate for small or slow change in volume in another compartment. For example, the intracranial contents of a patient with a slow-growing tumor compensate by shifting CSF from the cranium into the spinal subarachnoid space. Mild hyperventilation with a consequent low Pa_{CO_2} may further compensate by decreasing the volume of the intracranial vascular space. Only when compensatory mechanisms are exhausted does the ICP rise. Acute volume and ICP changes produce irreversible changes unless the pressure is promptly reduced. Surgical manipulations and anesthesia may alter this delicate intracranial balance, their potential minimized by full utilization of the monitoring techniques now available.

CEREBRAL BLOOD FLOW

Cerebral blood flow (CBF) measured by the Kety-Schmidt inert gas technique utilizing nitrous oxide estimates CBF to be 55 ml/100 gm/min and the $CMRO_2$ to be 3.3 ml/100 gm/min. Substitution of radioactive tracer gases (^{85}Kr and ^{133}Xe) for nitrous oxide, first by intracarotid injection and later by inhalation, has increased the accuracy of flow measurement and allowed for computation of regional CBF (rCBF). Currently accepted values for total CBF are about 44 ml/100 gm/min and for rCBF from 20 ml/100 gm/min for white matter to 80 ml/100 gm/min for gray matter. The recent development of positron emission tomography with its adaptation to measurement of CBF, $CMRO_2$, rCBF, and $rCMRO_2$ holds promise for rapid determinations in clinical situations.

Metabolic Regulation of CBF

Total CBF and $CMRO_2$ remain relatively constant during both consciousness and sleep, but considerable differences occur in rCBF. Activated states of neuronal function in sharply circumscribed brain areas such as the motor cortex increase rCBF and are accompanied by increased $rCMRO_2$. Increased activity is coupled with increased perfusion and elevated oxygen consumption, thought to be the result of elevations in H^+ and K^+ concentrations in extracellular fluid (ECF) bathing the cerebral resistance vessels in the area involved.

The Influence of Carbon Dioxide on CBF

Hypercapnia produces vasodilation and increased CBF, whereas hypocapnia causes constriction; the effect is rapid and linear (Fig. 27–1). For each torr CO_2 increase or decrease between Pa_{CO_2} 20 and 80, a 2-ml increase or decrease in CBF occurs within one minute.

The mechanism by which CO_2 promotes vasodilation is unclear, but alterations of H^+ concentration in CSF and brain ECF are likely explanations, as CO_2 diffuses freely across the blood brain barrier. The tissue H^+ concentration inside arteriolar smooth muscle cells is probably involved, but how this alters vasomotor tone is uncertain. Changes in perivascular osmolarity or concentration of ionized calcium may also play a role. Production of CSF alkalosis through hyperventilation increases transport of bicarbonate ions out of CSF, and pH returns to normal within 8 to 24 hours. All medications that depress respiration indirectly increase Pa_{CO_2}, induce cerebrovascular dilation, and increase CBF in the spontaneously breathing patient, actions that may lead to a rise in ICP in patients with head trauma or mass lesions.

The Influence of Blood Pressure on CBF

CBF is remarkably stable over a wide range of blood pressure levels. This phenomenon, termed autoregulation, refers to the ability of normal brain to maintain a constant CBF despite variations in cerebral perfusion pressure (CPP) and body position. CPP is the difference between mean arterial pressure and intracranial pressure, representing the pressure-head driving cerebral perfusion. In normal brain, a fall in CPP is accompanied by cerebral vasodilation, thus maintaining a constant blood flow, whereas vasoconstriction follows elevations in CPP. Autoregulation occurs in normal subjects over the range of 50 to 150 torr CPP (see Fig. 27–1); above or below these limits, CBF varies passively with CPP. In hypertensive patients, the upper and lower limits of this range are extended. Autoregulation is altered by volatile anesthetics and is dose dependent; at deep levels of anesthesia CBF is pressure dependent.

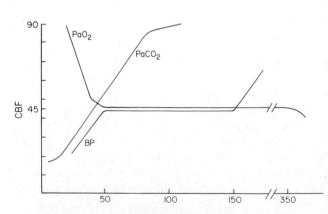

FIGURE 27–1. Changes in cerebral blood flow (ml/100/gm/min). Changes in the arterial partial pressure of CO_2 or O_2 or in the level of mean arterial blood pressure are indicated on the abscissa. The indicated line represents the resultant alteration in cerebral blood flow. (Reproduced with permission from Beal JM (ed): Critical Care for Surgical Patients. New York, Macmillan Co, 1981.)

Autoregulation may also be lost in the presence of brain tumors, infarct, subdural hematoma, hypoxia, hypercapnia above 80 torr, and drug therapy with ketamine or sodium nitroprusside. Changes in blood flow as a result of autoregulation may take several minutes before cerebrovascular resistance responds to altered CPP. The mechanism of autoregulation of CBF is unclear; metabolic, chemical, myogenic, and neurogenic mechanisms have been postulated. A probable explanation is that CBF autoregulation occurs as the result of an intrinsic response in arteriolar smooth muscle to distention or relaxation caused by changes in intraluminal pressure.

The Influence of Oxygen on CBF

Oxygen at concentrations clinically used exerts little effect on CBF (see Fig. 27–1). A measurable change occurs if Pa_{O_2} falls below 50 torr, whereupon CBF increases, reaching twice normal values at a Pa_{O_2} of 20 torr. That increases in cerebral lactate concentration also occur at low Pa_{O_2} values suggests that tissue H^+ concentration is the controlling factor. CBF will decrease by 10 to 15 per cent at 1 atmosphere and by 20 to 25 per cent at 2 atmospheres partial pressure of inspired oxygen. Brain tissue H^+ concentration does not appear to be involved in the cerebral vasoconstriction occurring at high inspired oxygen concentrations. Oxygen may have a direct vasoconstricting effect on cerebral vessels.

Drug Effects on CBF

Although many drugs are without effect on CBF, the list of directly or indirectly acting cerebral vasoactive drugs is impressive. The vasodilators include volatile anesthetic agents; acetazolamide (Diamox); drugs that can increase Pa_{CO_2}, such as the opioids; those that stimulate cerebral neuronal activity like the amphetamines, epinephrine, and ketamine; and directly acting substances, such as papaverine and nitroprusside. The vasoconstrictors, acting either directly or indirectly, include thiopental, etomidate, Althesin, and the xanthine derivatives. Norepinephrine, trimethaphan, and the alpha-receptor blockers are without direct effect on CBF except through blood pressure–mediated actions.

INTRACRANIAL PRESSURE (ICP)

Blood flow, intra-arterial blood pressure, and their interaction with intracranial contents regulate the level of ICP. Normally, ICP is in the 3- to 15-torr range in the supine position with the head in the midline and lower when in the sitting or standing position because of the effect of gravity. The composition of the three intracranial compartments is essentially aqueous and noncompressible but, as noted earlier, CSF and venous blood can be displaced from the skull. An intracranial compliance curve describes the relation between the volume of intracranial contents and the ICP, a nonlinear function (Fig. 27–2). An initial increase in volume causes little change in ICP through the compensatory responses of CSF and blood. Continued augmentation in volume mildly raises ICP as compensatory mechanisms approach their limits. Finally, even a small change in volume results in a large elevation in ICP. A further volume change may alter the shape or normal position of the brain; although noncompressible, the brain can be distorted in a plastic fashion. A shift occurs through the tentorium or foramen magnum, resulting in herniation and pressure on vital brain stem centers and imperiling survival before the primary process causing the increased ICP becomes the direct cause. Alternatively, cerebral ischemia may develop at high levels of ICP because of concurrent reduction in CPP.

The management of patients with head trauma or intracranial mass lesions requires monitoring of ICP. Measurement of the static value of ICP alone is inadequate, as it

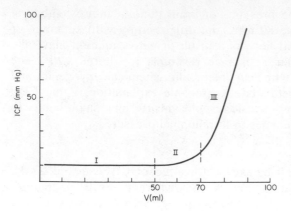

FIGURE 27–2. This curve represents the changes in intracranial pressure ICP (mm Hg) concomitant with changes in intracranial volume (V/ml). *I,* the zone of normal compliance; *II,* the zone of limited compliance as with an intracranial mass lesion; *III,* exhaustion of compensatory mechanisms and area of noncompliance. (Reproduced with permission from Beal JM (ed): Critical Care for Surgical Patients. New York, Macmillan Co, 1981.)

provides no information concerning the ability of compensatory mechanisms to tolerate further change in intracranial volume. A continuously recorded ICP can be obtained via an intraventricular catheter or by a device placed within the subarachnoid or epidural space. Techniques that utilize external transducers are preferred so that zero adjustment and recalibration checks can easily be made. Tracings of intracranial pressure waves have been classified by Lundberg as A (plateau), B, and C waves. The A waves occur during increased ICP, may last 10 to 20 minutes, and indicate that a patient is approaching the limits of volume compensation. A waves may be induced by painful stimuli, laryngoscopy, and tracheal intubation; during induction of anesthesia with vasodilating anesthetics; or by surgical stimulation during light planes of anesthesia. Compliance measurements are made by injecting a small volume of saline (0.1 to 2 ml) through an indwelling intraventricular catheter and then measuring the change in ICP. An increase of less than 2 torr that rapidly returns to baseline indicates that the pressure lies on the flat portion of the volume pressure curve. Large changes that persist or that return slowly to baseline indicate low compliance and danger of compression phenomena even though resting ICP is normal.

ANESTHESIA FOR PATIENTS WITH INTRACRANIAL MASS LESIONS

MONITORING

Intracranial trauma, mass lesions, induced hypotension, operations performed near the vital centers of the brain or done with a patient in the sitting position, and resection of vascular tumors are situations in which patient care may be improved by precise monitoring techniques. These include measurement of intra-arterial pressure, an electrocardiogram, and central venous pressure. Occasionally, pulmonary artery pressure monitoring, recording of minute volume ventilation and end tidal CO_2, intermittent blood gas analysis, monitoring of urinary output and esophageal temperature changes, assessment of neuromuscular function (see Chapter 15), and ICP monitoring are called for. Further monitoring may involve the use of a precordial Doppler ultrasound transducer (for detection of air embolism), an esophageal stethoscope, and a display of evoked cerebral potentials.

PREOPERATIVE ASSESSMENT AND PREMEDICATION

Preoperative evaluation should include a search for evidence of increased ICP. Nausea and vomiting, alterations in the level of consciousness, or pupillary dilation or decreased reactivity of the pupils to light may indicate the presence of elevated ICP. Retinal papilledema, bradycardia with hypertension, and disturbances in respiratory pattern definitely implicate raised ICP. X-ray or computerized axial tomography may provide evidence of displacement of the brain. If an intraventricular catheter has been inserted, intracranial compliance should be assessed. Opioids and long-acting barbiturates should be avoided, but diazepam and atropine are useful medicants. The safest course is to omit premedication when feasible.

INDUCTION AND MAINTENANCE OF ANESTHESIA

In patients with poor compliance or high ICP, measures to improve compliance include elevation of the head by tilting 10 to 15 degrees; administration of adrenocortical steroids, mannitol, or both; passive hyperventilation during induction; and avoidance of drugs and maneuvers that adversely affect compliance. In patients with closed head trauma or intracranial mass lesions in whom ICP measurements are not available and who show no evidence of elevated ICP, it is best to assume that compliance is at the knee of the curve (see Fig. 27–2, position II) and to take precautions against further volume changes.

Anesthetics that reduce or do not alter CBF are preferred, but choice is limited. All volatile anesthetics increase CBF and ICP and decrease $CMRO_2$ and CPP, although the effect is dose related. Thiopental and other intravenous agents used for induction, with the exception of ketamine, exert an opposite effect. We employ an induction dose of thiopental (3 to 5 mg/kg), followed by passive hyperventilation to a Pa_{CO_2} of 25 to 30 torr preceding administration of halothane, to avoid an increase in CBF and ICP. An alternative approach is to combine thiopental induction with intermittent intravenous doses of fentanyl (4 to 5 μg/kg) and droperidol (0.3 mg/kg) and to inject pancuronium (0.1 mg/kg) for neuromuscular blockade. Muscle paralysis is monitored while laryngoscopy and topical administration of 4 per cent lidocaine are delayed until relaxation is well established; the trachea is then intubated. Hyperventilation is again practiced when nitrous oxide (50 to 70 per cent) is used. Intermittent doses of fentanyl and pancuronium are then used for maintenance of anesthesia.

The head should be positioned to promote venous drainage. Infiltration of the scalp with 0.5 per cent lidocaine without epinephrine helps to prevent the hypertension sometimes seen with an incision. Minimal concentrations (0.5 per cent) of halothane may be used to prevent undesirable elevations of blood pressure. Osmotic and renal loop diuretics are used as indicated, and fluids are administered to maintain a slight negative fluid balance. Intravenous balanced salt solutions are preferred to avoid rebound cerebral edema, which is more common with the administration of dextrose in water. Colloidal solutions may be required to maintain normal osmotic pressure.

Upon dural closure, preparation should be made to awaken the patient without coughing or straining in reaction to the presence of the endotracheal tube. Thiopental (25 to 50 mg) or lidocaine (50 to 100 mg) given intravenously immediately before bandaging the head tends to promote smooth emergence and extubation. The airway is suctioned only if needed and then before reversing the neuromuscular block. Occasionally, naloxone is injected to reverse the respiratory depressant effect of opioids. Should pulmonary ventilation be inadequate at the end of the procedure, the endotracheal tube is left in place and ventilation continued mechanically. At some subsequent period, when ICP is within normal range, the orotracheal tube is exchanged for a nasotracheal tube if continued respiratory support is required.

PERIOPERATIVE EVALUATION OF NEUROSURGICAL PATIENTS

Improvements in monitoring and data management allow early detection of brain ischemia or elevation in ICP in the neurosurgical patient. Periodic evaluation and recording of vital signs (blood pressure, pulse, temperature, respiratory rate and pattern, and ICP level, pressure pattern, and compliance) and clinical neurologic function permit early recognition of complications. The Glasgow Coma Scale (Table 27–1) is used in some neurosurgical ICUs. Some also assign points to specific functions such as motor ability, phonation, shivering, muscle tone, level of consciousness, orientation, exercises of mental function, ocular muscle function, facial symmetry, tongue protrusion, finger-to-nose test, muscle strength, and reflex responses. Similar evaluations recorded regularly on special charts offer a sensitive and reproducible evaluation of neurologic status.

ANESTHESIA FOR PATIENTS WITH ANEURYSMS

Patients with intracranial aneurysms are usually seen following an acute subarachnoid hemorrhage and thereafter require control of blood pressure to prevent rebleeding, facilitate eventual clipping of the aneurysm, and avoid postoperative bleeding and vasospasm.

Most surgeons delay diagnostic studies for seven to ten days after the initial hemorrhage, as operative mortality during this period is high. Difficult operating conditions and persistent vasospasm complicate the operation, undertaken shortly after computerized tomography or angiography is completed. Others delay operation pending clinical and angiographic evidence of resolution of vasospasm.

Electrocardiographic abnormalities, probably induced by the acute hemorrhage, are seen preoperatively in about 60 per cent of these patients, resolving within ten days. Most frequently seen are T wave inversion or flattening, altered ST segments, U waves, prolonged QT interval, sinus bradycardia, premature ventricular contractions, and ventricular tachycardia. In the absence of a past history of ischemic heart disease, these are not contraindications to use of deliberate hypotension.

Induction of anesthesia must be carefully done to avoid alteration of transluminal pressure in the aneurysm and to minimize danger of rupture. Rupture during induction is more ominous than during craniotomy because a marked elevation of ICP occurs and cerebral ischemia may develop as CPP falls. Induction and maintenance of anesthesia follow the principles set forth earlier for management of patients with mass lesions. Controlled hypotension facilitates dissection and placement of clips, reduces the incidence of aneurysm rupture, and decreases rate of blood loss should rupture occur.

TABLE 27–1. Glasgow Coma Scale*

Eye opening	Spontaneous	4
	To speech	3
	To pain	2
	Nil	1
Verbal response	Oriented	5
	Confused conversation	4
	Inappropriate words	3
	Incomprehensible sounds	2
	Nil	1
Best motor response	Obeys	6
	Localizes	5
	Withdraws (flexion)	4
	Abnormal flexion	3
	Extensor response	2
	Nil	1

*Reproduced with permission from Teasdale G, Jennett B: Assessment of coma and impaired consciousness —a practical scale. Lancet 2:81, 1974.

There are no reliable data to indicate that one hypotensive technique is superior to another. We prefer the use of nitroprusside (see Chapter 31) during the period when the aneurysm is being manipulated and clipped or earlier should rupture occur.

Tracheal extubation should be delayed in patients obtunded preoperatively and in all patients with serious intraoperative complications. Tracheal extubation is done postoperatively when neurologic status is stable and adequacy of ventilation assured. Care is essential during application of the head dressing and in extubation of the trachea to avoid coughing or straining as earlier described.

ANESTHESIA FOR PATIENTS OPERATED ON IN THE SITTING POSITION

Many surgeons prefer the patient to be in the sitting position for operations performed in the posterior fossa, as this allows access to all parts of the fossa while blood drains from the operative site and arterial blood pressure is moderately reduced. The position interferes less with spontaneous respiration as compared with the lateral or prone position. Disadvantages include the possibility of air embolism, uncontrollable hypotension, demanding and time-consuming positioning, difficulty in returning the patient to the supine position in an emergency, and reduced cerebral blood flow, which may result from postural hypotension, intermittent positive pressure ventilation, or hypocapnia. The two most important problems in the sitting position comprise hypotension and venous air embolism (see Chapter 32). Blood pressure should be maintained near the preoperative level by avoiding or minimizing use of vasodilating agents, deep anesthesia, and hypovolemia. Elevating and wrapping the legs decreases venous pooling. Vasopressor drugs are seldom necessary to restore CPP.

Venous air embolism occurs in the sitting position, as the cerebral diploic veins are noncollapsible because of their bony attachments and venous sinuses in the skull remain patent through their dural attachments. Air entering the veins is rapidly carried to the right heart and pulmonary circulation, producing ventricular outflow obstruction and cardiac arrhythmias (see Chapters 32 and 33). Controlled ventilation during the operation decreases the incidence of air embolism.

ANESTHESIA FOR PATIENTS WITH SPINAL CORD INJURIES

Surgery on the spinal column may entail excision of a herniated intervertebral disc, correction of spondylosis, resection of neoplasms, drainage of infectious lesions, spinal fusion, correction of scoliosis, and stabilization of the spine after trauma to back and neck. Problems include any of the following.

Difficult Tracheal Intubation

Patients with unstable cervical fractures are at risk during attempted tracheal intubation owing to undue flexion or extension of the neck. Pressure on the cervical cord may occur, converting a minimal neurologic deficit into a major one. Conventional orotracheal intubation may be impossible. Usually a nasotracheal tube can be inserted during topical or general anesthesia. The fiberoptic bronchoscope has proved invaluable in this situation (see Chapter 16). Positioning the patient for operation requires particular care to avoid cervical cord damage.

Respiratory Disturbances

Pulmonary ventilation is often compromised by diaphragmatic or intercostal paralysis, preexisting chest disease, or kyphoscoliosis. Pulmonary function tests, such as vital capacity (VC) and forced expiratory volume (FEV), should be performed preoperatively and arterial blood gases obtained as guides to postoperative ventilatory management.

Vasomotor Instability

Precipitous hypotension may occur during positioning of a patient with high spinal cord transsection or a patient immobilized for a long period prior to operation. This results from a discrepancy between circulatory capacity and blood volume, which responds well to intravenous fluids and appropriate doses of phenylephrine or ephedrine.

Hyperkalemia

Succinylcholine administered to patients with neurologic motor deficits may produce precipitous hyperkalemia (see Chapter 15). Therefore, the drug is contraindicated in patients with acute or long-standing upper motor neuron lesions.

Evoked Potential Monitoring

Monitoring of somatosensory evoked potentials is useful during operations on the spine. Application of electrical stimuli to a peripheral nerve, such as the peroneal, and recording evoked responses via scalp electrodes placed over the appropriate area of the sensory cortex allow for continuous observation of spinal cord function. The impulse thus originating below the operative site is conducted over lateral afferent pathways through the spinal area of operation and recorded at brain level. Ischemia or cord compression changes the latency and amplitude of the recorded signal, which in general represents 30 to 50 evoked responses by computer averaging. The findings are immediately reported to the surgeon so that if corrective measures are instituted, cord injury may be avoided and the evoked response returns to the normal state.

Pulmonary Ventilation and Choice of Anesthesia

Impairment of ventilation is likely with high spinal cord injury, so that manually controlled or mechanical ventilation is usually necessary. A nitrous oxide–oxygen–neuromuscular block technique, with or without supplementation with low concentrations of a volatile agent, is our choice. Studies on the regulation of spinal cord blood flow suggest mechanisms that are the same as those that control cerebral blood flow. Because of the tenuous nature of the arterial supply to the cord, hypocarbia should be avoided. Similarly, arterial hypotension may lower perfusion pressure, especially in patients with recent cord trauma, in whom normal autoregulatory mechanisms are most often absent and tissue edema impedes cord perfusion.

REFERENCES

Albin MS, Carroll RG, Naroon JC: Clinical considerations concerning detection of venous air embolism. J Neurosurg 3:380, 1978.

Campkin TV, Turner JM: Neurosurgical Anesthesia and Intensive Care. Boston, Butterworth Publishers, 1980.

Cottrell JE, Turndorf H: Anesthesia and Neurosurgery. St Louis, CV Mosby, 1980.

English JB, Westenskow D, Hodges MR, Stanley TH: Comparison of venous air embolism monitoring methods in supine dogs. Anesthesiology 48:425, 1978.

Koht A, Cerullo LJ: Management of patients with elevated intracranial pressure. In Beal JM (ed.): Critical Care for Surgical Patients. New York, Macmillan Pub. Co., 1981.

Marsh ML, Marshall LF, Shapiro HM: Neurosurgical intensive care. Anesthesiology 47:149, 1977.

Shapiro HM: Intracranial hypertension. Anesthesiology 43:445, 1975.

Siesjo BK: Brain Energy Metabolism. New York, John Wiley & Sons, 1978.

Smith AL, Wollman H: Cerebral blood flow and metabolism: Effect of anesthetic drugs and techniques. Anesthesiology 36:378, 1972.

Trubuhovich RV: Management of acute intracranial disasters. Int Anesth Clin 17:3, 1979.

Chapter 28
GERIATRICS

Anesthetists are inclined to look upon the elderly as if they are diseased and often express surprise when the octo- or nonagenarian shows few abnormal physical or laboratory findings. The truth is that old age is not a disease but a fundamental biologic alteration, designated as the aging process, characteristic of all living matter. Alfred Worcester once said, "There are no diseases peculiar to old age and very few from which it is exempt." Nevertheless, we know that there are features of aging that can account for the well-documented higher morbidity and mortality in the geriatric surgical patient. No doubt these figures relate, in general, to a gradual deterioration in physiologic function with age (Fig. 28–1), estimated to be about a 0.8 to 0.9 per cent loss per year of the functional capacity present at age 30. Before going on to a description of these changes and their anesthetic implications, let us look at the profile of geriatric surgical practice as gathered from our own experience.

THE GERIATRIC POPULATION

The rate and expectation of dying are exponentially related to age. Although longevity remains constant for any species (approximately 100 years in man), the life expectancy is now about 73.8 years for men and 77.7 years for women. Most of the improvement, as compared with the lives of our ancestors, occurred between the years 1900 and 1950, with resolution of a large number of deaths before age 65, particularly in infancy. Thus, in 1970, the percentage of individuals in the population living over the age of 65 was 9.8 per cent. The median age of the population is now (1981) estimated to be 30 and possibly may be 40 by the year 2000. Therefore, one might expect those over the age of 65 to increase to about 52 million, or 16 per cent of the population, in the third millennium.

SURGICAL PROCEDURES

Operations performed on people over the age of 70 are usually major, more often than not emergencies of a kind, involving the gastrointestinal tract, the genitourinary system, orthopedics, the peripheral circulation, the heart, and the brain. Many of the elective operations pertain to malignancy and fewer to hernias and anorectal disease. Furthermore, the operations tend to take longer, and re-operations are common.

POSTOPERATIVE MORBIDITY AND MORTALITY

As might be expected, complications related to the heart and blood vessels head the list, including the cerebral circulation; followed closely by the lung with atelectases,

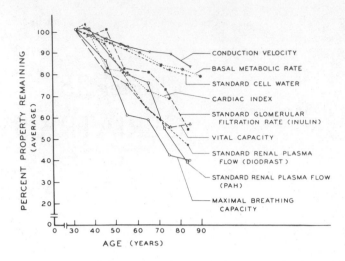

FIGURE 28–1. Percentage of various human functional capacities or properties remaining at various ages. (Reproduced with permission from Strehler BL: Q Rev Biol 34:117, 1959. Data from Shock et al.)

pneumonias, pulmonary emboli, and gastric aspiration; and then by indolent infections. The elderly patient in an intensive care setting often develops multi-organ system failure.

PHYSIOLOGIC CHANGES AND IMPLICATIONS FOR ANESTHESIA

As previously noted, medical personnel have a fairly clear notion of the characteristics of old age (Table 28–1). These impressions are confirmed by physiologic measurements, as will be seen in the following discussion.

THE CENTRAL NERVOUS SYSTEM

The aging of the human brain is the most crucial of the various effects of the passage of time because the senescence of this organ and other appended parts of the CNS produces both personal suffering and effects on other system performance.

BL STREHLER

Subtle Aspects of Loss of Cognition. Called *senility,* the common manifestations are confusion, memory loss, delusions, emotional instability, and puerile behavior. One should not overlook the possibility that any of these symptoms may relate to actual disease and that the symptoms are exaggerated in the institutional environment, by condescension or neglect on the part of attendants, and, most important of all, by the ill-advised use of drugs. Thus, in these people (let us say those over the age of 70), sedatives and tranquilizers might well be eliminated from preoperative and postoperative medication, used only in small dosages at best.

Altered Sleep Patterns. During sleep in the elderly, episodes of apnea and periodic breathing are common, probably related to cerebral arteriosclerosis. For the same

TABLE 28–1.   Characteristics of Old Age

High pain threshold	Dementia
Altered response to stress	Malnutrition
Arteriosclerosis	Anemia — low blood volume
Diminished autonomic tone	Diabetes
Edentia	Poor renal function
Emphysema	

pathologic reason, hyperventilation readily results in apnea. On the other hand, total sleep time in the aged is not greatly reduced. It may take longer to fall asleep, awakening is more frequent, the time spent abed while awake is longer, and the amount of time in the REM phase is reduced. Consequently, one should not be hasty in prescribing medications for sleep. In fact, many of the elderly decline this assistance; others proclaim that they get no sleep at all.

Neural Transmssion. In the aged, visually evoked responses (VER) in the brain show both a delayed latency and slower conduction velocity as compared with those in the young. Drugs would tend to enhance this tendency.

Susceptibility to General Anesthesia. Gregory showed that the minimum anesthetic concentration (MAC) declines progressively with advancing age, thus demonstrating a lesser need for high anesthetic doses with their attendant depressant effects on circulation and respiration (Fig. 28–2).

Altered Response to Drugs

Pain. Many physicians have the impression that the pain threshold is elevated in the aged. In this connection one notes that the incidence of postlumbar puncture headache begins to decline over age 70, perhaps a manifestation of a general reduction in neural elements and lesser distensibility of intracranial pain-sensitive blood vessels. Bellville and associates found that the mean sum of the intensity differences in pain relief after administration of morphine or pentazocine was significantly greater in the elderly. Thus, lesser amounts of opioids are required for analgesia, an important observation considering the respiratory and circulatory depressant actions of these drugs.

Anticholinergics. Dauchet and Gravenstein demonstrated a lesser degree of tachycardia following atropine administration in the elderly. Atrioventricular dissociation was also a common finding, whereas atrial chronotropic and conduction abnormalities were more prominent in the young. Pupillary responses to atropine were diminished.

Pharmacokinetics. The Boston Collaborative Drug Surveillance Group found that usual doses of diazepam produced a more profound and prolonged depression in the elderly as compared with the young. Relatedly, Malley and coworkers found that the half-lives of antipyrene and phenylbutazone were greater by 45 and 29 per cent, respectively, in an older age group as compared with a younger group.

Other available observations confirm the dictum that the older age group is more susceptible to the actions of all manner of drugs.

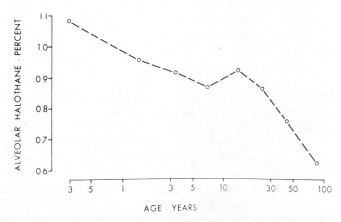

FIGURE 28–2. Mean alveolar halothane concentration versus age. (Reproduced with permission from Gregory GA, et al: The relationship between age and halothane requirement in man. Anesthesiology 30:488, 1969.)

THE CIRCULATION

Autonomic Nervous System. Duke and colleagues assessed the integrity of the autonomic nervous system in terms of baroreceptor reflexes. Performance of the Valsalva maneuver in the aged was marked by a more profound depression of mean arterial blood pressure during the positive thoracic pressure phase, and the subsequent "overshoot" was less as compared with a younger control group. Perhaps a chronic reduction in blood volume played a role in this response. Likewise, the slope of the curve relating an increase in the PR interval (bradycardia) on the electrocardiogram to a rise in mean arterial blood induced by intravenous phenylephrine was flattened and shifted to the right. These manifestations of diminished autonomic regulation bespeak instability of the circulation in the aged and the need for cautious anesthetic administration.

Regional Blood Flow. In measuring cerebral blood flow in the elderly with the nitrous oxide method, Kety found a progressive diminution in flow, cerebral oxygen consumption, and responsiveness of the cerebral vessels to a rise in Pa_{CO_2}. The reductions were most pronounced in those obviously senile. These findings, in conjunction with alterations in pulmonary function discussed later on, readily explain the prolonged induction of inhalation anesthesia and the susceptibility to stroke with a precipitous fall in blood pressure in the aged.

Liver and kidney function also become less efficient with aging. Acute tubular necrosis and liver failure readily occur after otherwise minor insults in the elderly.

Myocardial Performance. As depicted in Figure 28–1, cardiac output and the cardiac index slowly decline with advancing age. Thus, with progressive asymptomatic coronary arteriosclerosis, the performance of the heart is impeded, more readily affected by potent general anesthetics, and more susceptible to hypoxia and development of myocardial infarction. A recent study employing radionuclide angiocardiography has shown little influence of aging in the resting individual on the left ventricular ejection fraction, end diastolic volume, and regional wall motion. With exercise, however, a decline in the ejection fraction to less than 60 per cent of control was observed in 45 per cent of subjects over age 60 as compared with only 2 per cent in the younger group. Wall motion abnormalities were observed with increasing frequency in patients over age 50 during exercise. These age-related changes in ejection fraction during exercise were not associated with differences in end diastolic volumes or mean arterial blood pressure.

Respiration, Central and Peripheral. Note was made previously of the tendency toward abnormal breathing patterns and the ease of producing apnea via hyperventilation. These changes are accentuated by the opioids; carbon dioxide narcosis and apnea are fairly common occurrences in the aged when their susceptibility to respiratory depressant drugs is overlooked.

Years ago, Pontoppidan found a diminution in respiratory tract reflexes in the elderly, as demonstrated by a reduction in cough and breath holding in response to irritant concentrations of ammonia gas. Undoubtedly this phenomenon explains in part the frequent finding of silent aspiration of gastric contents in the elderly medical patient and the high incidence postoperatively.

Senile emphysema is a common radiologic diagnosis based on the increased diameter of the chest and heightened translucency of the lungs. However, this gross observation, often unconfirmed physiologically, is underscored by repeatedly confirmed data indicating that the elderly have an increase in the residual capacity of the lungs, a diminution in all static lung volumes, a decrease in forced expiratory volumes (FEV) and maximum breathing capacity (MBC), a diminution in the diffusing capacity of the lungs, and a progressive fall in Pa_{O_2} with advancing age (Fig. 28–3).

In view of these senescent respiratory changes, it is not unusual to experience

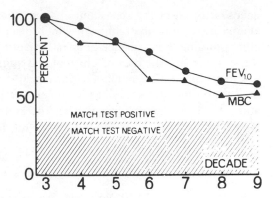

FIGURE 28–3. Percentage change in maximal breathing capacity (MBC) and forced expiratory volume (FEV) with age in normal subjects. (Reproduced with permission from Mithoefer JC, Karetzky MS: The cardiopulmonary system in the aged. *In* Powers JD (ed): Surgery of the Aged and Debilitated Patient. Philadelphia, WB Saunders, 1968.)

problems in induction of general anesthesia, difficulty in ventilation, and a high incidence of postoperative pulmonary complications. Respiration must not be further impeded by ill-considered drug usage.

Stress Response and Biochemical Alterations.   Although the usual tests for adrenocortical function or catecholamine secretion show no marked change with aging, little doubt exists in regard to the diminished response to stress; less resistance to infection, its indolent nature and muted febrile reactions; diminution in autonomic reflexes; and multi-organ system failure when one system gives way, as in hepatic failure after renal insufficiency or congestive heart failure with pulmonary infection. Biologists contend that the progressive increase in malignancy with age is a manifestation of diminishing immunogenicity, also explaining the infection phenomenon and refractoriness to chemotherapy in treatment of cancer and lymphomas.

In the elderly, the appearance of hyperglycemia is known as adult onset diabetes, whereas anemia and subtle signs of malnutrition are commonplace.

Physical Changes.   At this point it will suffice merely to list the changes of senescence, as they are so readily evident: 1) ocular changes: arcus senilis, cataract formation, glaucoma, sluggish pupils, presbyopia, retinal vessel arteriosclerosis; 2) generalized loss of elastic tissue and collagen: little subcutaneous tissue, tortuous fragile blood vessels, cutaneous pigmentation, keratosis (easy bruisability is demonstrated, so that one should not apply a face mask tightly, take great care in positioning for operation, and maintain surface pressure for some time after failed venipuncture); 3) tooth loss and loss of jaw substance conducive to poor mask fit and trauma during intubation; 4) osteoporosis: hip and wrist fractures, vertebral fractures and collapse, loss of disc substance, kyphoscoliosis, ossified spinal ligaments, diminution in body height, bone pain; 5) urinary tract obstruction in men, relaxation incontinence in women.

Every one of these structural alterations has bearing on anesthetic technique; mask fit for general anesthesia, difficulty in lumbar puncture for spinal and peridural anesthesia, plus altered dosage when employing these methods. In the immediate postanesthetic period, awakening is often delayed despite low anesthetic dosage; confusion, struggling, and attempts to get out of bed are also common. Rather than resort to the usual pharmacologic therapies, low dosage of opioids is the watchword. More important, however, are the understanding, reassurance, and constant surveillance provided by devoted and informed recovery room nurses and attendants.

APPRAISAL

Rather than supply a list of aphorisms, or do's and don't's, we have chosen to define the essence of good anesthetic care in the aged by listing some but not necessarily all of the senescent changes that bear upon the anesthetic process. These changes are the substratum on which disease in the elderly is superimposed, thereby compounding the problems of anesthetization. The picture might at first seem grim, but there are many degrees of chronologic aging, and age cannot be used as the sole criterion in anesthesia practice. Many a 70- or 80-year-old, normally active and in full possession of intellect, will fare nicely during and after a complex lengthy operation and attendant exacting anesthetic. The key would seem to lie in the recognition of the possibilities for harm in the technical and pharmacologic aspects of anesthesia.

REFERENCES

Bellville JW, Forrest WH, Miller E, et al: Influence of age on pain relief from analgesics. JAMA 217:1835, 1971.
Del Guericio LRM, Cohn JD: Monitoring operative risk in the elderly. JAMA 243:1350, 1980.
Duke PC, Wade JG, Hickey RF, et al: The effects of age on baroreceptor function in man. Can Anaesth Soc J 23:111, 1976.
Fries JF: Aging, natural death, and the compression of morbidity. N Engl J Med 303:130, 1980.
Hayflick L: The cell biology of human aging. N Engl J Med 295:1302, 1976.
Kennie DC, Moore JT: Management of senile dementia. AFP 22:105, 1980.
Port S, Cobb FR, Coleman ER, et al: Effect of age on the response of the left ventricular ejection fraction to exercise. N Engl J Med 303:1133, 1980.

Chapter 29

ANESTHESIA FOR OUTPATIENT SURGERY

At one time most physicians' offices contained a room where minor operations could be performed, a practice carried out in dentists' offices to this day. Whereas the latter chose general anesthesia, the former used local anesthesia for excision of cutaneous and superficially placed lesions, suture of lacerations, reduction of fractures, and endoscopy of the gastrointestinal and urological tracts. However, office treatments were not included in the development of third party payment plans for medical and surgical care. Therefore, minor operative procedures were moved to hospitals and operating suites where, naturally, the operations increased in complexity. As costs in the hospital setting increased, plans emerged whereby these procedures could be done essentially apart from hospital activities in general: in free-standing units not connected with a hospital; in units within hospital where operations were done in the major operating suite; and in separate, fully contained units within hospital. Regardless of the site, patients were to be admitted and discharged on the same day for surgical day care, ambulatory surgical care, outpatient surgery, or daytime minor surgery, as the plans were variously designated. For licensing purposes, all of these facilities had to rely on a general hospital for back-up care should the need arise.

Thus far, the performance in these units has been judged excellent with regard to safety and outcome, but health provider analysts still debate the matter of benefits if all indirect costs are taken into account. Nevertheless, savings seem to be largest in the free-standing unit, followed, in descending order, by the self-contained hospital facility and the hospital-incorporated operating room plan.

WHO BENEFITS

For the surgeon, the convenience is considerable; the schedule runs on time, nursing and anesthetic care is acceptable, re-imbursement is easily forthcoming, and there is no need for elaborate hospital office facilities and specialized staff. Insurers, both private and governmental, look upon this service as cost saving and readily accountable. The hospital may find that beds are more readily available when the census is high. Lastly and most importantly, the hospital stay is abbreviated and more acceptable to patients, financial and personal arrangements more easily settled, separation from family brief, and the aftercare at home more congenial and less institutionalized. Anesthetists appreciate the regular hours and predictable surgical outcome.

TABLE 29–1. Outpatient Operations

Dental	*Otolaryngology*
Extraction of teeth, restorations	Septoplasty
General	Myringotomy—drainage tube insertion/removal
Pediatric herniorrhaphy, orchiopexy	Otoplasty
Incision and drainage of abscess	Removal of foreign bodies
Suture of lacerations	Reduction of nasal fracture
Breast and node biopsy	Laryngoscopy
Nerve and muscle biopsy	T and A
Hemorrhoidectomy	*Plastic*
Fissure and fistula procedures	Excision of skin lesions
Gynecology	Augmentation mammoplasty
D and C, excision of cervical polyp	Scar revisions
Bartholin cyst excision	Rhinoplasty
Laparoscopy	Cosmetic procedures
Abortion	*Thoracic*
Ophthalmology	Esophagoscopy
Eye muscle procedures	Bronchoscopy
Tear duct probing	Esophageal dilation
Eyelid ptosis procedures	*Urology*
Iridectomy	Cystoscopy
Orthopedic	Meatotomy
Cast change, manipulations	Orchiopexy
Fracture reduction	Circumcision
Carpal tunnel procedures	Vasectomy
Removal of hardware	
Removal of plantar neuroma	
Trigger finger and De Quervain's disease repair	
Ganglion excision	
Arthroscopy	

KINDS OF OPERATIONS DONE

Although from an anesthesia standpoint no operation can be considered minor, the kinds of operation performed on an outpatient basis do indeed fall into that category. Table 29–1 presents a compilation of operations done in the various facilities from which reports have arisen.

ESSENTIALS OF PATIENT CARE

Almost without exception, patients fall into physical status categories I and II, the former predominating. An occasional emergency may be taken care of under strict regulations. The surgeon concerned will have sent to the facility, at least 24 hours beforehand, a complete history, physical examination, results of laboratory examinations, a signed consent, and orders for preoperative, intraoperative and postoperative care; all these details are easily handled on printed forms. With a day's notice, any possible contraindication to anesthesia may be detected before the scheduled time, additional data obtained, or the procedure cancelled without too much difficulty.

Given a packet of informational materials, patients will know when and where to report, how long the stay will be, and how to conduct themselves personally. Some of the essentials are listed in Table 29–2. Upon entry to the facility, credentials are checked; the patient admitted to a secluded bed; clothing changed; compliance with preoperative instructions reviewed; and temperature, pulse, respiratory rate, and blood pressure recorded.

Next, the anesthetist visits the patient, having first reviewed the records. Standard questions are asked and data recorded: state of health, prior anesthetic experiences, drugs ingested, allergies, familial responses to anesthetics and drugs, smoking and

TABLE 29–2. Directions for Patients

Time and place of registration, two hours preop
Calling in, URI, cancellations
NPO 10 hours
Escort to and from facility
Food service
Time and manner of discharge

Personal belongings (comb, brush, toothbrush, etc.)
Comfortable clothing easily stored
Light reading material
Valuables left at home
Remove nail polish, cosmetics, prostheses
Family waiting area, services
No driving, alcohol, major decisions postop
How and where to report complications
Possibility of longer stay
Cancellation: full stomach, late arrival, no escort, acute URI

alcohol habits, and occupation. Physical characteristics are noted, particularly body habitus, the airway and teeth, and physical deformities, and the heart and lungs are examined. An explanation of the anesthesia procedure is given including intravenous infusion, premedication, monitoring during anesthesia, kind of induction, maintenance with regional or general anesthesia, by mask or endotracheal tube, emergence, recovery, and expectation as to outcome. Acceptance of the procedure is assured and a physical status assigned.

ANESTHESIA

Although patients are admitted early in the day and the projected stay is considered to last from four to six hours postoperatively, the essence of this brand of anesthesia is rapid recovery. Thus, premedication given intravenously just before the start may consist merely of an opioid, e.g., fentanyl, and a tranquilizer such as diazepam or lorazepam. Most anesthetists avoid droperidol or droperidol plus fentanyl or ketamine as being relatively long lasting and possessing other well-known objectionable properties.

As indicated in Table 29–3, regional anesthesia is more common than general anesthesia. Although caudal and epidural anesthesia are employed, most practitioners avoid spinal anesthesia because of possible development of headache and problems in management later on as well as residual autonomic blockade at the time of discharge. In any case, short-acting local anesthetics are favored.

For general anesthesia, minimal amounts of short-acting intravenous barbiturates

TABLE 29–3. Anesthesia

Regional
Infiltration, field block
Digital, ankle block
IV regional
Brachial, cervical plexus block
Caudal, epidural
General
Mask or endotracheal
Balanced technique
Nitrous oxide, enflurane, forane

TABLE 29–4. Reported Complications

Hemorrhage (T and A, laparoscopy, mammoplasty)
Persistent nausea and vomiting
Infection
Perforated uterus (D and C)
Bowel burn, distention, pain (laparoscopy)
Airway edema
Delayed recovery from anesthesia
Chemical phlebitis
Psychotic reactions

are given for induction, followed by mask or endotracheal general anesthesia. Tracheal intubation, as in blind nasal insertion for dentistry or oral insertion for laparoscopy, is preceded by tubocurarine to block fasciculations produced by succinylcholine. Nitrous oxide is the mainstay, in conjunction with potent general anesthetics of lesser solubility, i.e., enflurane or forane. Anesthesia is maintained in the lightest plane, with opioid supplementation and succinylcholine infusion when required. Reversal of opioid and neuromuscular blocking effects can be done when larger amounts are used.

Monitoring of vital signs is practiced as for any regular anesthetic and a record kept of all events.

RECOVERY

This takes place in an area just like any recovery room that looks after postanesthetic problems. Many patients given regional anesthesia may be returned to the original entry site without a recovery room stopover. Rules for discharge to room are the same, with constant physician supervision. Complications occurring during operation and anesthesia may dictate an overnight stay in the hospital; perforated uterus, hemorrhage, need for accurate diabetic care or special drug therapy, cardiac arrhythmias, pulmonary aspiration of gastric contents, delayed pharmacologic recovery, protracted nausea and vomiting, psychiatric sequelae, and so on.

BACK TO THE ORIGINAL BED AND ENTRY SITE

Here the patient requires less supervision, is given medicines for discomfort or pain, is allowed to eat and drink if compatible, is assisted when standing to void or walk, is allowed to have visitors, and, when all signs are stable, is wheeled in a chair to the departing vehicle accompanied by a responsible adult. A final visit is made by the anesthetist.

OUTCOME

Although voluminous statistics are not available, mortality from this kind of surgical and anesthetic experience, if managed according to protocol, should be distinctly rare. Delayed complications might be anticipated according to the kind of operation done, as shown in Table 29–4.

APPRAISAL

Anesthesia care of ambulatory surgical patients can be provided safely and with cost savings. Acceptance by patients and physicians has been satisfactory, so that one might expect further expansion of this kind of service. Attention must be focused continuously on maintenance of high standards of safety when ambulatory care is elected.

REFERENCES

Berk AA, Chalmers CC: Cost and efficacy of the substitution of ambulatory for inpatient care. N Engl J Med 304:393, 1981.

Natof HE: Complications associated with ambulatory surgery. JAMA 244:1116, 1980.

Oosterlee J, Dudley HAF: Regular Review. Surgery in Outpatients. Br Med J 8 December 1979, p. 1459.

Reed WA, Ford JL: The surgicenter: An ambulatory surgical facility. Clin Obstet Gynecol 17:217, 1974.

Schmidt KF (ed): Outpatient Anesthesia. Int Anesth Clin 14(2), 1976.

Chapter 30

THE THERAPY OF PAIN

Pain is a complex problem beyond the domain of a single specialty. The knowledge and skills needed to evaluate and treat this symptom are best provided by a team of anesthesiologists, neurosurgeons, neurologists, orthopedists, psychiatrists, physiatrists, pharmacologists, and radiologists. Psychologists, sociologists, and physical therapists provide ancillary services.

An ideal pain clinic has a director, a clinic coordinator, consultants, nursing personnel, and administrative staff. The director provides leadership, whereas the coordinator plans daily clinical activities and teaching responsibilities. The clinic requires adequate space, equipment, and staff to permit physical examination and performance of diagnostic and therapeutic blocks for both outpatients and inpatients. Hospital beds should be available for complicated therapies and for the management of occasional complications that may arise. Patients are usually referred to the clinic by other physicians who summarize prior treatment, which is then evaluated by the coordinator, who schedules an appointment with clinic specialists and relevant consultants. Straightforward problems are then treated or recommendations made to the referring physician. More complex problems are evaluated by the group as a whole until a satisfactory solution can be presented to the patient and referring physician.

PAIN PATHWAYS

The reader is referred to standard texts for detailed information on the neuroanatomy of pain. However, the diagrams provided here (Figs. 30–1 through 30–3) should aid in understanding the therapeutic approaches to pain pharmacologically via nerve block and, perhaps, psychologically as well.

OPIOID RECEPTORS AND ENDORPHINS

Opioid receptors in neural tissue of invertebrates were first found in 1973 by binding-assay techniques and autoradiography. In vertebrates, these receptors are concentrated in the amygdaloid, corpus striatum, midline peri-aqueductal gray areas, locus ceruleus of the medulla, and substantia gelatinosa of the spinal cord. The medial thalamus has a fair number of receptors and cerebral cortex a lesser density. Their identification led investigators to suspect the presence of an endogenous substance that might bind to these receptors, a hypothesis supported when electrical stimulation of the peri-aqueductal gray area in the rat produced a high degree of peripheral analgesia, which was partially reversed by naloxone, a pure opioid antagonist. Electrical

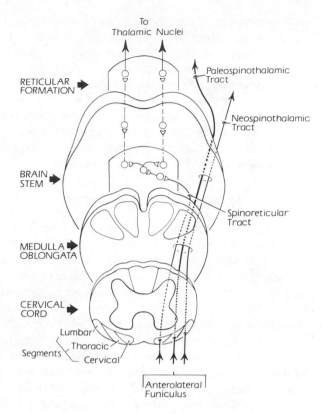

FIGURE 30–1. Ascending pain pathways from the spinal cord. The neospinothalamic tract processes information regarding the location of peripheral stimuli in space and time. The paleospinothalamic tract is involved in ventilatory, circulatory, and endocrine responses to pain. Extensive connections along the spinoreticular tract probably explain the failure of restricted cortical lesions to abolish pain. (Modified from Schmidt RF: Fundamentals of Sensory Physiology. New York, Springer-Verlag, 1978, p. 53.)

stimulation probably led to the release of morphinelike substances; two pentapeptides, met-enkephalin and leu-enkephalin, both possessing properties similar to morphine, have been isolated from brain extracts. Endorphin is a generic term referring to any brain peptide with opioid activity. Met-enkephalin, leu-enkephalin, and alpha-, beta-, gamma-, and delta-endorphins are specific peptides of the endorphin class.

Endorphins exert their activity by binding to opioid receptors. Nanomolar amounts of beta-endorphin injected into the cerebral ventricles of rats produce profound analgesia, whereas patients with chronic pain given minute doses of beta-endorphin intraventricularly invariably report pain relief. Yaksh injected opioids intrathecally in the rat and produced intense analgesia, the onset and duration predicted by the clinical effect of the drug when administered systemically. This analgesia was antagonized by intraperitoneal or intrathecal injections of naloxone. Morphine injected intrathecally in patients with chronic pain of cancer produces analgesia within 15 to 45 minutes, lasting some 12 to 24 hours with an average duration of 20 hours. Epidural placement of morphine has also been utilized to relieve pain; drugs injected epidurally diffuse through the dura to affect the spinal cord. Pain relief resulting from 100 mg meperidine injected epidurally occurs in five minutes, coinciding with concentrations of 0.5 to 2 mg/L in CSF, whereas meperidine concentrations in blood remain below analgesic levels. The analgesic effect of opioids injected intrathecally or epidurally has been ascribed to binding of the drug to receptors in the dorsal horn of the spinal cord.

Epidural morphine is effective in treatment of postoperative pain, rib fractures, and ischemic limb pain but is less effective in relief of labor pains and the acute localized pain of radiculitis and causalgia. When pain is the sole or major symptom, epidural opioids exert a considerable effect, but when pain is accompanied or caused by secondary muscle spasm or sympathetic hyperactivity, the effect is negligible. For postoperative pain, the advantages of epidural morphine include absence of sympathetic, motor, and proprioceptive blockade, which eliminates the problem of hypotension following local anesthetic blockade and allows a patient to perform postoperative deep breathing and leg exercises effectively. Undesirable side effects include pruritus, urinary retention, delayed somnolence, and respiratory and cardiovascular depression, the latter probably related to cephalad diffusion of opioid in CSF into the fourth ventricle, where respiratory and cardiovascular centers are located. Thus, close monitoring must be employed and provisions made for administration of naloxone to reverse adverse reactions. Whether these promising therapeutic maneuvers will lead to wide clinical application remains to be seen.

DIAGNOSTIC NERVE BLOCKS

The physical examination and history establish a baseline upon which the value of diagnostic and therapeutic blocks may be judged. Diagnostic "blocks" fall into the category of either the differential or the anatomic approach and are used to determine the neural pathways involved in the problem under scrutiny. These blocks differentiate somatic sensory pain from that mediated by sympathetic fibers or pain of central origin.

The differential approach takes advantage of sensitivities of the several nerve fibers to varying concentrations of local anesthetic; dilute concentrations block transmission in small unmyelinated fibers without affecting the larger nerves so that increasing concentrations progressively block sympathetic, sensory, and motor fibers, more or less in that order, thus providing the basis of differential spinal block. A lumbar puncture is done, the needle left in place, and the following solutions injected at 10- to 15-minute intervals: (1) 5 ml sterile saline (placebo); (2) 5 ml 0.2 per cent procaine (sympathetic block); (3) 5 ml 0.5 per cent procaine (sensory block); (4) 5 ml 1 per cent procaine (motor block).

Relief of pain upon needle insertion or with saline (without evidence of sympathetic or sensory block) suggests but by no means establishes a psychogenic basis for pain. Causalgia or reflex sympathetic dystrophy is presumed when complete pain relief occurs following sympathetic blockade. Pain mediated by somatic sensory pathways is diagnosed when pain is relieved by 0.5 or 1 per cent procaine. Partial pain relief after sensory block followed by complete relief with motor block is considered to be of organic origin, perhaps with psychological overlay. Central pain is suggested when there is no relief by a sensory block at a level ordinarily adequate to relieve the pain. Central pain can be psychogenically or organically mediated and includes any lesion arising along pain pathways, such as with a cerebrovascular accident, spinal cord injury, thalamic lesion, or brain tumor.

During performance of differential spinal block a patient is questioned as to the magnitude of pain relief. Blood pressure and pulse are recorded and signs of sympathetic and sensory blockade elicited. The procedure may be terminated at any time after relief of pain is complete.

Differential spinal block has shortcomings. Saline is not a true placebo when intrathecally given because segmental hypesthesia to pin prick or cold and partial sympathetic block with diminution of the psychogalvanic reflex may occur. A placebo may activate the endorphin-mediated analgesia system, thus clouding clinical interpretation.

The anatomic approach involves block of specific nerves or ganglia related to innervation of the area of pain. For pain of head, neck, and upper extremities, placebo injection followed by a stellate ganglion block is done to differentiate psychogenic causation and sympathetic dystrophy from somatic pain. If no relief results from stellate ganglion block, then the somatic sensory nerves involved in head and neck pain or the brachial plexus (upper extremity pain) are blocked. Saline injected into a stellate ganglion can produce Horner's syndrome, signs of sympathetic block of the arm, and partial relief of causalgia. For abdominal pain, celiac plexus block is useful in evaluating the role of the viscera, whereas intercostal block is done to evaluate pain of superficial somatic origin. For lower extremity pain, lumbar paravertebral sympathetic block at L1 to L2 and paravertebral somatic sensory block of the nerves innervating the area differentiate between pain of sympathetic and sensory origin. Successful sympathetic block of an extremity is suggested by vasodilation, anhidrosis, a two- to fivefold increase in pulse amplitude according to digital plethysmography, significant increase in skin temperature, and loss of the psychogalvanic reflex.

LOW BACK PAIN

Back pain may be referred from other areas or may relate to organic disease or mechanical disturbances of the back. Organic conditions to be ruled out include an enlarging or dissecting aortic aneurysm, osteoporosis owing to hyperparathyroidism, peptic ulcer, metastases from prostatic carcinoma, pancreatic lesions and kidney or other retroperitoneal disease. Disappointing results after surgical decompression or discectomy for pain owing to nerve root compression led to trials of steroids injected either systemically or into the intrathecal or epidural space for so-called protruded intervertebral disc. The rationale underlying steroid therapy is that inflammation in nerve roots contributes to or is the predominant cause of pain, for nerve roots often appear swollen and inflamed when surgically exposed. Diminution of edema in nerve roots in spite of persistent disc herniation has resulted in relief of symptoms. By contrast, mechanical pressure without inflammation of a nerve root does not necessarily cause pain.

Several reports of large numbers of patients reveal a 35 to 95 per cent incidence of relief of back pain with epidurally given steroids, the dose, type of steroid, and number of injections varying among clinics. Usually from one to three injections are given, the number depending on patient response. An 80-mg dose of dexamethasone has proved satisfactory for each injection. To achieve maximum benefit, injection should be made as close as possible to the involved root. Little benefit is derived from injecting steroids intrathecally if previous epidural injection has failed. The benefit derived from intrathecal steroids in the treatment of adhesive arachnoiditis is not established; on the other hand, caudal injection in patients with pain after laminectomy has relieved pain through lysis of epidural adhesions, a major cause for recurrence of pain after laminectomy.

Seven to twelve per cent of patients whose back pain is treated nonsurgically ultimately require operation, but a majority do not have recurrence or have only mild residual pain. Steroid therapy is only part of the recommended management for patients with back pain; exercises are prescribed, the patient instructed on proper body mechanics, and psychological problems addressed.

REFLEX SYMPATHETIC DYSTROPHY

Reflex sympathetic dystrophy usually results from prior nerve injury, trauma, cerebrovascular accident, or intervertebral disc disease. Signs and symptoms include hyperesthesia, burning pain, vasomotor and sudomotor disturbances, and trophic changes of skin, muscles, bones, and joints. In the advanced state, marked trophic

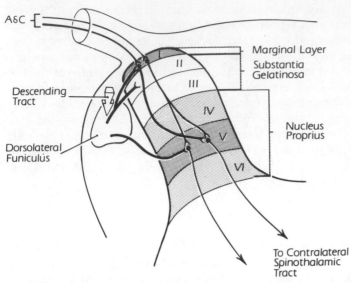

FIGURE 30–2. Interaction of the different pathways at the dorsal horn of the spinal cord. AδC fibers synapse at laminas I and V (occasionally at IV and VI) and form the spinothalamic tract. Descending inhibitory fibers through the dorsolateral funiculus inhibit the transmission of painful impulses at laminas I, II, and V. (Modified from Bonica JJ: Hosp Pract 9, 1979.)

changes of a hand may occur, the skin becoming smooth and glossy with flexion contracture of the fingers. The mechanism is not understood. One theory proposes that a nerve lesion initiates abnormal firing patterns, thus disturbing the internuncial neuron pool in the spinal cord. The abnormal activity spreads to neurons in the lateral and ventral gray matter to cause skeletal muscle spasm and sympathetic hyperactivity.

Treatment depends on the expertise of the managing physician, the preference of the patient, and the response to initial treatment. Corticosteroids given systemically or injected into a shoulder joint in patients with shoulder-hand syndrome can ameliorate symptoms. A series of sympathetic blocks accompanied by intensive physical therapy is most commonly practiced. Sympathetic nerve block may interrupt the self-perpetuating neuronal activity. As a finite period is required for abnormal sympathetic activity to resume and to affect a sufficient number of neurons to reproduce pain, relief of pain from a block should outlast the duration of the local anesthetic effect. Pain relief allows a limb to be exercised and allows both cessation and reversal of dystrophic changes. With successive blocks, a progressive increase in duration of relief occurs, accompanied by resolution of vasomotor signs. Although a series of five blocks has been recommended, this may be inadequate in some patients. Blocks are discontinued when pain is relieved and signs and symptoms disappear but is resumed if symptoms recur. Pain relief that consistently lasts only as long as the effect of the local anesthetic injected suggests the need for surgical or chemical sympathectomy. Injection of 50 per cent alcohol or 6 per cent phenol can be considered; surgical sympathectomy is the definitive alternative.

Guanethidine or reserpine injected intravenously into an exsanguinated limb has been recommended. As in intravenous regional anesthesia, the affected extremity is elevated and exsanguinated with an Esmarch bandage, the tourniquet inflated to one and one-half times systolic pressure, and 15 to 20 mg guanethidine or 1.25 mg reserpine in 20 to 50 ml saline injected into a previously catheterized arm vein (20 to 30 mg guanethidine or 2.5 mg reserpine in 50 to 100 ml diluent in a leg). Tourniquet time ranges from 10 to 20 minutes. Arterial hypotension or ECG changes on release of the tourniquet have not been observed. Reserpine reduces the re-uptake of catecholamines, whereas guanethidine accumulates in and displaces norepinephrine from intraneuronal storage granules at sympathetic nerve endings. A trial with this technique is recommended in those who refuse sympathetic block or who have had a bizarre reaction after block and before surgical or chemical sympathectomy.

Clinical and experimental results with transcutaneous electrical nerve stimulators are not uniform; both relief and aggravation of symptoms have been reported. Studies in volunteers and in patients with chronic pain provide conflicting results on the effect of transcutaneous nerve stimulation on autonomic responses. However, this therapy provides an alternative when more specific treatment fails.

ONCOLOGIC PAIN

The pain of malignancy may be caused by one or more of the following: tumor compression of nerve roots, trunks, or plexuses; infiltration of nerves and blood vessels by tumor; obstruction of a hollow viscus; occlusion of blood vessels by tumor; necrosis, infection, and inflammation of structures invaded by tumor; bony metastasis or expansion of a solid viscus stretching its capsule or peritoneal covering. Pain may arise in connection with therapy (chemotherapy or surgical or radiation treatment). The incidence of pain varies with site of the primary tumor. Primary bone tumors and cancer of the oral cavity and genitourinary tract carry a 70 to 85 per cent pain incidence; breast, lung, and gastrointestinal tumors 40 to 50 per cent; whereas only 5 per cent of patients with leukemia complain of pain. Treatment of the pain can be categorized according to measures directed at the neoplasm *per se* and symptomatic measures, the former beyond the scope of this text. Symptomatic treatment includes analgesics, nerve blocks, neurosurgical procedures, and psychologic therapy.

The majority of patients with pain of cancer can be treated with medicines. Initially, the least potent analgetic capable of relieving pain is given and continued as long as effective. Stronger analgetics are held in reserve as long as possible. By preference, oral medications are used for reasons of comfort, economy, and simplicity. Aspirin or acetaminophen is appropriate at the start regardless of severity of pain except in patients on methotrexate therapy, in whom aspirin is contraindicated. If aspirin or acetaminophen is ineffective, a combination of either drug with pentazocine, codeine, or oxycodone may be tried. Patients with severe pain ultimately require a major opioid. All are equally effective in relieving pain if the dose is adjusted to need. Dependence liability is the same while cross-tolerance occurs. It is hardly possible to predict duration of action of an opioid because of its dependence on dose given, severity of pain, criteria for satisfactory analgesia, previous opioid experience, and individual differences in pharmacokinetics. In the U.S., morphine is the analgetic of choice for severe pain of advanced cancer. There is no ceiling on its analgetic effect, no greater dependence liability than that following equianalgetic doses of other opioids, and no parenterally given analgetic offers a longer duration of action.

Brompton's cocktail, introduced in Great Britain and used in the treatment of cancer pain, consists of morphine or diacetylmorphine in variable dose and cocaine dissolved in alcohol, syrup, and chloroform water. Ethyl alcohol reduces contamination of the solution, prolonging its shelf life from one to three weeks. The addition of cocaine and use of diacetylmorphine in the cocktail are controversial. There is no convincing evidence that Brompton's cocktail is superior to adequate doses of morphine alone.

NEUROLYTIC BLOCKS

If cancer pain is localized, a nerve block is indicated before excessive doses of opioids are required and their adverse effects become limiting. Several blocks with local anesthetics of variable duration of action and comparison with placebo should be performed before neurolytic block is contemplated to assure effectiveness of the block and to observe the patient for signs of opioid withdrawal. Patient and relatives should be informed of the rationale, risks, and complications of the block, that pain relief is not always complete, and that relief may last only several weeks to months. Even partial improvement with a neurolytic block is helpful, because formerly ineffective analgetics may then provide satisfactory analgesia.

Gasserian ganglion block can relieve pain in the distribution of the trigeminal nerve. If the ophthalmic division is not involved, the maxillary and mandibular branches can be blocked peripherally, thus avoiding corneal anesthesia. Glossopharyngeal nerve block can also relieve pharyngeal pain.

Subarachnoid neurolytic blocks are indicated in cancer patients with severe pain confined to one side and related to a few specific spinal segments. These blocks require that the patient remain immobile in one position for an hour or so; the procedure should be performed in an operating room on an operating room table. Absolute ethyl alcohol, hypobaric, is usually used, but some prefer hyperbaric 6 per cent phenol. When alcohol is to be injected, the patient is turned semiprone at a 30- to 45-degree angle in relation to the horizontal with the affected side uppermost. The needle is inserted at the interspace where nerve rootlets coalesce to form the spinal nerve, not at the foramen of a vertebra where the spinal nerve exits. The intent is to interrupt conduction in the dorsal roots at the cord level and avoid involvement of other intrathecal structures. Dosage should not exceed 0.5 to 0.7 ml per interspace; larger doses may result in motor paralysis. The rate of injection is slow, 0.1 ml/30 sec. The patient remains in the same position for 30 to 45 minutes, then lies prone on a bed for two hours. Possible complications include weakness of the lower extremities and bowel or bladder dysfunction. The usual duration of pain relief is three to four months. When phenol is injected, the patient is positioned with the painful side down and the operating room table adjusted so that the area treated is at the lowermost point of the vertebral column. With this position, drug action is localized at the sensory posterior spinal nerve roots. Although the anterior root is predominantly motor, studies have shown that some afferent fibers enter the cord via this pathway, perhaps explaining the incomplete success with an otherwise well-executed intrathecal neurolytic block. Phenol is preferred for pain of pelvic and perineal cancer but is not very effective in treating leg, upper chest, and arm pain. Some advocate a mixture of phenol in glycerine whereby the phenol is gradually released to provide a longer lasting block. Attempts to produce long-lasting pain relief by intrathecal injection of hypertonic saline have proved both dangerous and unsuccessful.

The *celiac plexus* carries afferent sensory autonomic fibers from all abdominal viscera except the pelvic organs, so that block is effective for relief of pain in cancer of the upper abdomen. With the patient prone, 6-inch, 20-gauge needles are inserted on either side of the body of the first lumbar vertebra until the tips lie 1 to 1.5 cm anterior to the vertebral body. Accurate placement can be confirmed by fluoroscopy and injection of a small amount of water-soluble radiopaque substance. Fifty ml of 50 per cent alcohol or 6 per cent phenol are then injected into the area of the celiac plexus: a 91 to 94 per cent success rate eventuates with this block. The patient's appetite, sensorium, and spirit all improve with pain relief and discontinuation of opioids. Complications of the procedure include arterial hypotension owing to splanchnic vasodilation, inadvertent subarachnoid or intravascular injection, epidural or lumbar somatic nerve block, and perforation of viscera. Failure to relieve pain may relate to lack of diffusion of the drug in the retroperitoneal space because of tumor spread, metastasis to organs not innervated by the celiac plexus, opioid addiction, and injection of inadequate amounts of neurolytic solution.

Peripheral neurolytic blocks with either alcohol or phenol are not advised, as the subsequent high incidence of neuritis proves as disturbing as the original pain.

HERPES ZOSTER AND POSTHERPETIC NEURALGIA

Herpes zoster, an acute central nervous system infection caused by the same virus that causes chickenpox, involves sensory nerve roots, ganglia, dorsal columns, and corresponding cutaneous areas. The disease is more frequent in people over 50 years of age, especially those with malignancy or diabetes mellitus or those receiving immuno-suppressive drugs or radiation therapy. Herpes is characterized initially by a macular rash, followed by vesicular eruptions over one or adjacent dermatomes, and is accompanied by pain along the distribution of the nerve. The most common sites involve thoracic dermatomes T1 to T8, but the rash may appear anywhere on the body surface and is particularly dangerous when it involves the ophthalmic division of the trigeminal nerve. Pain or dysesthesia usually precedes the rash and persists for one to four weeks after the lesions heal. Postherpetic neuralgia, persisting for months to years, develops in approximately 30 per cent of patients, especially those over the age of 40.

Treatment of acute herpes is symptomatic, usually involving use of analgetics. Corticosteroids may shorten the period of acute pain but may promote dissemination of the lesions. Cytosine arabinoside, an antiviral agent, has been tried in therapy but prolongs the duration of acute lesions in some patients. Triamcinolone, a synthetic corticosteroid, when mixed with a local anesthetic and injected beneath the lesions provides excellent relief of pain and may prevent the occurrence of postherpetic neuralgia. On the whole, however, treatment of postherpetic neuralgia is unsatisfactory. Although pain may abate over months to years, it is refractory to analgetics; thus efforts should be made to prevent its onset. Stellate ganglion or epidural block when given during the early stages of the disease is effective in relieving pain and is accompanied by diminution of erythema and drying of the vesicles. Excellent results have been reported if the procedure is done within 24 days of onset of the lesions. If pain recurs, it is usually of lesser intensity and can be treated with additional sympathetic block. In patients with postherpetic neuralgia, relief has been reported with use of carbamazepine (Tegretol), 600 to 800 mg/day, together with nortriptyline, 50 to 100 mg in divided doses. Dosage is adjusted according to degree of pain relief and is continued for three to six months. Phenytoin, 300 to 400 mg/day, can also be prescribed for patients who do not tolerate carbamazepine. The results from transcutaneous nerve stimulation and surgical excision are poor; the latter, a mutilating procedure, is not indicated.

MYOFASCIAL SYNDROMES

Pain arising from skeletal muscle and ligaments produced by prior trauma, strenuous exercise, or postural abnormalities is often accompanied by psychogenic tension, resentment, and anxiety. Initially localized over the area of involved muscle, pain may later spread to other muscles, but usually not in the dermatomal distribution seen with the pain of herniated disc, vertebral facet syndromes, or spondylolisthesis. Neurologic deficit is not found on physical examination. Muscles are usually tender to palpation, and a localized and particularly tender trigger point exists where pressure reproduces distribution of the pain. Histologically, *trigger points* are associated with myofibrillar degeneration, acid mucopolysaccharide accumulation, and minor lymphocytic infiltration. The myofascial syndrome probably derives from muscle spasm following initial injury combined with decreased blood flow and accumulation of

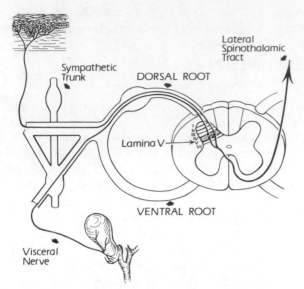

FIGURE 30–3. The phenomenon of referred pain. Noxious visceral impulses and innocuous cutaneous sensations terminate at lamina V of the dorsal horn of the spinal cord and synapse with the neurons of the spinothalamic tract. (Modified from Schmidt RF: Fundamentals of Sensory Physiology. New York, Springer-Verlag, 1978, p. 121.)

acid metabolites, leading to pain. These exaggerate the muscle contraction, and a self-perpetuating cycle is initiated. Trigger points associated with shoulder girdle and cervical myofascial syndromes are usually located at various points over the trapezius and major rhomboid muscles. Lumbosacral myofascial pain presents as trigger points in the paraspinal muscle, at the sacroiliac joint, and deep in the pyriformis muscle at the center of the buttock. On the anterior chest the pectoralis major and serratus anterior muscles are involved.

Treatment of this syndrome includes injection of the trigger point with a local anesthetic solution containing dexamethasone sodium phosphate (4 mg/50 ml) or 25 mg hydrocortisone. Pain may be exaggerated following injection but usually subsides after 8 to 12 hours, with injections repeated every four to seven days as necessary. Pain may be relieved by directing a spray of fluoromethane or ethyl chloride over the affected muscle from trigger point toward the reference zone, accompanied by passive muscle stretching of steady, gradually increasing force. Hot, moist packs are applied to the area and analgetics and muscle relaxants used for continued benefit. Amitriptyline hydrochloride or doxepin hydrochloride (Adapin) can be prescribed if psychogenic depression is a feature.

PHANTOM LIMB PAIN

Although most amputees report a persistent sensory feeling in the absent extremity immediately after amputation, only 5 to 10 per cent experience pain in the area of the phantom limb. Pain prior to an amputation increases the chances of experiencing a painful phantom. The pain appears shortly after amputation and is described as cramping, burning, shooting, or crushing. It usually diminishes and disappears with time but occasionally may become a severe and chronic problem. The mechanism of phantom pain is unknown, although sometimes a neuroma at the operative site is responsible. One suggestion is that the original trauma initiates abnormal firing patterns in closed, self-exciting neuron loops in the spinal cord, sending pain impulses to the brain. The abnormal activity spreads to neurons in the lateral and ventral horns, producing such autonomic and muscle symptoms as sweating and jerking movements of the stump. The abnormal cord activity can be self-sustaining, so that surgical excision of the peripheral stimulus may not terminate the process. Another theory suggests that limb amputation destroys a large number of sensory fibers, thus reducing the magnitude of input into the reticular formation and decreasing the inhibitory influence of the reticular formation. Pain results when the output of the self-sustaining neuron pools reaches a critical level.

Treatment of phantom limb pain is often frustrating. A painful neuroma can be injected with a local anesthetic or excised. Occasionally repeated anesthetic blocks of peripheral nerves innervating the stump may provide relief. Autonomic disturbances such as vasoconstriction and sweating can be treated with sympathetic blocks for relief of pain. However, sympathectomy rarely provides lasting relief, as in the case of causalgia. Phantom limb pain is sometimes triggered or aggravated by emotional disturbances; psychotherapy or hypnosis may decrease and occasionally abolish the pain. Use of transcutaneous electrical stimulators has been helpful.

NEUROSURGICAL CONTROL OF PAIN

Depending on the site and nature of the pain and the condition of the patient, surgical procedures may be useful in pain relief. Pain-conducting fibers can be interrupted at any point from the periphery to the cerebral cortex. Operations for pain relief include section of peripheral nerve, spinal dorsal sensory roots, the ascending spinothalamic tract, pathways in medulla oblongata, or mesencephalon; destruction of thalamic nuclei; ablation of the sensory cortex; interruption of thalamofrontal or limbic projections; and destruction of localized areas such as the pituitary gland. Electro-stimulation at various levels of the central nervous system has been tried.

Posterior rhizotomy is of value in relief of a well-circumscribed pain in areas innervated by one or several roots localized in the neck, chest wall, back, or perineum. Anterolateral cordotomy involves sectioning the spinothalamic tract contralateral to the pain site and is particularly effective in relieving the pain of cancer in a lower extremity. Complications arising from the procedure include urinary incontinence owing to destruction of sensory pathways in the lateral columns of the cord, bowel incontinence, and weakness of the ipsilateral extremity. Percutaneous cordotomy involves radiofrequency coagulation of the spinothalamic tract via a high cervical (C1 to C2) approach, a procedure done under local anesthesia and well tolerated by debilitated patients.

ELECTRICAL STIMULATION

The gate control theory of pain of Melzack and Wall proposes that the cell bodies in the substantia gelatinosa act as a gate modulating transfer of information from the periphery to the first central transmission (T) cells (Fig. 30–4). These target cells summate total input as well as descending impulses from higher brain centers. The inhibitory effect on afferent fiber terminals exerted by the substantia gelatinosa is enhanced by activity of large fibers, thereby decreasing pain perception. Pain control can be achieved by selectively influencing large fiber transmission through electrical stimulation. Stimulating electrodes are placed over the painful area, atop a peripheral spinal cord nerve supplying the painful area or within the epidural space, to stimulate dorsal columns containing the large fibers. Results of this therapy have been variable and are attributable, in part, to the psychological support that invariably accompanies use of electrical stimulation. Tracings of voltage and current fields resulting from dorsal column stimulation indicate that other structures such as the lateral spinothalamic tracts may be stimulated. Experimental placement of stimulating electrodes in the

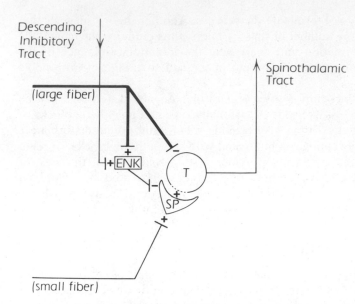

Descending
Inhibitory
Tract

Spinothalamic
Tract

(large fiber)

(small fiber)

FIGURE 30–4. Modification of the gate control theory. Impulses through the small fibers release substance P (SP), which excites the first central transmission cells (T). Large fiber impulses inhibit the opening of the "gate" and stimulate an enkephalinergic interneuron (ENK). Descending inhibitory tract also stimulates the enkephalinergic interneuron, which blocks the release of substance P. Fibers from the dorsal horn form the spinothalamic tract (ST).

central gray matter associated with the endogenous endorphin system yields results that offer promise in the treatment of chronic pain.

PSYCHOLOGICAL TECHNIQUES IN PAIN MANAGEMENT

OPERANT CONDITIONING

A patient in pain usually manifests a spectrum of actions to show others that pain is being experienced — grimacing, walking in a guarded manner, or asking for analgetics. This kind of behavior, called operant, is controlled by the consequences. If the operant behavior is followed by a favorable consequence as a positive reinforcer, behavior is likely to recur. If operant behavior is not thus followed, the behavior abates and ultimately disappears; punishment may have a similar effect. Operant conditioning involves both identification and elimination of positive reinforcers; thus, complaints of pain are ignored, whereas reduced intake of medication and increased activity are praised. Medications are given on a fixed time schedule and dosage gradually decreased, the color and taste of the medication masked to facilitate the reduction. The physical activity of a patient is gradually increased and a record made of improvement on a daily or weekly basis.

RELAXATION TECHNIQUES

Relaxation techniques have been used successfully in the treatment of anxiety states based on the observation that anxiety and deep muscle relaxation are incompatible. The cognitive and emotional factors accompanying pain are altered by a relaxation-meditation process involving several sessions with a therapist. The patient is made comfortable and simultaneously closes the eyes and concentrates on tensing and relaxing body muscle groups. Once relaxed, the mind is encouraged to drift slowly to a tranquil, pleasant memory and concentrate on it. The patient is deeply relaxed at this time; flickering of the eyelids and lateral scanning of the eyes are evident. This altered and relaxed state is maintained for at least one minute, a technique easily mastered after several sessions. Although aware of pain, patients usually state that they feel relaxed; they develop better control of their response to pain.

EMG BIOFEEDBACK

Biofeedback has been used to treat skeletal muscle spasm, anxiety, and autonomic responses to pain. The patient is taught to relax tense or spastic muscles while relaxation is quantitated via electromyography. The frontalis muscle is usually monitored, as tension there is a good indicator of anxiety and relaxation is considered an index of generalized muscle relaxation. A patient's mastery over the pain response is rewarding, and self-esteem is greatly improved.

HYPNOSIS

Hypnosis is a programmed state of focused attention on a specific site, object, sound, or image while all other peripheral input is blocked out. The patient develops a state of deep relaxation or trance while suggestions relating to analgesia are made in the form of symptom suppression or substitution. The painful sensation is altered in symptom suppression and then interpreted as an innocuous or comfortable sensation. In symptom substitution, the sensation of pain is transferred from one area to another. Time distortion is a hypnotic technique wherein time is psychologically altered. Painful times are moved faster and pain-free states moved slower. Age regression is another hypnotic technique in which the painful incident is recalled and fears and anxieties associated with the event are resolved.

Chronic pain, with its attendant financial and social pressures, changes the personality of the individual. The complaint is often used as a mechanism to escape responsibilities and to mask inadequacies. The intensity of pain is magnified and patients narrow their perspective of things and events to their own liking. The several psychological therapeutic techniques diminish anxiety, reduce pain intensity, restore patients to their former personalities, and prevent addiction. In highly suggestible patients, hypnosis is a significant adjunct in pain management.

The results of hypnosis (psychological techniques), alone or in conjunction with conventional treatment of pain, have not been critically investigated. However, personality changes as a result of chronic pain have been well established. These techniques are so innocuous that they should be added to the total control of pain symptoms.

APPRAISAL

We repeat the final two paragraphs of an article we published in Anesthesiology (15:98, 1954), which dealt with the problems of pain relief. The comments are still pertinent.

From our experience we have concluded that few residents in anesthesiology can be trained to treat painful syndromes in more than a technical manner. In a two-year residency program, there is insufficient time to train a physician to administer anesthetics and to give him adequate instruction and clinical experience in the diagnosis and treatment of painful syndromes. If, after his residency, he is willing to devote enough time, study, and clinical application to these problems, an anesthesiologist could become as well versed in the treatment of pain as any other physician.

When facilities, personnel, and time exist, anesthesiologists should take the initiative in establishing "pain clinics" staffed by physicians of the several specialties. Such clinics could accomplish much concerning the relief of pain, and the clinic could act as a teaching medium to students and residents as well as furnish much valuable data on the treatment of pain.

REFERENCES

Bowsher D: Pain pathways and mechanisms. Anaesthesia 33:935, 1978.
Brown BR: Diagnosis and therapy of common myofascial syndromes. JAMA 239:646, 1978.

Dilke TFW, Burry HC, Grahame R: Extradural corticosteroid injection in management of lumbar nerve root compression. Br Med J 2:635, 1973.

Hatangdi, VS, Boas RA, Richards EG: Postherpetic neuralgia: Management with antiepileptic and tricyclic drugs. *In* Bonica JJ, Albe-Fessard D (eds): Advances in Pain Research and Therapy. Vol 1, New York, Raven Press, 1976.

Magora F, Olshwang D, Eimerl D, Schorr J, Katzenelson R, Cotev S, Davidson JT: Observations on extradural morphine analgesia in various pain conditions. Br J Anaesth 52:247, 1980.

Melzack R: Central neural mechanisms in phantom limb pain. *In* Bonica JJJ (ed.): Advances in Neurology. Vol 4. New York, Raven Press, 1974, p. 319.

Stoelting RK: Opiate receptors and endorphins: The role in anesthesiology. Anesth Analg 59:874, 1980.

Swerdlow M: Sub-arachnoid and extradural neurolytic blocks. *In* Bonica JJ, Ventrafridda V (eds.): Advances in Pain Research and Therapy. Vol 2. New York, Raven Press, 1979, p. 325.

Thompson GE, Moore DC, Bridenbaugh LD, Artin RY: Abdominal pain and alcohol celiac plexus block. Anesth Analg 56:1, 1977.

Urban BJ, Mckain CW: Local anesthetic effect of intrathecal saline. Pain 5:43, 1978.

Winnie AP, Collins VJ: The pain clinic. I. Differential neural blockade in pain syndromes of questionable etiology. Med Clin North Am 52:123, 1968.

Chapter 31
CONTROLLED HYPOTENSION

Deliberate hypotension reduces bleeding into a wound, thereby providing the surgeon with both better visibility and technical freedom for a more definitive dissection; this is especially important in excision of malignancies. With less bleeding, the extent of ligated or cauterized tissue is reduced, the chance of infection is minimized, and wounds heal better, a prime concern of plastic surgeons. In radical dissections, the need for blood replacement is decreased. Attempts at reducing blood loss by deliberate hypotension have been used for over 40 years, first by Gardner, a neurosurgeon who, to lower the blood pressure, withdrew blood and subsequently re-infused it. The technique was unsuccessful because the hypovolemic hypotension and vasoconstriction approached shock and the margin of safety was low. Gillies used spinal anesthesia to lower the pressure, but the method was not quite controllable. Around 1950, Enderby and associates employed ganglionic blockers in conjunction with general anesthesia, the prototype of hypotensive techniques used today.

During the early 1950s, deliberate hypotension was widely and indiscriminately applied with a variety of techniques, for many different operations and in all categories of patients. The basis of the technique was not understood nor were its limitations; thus serious complications resulted and by 1960 few American anesthetists advocated its use. Because of continued favorable experience in a few centers abroad, mainly in England, and because reports appearing in the American literature defined the physiologic and pharmacologic background more clearly, interest quickened and deliberate hypotension is now commonly practiced.

THEORY

The physiologic basis of the technique is vasodilation, so that positioning the patient with the operative site uppermost allows blood to pool in dependent portions, thereby reducing venous pressure at the site and reducing venous return to the heart and the cardiac output. Therefore, hypotension is most helpful when positioning effectively pools blood peripherally, that is, for operations on the head, face, neck, and upper thorax. If blood is not sequestered, venous return and cardiac output cannot be reduced and the technique is ineffective. Thus, if a patient is anesthetized and operated on while supine, bleeding from a cervical operation may be considerable even though systolic blood pressure is at 70 torr. Similarly, if vasodilation is inadequate or the level of anesthesia insufficient to prevent subconscious perception of pain, cardiac output cannot be suppressed and conditions will be unsatisfactory.

The principal fear in using deliberate hypotension is the possibility of causing insufficiency of the coronary, cerebral, or renal circulations. As noted in Chapter 32, the circulation to brain and heart is not adrenergically mediated but responds intrinsically to metabolic demands of the myocardium and to hydrogen ion or baroreceptor alterations in brain. With deliberate hypotension, a reduction in blood pressure, heart rate, and cardiac output lessens the work of the heart and thus the metabolic demands of the myocardium; reduction in coronary blood flow is therefore acceptable. In the erect position, because of the height of the brain above heart level, the cerebral circulation is perfused at a mean pressure ranging from 50 to 55 torr. Consequently, a reduction in arterial pressure to that level in a supine, anesthetized individual breathing high concentrations of oxygen should be of little concern. It should be remembered that perfusion pressure is the result of arterial pressure minus resistance to flow across the capillary bed, minus venous pressure. A head-down position provides no protection during hypotension, because both cerebrospinal fluid pressure and cerebral venous pressure are elevated, thus retarding flow. When the body is tilted head up, perfusion pressure is higher in the kidney than at heart level.

These tenets presuppose the presence of normovolemia and a normally reactive vasculature. One would not contemplate using the technique in the presence of hypovolemia or if there were symptoms or signs of circulatory insufficiency in the vital organs.

TECHNIQUE

The technique is a combination of any of five components: general anesthesia, body tilt, vasodilation, positive airway pressure, and beta-adrenergic blockade. All are not necessary in every patient.

We have not found any particular regimen of preanesthetic medication better than another, although when dissections are prolonged, opioids facilitate maintenance of hypotension because of peripheral circulatory dilation. Anesthesia is usually induced with an intravenous barbiturate followed by nitrous oxide–oxygen and halothane or enflurane, both of which are excellent agents because of the myocardial depressant action and facilitation of peripheral blood pooling. Controlled ventilation with at least 50 per cent oxygen via an endotracheal tube is always used to counter the changes in ventilation-perfusion ratios that accompany hypotension and positioning.

The degree of tilt depends on the ease of lowering blood pressure and the ability of the surgeon to work with the patient in that position. In general, tilt is delayed until the patient is prepared, draped, and the surgeon ready to incise; otherwise positioning without the stimulus of pain may lead to excessively low blood pressure. Obviously, the steeper the tilt, the more readily blood pools. Some anesthetists more or less routinely use a 30-degree tilt; we aim toward 10 to 20 degrees. In many patients, particularly those in the older and less active age groups, the combination of potent halogenated anesthetics, controlled ventilation, and tilt are sufficient to produce appropriate conditions even in the absence of appreciable hypotension. In the healthy, robust, and physically active, it is usually necessary to use a vasodilator.

Two classes of vasodilator are available. The ganglionic blockers, trimethaphan and pentolinium, were once commonly used but now are largely replaced by a vascular smooth muscle relaxant, nitroprusside. The actions of trimethaphan and nitroprusside are rapid in onset and of short duration, and therefore are given in a continuous infusion; the effect disappears soon after the infusion is stopped. Doses of trimethaphan higher than 1 gm are not recommended because the action may persist, a direct vasodilator effect develops, histamine is released, and neuromuscular block may appear. The dose of nitroprusside should not exceed 100 mg/hr so that toxic metabolites, cyanide and thiocyanate, are not formed. Pentolinium is given intermittently in intravenous doses from 5 to 15 mg, the effect lasting 45 minutes or so depending on the level of anesthesia and degree of tilt. One fourth of the initial amount is repeated if needed. Pupillary dilation and lower than normal blood pressures may outlast the anesthetic; attendants must be cautioned about this. Pentolinium is preferred in lengthy operations in which hypotension is needed throughout and should be given before positioning. Nitroprusside is the choice when hypotension is needed for briefer periods only, as when ligating a cerebral aneurysm.

With a combination of general anesthesia, tilt, and a vasodilator, blood pressure can be further controlled, as dictated by surgical needs, by manipulation of airway pressure. Continuous application of end-expiratory pressure, 5 to 20 cm H_2O, further reduces venous return and lowers both cardiac output and blood pressure. Some hold that raised airway pressure increases venous bleeding in a cervical or facial wound, but this has not been our experience because blood is alternatively returned to the heart via the vertebral venous plexus.

An occasional patient may not respond to any of these measures, especially one who is robust and physically active. Tachycardia sometimes appears, preventing lowering of the cardiac output and increasing myocardial metabolic demands. Enderby utilizes a beta-adrenergic blocker, propranolol, 0.035 mg/kg intravenously, or practolol (not available in the U.S.), 0.14 mg/kg, to decrease heart rate and the velocity and force of myocardial contraction. Such therapy is to be used with extreme caution because of potential precipitation of heart failure or bronchial constriction.

A continuous infusion of an electrolyte and dextrose solution should be given to all patients. In the presence of vasodilation, some clinicians give too little fluid. In major dissections, blood loss should be measured and replaced as lost with a balanced salt solution, whole blood, or blood components as indicated.

OPERATIVE CONDITIONS

The purpose of deliberate hypotension is not to create a dry wound but to reduce bleeding and facilitate dissection. All visible vessels must be ligated even though bleeding is not brisk, because bleeding may occur when blood pressure returns to normal. There is no arbitrary level at which blood pressure is optimal. In the young and healthy, the usual level is 60 to 70 torr systolic, whereas in older individuals satisfactory conditions are attained at higher levels. Little is gained by depressing blood pressure more than necessary. Nor is there an absolute limit to the duration of hypotensive anesthesia. Blood pressure is not kept at a fixed level but is allowed to fluctuate within reason, depending on surgical needs. Obviously, operation should proceed with alacrity. Deliberate hypotension has been used successfully in children as young as five years and, to some extent, in the seventh and eighth decades of life.

MONITORING

Blood pressure should be monitored either by an oscillotonometer, which permits accurate beat by beat observations at low pressures, or via intra-arterial recording. The electrocardiogram and heart sounds are observed as usual. We have not gained worthwhile information through the use of electroencephalography. In procedures such as radical neck dissection and craniotomy, urinary output should also be measured.

POSTOPERATIVE CONDITIONS

At the end of the operation, or during operation if hypotension is excessive, the procedures heretofore outlined are reversed. Positive pressure ventilation is discontinued and spontaneous respiration allowed to resume. The operating table is leveled. Anesthesia is lightened or discontinued. If blood pressure does not return promptly to satisfactory levels, intravenous infusion is quickened and blood volume augmented. Rarely is a vasoactive drug indicated. Care should be exercised in moving patients from operating table to recovery bed and in subsequent transportation, as the circulation may be unstable. In the recovery room monitoring is continued and the nurses are specifically informed of the anesthetic procedure. The head of the bed should be raised only with caution, lest hypotension return. Urine output is checked. The majority of patients enjoy a remarkably smooth and uneventful recovery.

COMPLICATIONS

Unfortunately, there are far too few controlled studies of sufficient numbers of patients to draw valid conclusions as to the incidence of complications resulting from the use of this technique. The consensus of those most experienced in the use of deliberate hypotension is that complications in such patients are not more frequent, if indeed as frequent as those in similar patients operated on at normotensive levels. To obtain valid data, similar risks, the same kinds of operation, and comparable age groups with surgeons and anesthetists of equivalent skill should be compared. However, if one fails to discover circulatory insufficiency in vital organs preoperatively and employs deliberate hypotension, even the closest monitoring may not forewarn of trouble. There is no question that deliberate hypotension is a valuable technique, simplifying some complicated operations, making others possible, and causing the results of many to be superior. However, the technique should not be undertaken by the unwary or the casual clinician, nor by those who have not read the recent relevant literature.

REFERENCES

Eckenhoff JE, Rich JC: Clinical experiences with deliberate hypotension. Anesth Analg 45:21, 1966.
Enderby GEH: A report on mortality and morbidity following 9,107 hypotensive anaesthetics. Br J Anaesth 33:109, 1961.
Enderby GEH (ed): Symposium on Deliberate Hypotension. Postgrad Med J 50:555, 1974.
Fahmy NR, Laver MB: Hemodynamic response to ganglionic blockade with pentolinium during N_2O halothane anesthesia in man. Anesthesiology 44:6, 1976.
Leigh JM, Millar RA (eds): Symposium on deliberate hypotension in anaesthesia. Br J Anaesth 47:743, 1975.
Salem MR: Deliberate hypotension is a safe and accepted anesthetic technique. In Eckenhoff JE (ed): Controversy in Anesthesiology. Philadelphia, W B Saunders, 1979, p 95.
Vesey CJ, Cole PV, Linnell JC, et al: Some metabolic effects of sodium nitroprusside in man. Br Med J 2:140, 1974.

Chapter 32

ARTERIAL HYPOTENSION DURING ANESTHESIA

Experienced anesthetists view the significance of blood pressure somewhat differently from most of their medical colleagues, and with good reason. Physicians generally record blood pressure in individuals with normally functioning sympathetic nervous systems who are conscious, have normal muscle activity, and are breathing room air. The anesthetist supervises the supine, often paralyzed, unconscious patient whose sympathetic nervous activity is likely to be depressed and whose respiration is assisted or controlled using higher than normal concentrations of oxygen. Thus, the two situations are quite different. As recorded peripherally, blood pressure signifies the pressure driving blood through the circulation; considered as an independent observation, pressure means little except at extreme values. Of greater consequence is the resulting tissue perfusion.

Although many patients manage to maintain a relatively normal blood pressure during anesthesia and operation, a reduction from normal values is commonly observed. Hypotension *per se* is not so important; rather it is the degree and the cause that concern the anesthetist, for one can have adequate perfusion secondary to vasodilation, whereas at the same low pressure perfusion would be inadequate if vasoconstriction were present. One should learn to appraise the patient's overall condition. The initial reaction to hypotension is often one of alarm — blood pressure should not be so low and energetic treatment must be undertaken. The urge to respond irrationally must be suppressed. Is the skin warm and dry, is the color of blood in the wound satisfactory, and is the pulse full and regular, even though systolic blood pressure may be recorded at 70 torr? If the answers are yes, this hemodynamic situation is obviously different from one at the same level of blood pressure in which the skin is cold and blue, the pulse rapid and thready, and the blood in the wound dark.

We shall discuss some of the common causes of arterial hypotension, as follows: excessive premedication, influence of potent therapeutic drugs given prior to anesthesia, relative or absolute overdose of general anesthetics, circulatory effects of spinal and peridural anesthesia, raised airway pressure, hypovolemia and hemorrhage, surgical manipulation and stimulation, change in position of the patient, and cardiovascular problems. Incompatible transfusion, septic shock, and less common causes of hypotension will also be discussed.

GENERAL CONSIDERATIONS

Blood pressure is the circulatory sign most often recorded during anesthesia, perhaps because measurement is so simple. To evaluate the significance of any blood pressure reading, one must consider cardiac output, peripheral vascular resistance, blood volume, venous return, and heart rate. Except for heart rate, measurement of these variables is hardly practical during anesthesia, so they must be judged indirectly. We shall refer to these judgments throughout this chapter.

The circulation is regulated to maintain adequate blood flow to tissues but especially to the brain and heart, the two most vulnerable vascular beds because of their high metabolic demands. Thus, aspects of the coronary and cerebral circulations are worth noting. The coronary circulation responds to the metabolic demands of the work done by the heart, primarily determined by ventricular end-diastolic pressure (preload), the inotropic state of the myocardium, afterload (aortic diastolic pressure), and heart rate. Coronary vessels are not adrenergically controlled but dilate or constrict in response to oxygen need. Reduction in mean blood pressure or in rate decreases cardiac work, and even though accompanied by a lesser volume of coronary blood flow, the requirements of the heart can usually be met barring hypovolemia or myocardial disease. All these tenets presuppose normally reactive coronary vessels; however, in the presence of coronary arteriosclerosis, the vessels may be unable to respond to myocardial demand. Here blood pressure becomes the principal determinant of coronary flow, and a lowered pressure may be harmful.

The cerebral circulation is likewise essentially without autonomic influence, but flow is regulated by Pa_{CO_2} acting through changes in hydrogen ion concentration and also by mean perfusion pressure. In a supine individual mean perfusing arterial blood pressure can fall quite low, to 50 torr, and still be the equivalent of the perfusion pressure in an erect person with a mean pressure of 85 torr at the base of the heart and a 35-cm difference in height to the base of the brain. The brain normally extracts only about 25 per cent of the oxygen delivered to it, whereas the heart, a working muscle, removes nearly 80 per cent. The brain, therefore, has considerable oxygen reserves without a need to increase blood flow, whereas the heart must respond to a demand for more oxygen by either increasing the volume of coronary blood flow or decreasing myocardial oxygen requirements.

CAUSES OF HYPOTENSION

EXCESSIVE PREMEDICATION

The tendency of the opioids to lower arterial blood pressure is well known (see Chapter 5). The inference is that the opioids will reduce the ability to compensate for circulatory stress such as hemorrhage, trauma, or change in position and that they must be used with caution in ambulatory patients. Opioids administered intravenously during routine anesthesia or postoperatively before patients recover completely from general anesthesia may be followed by hypotension. For this reason it is best to reduce the dose of opioid (2.5 mg morphine, 25 mg meperidine, or 0.01 mg fentanyl), to give incremental doses, and to observe the blood pressure response.

Several of the barbiturates, secobarbital and pentobarbital, for example, disturb the circulation least when given in 50- to 150-mg doses intravenously or intramuscularly before anesthesia. However, larger doses may depress the circulation at several levels. Similarly, diazepam, now commonly used for premedication, rarely causes hypotension in the usual therapeutic doses. The incidence of complications rises sharply when opioids are combined with barbiturates, diazepam, or phenothiazine derivatives.

Although it is sometimes difficult to judge accurately the amount of premedication that will produce the desired tranquility without reaction, it is safer to err on the side of smaller doses than to seek marked sedation at the risk of arterial hypotension.

INFLUENCE OF POTENT THERAPEUTIC DRUGS USED PRIOR TO ANESTHESIA

Some drugs used in modern therapeutics can affect the course of anesthesia unfavorably, as discussed in Chapter 4. Although drugs with this potential do not invariably cause hypotension, it is important to obtain a history of all medications the patient has received. Of chief concern are the adrenal steroids, the antihypertensives, the beta-adrenergic blockers, and the tranquilizers, drugs that may potentiate the moderate reduction in blood pressure often seen with general anesthetics. Rarely, a patient may develop profound hypotension during or following anesthesia under these circumstances.

OVERDOSE OF GENERAL ANESTHETICS

Overdose of general anesthetics is a common cause of arterial hypotension. The overdose may be "absolute" or "relative"; in the former case, the amount of drug administered is in excess of that ordinarily tolerated by a normal patient. This may result from a sudden increase in the inspired concentration of an inhalation anesthetic or intravenous injection of a large amount of barbiturate.

Certain additional factors predispose to "absolute" overdose. As the patient's tissues approach saturation, a smaller increment of anesthetic is required to cause a rise in blood concentration. Overdose, therefore, tends to occur during prolonged anesthesia when large amounts of drug have been absorbed. Overdose with irritant volatile anesthetics occurs more easily if the trachea has been intubated, for the protective action of laryngeal closure is no longer present and pulmonary uptake can be considerable, especially if respiration is assisted or controlled. Overdose also tends to occur at the extremes of age and in the presence of hypothermia, as may develop during prolonged thoracic or abdominal operations when appropriate measures to maintain or monitor body temperature have not been applied.

In "relative" overdose the actual amount of drug given is acceptable for the age and weight of the patient but represents, at the time, a larger dose than is tolerable, a sensitivity more apparent than real. In the presence of reduced circulating blood volume the concentration of inhalation anesthetic increases more rapidly. If vasoconstriction in other body areas is present but blood flow to heart or brain is maintained, depression can result from addition to the blood of ordinarily innocuous amounts of anesthetic. Under either circumstance, a higher concentration of anesthetic is presented to the vital organs than expected from the small amount given.

Although we have referred to hypotension in the context of overdose, we remind the reader that the pharmacologic response to progressive deepening of anesthesia with all general anesthetics entails peripheral vasodilation and reduced myocardial contractility. With halothane and enflurane, the blood pressure response is a good guide to depth of anesthesia, especially when a neuromuscular blockade is not used (see Chapter 12). On the other hand, some studies show that the circulatory depressant actions of anesthetics tend to ameliorate with time.

Prevention of arterial hypotension resulting from overdose involves two principles: administering the least amount of anesthetic compatible with adequate surgical conditions, and taking the time to induce anesthesia gradually or to change from one level to another slowly. The surgeon should recognize that the optimal depth of anesthesia is that safest for the patient. A patient may tolerate a given blood concentration of anesthetic provided it develops slowly, whereas the same concentration rapidly produced may cause profound hypotension.

Treatment of overdose with inhalation agents comprises prompt reduction of the inspired anesthetic concentration, elimination of the anesthetic from the circuit, and, if necessary, assisted ventilation to facilitate lowering the concentration in blood. If the drugs concerned are eliminated in the main by routes other than the lungs, the general supportive measures listed at the end of this chapter are instituted.

VASCULAR ABSORPTION OF LOCAL ANESTHETICS

Rapid absorption of local anesthetics from mucous membranes or other highly vascular tissues may cause marked hypotension (see Chapter 18). Probable causes include depression of the myocardium and the vasomotor centers as well as dilation of peripheral vessels as a result of direct action. Prior administration of a barbiturate or diazepam does not protect against these effects and, indeed, may heighten circulatory depression.

Critically ill and elderly patients scheduled for local anesthesia are often unattended during operation; deaths have occurred under this circumstance. An anesthetist or other person trained in observing patients might well attend all patients, especially those in poor physical condition in whom extensive use of local anesthesia is planned.

Hypotension can be minimized by reducing the total quantity of anesthetic injected per unit time. Use of large volumes of concentrated solutions and rapid injection are chiefly responsible for dangerous elevation of blood levels of local anesthetic. When topical anesthesia is used, the same principles apply; application is done slowly to avoid rapid vascular absorption.

Treatment consists of the general supportive measures described at the end of this chapter.

SPINAL AND PERIDURAL ANESTHESIA

The reasons for the fall in blood pressure often observed after spinal and peridural anesthesia have been discussed (Chapters 19 and 20): briefly, a reduction in total peripheral resistance or a decline in cardiac output.

Several alternatives are available for prophylaxis or therapy. The first is to insert an intravenous cannula before lumbar puncture or peridural block and infuse 500 ml of lactated Ringer's solution rapidly to expand the vascular space and lessen the probability of hypotension. We prefer this technique in the young, active, and healthy patient. A second alternative is to inject a pressor drug such as ephedrine, 25 to 50 mg intramuscularly, three to five minutes prior to injection of the anesthetic. This technique is indicated in the elderly, in whom vascular reactivity may be diminished, and in patients in whom a decrease in systemic pressure may result in serious impairment of blood flow to heart or brain, as in patients with hypertension, coronary arterial disease, generalized arteriosclerosis, and a history of impaired cerebral blood flow. If effective spinal anesthesia does not result, the rise in systolic pressure resulting from the pressor drug rarely exceeds 40 torr, an elevation that probably occurs spontaneously in all patients from time to time.

A third alternative should be considered for patients in whom elevation in blood pressure or cardiac rate is to be feared. An intravenous infusion is begun before lumbar puncture. If hypotension appears after intrathecal injection, a previously prepared dilute solution of vasopressor is infused at a rate to approximate the patient's accustomed pressure (phenylephrine 20 mg in 250 ml of 5 per cent dextrose in water via minidrip). If the fall in blood pressure is precipitous, treatment may be too late.

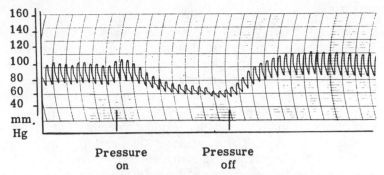

FIGURE 32–1. Arterial hypotension following the application of 20 cm H_2O pressure to the airway of a patient under general anesthesia.

To prevent a catastrophe associated with a sudden reduction in blood pressure, the anesthetist must recognize that hypotension can develop immediately upon intrathecal injection of the local anesthetic. Repeated measurement of blood pressure is therefore essential until anesthesia stabilizes; treatment must be prompt. If possible, the legs should be raised to provide autotransfusion. The entire body should not be tilted head down lest a higher level of anesthesia develop. Oxygen supplementation to respiration is begun. A vasopressor is given intravenously and fluids are infused rapidly unless otherwise contraindicated.

RAISED AIRWAY PRESSURE

Positive pressure applied to the airway may lower arterial pressure (Fig. 32–1), as the pressure is transmitted to the large intrathoracic blood vessels and pulmonary capillaries as well. The higher the mean pressure level the lower the blood flow through these vessels, and cardiac output diminishes in proportion to the degree of interference with venous return. As cardiac output and arterial pressure fall, compensatory vasoconstriction in both venous and arterial circulations is initiated via baroreceptor discharge. A normal individual can tolerate reasonable degrees of raised airway pressure through ability to constrict peripheral vessels, especially those of the venous capacitance system.

This phenomenon is more significant in the following circumstances: in hypovolemia, when the sympathetic nervous system is hypoactive, following use of ganglionic blocking drugs and general anesthetics; when positive airway pressure is maintained throughout the respiratory cycle; and when the patient is in the head-up position, so that blood is pooled in dependent portions of the body. Other changes occurring during anesthesia can either oppose or enhance the decrease in arterial pressure. Congested intrathoracic veins collapse less readily in response to external pressure than when venous pressure is normal. As halothane, enflurane, and isoflurane increase right auricular pressure secondary to myocardial depression, the hypotensive response to increased airway pressure would be depth dependent. The hypotensive response is muted in the presence of constrictive pericarditis, expanded blood volume, mitral stenosis, or congestive heart failure. If abdominal wall tone resists the transmitted intrapulmonic pressure, higher pressures are transmitted to intrathoracic structures. If the thorax is open, less pressure is transmitted to the great veins but pressure is still transmitted to capillaries.

Prevention or treatment of hypotension in this instance consists of decreasing the level and duration of pressure applied to the airway. If pulmonary ventilation thereby becomes inadequate, a return to spontaneous breathing should be permitted with respiratory assistance.

HEMORRHAGE

Arterial hypotension may follow either loss of whole blood or, in extensive operations, loss of plasma to the tissues. Unfortunately, estimation of the amount of blood lost during operation is faulty. The technique of weighing sponges and subtracting the dry from the wet weight permits a reasonably accurate appraisal of loss, allowing for blood replacement on a sounder basis. This does not, however, take into account "third space loss." Monitoring of central venous pressure is a fair guide to fluid and blood replacement requirements in most patients, but in those with left ventricular dysfunction a Swan-Ganz catheter will provide a more reliable guide (Chapters 9 and 23). A high degree of suspicion is essential when measured or estimated losses do not account for clinical evidence of hypotension.

Hypotension and tachycardia are often late signs of blood loss in the recumbent healthy patient, except in acute, major loss; bradycardia is common, especially in children and in the presence of hypoxia. A pale, moist skin and narrow pulse pressure are suggestive, as are restlessness and ischemic changes on the electrocardiogram. Urinary output is a sensitive guide, particularly so postoperatively when occult bleeding is the basis for progressive hypotension.

Hemodilution takes place slowly so that determination of hemoglobin or hematocrit values is of little immediate value. Determinations of blood volumes are not useful unless preoperative measurements are available for comparison and bleeding has ceased. Occasionally, the presence of blood intraperitoneally can be demonstrated by culdotomy or peritoneal tap.

If considerable blood loss is anticipated, one or more 14- to 16-gauge intravenous catheters are placed so that blood can be administered rapidly, under pressure if necessary. Hazards involved are discussed in Chapter 23.

The necessity of having sufficient whole blood typed, crossmatched, and available prior to elective major operation is obvious. In an emergency, type O universal donor blood of low A or B titer can be used, although a 10-minute saline crossmatch is preferred. On the other hand, considerable hemodilution with lactated Ringer's solution is well tolerated, as witnessed during extracorporeal circulation and in operations on Jehovah's Witnesses who will not accept blood products. One should not overlook the value of blood component therapy or dextran or albumin in moderate quantities as plasma expanders (see Chapter 22).

SURGICAL MANEUVERS

Surgical manipulation in the neck, thorax, or abdomen is a common cause of arterial hypotension, explainable on a mechanical or reflex basis. Venous return to the heart may be obstructed by surgical packs, torsion or compression of large veins by retractors, gallbladder or kidney rests, or pressure of the gravid uterus or large abdominal tumors on the inferior vena cava. Rapid release of increased intra-abdominal pressure during drainage of ascites or delivery of a large abdominal tumor may be followed by hypotension as a result of blood pooling in dilated veins. Rapid decompression of a distended urinary bladder can also cause hypotension.

Hypotension may reflexively follow traction on the gallbladder, bowel, uterus, or mesentery or stimulation of the parietal peritoneum in the upper abdomen (Fig. 32–2). If the patient is conscious during regional anesthesia, such manipulation may also cause pain, nausea, vomiting, and breath holding. Reflex hypotension is not limited to stimulation intraperitoneally but may follow manipulation in the chest or stimulation of periosteum or joint cavities. It is presumed that the autonomic nervous system is involved in these reactions, but whether afferent impulses ascend via sympathetic, phrenic, or vagal pathways is unclear. In the upper abdomen the intercostal nerves are

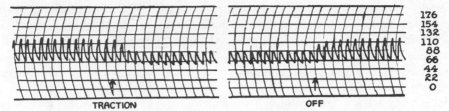

FIGURE 32–2. Continuous intra-arterial pressure tracing showing abrupt reduction of pulse pressure with traction on the mesentery of the colon of an anesthetized patient. Numbers at right represent torr.

believed to carry some of these impulses. As a result of afferent impulses, both inhibition of sympathetic activity and increased vagal tone on the heart have been shown. Atrial contraction contributes to ventricular filling, and vagal-induced reduction in contractility may participate in the diminished stroke volume observed. A puzzling aspect of the hypotension observed during surgical activity is the absence of bradycardia on some occasions and its presence at other times. Atropine given intravenously is useful in treatment. Peripheral vasodilation may play a role in some instances.

Some evidence suggests that reflexes are more active during lighter planes of general anesthesia and may be partially or completely blocked in the deeper planes or inhibited by neuromuscular blockers that interfere with ganglionic transmission (see Chapter 15).

Serious hypotension may result when a surgeon removes a clamp from the aorta or if both aorta and vena cava are occluded simultaneously, obstructing venous return. Hypoxemia, hypotension, and even cardiac arrest have followed total hip replacement owing to absorption of monomeric methyl methacrylate, a component of the bone cement. More care in preparation of the cement at operation has practically eliminated the incidence of this complication. Carotid sinus stimulation may occur during operations on the neck, resulting in vagal-induced bradycardia and hypotension; local anesthetic infiltration or atropine given intravenously mutes this response.

Gentleness on the part of surgeons and awareness of the consequences of their maneuvers constitute the basis for prevention and treatment of hypotension resulting from surgical manipulation. The anesthetist must be aware of the surgeon's actions at all times and must remain in constant communication.

CHANGE IN POSITION OR MOVING THE PATIENT

The circulation of the anesthetized patient is less able to compensate for stress than that of the unanesthetized one, particularly in those critically ill. Positional changes should be accomplished slowly and gently and blood pressure observed throughout.

Certain operative positions may be poorly tolerated; the lateral decubitus position and flexion required for exposure of the kidney or adrenal gland are good examples. Operations performed with the patient in the sitting position are often complicated by hypotension. Here the legs should be wrapped in Ace bandages beforehand. In patients in poor physical condition it is helpful to test the cardiovascular response to the anticipated position before anesthesia is induced.

CARDIOVASCULAR DISEASE

Myocardial ischemia or infarction during anesthesia may be followed by a profound fall in blood pressure. Diagnosis is usually difficult and is rarely established until the ischemia is of several hours duration. Hypotension may accompany ventricular tachycardia in patients with mitral stenosis who are not adequately digitalized.

Multifocal ventricular tachycardia may compromise diastolic filling of the heart; blood pressure then declines. Nodal rhythm, through alteration of the auricular-ventricular filling pattern, may reduce cardiac output and cause hypotension.

Embolism to any of several vascular beds may lead to hypotension, the cause not readily recognized. Cerebral air embolism is a precipitating factor in hypotension as seen during open heart surgery. Usually this involves the brain stem, and other neurologic signs are present. Pulmonary embolism from peripheral veins may occur, as may fat embolism from fracture sites, amniotic fluid emboli during delivery, and venous air entrainment during cervical operations or craniotomy. Massive embolism is suspected with appearance of an electrocardiographic pattern of acute cor pulmonale.

Hypovolemia may be present prior to operation. Dehydration, hemorrhage, loss of gastrointestinal secretions, and plasma loss in extensive burns contribute to this state. If hypovolemia is unrecognized, dilation of the vascular bed associated with induction of anesthesia is often followed by hypotension. Deficits of both extravascular and intracellular fluid can be factors in circulatory inadequacy. This is inextricably related to sodium concentration, so that both fluid and electrolyte imbalance can be associated with hypotension. Furthermore, the electrolyte environment of the peripheral circulation is a major influence in the response to endogenously secreted catecholamines and adrenal steroids.

Cardiac tamponade following penetrating injury of the heart, cardiotomy, or anticoagulant therapy may be an unsuspected cause of hypotension.

Heart failure may develop during anesthesia as a result of excessive fluid replacement or in relation to the circulatory complications previously noted. Failure is relatively easily diagnosed by a rising central venous pressure in the face of a falling arterial pressure, engorgement of neck veins, and the presence of rales on auscultation of the lungs. If the diagnosis of fluid overload is suspected, furosemide is first administered intravenously and urinary output measured; on the other hand, if left heart failure seems more likely, a Swan-Ganz catheter is inserted, pulmonary wedge pressure measured, diagnosis confirmed, and then dopamine infused, with furosemide subsequently if needed (see Chapter 23).

In refractory cardiogenic shock, intra-aortic balloon counterpulsation may tide a patient over until blood pressure can be maintained spontaneously.

SEPTIC SHOCK

Septic shock rarely appears for the first time during anesthesia; it is either present preoperatively and operation is attempted in the hope of eliminating the source of infection, or it develops postoperatively owing to spread of a previously contained infection or contamination of a wound.

Septic shock is commonly caused by *Escherichia coli, Aerobacter aerogenes, Pseudomonas aeruginosa,* clostridia, or *Staphylococcus aureus* and is related to the release of endotoxins that potentiate the action of catecholamines, eventually causing major plasma loss in tissues. In the fully developed syndrome, severe hypotension is accompanied by tachycardia, cold and blanched skin, and inadequate tissue perfusion. But early in the course the skin may be hot and dry. Whether endotoxins depress the central nervous system by direct action in addition to depressing the myocardium and smooth muscle of blood vessels is not known.

Treatment of septic shock varies. In addition to standard supportive therapy, control of fever, and use of antibiotics, vasodilator therapy with concomitant use of large volumes of plasma or balanced salt solution is also instituted. This treatment is predicated on a significant element of vasoconstriction. Massive steroid therapy has been advised, with repeated doses of 2 gm or more given intravenously; the pharmacologic actions are debatable, but steroids presumably establish a better balance at peripheral vascular sites among catecholamines, steroids, and electrolytes. As myocardial failure may occur, digitalis is indicated, perhaps dopamine, and certainly respiratory assistance with oxygen. A Swan-Ganz catheter will provide data to guide therapy, but the observation must be correlated with systemic blood pressure, urinary output, and periodic testing with intravenous infusions, as outlined in Chapter 23.

INCOMPATIBLE TRANSFUSION

Major blood group incompatibility reactions may be accompanied by hypotension. Indeed, together with generalized cyanosis and oozing at the operative site, unexplained hypotension should suggest the possibility of a hemolytic transfusion reaction (see Chapter 23).

ANAPHYLACTIC REACTIONS

One kind of allergic reaction to extrinsic antigens involves the presence of circulating antibodies in the serum of the host. Anaphylaxis is an example of this response, which also includes serum sickness, allergy involving the wheal and flare reaction, angioneurotic edema, urticaria, asthma, and certain drug reactions. The reactions observed are referred to as "immediate." This is perhaps the least common cause of hypotension observed by anesthetists, but an anaphylactic reaction with severe hypotension has been reported during spinal anesthesia upon administration of a small amount of dextran (a macromolecular polysaccharide of bacterial origin) and after injection of penicillin. Some degree of protection against anaphylaxis by general anesthetics has been demonstrated, but as there are varying degrees of reaction, it is reasonable to assume that general anesthesia offers protection only against the mild reaction. Treatment consists of administration of oxygen by positive pressure to overcome bronchospasm, administration of epinephrine intramuscularly or intravenously, and infusion of theophylline ethylenediamine followed by hydrocortisone. Antihistamines are of little value once the reaction has occurred.

MANAGEMENT OF HYPOTENSION

DIAGNOSIS

The standard means of diagnosing inadequacy of circulation include measurement of arterial blood pressure and pulse and estimating the pulse volume as an index of the volume of cardiac ejection or run-off in the peripheral circulation. In healthy young adults a systolic blood pressure of 80 torr may require no treatment, whereas a similar finding in an elderly patient with arteriosclerosis and a history of hypertension constitutes a threat to life. A conscious patient in whom cerebral ischemia develops secondary to a decrease in blood pressure will be restless, anxious, and even disoriented. One can occasionally detect waxing and waning of mental acuity in such patients during alterations in the rate of infusion of a pressor drug. Pallor, cold wet skin, and dilated pupils suggest circulatory inadequacy, as does peripheral cyanosis. The rate of capillary refill upon application of pressure to the skin is sometimes used as an index of the state of the peripheral circulation. Deep sighing respirations or air hunger in a conscious individual suggests a severe degree of shock. Presumably, respiratory stimulation is initiated via carotid sinus pressor receptors. Delayed onset of anesthesia after injection of intravenous anesthetics suggests a sluggish circulation. If an intravenous infusion slows, venoconstriction is suggested as compensating for circulatory inadequacy. Similarly, a reduction in bleeding in the operative field, unusually dark venous blood, and pallor of organs reflect hypotension and compensatory vasoconstriction. Urine output is closely related to the adequacy of renal circulation.

GENERAL THERAPEUTIC MEASURES

The aim of treatment should be to augment perfusion of vital organs, which usually do not require a systolic pressure higher than 70 torr so long as other factors impeding oxygen and carbon dioxide transport are not operative. If circumstances permit, elevation of the legs may increase blood pressure through mobilization of pooled blood, especially after sympathetic blockade. One must also consider relief of pain in the traumatized patient, remembering that opioids may produce hypotension.

Fluid Therapy

Rapid intravenous administration of any of a variety of solutions may be lifesaving during severe hypotension. The volume of fluid given rather than its composition is vital in the early moments, especially if hypotension is the result of trauma or blood loss. The initial selection is based on what is immediately at hand. Physiologic saline, 5 per cent dextrose in water, a balanced salt solution, or a plasma expander such as albumin or 6 per cent dextran is given until whole blood becomes available. Consult Chapters 22 and 23 for further details.

Oxygen Therapy

Oxygen should be breathed while a diagnosis is being established and continued as therapy. To assure adequacy of ventilation, respiration must be assisted, with care to prevent excessive airway pressure. If general anesthetics are being administered, they should be discontinued or sharply reduced in concentration. If the patient remains hypotensive at the end of operation, oxygen should be continued.

Vasopressor Drugs

These agents are indicated in the therapy of hypotension if the systolic blood pressure has not responded to the measures already outlined or when signs of inadequate perfusion to vital organs persist. The commonly used pressor drugs are sympathomimetic amines that exert a vasoconstrictor action through stimulation of alpha receptors of the sympathetic system or via increase of myocardial contractile force and heart rate by activation of beta receptors. Vascular responses induced by the two kinds of receptors are as follows: alpha constriction of vascular smooth muscle, cutaneous vessels, mucosa, kidney, and splanchnic circulation; beta positive inotropic activity, stimulation of sinoatrial node, and dilation of blood vessels in skeletal muscle and splanchnic bed.

Selection of the most appropriate pressor drug for therapy of hypotension is not easy. Some drugs have been studied in individuals with normal blood pressures, but few have been completely evaluated in the treatment of hypotension observed under clinical circumstances. As it is in the latter situation that these substances find most use, selection is empiric. Drugs in use today and suggested doses are listed in Table 32–1.

Cardiac Effects. Three cardiac actions are of importance: effect on the force of ventricular contraction, effect on the sinoauricular node and conduction system, and production of ventricular irritability. With the following exceptions, the drugs listed increase myocardial contractile force: methoxamine lacks this action entirely, and it is not a prominent characteristic of phenylephrine. So far as alteration in sino-atrial nodal activity is concerned, epinephrine, ephedrine, levarterenol, isoproterenol, and methamphetamine produce tachycardia by direct action. Slowing of the

TABLE 32–1.   Dosages of Pressor Drugs

	Single Dose (mg)		Continuous IV (mg/500 ml of 5% glucose in water)
	IM	IV	
Dopamine	–	–	400*
Ephedrine	25–50	10–15	–
Epinephrine	–	–	1.0
Isoproterenol (Isuprel)	–	–	0.4–0.8
Levarterenol (Levophed)	–	–	4 ml†
Mephentermine (Wyamine)	15–30	5–15	–
Metaraminol (Aramine)	2–10	0.5–5.0	20–40
Methoxamine (Vasoxyl)	10–20	3–5	–
Phenylephrine (Neo-Synephrine)	1–3	0.2–0.4	10–30

*One ampule of Intropin, 5 ml, contains 200 mg dopamine HCl.
†One ampule contains 4 ml of 0.2% levarterenol bitartrate (0.1% free base).

heart after injection of levarterenol, phenylephrine, or methoxamine is reflexly produced by activation of baroreceptors secondary to the rise in pressure, an effect useful in treating supraventricular tachycardia. Ventricular arrhythmias are common after administration of epinephrine, ephedrine, levarterenol, isoproterenol, and methamphetamine and their incidence and severity enhanced in the presence of hypoxia, hypercarbia, or acidosis. Mephentermine shows relatively little tendency to cause ventricular arrhythmias. Dopamine in 1 to 2 μg/kg/min doses increases myocardial inotropism and blood pressure while acting as a peripheral vasodilator via so-called dopaminergic receptors.

Peripheral Vascular Effects.   All the drugs listed cause vasoconstriction except isoproterenol and dopamine, and the effect with epinephrine is mitigated by vasodilation in muscle. Constriction is prominent in renal, cutaneous, and splanchnic vessels. A powerful action is exerted upon venules and veins, constricting the large venous reservoir and returning to active circulation blood pooled in this area, important in increasing cardiac output. As the dose of dopamine is increased above that mentioned, to 5 to 15 μg/kg/min, the inotropic and vasodilator actions become predominantly those of beta-adrenergic stimulation. With greater than 20 μg/kg/min doses, alpha-adrenergic stimulation occurs.

Apart from angiotensin, which is not used clinically, levarterenol is the most potent vasoconstrictor but also the shortest acting; it is administered exclusively by intravenous infusion, preferably through a centrally placed catheter. Slough of skin, subcutaneous tissue, and muscle has occurred at the site of superficial intravenous injection. Treatment for extravasation consists of local infiltration with phentolamine. At one time levarterenol was so popular that few patients with serious hypotension escaped its application. Now, treatment is directed more toward the cause, and levarterenol is less frequently employed.

Factors Limiting the Effectiveness of Pressor Drugs.   For an optimal pressor effect, blood volume must be sufficient to fill the vascular space in its changing capacity. The response of peripheral vessels depends on a proper balance among endogenous catecholamines, adrenal steroids, sodium, potassium, and hydrogen ion concentration. Imbalance leads to poor reactivity. Either respiratory or metabolic acidosis may counter the action of pressor drugs. Therefore, blood gas measurements should accompany treatment.

Selection of Drug.   With coincident hypotension and bradycardia, it seems reasonable to administer a drug that stimulates the sinoauricular node. When vasodilation exists, as after spinal anesthesia, a pressor drug with an action primarily on peripheral blood vessels is considered the drug of choice. If an inotropic drug is needed in the presence of peripheral vasoconstriction and hypotension, then dopamine seems appropriate.

REFERENCES

Due TL, Johnson JM, Wood M, et al: Intraoperative autotransfusion in the management of massive hemorrhage. Am J Surg 130:652, 1975.

Gelin LE, Davidson I, Haglund U, et al: Septic shock. Surg Clin North Am 60:161, 1980.

Goldberg LI: Dopamine — clinical use of an endogenous catecholamine. N Engl J Med 291:707, 1976.

Jakschik BA, Marshall GR, Kourik JL, et al: Profile of circulatory vasoactive substances in hemorrhagic shock and their pharmacologic manipulation. J Clin Invest 54:842, 1974.

Shoemaker WC, Brown RS: Dilemma of vasopressors and vasodilators in therapy of shock. Surg Gynecol Obstet 132:51, 1971.

Smith LL, Moore FD: Refractory hypotension in man — Is this irreversible shock? Clinical and biochemical observations. N Engl J Med 267:733, 1962.

Smith NT, Corbascio AN: The use and misuse of pressor agents. Anesthesiology 33:58, 1970.

Theye RA, Perry LB, Brzica SM, Jr: Influence of anesthetic agent in response to hemorrhagic hypotension. Anesthesiology 40:32, 1974.

Vandam LD: Drugs for arterial hypotension and shock. In Modell W (ed): Drugs of Choice. St Louis, C V Mosby Co., 1980.

Chapter 33

UNUSUAL COMPLICATIONS OF ANESTHESIA AND MORTALITY

Many complications may arise during the course of anesthesia. These occur because of certain physical or pathologic characteristics of the patient, the drugs or the techniques of anesthetic administration employed, or the supportive measures used. Most of these complications have been discussed in other sections of this text, included under specific agents, or techniques. Those discussed here occur with sufficient frequency and serious consequence to warrant emphasis.

ASPIRATION OF GASTRIC CONTENTS

Throughout this text we have hinted at the serious consequences of aspiration of gastric contents into the lungs, but further emphasis is needed at this point. The possibility of a full stomach exists in any surgical or medical patient; hence the dictum of withholding oral intake of food or drink during the eight to ten hours prior to anesthetization. Obviously aspiration is always a threat in emergency operations, in the presence of pyloric or intestinal obstruction, when diaphragmatic hernia or esophageal diverticula exist, and in those patients with diminished pharyngeal reflexes owing to neurologic or debilitating disease. Above all, the parturient is at highest risk because of the unpredictable time of delivery and the delay in gastric emptying time caused by the processes of labor.

The pulmonary consequences of aspiration relate to both the volume and the character of the material inhaled. Large amounts of fluid will inundate the lungs, whereas particulate matter may result in obstruction at any level; either will cause varying degrees of asphyxiation. Pathogenic bacteria and colon bacilli in stagnant secretions or feculent matter will produce infection, but perhaps the most serious consequences result from the relative acidity of gastric secretions. Inhalation of material with a pH less than 2.5 causes an immediate intense bronchoconstriction and destruction of the tracheal mucosa; within hours, a spreading and patchy pneumonitis appears as a fluffiness or "whiteout" on chest x-ray. As a result of obstruction and atelectasis, a major degree of pulmonary shunting occurs, with a widening of the A-a oxygen gradient. Pulmonary edema may develop as a consequence of the chemical insult alone or secondary to heart failure. Eventually, the full-blown pathogenic picture resembles that of the so-called adult respiratory distress syndrome. The syndrome bears the eponym of Mendelsohn, who first called attention to the problem in obstetric patients.

As in all complications of anesthesia, prevention is the key. If feasible before general anesthesia, an attempt should be made to empty the stomach via gastric drainage, a method that is hardly effective when solid food is present. Furthermore, upon induction of anesthesia, with relaxation of the pyloric and gastroesophageal sphincters, reflux of secretions continues in the presence of intestinal obstruction. Thus, sealing off the trachea at the start of general anesthesia is essential. With the aid of topical anesthesia, the trachea may be intubated in cooperative patients while still awake, but aspiration may still take place during the process. Otherwise, a rapid induction is done bearing in mind the hazards of drug overdose in these usually ill patients. With the patient's head elevated about 45 degrees and following oxygenation, a small dose of induction agent is given intravenously followed by succinylcholine after fasciculations have been eliminated by a competitive neuromuscular blocker. As unconsciousness ensues, an assistant should occlude the esophagus via gentle backward pressure on the cricoid cartilage (Sellick's maneuver). The trachea is intubated as quickly as possible, the cuff on the tube immediately inflated, and induction of general anesthesia begun, although gradually. Gastric drainage is continued throughout and, at termination, unless otherwise indicated, extubation is accomplished when pharyngeal reflexes are once again active, with a large-tipped suction device at hand and the patient in the lateral decubitus position.

When aspiration occurs or is suspected before the trachea has been sealed, rapid intubation is still indicated and the trachea suctioned. The pH of the aspirate should be tested by means of litmus paper or one of the commercially prepared papers, even though dilution with alkaline material may already have occurred. Tracheal lavage with saline, 5 ml at a time, followed by suction, is advocated even though the inspiration preceding a cough serves to spread the material throughout the lungs. If large particulate material is present, bronchoscopy and removal are necessary. At one time tracheal instillation and parenteral administration of a corticosteroid were practiced to diminish the mucosal inflammatory response, but subsequent studies have cast doubt on the efficacy of these measures. Undoubtedly the most effective therapy is that employed for any kind of acute pulmonary insufficiency whether the result of aspiration, drowning, or infection. In all studies the use of PEEP (see Chapter 37) has proved most effective in reversing the pathophysiologic changes. Antibiotics may be given when there is bacterial contamination and a bronchodilator such as aminophylline used to combat spasm.

THE MALIGNANT HYPERTHERMIA SYNDROME

Malignant hyperthermia syndrome (MHS) is defined as a potentially fatal hypermetabolic syndrome induced by practically all of the currently used inhalation anesthetics and usually triggered by injection of succinylcholine. More people may have had MHS than hitherto realized, perhaps induced by major stress, trauma, emotional upheaval, or strenuous exercise.

HISTORY

Denborough of Australia deserves credit for calling attention to the problem in the 1960s, when he encountered a 21-year-old student with a leg fracture. The patient was concerned not so much about the fracture as by the knowledge that ten relatives had died as a consequence of diethylether anesthesia; all had had high fevers, the first familial death occurring in 1922. His physical examination and all biochemical tests were normal. Study of the family history revealed that he had probably inherited this previously unrecognized anomaly of metabolism as a mendelian dominant characteristic. This discovery raised the question that some of the sudden deaths occurring perhaps over a century during or immediately after anesthesia and associated with high fever and convulsions might have been caused by MHS.

ETIOLOGY

The basis of MHS is an underlying pathophysiologic disorder of muscle that may affect body membranes in general. Theoretical considerations are based on the results of experiments on MHS-susceptible species of pigs (Dutch Landrace, Poland China, and Pietrain). These species may succumb to stress alone, a syndrome well known in veterinary medicine in the dog, cat, and horse. Two predisposing kinds of myopathy seem to exist in man. In one, MHS is a dominantly inherited variety not apparent until the syndrome is triggered. The other is a disease of young men with any of a galaxy of physical deformities: short stature, cryptorchidism, pectus carinatum, ptosis, low-set ears, kyphosis, lordosis, weak serrati muscles, and antimongoloid slant of the palpebral fissures. A nonpyrexic variety of the disease has been described that might explain an occasional enigmatic cardiac arrest during anesthesia.

Development of MHS depends on a combination of myogenic, neurologic, and endocrinologic derangements as well as generalized membrane dysfunction. Hyperactivity of the sympathetic nervous system, with release of catecholamines and thyroid hormone, has been implicated in the progression of MHS through their effects on mitochondria. Thus, candidates for operation with undue anxiety, fever, and acrocyanosis before anesthesia may develop MHS. The distinction between causative and secondary events is unclear.

MYOGENIC ORIGIN

In addition to musculoskeletal abnormalities, development of muscle rigidity after intravenous injection of succinylcholine, although by no means universal, is considered a prime sign of onset. In susceptible patients an elevation of serum creatine phosphokinase (CPK) is sometimes found, and, at the height of the syndrome, CPK rises markedly along with the appearance of myoglobinuria. Muscle biopsy reveals depletion of adenosine triphosphate and CPK. Although the concept is not accepted by all, a rise in skeletal muscle oxygen consumption is said to precede the generalized rise in somatic oxygen utilization with subsequent elevation in body temperature. In susceptible patients muscle biopsies yield no specific structural abnormalities as indicated by either light or electron microscopy.

BIOCHEMICAL THEORY

The most reliable diagnostic laboratory test is the development of contracture in isolated muscle exposed to both caffeine and halothane. Caffeine in a concentration of 2.5 mM induces influx of calcium into the myoplasm from the sarcoplasmic reticulum (SR) in response to muscle depolarization, whereas re-uptake of calcium into the SR is blunted at higher caffeine concentrations. Halothane augments the contracture. Two processes are involved in excitation-contraction. First, depolarization of the motor end plate occurs in response to acetylcholine released from the nerve ending. A transient alteration of membrane permeability results in influx of sodium and efflux of potassium. As the electric potential is propagated in muscle, calcium is released into the myoplasm of the muscle fiber. Calcium causes actin or myosin filaments to slide past each other to produce contraction. The bulk of the calcium is thought to lie within the muscle fiber, probably the SR.

Isolated muscle from susceptible patients shows increased sensitivity to caffeine contracture when exposed to halothane. One theory holds that a defect in regulation of myoplasmic calcium exists, so that on exposure to a triggering agent muscle is unable to control the level of intramyoplasmic calcium. As a result of inability to strike a balance between the amount of calcium needed to sustain contraction and that sequestered, hypermetabolism develops. Dantrolene seems to act on the excitation-contraction mechanism, which couples depolarization of the sarcolemma membrane with release of calcium from SR.

CLINICAL SYNDROME

The clinical course of MHS probably begins with a hypermetabolic state of muscle, followed by a rapid rise in temperature, as high as 108°F. Development of sustained contracture after succinylcholine administration is a warning sign. On rare occasion, some of the opioids cause muscle contracture apart from the MHS syndrome. Often, the first sign of MHS is tachycardia, secondary to fever and metabolic and respiratory acidosis. The skin feels hot, and venous blood in the operative field is dark as a result of the high oxygen consumption. Tachypnea is observed in the spontaneously breathing patient owing to excess carbon dioxide production but is obviously not present in paralyzed patients.

TREATMENT

When MHS is suspected, anesthesia and operation should be terminated as quickly as possible and cooling begun by one or a combination of measures: lavage of stomach and body cavities with iced saline, body immersion in iced water, surface cooling with ice packs (the least effective step). With cooling it is important to avoid drift into the hypothermic range. Pulmonary hyperventilation is instituted and sodium bicarbonate given intravenously to combat both respiratory and metabolic acidosis. Monitoring of arterial blood gases and acid-base status is necessary in treatment, and the bladder is catheterized. An osmotic diuretic should be given to avert vasoconstrictive nephropathy (ATN). Cardiac arrhythmias or arrest may comprise the initial signs of MHS. Choice of treatment for arrhythmias is not lidocaine, which seems to aggravate the biochemical alteration, but procaine and preferably procainamide. Hyperkalemia is treated with insulin and glucose infusion. Because of the damage to cell membranes, fluid extravasates from the circulation; therefore, large volumes of crystalloids may be required to maintain circulatory adequacy. One mg/kg body weight of dantrolene up to a dose of 10 mg/kg is given as soon as possible.

All of these measures are continued postoperatively in the intensive care setting, as relapse may occur. Commonly reported late complications include disseminated intravascular coagulation and ATN. Coma, when present, may be irreversible, a manifestation of ischemia secondary to hypoxia.

PREVENTION

Whatever the outcome, relatives of the victim should be examined for MHS potential and those found susceptible advised to wear a Medic-Alert bracelet. Although CPK determinations are not reliable, the *in vitro* caffeine-halothane contracture test is acceptable, but muscle biopsy is required. When faced with the need for anesthesia, susceptible patients should be given dantrolene prophylactically. Although no single anesthetic regimen is considered safe, the barbiturates (pentobarbital and thiopental), a neuroleptic (droperidol), and a nondepolarizing neuromuscular blocker (tubocurarine and pancuronium) are least likely to induce MHS. Regional anesthesia is a good choice, with use of one of the ester local anesthetics (procaine or tetracaine) rather than lidocaine, plus heavy sedation to avoid stress. A history of family anesthesia problems, emotional status, and certain physical defects as well as a concern for the heavily

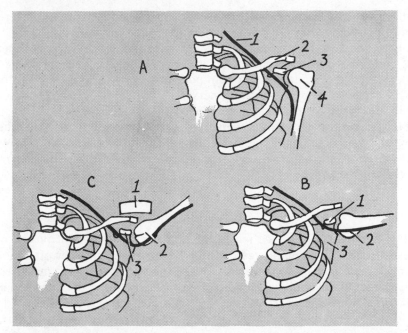

FIGURE 33–1. Traction on brachial plexus. *A*, Arm at side: *1*, brachial plexus; *2*, clavicle; *3*, coracoid process of scapula; *4*, head of humerus. *B*, Arm at right angle: scapula (*3*) rotates and brachial plexus is stretched beneath coracoid process (*1*) and around head of humerus (*2*). *C*, Arm hyperextended with shoulder brace (*1*) depressing scapula (*3*). Brachial plexus stretched beneath coracoid process and around head of humerus.

muscled, injured person are among the important details for the anesthetist's consideration.

NERVE INJURY

Peripheral nerves can be injured during anesthesia through stretch or compression because the anesthetized patient does not perceive pain and lacks protective muscle tone. Among the nerves commonly injured are the several divisions of the brachial plexus and the ulnar, radial, common peroneal, and, rarely, facial nerves.

The nerves comprising the brachial plexus arise centrally at the transverse processes of the vertebrae and terminate peripherally at the point of entry into the arm. Separation of these points may stretch the nerves with resulting molecular damage, hemorrhage or ischemia, and development of palsy (Fig. 33–1). Flexion of the head to the opposite side with coincident downward displacement of the shoulder places tension on the nerves. Several anatomic fulcrums, such as the scalene muscles, the attachment of the pectoralis minor muscle to the coracoid process of the scapula, and the rounded head of the humerus, provide additional possibilities for stretch; hyperabduction, extension, and external rotation of the arm stretch the brachial plexus around these fulcrums. A supporting brace improperly applied to the shoulder may act not only as an artificial fulcrum but may compress the brachial plexus against the first rib. A shoulder brace should not be used when the arm is extended on an arm rest. The plexus may also be pinched between the clavicle and first rib.

To avoid brachial plexus injury one must bear the possibility in mind and avoid extremes of position of the head and arm. When palsy develops a careful neurologic examination should be recorded and measures for restoration of function immediately begun with support of the paralyzed muscles and physiotherapy. In severe injury, restitution of normal function, if at all, may require up to a year.

The ulnar, radial, and common peroneal nerves are superficially placed, hence they are easily compressed against bone, stirrups, or the sides of an operating table or stretched around bony eminences. Certain positions, such as lithotomy or the lateral decubitus, predispose to injury of these nerves. If paralysis occurs, treatment is the same as that described for brachial plexus injury.

The facial nerve may be injured by overenthusiastic attempts to elevate the jaw via pressure on the rami of the mandible or by tight application of a head strap. Weakness of the muscles about the mouth or eyes is a manifestation of injury usually reversible within a week or two.

OCULAR INJURY

Careless application of a face mask, the position of the patient on the operating table, anesthetic technique employed, or preparation of the skin for operation on the head and neck may predispose to ocular injury. The once used open mask techniques for administration of volatile anesthetics were especially prone to cause conjunctivitis or corneal abrasion. Liquid anesthetic or vapor reaching the eye directly could produce corneal ulceration. However, ulceration is more likely to be the result of trauma or drying of the cornea. Large masks pressing on the eyes have resulted in retinal detachment, periorbital edema, and numbness in the distribution of the supraorbital nerve. Patients with prominent eyes or exophthalmos and those with neurologic disease such as Bell's palsy are at greater risk of corneal injury.

The best precaution against corneal injury is to keep the lids closed. One should not elicit the corneal reflex to determine depth of anesthesia. When the eyes are to be covered by surgical drapes, the lids are best kept closed with a plastic eye shield or adhesive tape. The same precautions apply when the patient is in the prone position or the head is face down on a cerebellar head rest; the head should be raised periodically to prevent pressure necrosis of the forehead and cheeks. Instillation of sterile mineral oil into the conjunctival sac prevents desiccation of the cornea.

The eyes should be inspected at the conclusion of anesthesia. If injury is detected, ophthalmologic consultation should be sought. Simple conjunctivitis is best treated with topical antibiotics such as Neosporin, erythromycin, or tetracycline. Corneal abrasions are not only painful but may progress to inflammation of the uveal tract. If treated early with an antibiotic or one of the sulfonamides, locally instilled, abrasions usually re-epithelialize within 24 hours. Topical steroids should be avoided. During this time the eye is securely patched with a sterile ocular pad. Atropine is used for mydriasis to prevent formation of synechiae when inflammation is present and to relieve the pain associated with spasm of the iris and ciliary muscle. Topical local anesthetics for relief of pain should be avoided since they retard corneal epithelial regeneration.

INJURY TO THE LUNGS

EXCESSIVE PRESSURE

Because the gases used in anesthesia are delivered from cylinders and wall outlets at higher than atmospheric pressure, the possibility of damage to the lungs is ever present. Injury can occur not only during anesthesia but whenever inhalation therapy or resuscitation is practiced. The exact limits of pressure that can be safely applied to the lungs have not been defined. Generally, pressure should not exceed 20 to 30 cm H_2O; however, higher pressures may be required to inflate the lungs after collapse. Whether or not damage occurs depends on the rapidity of the rise in pressure, the pattern of

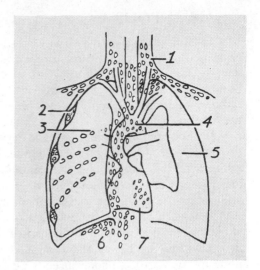

FIGURE 33–2. Escape of air following rupture of lungs. *1*, Subcutaneous emphysema; *2*, subpleural bleb; *3*, pulmonary interstitial emphysema; *4*, mediastinal emphysema; *5*, pneumothorax; *6*, pneumoperitoneum; *7*, air embolism to heart.

distribution, and whether the thorax is open at the time. Furthermore, high pressures applied at the nose and mouth are not necessarily transmitted to the alveoli.

When high pressure is transmitted to the alveoli, rupture may take place, with hemorrhage and capillary air embolism or dissection into the interstitial tissues (Fig. 33–2). Air in the interstitial tissues of the lungs may collect beneath the pleura, forming blebs and rupturing into the pleural cavity, or it may dissect back via the hilum into the mediastinum (pneumomediastinum). The lungs become distended with air trapped in the interstitium (pulmonary interstitial emphysema), and venous return to the heart may be blocked by collection of air in the mediastinum (air block). Mediastinal emphysema and air block can be recognized by distinctly audible churning sounds synchronous with the heart beat, the so-called mill wheel murmur (Hamman's sign). Air in the mediastinum can dissect downward retroperitoneally or escape into the subcutaneous tissues of the neck or into the pleural cavities when the superior mediastinal pleura ruptures.

Alveolar rupture may occur when there is free transmission of high pressures to the alveoli, as when the trachea is intubated. In the presence of subcutaneous emphysema or otherwise unexplained respiratory distress and hypoxia, pneumothorax, mediastinal and pulmonary interstitial emphysema, and capillary air embolism must be suspected and treated at once if the patient is to survive. In the extreme case there may be little one can do, but the following treatments are suggested.

Pneumothorax. With the patient upright, entry is made into the pleura at the midclavicular line in the second intercostal space anteriorly, with a large gauge needle attached to a 50-ml syringe and a two-way stopcock. Air is aspirated fractionally and underwater drainage instituted. At the same time, pressure is applied to the airway to re-expand the lungs. If tracheal rupture has occurred as a result of trauma or prolonged pressure from a cuffed tracheostomy or tracheal tube, it may be possible to pass a tracheal tube beyond the site to prevent continued escape of air. A double lumen tube at the bifurcation may be useful.

Mediastinal and Subcutaneous Emphysema. Superior mediastinotomy may be performed using local anesthesia if the trapped air is under pressure and is causing respiratory or circulatory embarrassment; unfortunately, this is not of much value.

Protection against high pressure injury to the lungs can be assured only by careful actions and the obligatory placement of safety valves between the pressure source and the patient's airway. As a general rule, gas cylinders or wall outlets should be opened and flows adjusted before connection to the patient is made.

AIR EMBOLISM

In addition to positive airway pressure, air embolism may occur as a result of air entrained in the diploic veins during craniotomy or as a complication of cardiopulmonary bypass, thyroidectomy, or intrauterine manipulation. Concurrent administration of nitrous oxide anesthesia increases the lethality of air embolus by diffusion into the air bubble, enlarging the volume. One hundred per cent oxygen should be substituted immediately.

In suboccipital craniectomy and cervical laminectomy with the patient in the sitting position, prior placement of a catheter in the right ventricle permits immediate withdrawal of trapped air. Air embolism is suspected on appearance of cardiac arrhythmias or unexplained hypotension. A precordial stethoscope or Doppler device will detect the characteristic bubbling or mill wheel sounds.

When feasible, the patient is placed in a steep head-down position with the right side uppermost to prevent tamponade in the outflow tract of the right ventricle. If air is heard within the heart, an attempt is made to aspirate it by means of ventricular puncture or via the catheter already placed. If heart action stops, cardiac resuscitation as described in Chapter 35 should be undertaken. Closed chest manual systole helps the passage of air emboli lodged in the coronary arteries. Hyperbaric oxygenation has been beneficial in effecting recovery of patients with extensive neurologic damage resulting from massive air embolus occurring during cardiopulmonary bypass. Exposure initially to 6 atm, absolute, is followed by prolonged decompression, more or less as practiced in other kinds of barotrauma.

MISCELLANEOUS ACCIDENTS

An infinite number of accidents may happen during or following anesthesia. The following is a partial list of complications observed by the authors:

1. A child, left unattended, fell from an operating table, sustaining lacerations of the scalp.

2. A man carelessly positioned in the lateral position for lumbodorsal sympathectomy awoke with pressure contusions of the genitalia.

3. A patient developed marked swelling of the neck resembling parotitis because of manual efforts to elevate the mandible during respiratory obstruction.

4. A unit of blood was permitted to extravasate into the tissue of a patient's leg that was out of sight beneath surgical drapes.

5. The hand of an unconscious patient was crushed during elevation of the foot of an operating table.

6. A patient with severe generalized osteoporosis sustained a fracture of the humerus during transfer from operating table to litter.

7. Vigorous tracheal suction with repeated cough at the termination of anesthesia led to rupture of abdominal sutures and wound dehiscence.

8. A bottle containing intravenous fluid fell from its stand, striking the patient's head and causing laceration of the scalp.

ANESTHETIC MORTALITY

One observer claims that there is no accurate definition of anesthetic death, that in the past we have focused on presumed errors in anesthetic administration and have overlooked risk-benefit aspects. Anesthetics are not considered in the same context as other pharmacologic agents; there are large variations in response, and untoward reactions may simply signify interaction with other drugs. Induction of hepatic microsomal enzymes may possibly be a more important factor in adverse reactions than hitherto realized.

For many years the term "anesthetic death" has been applied out of ignorance. For example, administration of succinylcholine for muscle relaxation in the burned patient led to excessive release of potassium, resulting in cardiac arrest. Such an occurrence was an unexplained anesthetic death until the cause was found years later. Similarly, a death on the operating table might have been a consequence of malignant hyperthermia. Prolonged respiratory depression after the use of succinylcholine was misunderstood until an abnormal pseudocholinesterase level or its absence explained failure of hydrolysis of the compound. Moreover, as 250,000 sudden deaths occur each year in the U.S., including death from acute arrhythmias, mitral valve prolapse, and Prinzmetal's angina, some deaths in the perioperative period might well be of a coincidental nature.

The concept of preventable anesthesia death was entrenched by the establishment of an Anesthesia Study Commission in Philadelphia in the 1940s, when hospital departments were encouraged to report operating room deaths anonymously. Anesthetists were assumed to be responsible for all factors related to death other than surgical care, and deaths were classified by vote as preventable or nonpreventable. In a 1944 report, 47 per cent of 306 deaths were deemed preventable, 38 per cent nonpreventable, and the remainder indeterminate. The highest percentage of preventable deaths was found in the good risk category, and death was ascribed to inadequate management, poor oxygenation, drug overdose, or error in judgment. Forty three of 59 spinal anesthetic deaths were deemed preventable. Except for inadequate oxygenation, the other judgments were probably subject to interpretation. The patterns of mortality established then still exist today.

The only prospective study of anesthetic deaths was reported in 1954 by Beecher and Todd, who tried to establish exact operative death rates, why such deaths occurred, and whether they could be attributed to anesthesia. From 1948 to 1952, all operative deaths at 40 medical school–associated hospitals were subjected to scrutiny. Cause was determined by an independent committee of surgeons, anesthesiologists, and internists. Deaths were then ascribed to error in diagnosis or surgical judgment and technique; deaths related to anesthesia were ascribed to choice of anesthetic, toxicity, abnormal sensitivity, error in administration, inadequate supervision, error in postoperative care, and miscellaneous reasons. The death rates derived are shown in Table 33–1, along with data from subsequent studies.

TABLE 33–1. Estimates of Anesthetic Risk*

| | | | Incidence of Death | |
Author	Year	Number of Anesthetics	Anesthesia Primary	Anesthesia Primary and Contributory
Beecher and Todd	1954	599,584	1:2,680	1:1,560
Dornette and Orth	1956	63,150	1:2,429	1:1,344
Dripps et al†	1961	33,224	1:852	1:415
Clifton and Hotten‡	1963	205,640	1:6,048	1:3,955
Memery	1965	69,291	1:3,145	1:1,082
Harrison§	1968	177,928	—	1:3,007

*Reproduced with permission from Goldstein A Jr, Keats AS: The risk of anesthesia. Anesthesiology 33:130, 1970.
†Considered only spinal anesthesia and general anesthesia with muscle relaxants.
‡Considered only deaths during anesthesia or without return to consciousness.
§Considered only deaths within 24 hours of anesthesia or without return to consciousness.

Although the report was accepted for most of the data given, a major controversy erupted over the contention that death rates were significantly higher when curare was part of the anesthetic technique, explained by Beecher and Todd as an inherent toxicity. But one might recall that the study was carried out at a time when techniques of administration of curare were in a state of flux, monitoring of neuromuscular transmission was unknown, and muscle paralysis was not routinely reversed with atropine and prostigmine. Very likely, the higher death rate resulted from undetected prolonged respiratory paralysis. Overall, Beecher and Todd concluded that unsubstantiated clinical impressions of the causes of anesthetic death abounded, that anesthetic practices were unsettled, and too often there was too much haste to blame or praise. Nevertheless, the anesthetic death rate decreased from 1:1440 to 1:1880 anesthetics given during the years of the study.

For the years 1959 to 1962, surgical death rates were ascertained in the National Halothane Study as part of a retrospective attempt to discover the incidence of fatal hepatic necrosis. Rates were based on necropsy reports of deaths occurring within six weeks of operation in 34 hospitals. Only 11,289 of 16,840 deaths were subject to necropsy, and in 10,141 cases the abdominal cavity was examined. Aside from the problem of hepatic necrosis, halothane emerged as the anesthetic with the best overall death rate, 1.8 per cent, other anesthetic choices had a death rate of 1.93 per cent, and cyclopropane had the poorest record. Perhaps the most provocative statistic was a tenfold difference in institutional death rates, a matter yet to be rationalized.

We have the distinct impression that, in modern anesthetic practice, mortality is related to human error, faulty design and use of apparatus, and errors in administration of reliable drugs. The overall death rate seems to be on the decline in spite of the increasing number of complicated major operations on people of ever-increasing age and severity of disease. Improvement has come from a better understanding of preoperative factors in anesthetic deaths; the use of predictive indices in certain categories of illness such as arteriosclerotic heart disease and myocardial infarction; more exact monitoring of physiologic functions during anesthesia; improved understanding of the pharmacokinetics and pharmacodynamics of anesthetics and other drugs; and a better knowledge of pharmacogenetics in relation to anesthesia. Still the nagging questions remain. How do we prevent deaths? Are all anesthetic deaths preventable? Why do death rates differ from institution to institution? In this context two final recommendations of the National Halothane Study are worth repeating. Limited randomized studies of anesthetics, particularly the newer ones, ought to be instituted and a group of institutions ought to be established to serve as a panel laboratory for the acquisition of trustworthy information on new drugs, not merely anesthetics alone.

REFERENCES

Aldrete JA, Britt BA (eds): Malignant Hyperthermia. The Second International Symposium (1977). New York, Grune and Stratton, 1978.

Brooks GZ, Vandam LD: Ocular complications of anesthesia. Weekly Anesthesiology Update 2(13), 1979.

Chapman RL: Treatment of aspiration pneumonitis. Int Anesth Clin 15:85, 1977.

Cullen DJ, Caldera DL: Incidence of ventilator-induced pulmonary barotrauma in critically ill patients. Anesthesiology 50:185, 1979.

Martin JT: Positioning in Anesthesia and Surgery. Philadelphia, WB Saunders Co, 1978.

MORTALITY

Goldstein A Jr, Keats AS: The risk of anesthesia. Anesthesiology 33:130, 1970.

Keats AS: The ASA classification of physical status — a recapitulation. Anesthesiology 49:233, 1978.

Keats, AS: What do we know about anesthetic mortality? Anesthesiology 50:387, 1979.

Vandam LD: To Make the Patient Ready for Anesthesia. Medical Care of the Surgical Patient. Menlo Park, CA, Addison-Wesley, 1980.

Chapter *34*

ELECTRIC HAZARDS, FIRES, AND EXPLOSIONS

The hazard from combustion of flammable anesthetics has lessened with their virtual abandonment and with the acceptance of halogenated agents, but the dangers from shock and electrocution have increased because of the widespread use of electric equipment in patient care areas. Monitors for assessing vital signs, cardiac pacemakers, electrically operated beds, respirators, and even television sets have increased the potential for electric injury to the patient. These problems are compounded by the increasing use of invasive techniques in which the protective skin barrier is interrupted and the patient becomes more susceptible to injury.

ELECTRIC HAZARDS

When the patient completes an electric circuit, sufficient current may flow to produce tissue damage such as a burn, sustained muscular contraction producing asphyxia, impairment of central nervous system function, or, more commonly, ventricular fibrillation (VF). The specific injury depends on the kind of electric current and the site of application to the body.

The ability of an electric current to induce VF depends on several factors. As current must flow through the heart, the conductive properties of blood favor induction of a cardiac current when an electric potential is applied to the body. This current must be of sufficient magnitude and duration to interrupt the normal electrophysiology of the cardiac cells to produce fibrillation. Minimal currents can usually be accommodated by the cell enzyme systems that normally regenerate the membrane electric potential. Cells normally recover from short-duration impulses of less than 10 msec (i.e., as with pacemakers); however, when impulses occur during the vulnerable period (upstroke of the T wave) or persist for longer than 10 msec, VF can be produced if current density and frequency are sufficient. With respect to frequency, the heart is most susceptible at 50 to 60 Hz, but the fibrillation threshold is markedly elevated at lower (direct current) and higher (electrocautery units) frequencies. Fibrillation can be induced with as little as 20 μA (.00002 A) of 60 Hz when applied directly to the ventricular endocardium; 200 μA when applied to the epicardium and 100 mA to 3 A when applied to the skin. These currents can easily be achieved with 10 mV applied to the chambers of the heart via a metallic electrode or 1V via an electrolyte-filled cannula. Larger voltages are required when more body tissues, particularly the high

391

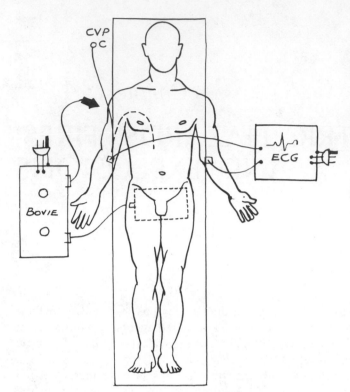

FIGURE 34–1. Some potential hazards to a patient in the operating room. The patient lies on a conductive mattress on a metal table on a conductive floor. Electrocardiograph electrodes are connected to the arms, and the ground plate from an electrocautery is under the buttocks. If a break occurs in the electrocautery grounding line and if the ECG electrodes are grounded or if the patient is grounded at a small area to the table, a burn may result when the cutting current is applied. If the ground to a cardiac monitor is broken, as through faulty connection in the plug, and a fault occurs in the monitor, current could be conducted through one of the arm leads to either the cautery ground or the table and result in electrocution. A central venous pressure catheter could also provide a conducting path to the heart.

resistance of the integument, are included in the circuit. However, since the resistance across the trunk is reduced from 100,000 ohms to approximately 1,000 ohms by sweat, electrolyte solutions, or conductive gels, the 120-V line voltage may easily induce fibrillation. Large voltages producing currents of 6 A or greater induce sustained myocardial contraction, with resumption of sinus rhythm when interrupted (defibrillation).

Prevention of electric injury is aimed at eliminating extraneous voltage sources and avoiding connections that result in complete circuits through tissue. Electric energy cannot be completely excluded, as it is used to operate devices essential or useful in patient care. Good practice can, however, eliminate extraneous voltage sources. Circuits may be completed through wires, conducting liquids such as body fluids or saline, or "ground." One of the current-carrying wires of hospital (or household) electric systems is at ground potential where it enters the hospital (or home). However, small voltages can exist between this "cold" lead and the patient's bedside if leakage currents are large. The metal conduit that carries these wires and a third, noncurrent-carrying ground wire are also at ground potential, as are the metal cases of many electric devices, water and heating pipes, bed frames, and operating tables. Thus, the patient is likely to be grounded and to supply one side of an electric circuit. To avoid electric injury, a voltage source should not be connected to the patient.

What are the potential sources of current leakage and how may they be eliminated (Fig. 34–1)? Improper design or malfunction may induce voltages in leads from monitoring equipment or virtually any other electric device connected to the patient. Instruments containing transformers or motors or other electromechanical devices harbor inherent leakage currents, which must be isolated from the patient. Instruments must be so designed that these currents are conducted to the ground and not to the patient via electrodes or to chassis components that can be touched by anyone in the vicinity. Instruments should be ruggedly built so that physical or electric damage or high humidity is unlikely to cause failures that can result in dangerous voltages in patient leads.

Furthermore, design should include the precaution that two faults must occur before a dangerous current is permitted. All instruments should be equipped with three-wire power cords and grounding plugs as well as grounding terminals by which they may be interconnected by a common bus bar to ensure that all devices are at an equipotential ground and to avoid possible voltage differences between grounds, which can occur with varying resistances and with leakage currents. In anesthetizing locations, the National Fire Protection Association (NFPA) requires that the bus be of highly conductive bare metal with terminals for grounding each electric receptacle in the room as well as all metal furniture. The bus must be isolated from all other grounds in the building except at a single common grounding point.

Current flow to a patient through instrument leads can be limited by an electric gap utilizing telemetry or nonconductive coupling transducers (optical, acoustic, or mechanical coupling). The use of simple fuses or other current-sensing devices cannot protect from the extremely small currents that cause intracardiac injury.

BURNS

Burns constitute another electric hazard. Ordinarily, if a 60-Hz current of sufficient intensity to cause thermal burns passes through the trunk, fibrillation or sustained myocardial contraction will occur. However, a burn alone may result if the same current passes through an extremity without an electrical path to the heart. High-frequency current from electrocautery apparatus is a common cause of burns. The active electrode of the cautery cuts or cauterizes with intense heat because all current flows through a small area. When this current leaves the body through the large ground plate, the current density is small and significant heating is not produced. If, however, the ground wire is broken or disconnected and the current exits through an ECG electrode, via a conductive face mask, or by contact with a metal table, a burn may result. Current densities higher than 100 mA/cm² can result in burns. Large ECG electrodes provide a greater surface area, and burns are less likely to result when currents accidentally pass through them. The anesthetist, who may be grounded through conductive shoes, may also be shocked or burned.

CHEMICAL BURNS

Chemical burns resulting from the use of direct current have also occurred. If a few volts are applied to saline solution, electrolysis occurs with sodium hydroxide formed at the cathode and chlorine at the anode; the hydroxide thus formed is caustic. In some electrosurgical units a small direct current voltage is applied to the ground plate to detect ground failures; faults occurring in this circuit can also cause electrolysis.

OPTICAL LASERS

Optical lasers are now commonly used as surgical instruments. Their intense, coherent beams of light carry large amounts of energy that focus on small areas of tissue and therefore act as a scalpel by desiccating, vaporizing, and coagulating tissue, thus cutting and providing hemostasis. Papillomas of the larynx, for example, may be vaporized by a carbon dioxide laser beam; this laser operates in the infrared spectrum at 10.6 μm. The energy of its beam can obviously cause deep burns and can ignite or puncture endotracheal tubes, which must therefore be protected by a reflecting metal tape or foil cover. Laser beams of visible light are transmitted by glass as well as by the ocular lens. Operating room personnel must wear appropriate lenses to protect against stray reflections; patients' eyelids should be taped shut.

MAINTENANCE OF EQUIPMENT

Electric equipment must not only be well designed but properly maintained. Maintenance is ordinarily beyond the ability of physicians and should be delegated to experts. In small hospitals it is usually not possible to employ a full-time electronic technician or engineer; hence, it may be necessary to rely on the manufacturer or a maintenance firm. Certain faults, however, should be obvious even to the unsophisticated. Equipment with frayed or broken cords, plugs that do not seat firmly in outlets, and damaged instruments should not be used but set aside for repair. If the operator of an instrument receives a shock, use of that instrument for a patient should be avoided. A regular maintenance program is essential, not simply repair when a fault occurs.

POWER DISTRIBUTION IN HAZARDOUS AREAS

A three-wire grounded distribution system, as in patient rooms, has one "hot" wire and one wire at ground potential with an additional, separate ground wire. If contact is made with the hot wire and ground, current passes through the body (see Fig. 34–1). The ungrounded system in the operating room incorporates an isolation transformer that eliminates the ground connection of the usual power distribution system so that neither electric lead is at ground potential. In this system, contact between either the secondary wire or the transformer and ground will ordinarily not allow current to flow. Current flows only if contact is made between both secondary wires. Personnel and objects in the operating room may be grounded to reduce the electrostatic spark hazard without danger of shock. Excessive leakage currents to ground from equipment connected to an ungrounded secondary winding of the isolation transformer can complete the electrical circuit, so that contact between a second-

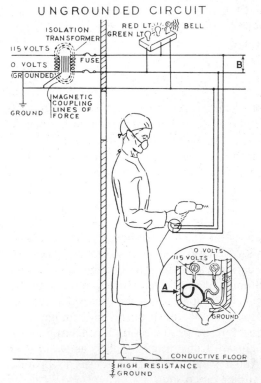

FIGURE 34–2. The ungrounded circuit and the isolation transformer. Spark or shock occurs only when both live conductors are in circuit. Insulation failure (*A*) permits a current of 2 milliamperes to flow to ground. The ground contact indicator is activated to warn of the failure. No spark or shock hazard is established. (Reproduced with permission from Walter CW: Anesthesiology 25:505, 1964.)

ary winding and ground could allow a lethal current to flow. To monitor this leakage, the line isolation monitor (LIM) is incorporated in the isolated system to sound an alarm when leakage currents cause a secondary winding to be effectively at ground potential on the otherwise isolated side, such as when faulty equipment is connected to the power distribution system. The ground warning not only protects personnel but also indicates the need for repair. The warning system relies on a high-resistance, current-limiting relay, activated when a ground connection occurs on the isolated side. This completes a circuit through the secondary winding of the transformer, and the relay activates a warning light and buzzer (Fig. 34–2). A green light indicates safe conditions, whereas red warns of a ground in the system.

CODES AND STANDARDS

The applicable codes and standards of the NFPA are prepared by committees representing industry, health care facilities, medical societies, and standards groups. The codes are continually being analyzed and revised to keep abreast of advancing technology and to resolve controversy. In many jurisdictions the standards are incorporated into local building codes and therefore are of legal significance. Some older installations, however, may not have construction consistent with current standards. Anesthetists who become involved in the design or administration of health care facilities must be aware of safety practices and local regulations; technical consultation should be sought when needed.

FIRES AND EXPLOSIONS

In comparison with other hazards of anesthesia, explosions occur so infrequently as to be relatively insignificant. When ether and cyclopropane were in common use, the mortality from explosions was estimated at about one in 1,500,000 anesthetics. The overall death rate attributable to anesthesia is difficult to determine, but probably lies somewhere between one in 350 and one in 4000, depending on the physical condition of the patient. However, the emotional upheaval created by an anesthetic explosion and the resulting publicity once caused consternation far out of proportion to the incidence. Most anesthetists in developed countries believe that there is no longer a place for flammable agents in anesthesia since there are no absolute indications for the use of ether or cyclopropane and since adequate alternatives are available. The rare use of these agents does not justify the high cost of installing and maintaining isolated electric circuits and conductive floors. However, ether does remain an important anesthetic agent in developing countries.

Fires and explosions are combustion processes differing in speed of reaction and magnitude of forces released. Three elements are necessary for combustion: a combustible substance or fuel, an oxidizing agent, and a source of ignition. For a fire or explosion to occur, the fuel and the oxidizer must be present in appropriate proportions; too little fuel or too little oxidizer will not permit combustion. All flammable anesthetics are fuels; oxygen and nitrous oxide are oxidizers, and sparks, flames, or heated surfaces are the common sources of ignition. The lower explosive limits in oxygen (too little fuel) are 2.0 vol per cent for ether and 2.5 vol per cent for cyclopropane. The upper explosive limits (too little oxygen) are above the clinically useful anesthetic concentrations. For all practical purposes any anesthetic given with ether or cyclopropane will lie in the flammable range.

Measures for prevention of fires and explosions have been suggested by engineers, fire insurance underwriters, manufacturers, and physicians. The most complete set of recommendations is found in the Standard for the Use of Inhalation Anesthetics of the NFPA, revised periodically since first promulgated in 1941. We endorse the application of all protective measures that can be adopted within the limits of practicality, unless their adoption involves substitution of a greater hazard.

REFERENCES

Brunner JMR: Common abuses and failures of electrical equipment. Anesth Analg 51:810, 1972.

Duncalf D: Survey of the use of flammable anesthetics. Anesthesiology 48:298, 1978.

Hull CJ: Electrocution hazards in the operating theatre. Br J Anaesth 50:647, 1978.

Leeming MN: Protection of the "electrically susceptible patient." Anesthesiology 38:370, 1973.

National Fire Protection Association, 470 Atlantic Avenue, Boston, MA 02110:
    NFPA 56A Inhalation Anesthetics, 1978.
    NFPA 70 National Electrical Code, 1981.
    NFPA Essential Electrical Systems for Health Care Facilities, 1977.

Prevoznik SJ: Flammable anesthetics are outmoded. *In* Eckenhoff JE (ed): Controversy in Anesthesiology. Philadelphia, WB Saunders, 1979, pp 19–25.

Snow JC, Norton ML, Saluja IS, et al: Fire hazard during CO_2 laser microsurgery of the larynx and trachea. Anesth Analg 55:146, 1976.

Spooner RB: Hospital Electrical Safety Simplified. Research Triangle Park, NC, Instrument Society of America, 1980.

Vickers MD: Fire and explosion hazards in operating theatres. Br J Anaesth 50:659, 1978.

Section 4
ANCILLARY ANESTHESIA CARE

Chapter 35

CARDIOPULMONARY RESUSCITATION

Cardiopulmonary resuscitation extends far back into the history of mankind. Thumping on the chest and mouth-to-mouth breathing were utilized in antiquity, the latter cited in the Bible. However, no concerted attempts at resuscitation were made until the present century, when the prone pressure technique of artificial respiration was widely taught in the United States and other techniques were used abroad. During World War II these techniques were re-evaluated, and the advent of operations on the heart brought cardiac resuscitation into focus. In the 1950s, thoracotomy and manual compression of the heart, use of resuscitative drugs, and electric defibrillation gained wide acceptance. Mouth-to-mouth breathing was shown to be far more effective for pulmonary ventilation than manual methods. In the 1960s closed chest manual compression of the heart largely supplanted the open technique.

Respiratory and circulatory resuscitation are treated here as one, for the two are inseparable. When respiration ceases, cardiac arrest soon follows, whereas circulatory standstill as a primary event is almost coincident with cessation of breathing. In this chapter we present in outline form the currently accepted standards and guidelines for cardiopulmonary resuscitation (CPR), which are also applicable to the drowning victim.

RESPIRATORY RESUSCITATION

Respiratory standstill is easily diagnosed, but not so the subtle degrees of ventilatory inadequacy. Both are synonymous with hypoxia and carbon dioxide retention. Cessation of respiration, even for brief periods, may result in irreversible cerebral damage, hence the need to restore gas exchange as rapidly as possible. The duration of permissible apnea varies with the adequacy of oxygenation prior to onset and the body's metabolic demands. In a denitrogenated, well-oxygenated patient, the safe period of apnea may extend up to five minutes, whereas in hypoxic persons, apnea for 20 to 30 seconds may be fatal.

The causes of respiratory failure may reside in the inhaled atmosphere, the airways and lungs, the oxygen transport system, or the control of respiration. Anesthetists encounter all of these problems in their daily activities.

Inhaled Atmosphere. Decreased oxygen tension in inhaled gas may be the result of lowered oxygen concentration at ambient pressure or reduction in the partial pressure of oxygen at high altitudes.

399

Airway Obstruction or Pulmonary Disease.   Obstruction may be caused by soft tissues in the head and neck, tumor, bronchoconstriction, secretions, or solid material; disease such as pneumonia; structural alterations in alveoli, as occur in severe emphysema; mechanical interference with ventilation, as seen in the fixed chest, paralyzed diaphragm, or flail chest; or impaired diffusion, as found in pulmonary edema or fibrosis.

Transport System.   Alterations in blood flow may occur in the lungs or the systemic circulation, or deficient oxygenation may result from anemia or carbon monoxide poisoning.

Control of Respiration.   This is influenced by central nervous system disease; drugs causing central respiratory depression, such as anesthetics and opioids; respiratory acidosis; and trauma to brain.

An essential criterion of respiratory resuscitation is that the method be immediately available and effective. Mouth-to-mouth breathing bears these characteristics.

EXPIRED AIR TECHNIQUES

A sufficient amount of oxygen is present in expired air to assure oxygenation of a victim's blood. Almost all the disadvantages of manual pressure techniques are overcome by positive pressure applied to the airway with expired air via mouth-to-mouth or mouth-to-nose breathing. With either, the resuscitator supports the head and mandible, the adequacy of gas exchange is judged by rise and fall of the chest, and tidal volume is thus estimated. In addition, accumulation of secretions or vomitus and obstruction of the airway can be detected. Little expenditure of energy is required to ventilate the lungs in this manner.

The patient lies supine, the upper airway cleared of obstructing secretions or foreign material. The resuscitator kneels at the side of the patient's head, which is tilted maximally backward with the mandible held forward (Fig. 35–1). This maneuver carries the base of the tongue out of the pharynx and brings the oral cavity and oropharynx into line with the larynx and trachea. With a suspected cervical injury, head tilt should not be employed. In mouth-to-mouth breathing the patient's nostrils are closed by the fingers of one hand while the other maintains backward tilt of the head; alternatively, leakage of air from the nose can be prevented by application of the operator's cheek against the nostrils. The operator's mouth is opened widely, and the lips are placed firmly around the patient's open mouth, followed by a forceful expiration. The effect is gauged by observing movement of the chest wall. It may be necessary to approach jaw dislocation to assure an unobstructed airway by pulling the mandible forward with the fingers in the mouth or by upward traction at the angles of the jaw. In mouth-to-nose respiration the patient's lips are closed and air is blown into the nose. After inflation of the lungs, the operator removes the mouth from the patient's nostrils to allow passive expiration. The patient's mouth should be open during expiration in the mouth-to-nose technique, because the uvula and soft palate may obstruct escape of air through the nose.

A tidal volume of 800 to 1000 ml with a rate of 10 to 12/min is sought, to yield a minute volume of 10 to 12 L in the adult. If the airway is satisfactory, one hand of the operator is placed over the epigastrium to prevent distention of the stomach with air. In the infant or child the operator's mouth is easily placed over both nose and mouth. In single-rescuer CPR two quick breaths are given after each cycle of 15 chest compressions: one breath every five strokes during two-rescuer efforts.

Various refinements of the technique have been suggested. These include use of a double oropharyngeal airway, an esophageal obturator airway, an airway with a one-way valve to avoid return of expired air to the operator's mouth, and a face mask into which the operator breathes rather than making direct contact with the patient's

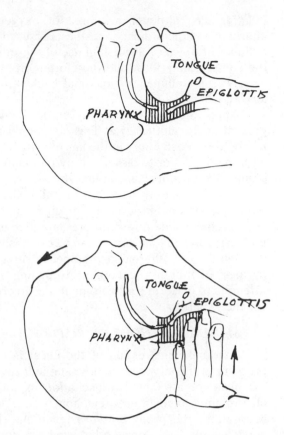

FIGURE 35–1. Position of the head for mouth-to-mouth breathing.

mouth. Although an airway may improve ease of expansion of the patient's chest, it is not always readily available. Placement of a handkerchief over the patient's mouth for aesthetic reasons interferes with gas exchange.

Expired air resuscitation requires no extensive period of training for efficient use. The disadvantages relate principally to contact with the patient's nose or mouth. This is a minor objection, although resuscitation of an apparently drowned or intoxicated individual is not a pleasant prospect. Greater concerns are the possibility of inflation of the patient's stomach with air followed by regurgitation, transmission of infection to the operator, or rupture of the patient's lungs.

BAG AND MASK TECHNIQUE

In expired air techniques, the resuscitator's diaphragm acts as the source of power to expand the patient's lungs. The same effect results from use of a mask attached to a self-inflating reservoir bag intermittently compressed by hand (Fig. 35–2). Air is the

FIGURE 35–2. Diagram of the Ruben-Ambu resuscitator, *1,* Reservoir bag with sponge rubber lining; *2,* Ruben inflating valve; *3,* one-way valve. (Reproduced with permission from Mushin WW, Rendell-Baker L, Thompson PW, et al: Automatic Ventilation of the Lungs. London, Blackwell Scientific Publications, 1959.)

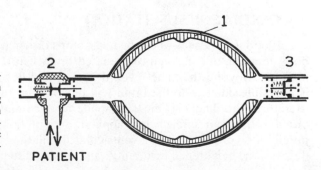

PATIENT

inflating gas, although a source of oxygen can be attached when available. An alternative is the ordinary anesthesia reservoir bag and mask, with gas supplied from a cylinder of oxygen. Successful use of these techniques requires a tight mask fit during the compression phase and therefore more training for the lay person. Patency of the airway is maintained by maximal backward head tilt and insertion of a pharyngeal airway when available.

Application of positive pressure at the mouth is not effective when obstruction is present at the glottic level. This commonly results from lodgment of a foreign body, rarely from crush injury to the larynx. An attempt should be made to extract the object with the fingers or to dislodge it by pounding the back between the shoulder blades or giving several upper abdominal thrusts while turning the victim head down. This is more easily done in the infant or child. If an object, a chunk of food, for example, lodges at the cricoid level, Heimlich recommends embracing the victim from behind and exerting sudden, forceful high in the abdomen to dislodge the material. If both measures fail, an airway can be established with a large gauge needle or by incision through the cricothyroid membrane. Positive pressure respiration by means of a large syringe, or mouth-to-cricothyroid opening, is then carried out. We do not advocate attempts to perform tracheotomy in the emergency situation, a difficult procedure even for the expert.

MANUAL METHODS OF RESPIRATION

External compression of the chest is employed in situations in which positive pressure at the airway cannot be applied: severe maxillofacial injury, inaccessibility of the head, or attempted resuscitation in unusual locations, such as treatment of an electrocuted lineman on a telephone pole. The once widely taught method of artificial respiration, the prone pressure technique, is the least effective in moving air and consequently is no longer advocated. Its only advantage is the prone position, which offers a better chance of a clear airway and escape of gastrointestinal contents from the mouth.

Posterior or anterior chest compression may be combined with displacement of the patient's hips or shoulders to expand the thoracic cage. With the patient prone, this is accomplished by elevation of the hips or by lifting the flexed arms over the head. Either maneuver increases chest volume by relieving pressure on the ribs, allowing the abdominal cavity to expand, and pulling the diaphragm downward. When the patient is supine, lung volume is increased by hyperextension of the arms. This maneuver increases the anterior-posterior diameter of the chest through traction on the shoulder girdle. A nearly adequate volume of air can be moved with these methods if the trachea is intubated. However, in the usual emergency the resuscitator cannot be certain of a patent airway, and it is difficult to gauge the proper degree of chest compression. Furthermore, these methods are ineffectual when the patient is lying on a soft mattress that yields to pressure.

CARDIAC RESUSCITATION

Blood flow ceases when the heart stops or when the ventricles fibrillate. At normal body temperature the well-oxygenated brain will tolerate ischemia for less than four minutes. Beyond this time, even though blood flow is restored, major and frequently irreversible damage to the brain will have occurred. Should circulatory arrest occur, therefore, the diagnosis must be made at once and a method of moving oxygenated blood to the brain immediately applied. Several factors, singly or in combination, may precipitate cardiac arrest or ventricular fibrillation: complete heart block, myocardial depression, heightened irritability, and inadequate coronary blood flow.

Myocardial Depression or Increased Irritability. The common causes are hypoxemia; effects of drugs such as general and local anesthetics, digitalis, quinidine, and procainamide; reflex vagal effects arising from stimulation of the carotid sinus, from pulmonary receptors giving rise to the von Bezold-Jarisch reflex, or attendant upon surgical manipulation of the head, neck, thorax, and upper abdomen; major electrolyte disorders resulting from potassium, sodium, or calcium imbalance, occurring during digitalis therapy, in association with diuresis, following massive transfusion, in uremia, and in intestinal obstruction with vomiting or severe diarrhea; and electrocution through use of ungrounded or faulty electric equipment used in diathermy, x-ray, cardiac catheterization, implantation of cardiac pacemakers, or monitoring of physiologic function (ventricular fibrillation may occur in these situations).

Inadequate Coronary Blood Flow. This may involve decreased blood flow to the myocardium or may result from increased cardiac work or a demand for oxygen that cannot be met. In the former instance, common factors are hypotension from hemorrhage, spinal or peridural anesthesia, overdose of premedicant drugs or local or general anesthetics, traction reflexes, a Stokes-Adams attack, and coronary artery thrombosis. So far as increased demand is concerned, epinephrine, isoproterenol, or aminophylline may cause an increase in cardiac work and a high oxygen requirement. Cardiac work is increased by elevation of heart rate and a heightened myocardial tension and contractile state as well as impedence to ventricular ejection.

Anesthetists may encounter cardiac arrest at any time during anesthesia or postoperatively. Arrest is more likely in the elderly and the neonate, in patients with previously diagnosed paroxysmal arrhythmias, in digitalis toxicity, following massive hemorrhage, in patients with myocarditis or heart block, and during operations on the heart. A preconceived treatment plan should be ready for implementation at a moment's notice.

DIAGNOSIS

The following signs are suggestive or diagnostic of circulatory arrest.

1. Absent radial, carotid, or femoral pulses
2. Inaudible heart sounds
3. Sudden pallor or cyanosis
4. Sudden pupillary dilation
5. Respiratory standstill or apneustic gasps
6. Seizures, convulsions, or loss of consciousness
7. Absence of bleeding and dark blood in the operative field
8. Electrocardiographic evidence of asystole or ventricular fibrillation
9. Electric silence on the electroencephalogram

Most of these signs are unreliable, for they may be present during severe hypotension alone. It must be emphasized, however, that if the blood pressure is not audible, one should not make the error of re-adjusting the cuff and wasting time in the process.

EXTERNAL MANUAL CARDIAC SYSTOLE

Before initiating chest compression, a sharp blow is given to the midsternum. This may induce the minimal electric current sufficient to start a heart in asystole or to terminate certain arrhythmias. The external approach to cardiac arrest involves intermittent application of manual pressure to the sternum just above the xiphoid with the heel of one hand on top of the other and the fingers held straight in the long axis of the sternum. The shoulders of the resuscitator should be directly over the sternum, and the elbows should be straight (Fig. 35–3). The sternum is depressed 4 to 5 cm toward the

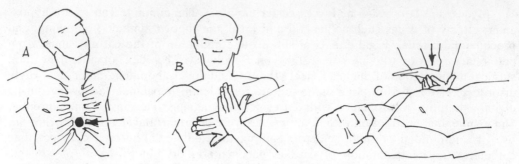

FIGURE 35–3. External manual systole. *A*. Point of application of the lower hand to the sternum, just above the xiphoid. *B*. Use of two hands, the heel of one hand atop the other, fingers held straight. *C*. Depression of the sternum from above, about 4 to 5 cm toward the vertebral column.

vertebral column, not easily done in the elderly in whom the chest lacks resiliency. For this to be done effectively, the victim must lie on a unyielding surface, either on the floor or on a board placed beneath the chest. Sixty down strokes per minute are necessary to yield a minimally effective cardiac output and blood pressure with a 60:40 ratio of compression to relaxation. In the infant or child, mere compression with the fingers or with the chest held between the fingers is effective. (see Chapter 25). The legs should be raised to increase venous return to the heart. Adequacy of chest compression is judged by re-appearance of peripheral pulses, disappearance of pupillary dilation, and improvement in skin color.

As manual systole continues the lungs are simultaneously ventilated, for even if sternal pressure results in effective circulation, oxygenation must proceed apace; intermittent sternal pressure alone does not accomplish this. If equipment is not available, mouth-to-mouth or mouth-to-nose ventilation is essential. With bag and mask at hand, 100 per cent oxygen is given by intermittent positive pressure. Tracheal intubation, not an essential immediate step, can be carried out after oxygenation has been established. Lung inflation is coordinated with sternal compression: five compressions alternating with one lung inflation is the recommendation. When only one resuscitator is available, two quick breaths are given after each cycle of 15 chest compressions.

The manual method of cardiac resuscitation has met with considerable success; of great value is its immediate applicability and avoidance of thoracotomy. Rib fracture, costochondral separation, laceration of the liver or spleen, and fat embolization, all noted occasionally following sternal compression, are a small price to pay if circulation is resumed. Mechanical devices manually operated or motor driven have a place in the hospital or ambulance after manual compression has been instituted and when resuscitation is prolonged. A stiff pad at the end of a metal rod is applied rhythmically via pump handle action as a piston to the precordium.

RECOMMENDED PROCEDURE IN CARDIOPULMONARY RESUSCITATION

In teaching resuscitation, the order of treatment is best remembered by the first four letters of the alphabet: *A* for airway; *B* for breathing; *C* for cardiac compression; and *D* for definitive therapy. These procedures can be done simultaneously but require the presence of at least three individuals once initial measures have been instituted. A list of drugs required for resuscitation appears in Table 35–1. Resuscitation may proceed along one of several lines: immediate success; an intervening period of trial with ultimate success; or trial with ultimate failure.

TABLE 35-1.   Drugs for Use in Cardiopulmonary Resuscitation

Drug	Initial Dose	Route	Indication
Atropine sulfate	0.5 mg	Intravenous	For sinus bradycardia and to improve A-V conduction
Epinephrine (Adrenalin)	0.5–1.0 mg	Intravenous or intracardiac	Asystole: To initiate heartbeat Ventricular fibrillation: To improve myocardial tone and induce coarse fibrillation
Sodium bicarbonate	40–50 mEq	Intravenous	Circulatory insufficiency: To correct metabolic acidosis caused by tissue hypoxia
Lidocaine (Xylocaine)	60–80 mg 1 mg/kg	Intravenous Infusion (1–4 mg/min)	Ventricular fibrillation: To depress ventricular irritability, facilitating defibrillation
Procainamide	100 mg q 5 min	Intravenous	To suppress ventricular ectopy
Bretylium tosylate (Bretylol)	5 mg/kg	Intravenous	For ventricular tachycardia and fibrillation
Propranolol hydrochloride (Inderal)	1.0 mg q 5 min	Intravenous	For atrial and ventricular tachyarrhythmias
Calcium chloride	1000 mg	Intravenous or intracardiac	Inadequate force of contraction: To increase myocardial contractility
Levaterenol (Levophed)	8 mg in 500 ml	Intravenous drip	Hypotension: To increase myocardial contractility and produce peripheral vasoconstriction
Isoproterenol (Isuprel)	1 mg in 500 ml	Intravenous drip	Bradycardia and inadequate force of contraction: To increase rate and strength of heartbeat
Dopamine (Intropin)	200 mg in 500 ml	Intravenous drip	Hypotension and inadequate force of contraction: To increase myocardial contractility and improve renal blood flow by renal vasodilatation

Note: Other drugs used in resuscitation include digitalis preparations, sodium nitroprusside (Nipride), diuretics (furosemide [Lasix]), and corticosteroids (methylprednisolone sodium succinate, 5–30 mg/kg IV for cerebral edema).

The following steps are taken in resuscitation from cardiac arrest:

1. Establish diagnosis: best signs are apnea, collapse, absence of pulse, pupillary dilation, and absence of heart sounds.
2. Note time. Thump chest sharply two or three times (to counter vagal arrest).
3. Summon help. Sound the alarm for cardiac arrest (hospital alert signal, confirm location).
4. Place support under patient's back and begin mouth-to-mouth breathing and closed chest compression.
5. With the arrival of others, one physician assumes command; resuscitators are relieved as necessary.
6. Arrival of emergency cart:
   a. Start intravenous infusion by needle or cutdown and establish an intra-arterial line.
   b. Attach cardiac monitor; prepare defibrillator. If fibrillation is present, shock

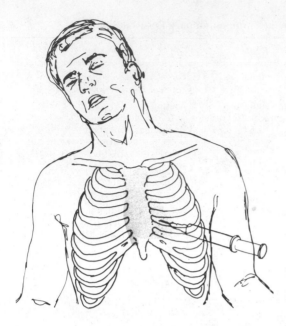

FIGURE 35–4. Intracardiac injection is made with a 7.5-cm needle through the fourth or fifth interspace, about 5 cm to the left of the midline.

externally as soon as possible. (DC shock 200 to 300 joules in adults, less than 100 watt-seconds in children.)

c. Inject 44.6 mEq of bicarbonate intravenously to counter metabolic acidosis.

d. For cardiac standstill, primary or postdefibrillation, inject epinephrine (0.5 to 1.0 mg or 0.5 to 1.0 ml of a 1:1000 solution) into left ventricle (parasternally, fourth or fifth interspace) (Fig. 35–4). Similar doses of epinephrine have been effective when given intratracheally.

e. With appearance of cardiac rhythm, support blood pressure with a vasopressor intravenously (phenylephrine).

f. When feasible, intubate trachea; give oxygen by intermittent positive pressure. Sample arterial blood for Pa_{O_2}, Pa_{CO^2}, and pH; give bicarbonate as necessary. Defibrillate again if needed. Inject lidocaine to control ventricular irritability, isoproterenol by intravenous infusion if blood pressure is not maintained by vasopressors, or calcium gluconate to improve myocardial tone. Administer fluids intravenously to increase blood volume and venous return.

7. Continue with resuscitative efforts so long as there is hope and the patient is salvable. Consider open chest compression under proper circumstances (see following section). The final decision to continue or desist rests with the physician in charge.

When signs of a good circulation are not immediately evident, the question arises as to how long to persist before opening the thorax. In several situations closed chest compression may be ineffective: the flail or crushed chest, aortic or mitral valvular insufficiency preventing propulsion of blood, pericardial tamponade owing to hemorrhage or effusion, massive myocardial infarction with a toneless ventricle, exsanguinating hemorrhage, and massive pulmonary embolization. It seems reasonable that direct cardiac massage should be more effective in these situations, permitting establishment of the diagnosis at the same time. With the indirect technique the pulse felt peripherally is merely a shock wave, the mean arterial pressure low, and the central venous pressure high as blood is forced in both directions with compression.

For these reasons we believe there is a place for thoracotomy and direct compression of the heart, for we have experienced success when the indirect method has failed. But the conditions are sharply defined. Closed chest systole is used to gain time. If not successful within five minutes, if the patient is salvable and if circumstances permit management of the open chest, thoracotomy should be done at once. This may be done in the operating room, emergency room, recovery room, intensive care area, but rarely on the ward.

OPEN CHEST COMPRESSION OF THE HEART

An incision is made in the fourth or fifth left intercostal space, not extending to the sternum lest the internal mammary artery be severed and not too hastily to avoid lacerating the lung. The pericardium need not be opened at first but should be opened as soon as possible after first compression of the heart, avoiding injury to the phrenic nerve. A rib spreader is placed to avoid cramping the operator's hands. The heart is cradled in the operator's hands, with the ventricles compressed between the thumb and fingers of one hand or the fingers of both hands (Fig. 35–5). Compression is done at a rate of 60/min to ensure a sufficient cardiac output. Because of the fast rate, fatigue occurs rapidly, so an alternate operator should be ready to take over.

As in the closed chest technique, adequate venous filling is necessary to supply an adequate stroke volume; all of the ancillary measures advocated for closed chest resuscitation are applicable when the chest is open. In addition, the aorta can be occluded below the carotid artery to improve coronary blood flow. At the risk of sounding repetitious, we again list those signs that suggest effective cardiac compression: full heart, palpable peripheral pulse, constricted pupils, and improvement in color of skin, mucous membranes, and blood.

If the ventricles fibrillate, the first measure is to effect myocardial oxygenation via manual compression. With oxygen ventilating the lungs and circulation through the coronary vessels re-established via compression, the myocardium should lose its dusky color. Defibrillation is then attempted. For internal defibrillation, in contrast to external

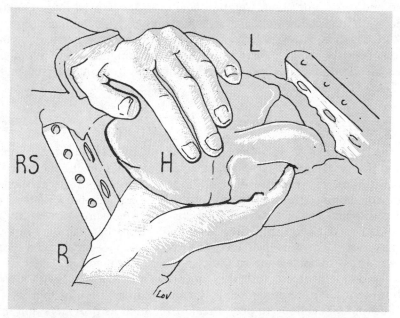

FIGURE 35–5. Method of performing open chest manual systole. *R*, Right hand; *L*, left hand; *H*, heart; *RS*, rib spreader. (After M. Codding.)

defibrillation, DC shocks of 30 to 60 watt-seconds are applied by means of disc electrodes at opposite sides of the heart. The larger the mass of the ventricles, the higher the voltage required. Defibrillation is usually followed by asystole, so the pharmacologic treatment already outlined is applied. To prevent electrocution, surgeon and anesthetist must avoid contact with the patient as the shocks are applied. When a drug is injected, the aorta is occluded distally to direct the drug through the coronary system.

PROGNOSIS

Damage to the brain as a result of hypoxia is the determining factor in prognosis when restoration of circulation has been accomplished. If hypoxemia has preceded cessation of cerebral blood flow associated with cardiac arrest, the capacity of the brain to survive the insult will almost certainly have been reduced below the four-minute figure. There are few measures that can prolong survival time. Hypothermia may be protective but only if induced immediately and in the right temperature range (30°C). General anesthesia, by reducing cerebral metabolism, may afford slight protection.

The signs presaging recovery include prompt reversal of pupillary dilation, pupillary reaction to light, prompt return of spontaneous respiration, and rapid return of consciousness and orientation. Under these circumstances complete recovery can practically be guaranteed, although delayed relapse and death have occurred on occasion. When there is severe brain damage, decerebrate rigidity convulsions, hyperpyrexia, and persistent coma are the manifestations of cell destruction. Continued apnea and hypotension resistant to treatment are ominous, both indicative of brain stem damage. Prognosis is guarded, because the longer these conditions persist the more hopeless the outlook. Serial electroencephalograms offer a means of determining the degree of damage and improvement.

Further anoxia resulting from repeated convulsions should be prevented by the administration of barbiturates or phenytoin. Tracheostomy and assisted or controlled respiration may be necessary. Temperature should be reduced to decrease tissue metabolism and oxygen demand. Cerebral edema and increased intracranial pressure are treated with dexamethasone and osmotic diuretics. Continued intensive surveillance of the patient is necessary until recovery is assured because recurrence of cardiac arrest is not uncommon. Currently, the prompt application of hypothermia and large doses of barbiturates to improve brain survival are controversial matters (see Chapter 27).

CPR IN THE COMMUNITY

With the advent of large numbers of individuals trained in cardiopulmonary resuscitation (CPR), reports suggest both a higher survival rate and increased numbers of persons with a better quality of life following resuscitation from cardiopulmonary arrest in the community. Resuscitators who have been trained and periodically retested in the prompt application of basic life support (BLS) measures as well as advanced cardiac life support (ACLS) techniques have obtained the best survival rates. At least one study has shown the following factors to be conducive to success: the shortest time interval from arrest to application of CPR and from arrest to onset of ACLS. These results may seem self-evident, but they do prove that cardiac resuscitation in the community benefits from program planning and rapid provision of therapy. Anesthetists have and should continue to play a major role both as providers and teachers of CPR.

APPRAISAL

Cardiopulmonary resuscitation has saved and will save many lives, but it is a dramatic form of therapy that should be thoroughly understood before one is called upon to apply it. Planning is essential. Closed and open chest compression and defibrillation should be practiced in the animal laboratory to develop self-confidence. Personal conviction of the need for prompt diagnosis and immediate action are the keys to success.

Heroics in therapy are inappropriate when a favorable outcome cannot be expected. It is poor medical judgment to attempt cardiac resuscitation when the heart has stopped beating in a patient with terminal cancer. Success is less likely if cardiac arrest occurs outside the operating room, although a number of successful resuscitations have been reported under this circumstance. The full gamut of resuscitative measures should be attempted outside the operating room only when conditions for success are optimal, that is, when the patient is salvable and individuals who understand the principles of resuscitation are present.

REFERENCES

Bishop R, Weisfeldt ML: Sodium bicarbonate during cardiac arrest. Effect on arterial pH, $PaCO_2$ and osmolality. JAMA 235:506, 1976.

Bryson TK, Benumof JL, Ward CF: The esophageal obturator airway: a clinical comparison to ventilation with a mask and oropharyngeal airway. Chest 74:537, 1978.

Eisenberg MS, Bergner L, Hallstrom A: Cardiac resuscitation in the community. Importance of rapid provision and implications for program planning. JAMA 241:1905, 1979.

Luce JM, Cary JM, Roso BK, et al: New developments in cardiopulmonary resuscitation. JAMA 244:1366, 1980.

Redding JS: The choking controversy: critique of evidence on the Heimlich Maneuver. Crit Care Med 7:475, 1979.

Rudikoff MT, Maughan WL, Effron M, et al: Mechanisms of blood flow during cardiopulmonary resuscitation. Circulation 61:345, 1980.

Standards and guidelines for cardiopulmonary resuscitation (CPR) and emergency cardiac care (ECC). JAMA 244:453, 1980.

Taylor GJ, Tucker WM, Greene HL, et al: Importance of prolonged compression during cardiopulmonary resuscitation in man. N Engl J Med 296:1515, 1977.

CHAPTER 36

THE IMMEDIATE POSTOPERATIVE PERIOD: RECOVERY AND INTENSIVE CARE

HAZARDS OF THE IMMEDIATE POSTOPERATIVE PERIOD

As an operation draws to a close, there is a tendency for all concerned to "let down." Pressures associated with the surgical procedure are over, and there is an understandable need for those involved to relax; therefore attention is partially diverted from the patient. The senior surgeons often depart the operating room, leaving the anesthetist without help, although at this time events may occur that threaten the patient's life. Upon emergence from general anesthesia, laryngospasm, retching and vomiting, and excitement may occur or there may be failure to resume adequate breathing.

An anesthetized patient being moved from the operating table to litter or bed must be protected against bodily harm. Poorly attended patients have fallen to the floor and been injured. Following abrupt transfer, they have suffered muscle and ligament strain, brachial plexus injury, or dangerous degrees of hypotension. A sufficient number of individuals must assist in the transfer to avoid incidents of this kind. For very heavy patients, roller devices are available to move them onto the litter. Once the patient is moved, the sides of the litter or bed must be elevated or a restraining strap put in place and the patient constantly attended. The unconscious patient is positioned in the lateral decubitus position, when possible, to protect the airway.

CIRCULATORY COMPLICATIONS

Hypotension

While the anesthetist is busy disconnecting apparatus from the anesthesia machine, turning off the gas supply, and preparing to move the patient from the operating room, blood pressure or pulse may not be observed for a time, even if monitoring devices are in place. Hypotension may reach serious proportions before being recognized. Chapter 32 lists the causes and treatment of hypotension during and following anesthesia. With a few obvious exceptions, these also apply to the postoperative patient, including residual effects of premedication, anesthetics, and neuromuscular

410

blockers; unreplaced blood loss; motion and change of position; cardiac arrhythmias; hypoxia; metabolic acidosis; and electrolyte imbalance.

Hypertension

Although one tends to emphasize the dangers of a decrease in arterial pressure, a certain number of patients become hypertensive. If the rise in pressure is sufficient, cerebrovascular accident may result, particularly in the arteriosclerotic or hypertensive patient. The more common causes of hypertension are pain, hypercarbia, hypoxia, residual effects of vasopressor drugs, and over-replacement of fluid losses. Treatment is obvious: namely, analgetics, improved alveolar gas exchange, and oxygenation. We have seen marked hypertension after aortic grafts or prolonged abdominal or thoracic operations; the skin appears mottled and cold, and the patient is restless and complains of headache. Whether a rise in pressure represents excessive mobilization of catecholamines is not known, but whatever the cause, if dangerously high levels of pressure exist, use of antihypertensive medication is indicated. Sodium nitroprusside titrated carefully by slow intravenous infusion or fractional administration of chlorpromazine has proved useful under these conditions.

RESPIRATORY PROBLEMS

Hypoxemia

Airway obstruction, laryngospasm, and inadequate gas exchange may be present. Perhaps the most common postoperative respiratory problem today is the result of residual neuromuscular block (Chapter 15). Hypoxemia is a threat. Because of the unreliability of recognition of cyanosis and the knowledge that Pa_{O_2} is usually decreased, particularly in the elderly or after major operation, patients are transported to the recovery room with oxygen given via mask plus assisted ventilation. Portable oxygen cylinders are easily suspended from litter or bed.

Hypoxemia in the immediate postanesthesia period is related more to the effects of anesthesia than to the effects of operation on pulmonary function. Factors in the genesis of this initial hypoxemia include alveolar hypoventilation, ventilation:perfusion ($\dot{V}_A/\dot{Q}$) mismatch, intrapulmonary right to left shunting, decreased cardiac output, increased oxygen consumption, and diffusion hypoxia (see Chapter 37).

Hypoventilation due to depression of the respiratory centers by residual anesthetic effects is commonly observed. Anesthetics also depress the pulmonary vasoconstrictor reflexes that maintain perfusion of ventilated alveoli, thus exacerbating $\dot{V}_A/\dot{Q}$ mismatch. Hypoventilation should be sought and promptly treated. We recommend that oxygen be given to all patients in the recovery room who have had general anesthesia unless the anesthetist states otherwise. Giving oxygen routinely in the absence of orders to the contrary emphasizes our concern with the possibility of postoperative hypoxemia.

This approach also minimizes the transient diffusion hypoxia that occurs at termination of nitrous oxide administration. When room air is inhaled, nitrogen diffuses into blood and nitrous oxide into alveoli. Because of higher solubility in blood, the volume of nitrous oxide available for diffusion into the alveoli is greater than the volume of nitrogen entering the circulation. Residual oxygen in the alveoli is therefore diluted and Pa_{CO_2} decreased. Provision of a high oxygen concentration for three to four minutes as nitrous oxide is eliminated avoids the hypoxemia. Although diffusion hypoxia is well tolerated by normal individuals, it can combine with other factors to decrease tissue oxygenation. Oxygen must be administered with caution to patients with chronic pulmonary disease and elevated Pa_{CO_2}. These patients invariably depend on an hypoxemic drive to maintain ventilation, and hyperoxia leads to acute ventilatory failure (see Chapter 37). Preoperative arterial oxygenation is usually compromised, and patients are at risk of developing severe hypoxemia postoperatively. Therefore, they need to receive oxygen, but titrated carefully against Pa_{O_2}. Knowledge of preoperative blood gas values is of great assistance. We recommend giving oxygen via a high flow system starting with 24 per cent and increasing the FI_{O_2} after measuring arterial blood gases. The aim is to maintain Pa_{O_2} close to the preoperative value. Abdominal and thoracic operations derange pulmonary function in the first few hours postoperatively, progressing to a maximum at 12 to 18 hours and slowly returning to normal over several days. Patients show a pattern of restrictive pulmonary function with reduced inspiratory capacity, vital capacity, and, to a lesser extent, functional residual capacity (FRC). This leads to decreased pulmonary compliance, increased airway resistance, and increased work of breathing (see Chapter 37). Patients breathe rapidly and shallowly, do not take deep breaths, and have an ineffective cough. Thus, a tendency exists for secretions to accumulate and atelectasis to develop. The mechanisms of this restrictive pattern are incompletely understood, although pain is a major factor. In addition to pain, the surgical incision interferes with chest and abdominal wall function. Measures that maintain FRC, used in conjunction with appropriate analgesia, minimize these effects.

In addition to deliberate elevation of FI_{O_2}, the aim today is to reduce the work of breathing and provide better gas exchange through mechanical ventilation or positive airway pressure therapy for critically ill patients. In high risk patients, prophylactic use of 5 to 10 cm/H_2O positive airway pressure reduces the incidence of pulmonary complications, probably by maintaining FRC at levels closer to normal. A tracheal tube is often left in place and support provided for hours or days, according to need (see Chapter 37).

Pneumothorax

We have witnessed the development of pneumothorax following brachial plexus or intercostal nerve block, as a result of spontaneous rupture of an emphysematous bleb, during dissection in the neck, or following operation performed just beneath the diaphragm, as for nephrectomy. Listening to the chest for breath sounds and determining that the trachea is in the midline usually establishes the diagnosis, which is then confirmed by x-ray. Should tension pneumothorax be present, prompt aspiration of air and institution of underwater drainage are essential (see Chapter 33).

Restrictive or Obstructive Dressings

Inadequate ventilation may be caused by excessively tight surgical dressings, as after radical mastectomy, and respiratory obstruction may follow application of dressings or plaster jackets about the head and neck.

ASPIRATION OF VOMITUS

This subject is discussed in Chapter 33.

SHIVERING

Shivering has two components, one neurologic and the other relating to temperature control. Pyramidal tract signs are commonly seen as the patient emerges from light planes of general anesthesia, gross clonus sometimes mimicking a convulsion. This can be controlled with methylphenidate given intravenously. Many patients emerge from anesthesia with lowered body temperatures; shivering can be marked, thus increasing heart rate and work and oxygen consumption, all of which can lead to hypoxemia. Heat loss is engendered in the use of semiclosed and open anesthesia systems, by failure to warm infused fluids, by the presence of open body cavities, during deep planes of anesthesia, and in the child, elderly, and cachectic; but the major factor is the air-conditioned operating room. Reduction of body temperature is minimized by maintaining room temperature at least at 21 C.

PAIN

Pain is inevitable after operation, the degree, duration, and effect varying enormously. The very young, the emotionally stable, and the elderly tend to show lesser responses. Superficial operations are accompanied by less pain than following intrathoracic or intra-abdominal procedures or those associated with bladder or anal spasm. Muscle splinting, inadequate ventilation, and diminished cough predisposing to atelectasis are some of the respiratory sequelae of pain, whereas tachycardia and hypertension are common circulatory reactions.

The patient who has recovered incompletely from general anesthesia is given less than the usual dose of opioid to avoid re-anesthetization, hypotension, respiratory depression, and hypoventilation. Intravenous titration of small doses of opioid is the safest, quickest, and most reliable means of achieving adequate analgesia without encountering undesirable side effects, especially for patients with cardiorespiratory disease. However, morphine, 5 mg, or meperidine, 50 mg, given intramuscularly, is generally satisfactory for the average adult without significant cardiopulmonary disease. Regional nerve block is an excellent alternative to systemic analgesics.

RESTLESSNESS AND EXCITEMENT

Agitation during emergency from general anesthesia may be so severe as to occupy several attendants and require mechanical restraint. In addition to pain, a number of factors contribute to the phenomenon. Patients with psychomotor disturbances, those fearful of the findings at operation, or those who confess that they cannot tolerate pain are likely candidates. Prolonged maintenance of an uncomfortable position or a distended urinary bladder are additional influences. Excitement as a result of hypoxia occurs after thoracic, head and neck, or upper abdominal operations and in the presence of pneumothorax, tracheal collapse, vocal cord paralysis, or respiratory depression from any cause. Arterial hypotension contributes through production of cerebral hypoxia. Scopolamine or the phenothiazines and barbiturates as premedicants are associated with a higher incidence of excitement. However, when these drugs are combined with an opioid, postoperative restlessness is less likely. The role of ketamine in causing postoperative confusion and hallucinations has been discussed in Chapter 14.

Prevention of excitement is apparent from a consideration of the causes. Should agitation develop, however, the following measures are helpful. If the patient has remained in one positon on a recovery room bed for a long time, position should be changed. If pain is a factor, an opioid is effective, in small doses by vein if there is delirium, otherwise given intramuscularly. If hypoxemia exists, the underlying causes should be treated, if possible while $F_{I_{O_2}}$ is increased. As the anesthetic is eliminated and self-control returns, the patient becomes quiet. Time, therefore, is of the essence, but the experience is upsetting for other patients in the area, for attendants, and for the patient as well.

THE RECOVERY ROOM

A postoperative recovery room serves to care for patients until they are sufficiently recovered from the physiologic derangements produced by operation and general anesthesia. Close monitoring is permitted to central neurologic, cardiovascular, respiratory, and renal function, and immediate therapy is available. A centralized recovery room offers the following advantages: (1) maximal safety for patients; (2) alleviation of the burden of immediate postanesthetic care for the general nursing staff and economy in distribution of nurses; (3) concentration of monitoring and resuscitation equipment; (4) immediate availability of surgeons and anesthetists; (5) opportunity for study of problems associated with the immediate postanesthetic period.

PERSONNEL

Successful operation of a recovery room depends in great measure on the skill and devotion of the nursing staff. These individuals must be dedicated to their work, for in few other branches of nursing is attention to detail so vital and the need for immediate, intelligent action so necessary. At any moment a patient's condition may worsen. Instant recognition of the change, appraisal of its significance, and prompt application of corrective measures are demanded. The luxury of being able to assign a physician to full-time recovery room duty is denied most hospitals, but an anesthetist should be immediately available. In some institutions student nurses obtain their only experience in the care of unconscious patients while on assignment to the recovery room. Under close supervision they learn the problems and management of the unconscious patient: respiratory obstruction, hypotension, emergence excitement, and pain. Orderlies, housekeeping personnel, and respiratory therapists play a major role in the day-to-day operation of the area.

DESIGN AND FACILITIES

The design and facilities of a particular recovery room vary with the nature and volume of operations performed. Certain design features are desirable. Air conditioning is essential, and lighting should be uniform and sufficiently bright to permit appraisal of change in color of a patient's skin and mucous membranes. Individual bed lights are helpful for the times when special procedures must be performed. The nurses' station should command a view of all patients, as constant surveillance is essential. The unconscious patient should lie in the lateral decubitus position to minimize possibility of aspiration of vomitus, if possible facing the nurses' station. During the postanesthetic period, separation of sexes is not essential, but care should be taken not to expose patients unnecessarily. Cubicles and curtains can be utilized if an attendant can be assigned to each patient and if the patient can be observed from the central station. At least two telephones are required in the area to be sure that an open line is available in an emergency. A call system permitting nurses to summon additional help is necessary.

An area for assembling, cleaning, and sterilizing equipment and for storing infrequently used apparatus should adjoin the patient area; a clinical diagnostic laboratory nearby is a necessity. The recovery room should be adjacent to the operating rooms. If a blood bank is not nearby, a substation is established in the vicinity as well as a storage area for respiratory therapy equipment. It is wise to stock equipment of uniform design so that all understand its use and function. A portable x-ray machine is frequently needed.

Wash basins, adequate electric outlets, bedside tables, work counters, and ceiling suspension of equipment add to the efficiency. The psychological aspects of patient care should not be overlooked. Noise is kept to a minimum; indeed, piped-in music sometimes provides distraction. Conversation about a patient's condition and prognosis should not be audible to the patient.

Oxygen and suction outlets are provided for each patient. Oxygen therapy equipment capable of providing an FI_{O_2} from 25 to 100 per cent is required (see Chapter 38). Mechanical ventilators should be at hand or on call from the respiratory therapy service. All kinds and sizes of pharyngeal airways, endotracheal tubes, laryngoscopes, a bronchoscope, and tracheostomy sets are stocked. Few drugs are useful as respiratory stimulants; however, doxapram is effective if one is needed. Bronchodilating agents should be at hand for patients with asthma or bronchoconstriction of other cause; epinephrine, isoproterenol, and aminophylline are used for these conditions.

For hydration and support of the circulation, saline, glucose in water, and one of the plasma expanders such as albumin or Hetastarch must be at hand. Several units of type O, Rh negative whole blood are stored in the blood bank for emergency transfusion; these are given until properly crossmatched blood or blood components are available. In addition to the usual intravenous sets, provision is made for administering intravenous fluids or blood under pressure. Venous cutdown trays, cannulas, and plastic tubing of various sizes are part of resuscitative paraphernalia. To support blood pressure, phenylephrine, metaraminol, dopamine, ephedrine, and levarterenol are often used. A fully constituted cardiopulmonary resuscitation cart is a requisite. A cardiac kit with scalpel and thoracic retractors should also be stored. Devices to monitor blood pressure, central venous and pulmonary artery pressures, and body temperature are at hand as is the electrocardiogram. Cooling blankets are essential in the treatment of hyperpyrexia.

Heart failure may occur. Digoxin, more rapidly acting inotropic agents, diuretics, and antiarrhythmic drugs such as quinidine, procainamide, and lidocaine are stored. A recording electrocardiograph permits accurate diagnosis of arrhythmias or myocardial ischemia.

Facilities for management of all types of drainage are needed: gastrointestinal suction apparatus, bladder irrigating sets, underwater chest drainage units, and sump pumps.

Restraining straps, wristlets, armboards, and side rails for beds are needed in the management of restlessness. Opioids, barbiturates, tranquilizers, chlorpromazine, and phenytoin are stocked. In case of overdose of opioids, naloxone is a necessity. A locked cabinet for opioids is needed, and an accurate record of usage must be kept.

Standard equipment such as blood pressure cuffs and manometers, stethoscopes, syringes and needles, thermometers, urinary bladder catheters, emesis basins, and urinals and bedpans are always available. A supply of linen and blankets is stocked; a blanket warmer is a useful device. A refrigerator is needed for storage of perishable drugs.

Drugs stocked in the authors' recovery areas are listed in Table 36–1.

Patients with radium implantations for treatment of malignancy are separated from other individuals in the recovery room so that radiation hazards are minimized. Patients with transmissible infections should not be admitted to the recovery room unless isolation techniques are practiced. Strict infection control to minimize transmission of organisms between patients must be exercised.

RECORDS

An accurate record of the patient's course in the recovery room is kept; two such records are shown in Figures 36–1 and 36–2. Vital signs are recorded. Some anesthetists assign a numerical value to the patient's condition on entry, graded in much the same fashion as the Apgar score for newborns. Criteria include reflex activity, respiration, circulation, state of consciousness, and color. All therapeutic measures are listed in the order administered. Pertinent observations on the patient's appearance and reactions are noted. The record eventually becomes part of the permanent hospital record

TABLE 36–1. Drugs Stored in The Recovery Area

Amphetamine	Metaraminol
Atropine sulfate	Methoxamine
Bethanechol chloride	Nalorphine
Bretylium tosylate	Naloxone
Bupivacaine	Neostigmine
Calcium chloride	Nitroglycerin
Calcium gluconate	Opioids
Chlorpromazine	codeine
Cocaine	fentanyl
Cortisone	meperidine
Dexamethasone	morphine
Diazepam	Oxytocin
Digitoxin	Pentobarbital
Digoxin	Phentolamine
Diphenhydramine	Phenylephrine
Dobutamine	Phenytoin
Dopamine	Physostigmine
Doxapram	Phytonadione
Droperidol	Potassium chloride
ε-Aminocaproic acid	Procainamide
Edrophonium	Procaine
Ephedrine	Prochlorperazine
Epinephrine	Promethazine
Fibrinogen	Propranolol
Furosemide	Protamine
Glucagon	Quinidine
Glucose, 50 per cent	Secobarbital
Glycopyrrolate	Sodium bicarbonate
Heparin	Sodium iodide
Hydralazine	Sodium lactate
Hydrocortisone	Sodium nitroprusside
Insulin	Succinylcholine
Isoproterenol	Theophylline ethylenediamine
Lanatoside C	Thiopental
Levarterenol	Trimethaphan
Lidocaine	Tripelennamine
Magnesium sulfate	Water for injection, sterile
Mannitol, 25 per cent	

and is of value to personnel who subsequently assume responsibility for the patient, providing as it does a summary of the early postoperative period. A yearly statistical report for the recovery room should include numbers of admissions, length of stay for each patient, mortality, special procedures performed, and unusual problems encountered.

Although complications anticipated in the postoperative period have been listed earlier in this chapter, a few comments on special situations indicate the breadth of problems demanding attention in hospitals providing this kind of care. A neurosurgical patient may develop systolic hypertension, bradycardia, Cheyne-Stokes respiration, unequal pupils, fixed and dilated pupils, loss of consciousness, and aggravation of hemiparesis as indices of increased intracranial pressure. Transurethral resection of the prostate may be associated with absorption of a large volume of irrigating fluid through the prostatic bed, resulting in water intoxication, mental confusion, and hypertension. Obstruction of urinary bladder catheters is not uncommon, requiring irrigation. These and other challenging situations require the best in diagnostic acumen and therapy.

GENERAL POLICIES FOR ADMISSION AND RELEASE OF PATIENTS

Admission to and release from the recovery area are the joint responsibility of the services that supervise the recovery area, usually anesthesia, surgery, and nursing,

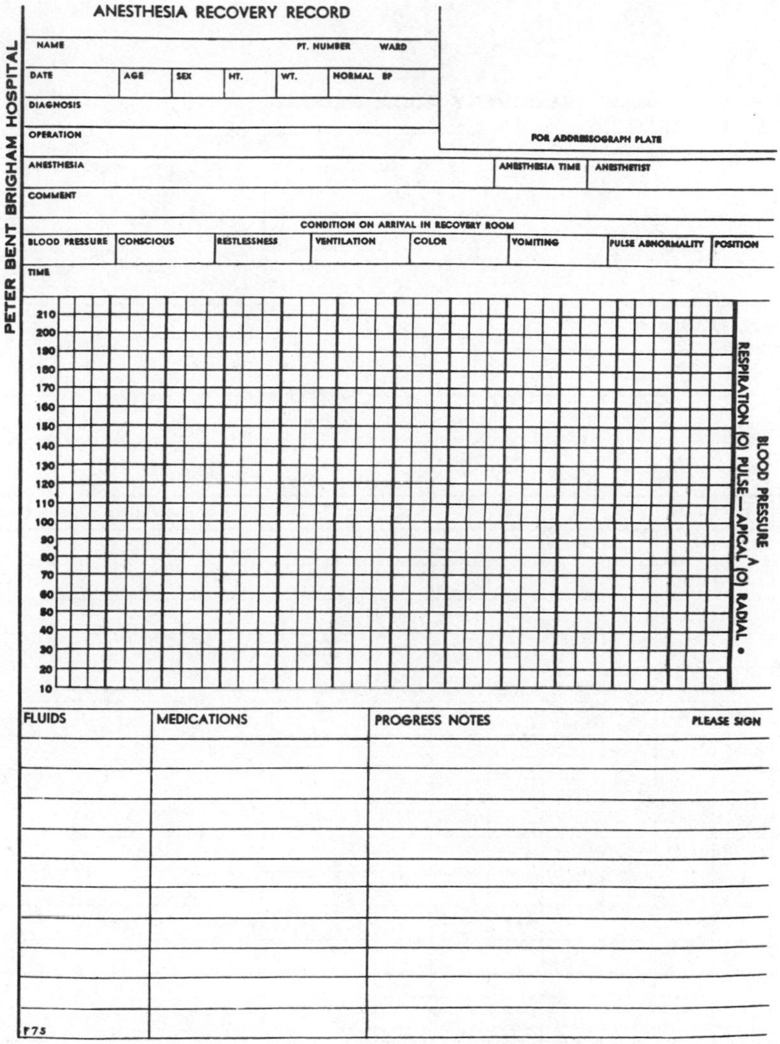

FIGURE 36–1. An example of an anesthesia recovery record.

under the overall guidance of hospital administration. This group establishes the rules for conduct in the area: hours of use, admission of visitors, aseptic procedures, hiring of personnel, and charges for services. Only good judgment on the part of the responsible physician and nursing staff can determine when a patient should be discharged from the recovery room. The following criteria are useful: stability of vital signs, control of prior bleeding, sufficient reflexes to prevent aspiration of vomitus, orientation of patient as to time and place, and ability to maintain a safe position in bed, e.g., the optimal position for chest drainage or unobstructed breathing.

Discharge of patients depends on the primary reason for admission; e.g., outpatients are kept until they can walk without dizziness or nausea. Patients who have had spinal anesthesia are detained until the level of anesthesia recedes and blood pressure is stable. Some recovery rooms are open only during the day, others are prepared to keep patients overnight only under exceptional circumstances, whereas still others retain patients for several days. Ambulatory care surgical units usually maintain their own recovery areas, as do obstetric divisions.

Northwestern Memorial Hospital | **RECOVERY ROOM RECORD**
Form No. 404798   Rev. 7/81

PROCEDURE: _____

ANESTHETIC AGENTS: _____

PRE-OP PROBLEMS: _____

INTRA-OP PROBLEMS: _____

ANTICIPATED POST-OP PROBLEMS: _____ DATE: _____

O.R. INTAKE - FLUIDS: _____ O.R. URINE OUTPUT: _____

BLOOD: _____ BLOOD DERIVATIVE: _____ EBL: _____

TIME ADMITTED: _____   TIME RESPONDED: _____   TIME DISCHARGED: _____   SIGNATURE OF ANESTHESIOLOGIST: _____

TIME	BP CUFF	BP SCOPE	MEAN	P	R	TEMP.		SWAN GANZ	URINE OUTPUT	NURSING OBSERVATIONS AND NOTES

A

SIGNATURE OF DISCHARGING M.D.

SIGNATURE OF DISCHARGING R.N.

FIGURE 36–2.   An example of an anesthesia recovery record.

Illustration continued on opposite page

RECOVERY ROOM RECORD

Patient Name: _____ Hospital No. _____

	MEDICATIONS				
TIME	DRUG	DOSE	ROUTE	SIGNATURE	

			LAB RESULTS			
TEST	TEST	TEST	TEST	TEST	TEST	TEST
TIME	TIME	TIME	TIME	TIME	TIME	TIME
SX. NOTIFIED	SX. NOTIFIED	SX. NOTIFIED	SX. NOTIFIED	SX. NOTIFIED	SX. NOTIFIED	SX. NOTIFIED
M.D. NAME	M.D. NAME	M.D. NAME	M.D. NAME	M.D. NAME	M.D. NAME	M.D. NAME

RECOVERY ROOM INTAKE FLUIDS/BLOOD PRODUCTS			RECOVERY ROOM OUTPUT FLUIDS		
TIME	IV		URINE		
			NG.		
			WOUND		
	IVPB		EMESIS		
	BLOOD				
	BLOOD PRODUCTS				
		TOTAL		TOTAL	

MONITOR STRIP:

B

FIGURE 36–2 *Continued*

INTENSIVE CARE

Critically ill patients can be defined as those having life-threatening or potentially life-threatening illnesses whose condition is unstable and who is liable to rapid and frequent change. Therefore, they require close surveillance and frequent therapeutic interventions. When such specialized care is needed for days rather than hours, a more versatile unit that provides facilities for highly sophisticated monitoring, diagnostic procedures, and therapy is necessary. In addition to the large number of specially trained personnel and equipment, provision of meals, a waiting area for relatives, a changing area for nurses, sleeping quarters for physicians on call, a clinical laboratory, an x-ray diagnostic unit, and a conference room are required.

Depending on the size and function of the hospital, there may be one or several intensive care areas. Individual units have been established for the neonate, the child, and patients with suspected or proved myocardial infarction, trauma, burns, and respiratory failure. In a medical intensive care unit one finds patients with such varied problems as cardiac, pulmonary, renal, or hepatic failure; gastrointestinal hemorrhage; and neurologic disease; whereas surgical intensive care wards house a wide spectrum of critically ill patients both prior to and following operation. Whether all intensive care areas should be physically adjacent and whether personnel should rotate among them are in dispute.

Most of the features and the philosophy of the recovery area pertain to intensive care units, with about 10 per cent of hospital bed capacity devoted to the latter function.

Philosophic and Psychological Problems Posed by Intensive Care

Intensive care can be an effective means of maintaining life as evidenced by reduced mortality, but it is also a costly practice. It is vital, however, that the criteria for instituting care be determined by the implied consent of all involved. Death is no longer defined by absence of spontaneous breathing or heart beat. Thus it is reasonable that selection of patients for prolonged respiratory support should be done with the hope of ultimately providing a useful existence. In addition to such criteria as measurement of blood gases and physical findings, considerable judgment and knowledge of the patient's problems are required for selection, and it is by no means certain who should make the final decision for cessation of treatment.

Intensive care medicine is often unnecessarily dehumanizing. Patients with tracheal intubation or a tracheostomy have difficulty in communicating. They are exposed to the observations and ministerings of many individuals and are surrounded by strange and monotonously noisy machinery. Unfortunately, physicians and others occasionally talk carelessly before these people. They may be keenly aware of the critical nature of their illness, and death is all around them. They are deprived of such normal experiences as sleep and awareness of night and day, while tubes are constantly suctioned, and are turned and subjected to investigative procedures.

It is not surprising that such patients frequently develop disorientation, delirium, and psychoses. Thus it is essential that people involved in their care make every effort to minimize noise and discomfort and to provide reassurance and psychological support. The experienced nurse serves a vital function in this respect, because constant attendance at the bedside provides a calm, friendly, and human approach in this highly charged atmosphere.

REFERENCES

Beal, JM (ed.): Intensive and Recovery Room Care. New York. The Macmillan Co, 1982.
Becker, ID, Paulson BA, Miller RD, et al: Biphasic respiratory depression after fentanyl-droperidol or fentanyl alone used to supplement nitrous oxide anesthesia. Anesthesiology 44:291, 1976.
Craig DB: Postoperative recovery of pulmonary function. Anesth Analg 60:46, 1981.
Gal TJ, Cooperman LH: Hypertension in the immediate postoperative period. Br J Anaesth 47:70, 1976.
Lisbon A (ed): Anesthetic consideration in setting up a new medical facility. Int Anesth Clin 19:63, 1981.
Masson AHB, Millar RA: Symposium on the postoperative period. Br J Anaesth 47:89, 1975.
Schmidt FB, O'Neill WW, Kotb, A, et al: Continuous positive airway pressure in the prophylaxis of the adult respiratory distress syndrome. Surg Gynecol Obstet 143:613, 1976.

Chapter *37*

RESPIRATION AND
RESPIRATORY CARE

Well-functioning lungs are among the anesthetists' most important allies in the operating suite and recovery rooms. Therefore, we believe that emphasis on the quantitative aspects of gas exchange is of importance not only in reference to the respiratory gases, O_2 and CO_2, but in uptake and elimination of volatile anesthetics. The mechanical properties of the respiratory system are literally felt by the anesthetist whenever the breathing of an anesthetized patient is controlled or assisted; hence, knowledge of respiratory mechanics is essential for good management. Again, because the anesthetist is responsible for maintenance of the patient's fluid balance during operation, understanding of the fluid exchange in the lung and the mechanisms that can derange it cannot be overemphasized.

This chapter is not meant to be a comprehensive text on the physiology of respiration or respiratory failure. A list of monographs and review articles is given in the references to guide readers to further information and to refer them to original articles.

LUNG FUNCTION AND STRUCTURE

The primary function of the lungs is the exchange of the respiratory gases between blood and atmosphere. The ultimate destination of oxygen is the mitochondrion in the cells, where it serves as a proton acceptor in oxidative metabolic pathways and yields "metabolic" water; CO_2 is produced in cells via the various kinds of decarboxylation. Thus the gas exchange between atmosphere and blood that occurs in the lungs is only one step in the transport of O_2 and CO_2 between atmosphere and cells.

The structure of the lungs is exquisitely suited to their function as a gas exchanger: in an adult man mixed venous blood is exposed to gas within the lungs at an internal surface of 50 to 100 sq m (approximately the size of a tennis court). The gas-exchanging membrane consists of about 300 million alveoli with capillary networks in their walls. The membrane separating gas and blood is thin, on the average about 1 μm, and the diameters of alveoli are small, about 150 μm. With this large surface area and the small distances involved, conditions are favorable for efficient diffusional exchange of O_2 and CO_2 between the gas phase and blood.

Gas is transported to the alveoli by mass movement through conducting airways. The function of the upper airways — nose, mouth, pharynx, and larynx — is to filter out particles of large size, to warm and humidify inspired gas, and to conserve water vapor in expired gas. These conditions are eliminated when the upper airway is bypassed with tracheal intubation or tracheostomy. The lower airways begin at the trachea and its division at the carina, into two main stem bronchi, with subsequent irregularly dichotomous branching for over 20 generations of division. The diameter of each new generation of tubes decreases; however, the total cross-sectional area increases sharply at the level of the terminal bronchioles, about 90 times that of the combined main stem bronchi. Thus, the velocity of gas flow decreases toward the periphery.

The airways consist of an epithelial layer with a basal membrane and supporting connective tissue containing cartilage and smooth muscle. The cartilages are U-shaped in the trachea and main stem bronchi and are more irregular beyond, disappearing at the level of the bronchioles (about 1 mm in diameter, at the 10th or 11th generation). Maintenance of patency in the small airways depends on the elastic recoil of lung tissue. Smooth muscle is present throughout the tracheobronchial tree down to terminal bronchioles. Upon constriction, as in asthma, airway resistance increases. However, in normal lung the physiologic role of smooth muscle is not understood. Epithelium is of the pseudostratified columnar type in large airways, the thickness progressively decreasing to a layer of cuboidal cells in terminal bronchioles. Most prominent are the synchronously beating ciliated cells, with mucin-producing goblet cells and serous cells interspersed; large and intermediate bronchi contain glands that penetrate the basal membrane. In chronic bronchitis, the thickness of the glandular layer increases. Ordinarily, secretions produced by the epithelial elements form a mucous carpet that is propagated toward the pharynx by the cilia. Because of a functional "blood-bronchial barrier" the liquid component of the mucus is not a simple ultrafiltrate of plasma. One of the consequences of the barrier is that most antibiotics systemically administered appear in bronchial secretions in appreciably lower concentrations than in plasma. Nutrition of the airways derives from the bronchial circulation, which extends to the terminal bronchioles. Bronchial veins drain into pulmonary veins.

Inhaled particles (including bacteria) that are not trapped in the upper airways are deposited on the mucous carpet and removed by continuous motion toward the pharynx. The efficiency of mucociliary clearance depends on the viscosity of the bronchial secretions and on ciliary action. The latter is depressed by irritants such as tobacco smoke or anesthetics. The smallest inhaled particles, less than 3 μm in diameter, upon reaching the alveoli are engulfed by pulmonary macrophages, which digest particles or microorganisms and clear them via pulmonary lymphatics and capillary blood vessels.

The airways, from nose to terminal bronchioles, are not endowed with gas-exchanging membranes, thus constituting the anatomic dead space. The respiratory zone, representing some 90 per cent of the lung, begins at the respiratory bronchioles with outpocketings of single alveoli, followed by alveolar ducts and sacs.

MECHANISMS OF PULMONARY GAS EXCHANGE

These are grouped under three categories: pulmonary ventilation, blood flow through the lung, and diffusional exchange of O_2 and CO_2 between gas and blood. For effective diffusional exchange, it is essential that ventilation and blood perfusion match throughout the lung. Ideally, the most efficient arrangement would be a perfectly homogeneous distribution of both ventilation and blood flow, and in the first approach to a quantitative evaluation of gas exchange we shall assume this to be the case. However, even in healthy lungs, ventilation and perfusion are not homogeneously distributed, owing to the effect of gravity. In the diseased lung, matching of ventilation and perfusion is further disturbed, with important consequences for gas exchange.

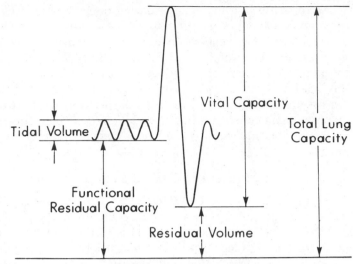

FIGURE 37–1. Volumes in the lungs.

PULMONARY VENTILATION

Distances in the conducting airways are so great that no significant amount of gas can be transported via simple diffusion from atmosphere to alveoli. Thus mass movement of gas, or pulmonary ventilation, is essential. In dealing with mechanisms of pulmonary ventilation, we first describe the static volumes of the lungs, then concentrate on the mechanics of respiration, factors that determine bulk movement of gas between the atmosphere and the respiratory zone. Finally, we deal with quantitative aspects of exchange of individual respiratory gases and with the consequent effect on composition of alveolar gas and arterialized blood.

LUNG VOLUMES

Figure 37–1 shows typical values for static volumes in the normal human lung. Tidal volume and vital capacity can be measured with a simple spirometer. Absolute volume of gas present in the lung at functional residual capacity, at residual volume, and at total lung capacity can be determined by gas dilution techniques or with a body plethysmograph.

RESPIRATORY MECHANICS

The tidal volume (V_T) is the volume of gas moved in and out of the lungs in a single breath. At rest, the average V_T is about 500 ml. The product of tidal volume and frequency of breaths per minute is the minute ventilation, usually measured as the expired volume, $\dot{V}_E$ L/min. Respiratory rate at rest is about 14 breaths/min; thus a typical resting $\dot{V}_E$ would be 7 L/min.   *100 ml / kg/min.*

To produce a flow of gas between the atmosphere and lungs, a pressure difference must exist between mouth and nose (Pao) and that in alveoli (P_A). In spontaneous breathing, P_A is lowered below atmospheric pressure by the action of inspiratory muscles; during artificial ventilation, the pressure difference (Pao − P_A) is created by applying positive pressure to the airways, or positive pressure ventilation (PPV).

The diaphragm is the essential inspiratory muscle, innervated by the phrenic nerves. As the diaphragm contracts, the volume of the chest is increased by both descent of the diaphragm and elevation of the distal margins of the rib cage. The ribs are also elevated by contraction of the external intercostal muscles, segmentally innervated from the thoracic spinal cord. In forceful inspiration, accessory muscles of inspiration are recruited (shoulder-girdle and neck) to elevate the rib cage.

Expiration is a passive act during quiet breathing owing to elastic recoil of the respiratory system as it returns to resting volume. During the hyperpnea of exercise or in voluntary hyperventilation, expiration becomes active. The important expiratory muscles are those of the abdominal wall, which increase intra-abdominal pressure, thrusting the relaxed diaphragm into the chest and exerting traction on the rib cage. The internal intercostals also assist expiration by downward traction. Expiratory muscles are essential for forceful expiration during cough. In tetraplegics, residual sparing of diaphragmatic contraction may be enough to develop adequate inspiratory force during resting ventilation; however, efficient cough is impossible owing to loss of expiratory muscles.

Mechanical Properties of the Respiratory System

Most of the work of breathing is spent in expanding the chest wall and lungs, not on moving air. Recall that in spontaneous breathing the pressure difference between Pao and P_A required to move air is low, about 1 cm H_2O during quiet breathing. Mechanical properties of the lungs determine the distribution of the volume of gas to various parts of the lungs; this, together with regional perfusion, determines the efficiency of gas exchange and the composition of alveolar gas and arterialized blood. Changes in the mechanical properties of the lung are prominent in most pathologic conditions.

Elastic Properties of the Lungs

The isolated, excised lung changes volume like an elastic balloon; volume increases when the pressure inside increases over that outside, and deflation is spontaneous as a result of elasticity. Static elastic properties of the isolated lung can be described by studying the static pressure-volume relation. The relevant pressure is the transpulmonary pressure (P_L) or the difference between P_A and the pressure at the surface of the lung. When P_L increases, volume increases, and vice versa. In the excised lung, surface pressure is the barometric pressure (P_B). To maintain an excised lung at a given volume, P_L must be positive, P_A higher than P_B. With the lung in the chest with no gas flow and the airway open, P_A equals P_B and a positive distending pressure (P_L) results from a subatmospheric negative pleural pressure (P_{pl}) exerted by traction of the chest wall. Figure 37–2 shows a pressure-volume plot of a normal dog lung. Note that the curve during inflation differs from that obtained on deflation, a phenomenon called hysteresis. The slope of the pressure-volume curve at any lung volume is the lung compliance (C_L). Within the range of normal tidal breathing, C_L is about 200 ml/cm H_2O. At high lung volumes, compliance decreases markedly and the lung becomes very stiff.

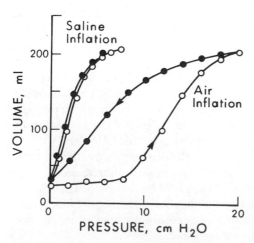

FIGURE 37–2. Pressure-volume curve of an excised lung showing hysteresis of a gas-filled lung. Open circles, inflation; closed circles, deflation. Note the greater compliance and reduced hysteresis when the lung is filled with saline. (Reproduced with permission from Remington JW (ed): Tissue Elasticity. Bethesda, Md, American Physiological Society, 1957.)

The elasticity of the lungs is a result of two factors: the presence of a fibrous network in parenchyma, and the effect of surface tension at the gas-liquid interface within alveoli and small airways. The fibrous network consists of elastin, an extensible protein, and collagen, a rigid material. Elastin probably functions over the whole range of lung volumes, whereas collagen fibers may act as an inextensible net that becomes tense at high lung volumes, not unlike a net around an inflated balloon. Presumably collagen fibers are responsible for the low lung compliance at high lung volumes.

Surface tension is the major component of elastic recoil. When the lungs are filled with saline (no gas-liquid interface), lung compliance is greater and the pressure-volume curve shows little hysteresis (see Fig. 37–2). Considering the very small diameter of alveoli, it is surprising that the contribution of surface tension to lung elastic recoil is not greater. This is explained by the presence of surfactant, a dipalmitoyl-lecithin bound to a protein, lining the alveoli and terminal airways. Its surface tension is low, about 5 dynes/cm, as compared with plasma surface tension of about 50 dynes/cm and saline surface tension of about 70 dynes/cm. In addition to the low surface tension, surfactant exhibits marked hysteresis, that is, surface tension increases on expansion and decreases on diminution of the surface area. The advantages of surfactant entail increased lung compliance, especially at low volumes.

Surfactant probably also contributes to the inner stability of alveoli. An arrangement of 300,000,000 intercommunicating "bubbles" is very unstable, the smaller bubbles tending to empty into the larger as pressure within a bubble is inversely proportional to its radius. The variable surface tension of surfactant, decreasing with diminishing radius and increasing with expansion of the alveolus, tends to stabilize the lungs by keeping alveoli open. Another, and perhaps more important mechanism contributing to stability of the alveoli is their interdependence. Any lung region less distended than the surrounding tissue does not collapse because it cannot move independently of contiguous units.

Mechanical (Elastic) Properties of the Chest Wall

The chest wall comprises the rib cage, the diaphragm, and the abdomen. In the chest wall both passive components, with intrinsic elasticity, and active components, the respiratory muscles, exist. In the resting state, the chest wall harbors a certain volume and resists deformation, that is, compression by expiratory muscles or expansion by inspiratory muscles. Elastic properties of the passive chest wall can be described by the relation between distending pressure and volume. The distending or transthoracic pressure is the difference between the pressure inside the chest wall (P_{pl}) and the pressure outside (atmospheric pressure, P_B). P_{pl} is measured in the esophagus using a balloon-tipped catheter. Figure 37–3 shows a pressure volume plot of the

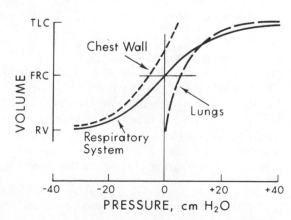

FIGURE 37–3. Schematic pressure-volume curves of the chest wall, the lungs, and the total respiratory system.

passive chest wall together with that of the lungs, the two contributing to the plot for the total respiratory system. The plot is best described as if it were obtained in a paralyzed subject. Starting from the resting position, known volumes of air would be injected into or removed in steps from sealed airways with the pressures measured statically at the airway opening (Pao) with no gas flow. It can be seen that the compliance of the chest wall over most of the range of vital capacity is similar to that of the lungs, about 200 ml/cm H_2O; only at very low volumes does the chest wall become stiff. If no deforming force is applied to the system (Pao = 0 in our experiment on a paralyzed subject), the tendency of the lung to collapse is equal and opposite to the tendency of the chest wall to expand, a point reached at the end of a quiet passive expiration, the functional residual capacity (FRC). It is also apparent in Figure 37–3 that the lung becomes stiff at high volumes, whereas the chest wall becomes very stiff at low volumes.

The total compliance of the respiratory system results from the combined compliance of lungs and chest wall. With the lung within the chest, their elastic resistances, reciprocals of compliances, act in series:

$$\frac{1}{C_L} + \frac{1}{C_{CW}} = \frac{1}{C_{RS}}, \text{ i.e., } \frac{1}{200} + \frac{1}{200} = \frac{1}{100}$$

Thus, the normal compliance of the whole respiratory system (C_{RS}) is 100 ml/cm H_2O.

P_{pl} in the relaxed state is subatmospheric owing to the inward pull of the lungs and outward traction of chest wall. Upon contraction of inspiratory muscles P_{pl} becomes more negative, and with compression of the chest P_{pl} becomes less negative, reaching positive (higher than atmospheric) values with active compression of the chest by the expiratory muscles. Note that during spontaneous breathing P_{pl} is determined by the elastic properties of the lungs, whereas with PPV the elastic property of the chest wall is the determinant.

In the upright position intrapleural pressure is less negative at the base of the lungs than at the apex, with a continuous gradient of pressure presumably owing to the weight of the lungs. Thus, along this gradient in P_{pl}, the lungs are more expanded at the apex than at the base and, during tidal breathing, the various parts of the lungs operate along different segments of their pressure-volume curves. With lowering of pleural pressure during inspiration, the lower lung receives more ventilation than the upper; the mechanism is responsible for a gradient of uneven pulmonary ventilation, more ventilation going to the base than to the apex. In the supine position the gradient from apex to base is abolished, and now there is a gradient between the upper and lower parts of the lung.

Airway Closure

Small airways without cartilaginous support in their walls depend on the elastic recoil of lung parenchyma for patency. With low elastic recoil of surrounding tissues the small airways close, mostly in the dependent regions because of the deforming effect of gravity. If perfusion with blood continues in those regions, shunting results. Airway closure occurs in young, healthy individuals only when the lung volume is very low, close to RV; in elderly persons and in those with emphysema, owing to loss of elastic recoil, airway closure occurs at higher lung volumes and may exist during tidal breathing. The lung volume at which closure occurs is called closing volume. The principle of measuring closing volume is as follows:

When inspiration begins at a very low lung volume, near RV, the distribution of inspired gas is such that none initially goes to closed regions; only later, during inspiration at a higher lung

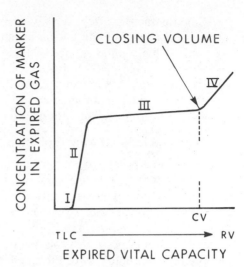

FIGURE 37–4. Idealized tracing of helium concentration in expired gas during a slow exhalation from total lung capacity (TLC) to residual volume (RV) after the previous breath has been labeled with a bolus of helium. Explanation in the text.

volume when the closed regions re-open, are they filled with inspired gas. A bolus of a poorly soluble marker gas, such as helium or xenon, is inhaled at the beginning of inspiration starting at RV, followed by inspiration of room air to TLC. Thus, the regions that were closed as the marker gas was being inhaled will contain no marker and will fill with nonmarker gas later during inspiration when opened at a higher lung volume. During subsequent expiration, the concentration of marker gas is measured in exhaled air in the course of a slow expiration from TLC to RV. The concentration of marker gas in exhaled air varies, reflecting the pattern of regional emptying of the lungs. A schematic record is shown in Figure 37–4. Phase I represents gas from the dead space; phase II is a mixture of dead-space gas and alveolar gas; phase III, the "alveolar plateau," represents mixed alveolar gas; and phase IV, with a sudden increase in He concentration, marks the lung volume at which the dependent lung regions, containing a lower He concentration, begin to close and cease to contribute to exhalation. Closing volume is defined as that part of the vital capacity left in the lungs at the turning point between phases III and IV. Closing capacity is the closing volume plus residual volume, RV, usually expressed in per cent of TLC (CC/TLC per cent).

Airway Resistance

A measure of airway resistance is the pressure difference required to produce a given flow of air through the entire system. The driving pressure is $Pao - P_A$, pressures that can be measured by a body plethysmograph. Physiologically important determinants of airway resistance are the geometry of the airways, including diameter, length, and branching, and the kind of gas flow, whether laminar or turbulent. Recall that resistance increases linearly with the length of a tube, is indirectly proportional to the fourth power of the radius of the tube if flow is laminar, and increases approximately with the fifth power of the radius during turbulent flow. Turbulence is promoted both by high velocity flows and by a large diameter of a tube or its irregularities. In the lungs, laminar flow probably occurs in smaller airways where air flow is slow; flow is turbulent in the trachea, and in intermediate airways the pattern is probably mixed. A typical value for normal airway resistance in the adult is 1 cm H_2O/L/sec of air flow. In the most severe attack of asthma, resistance can approach values of 50 cm H_2O/L/sec.

About 60 per cent of total airway resistance is contributed by the upper airway, nose to larynx. Small airways, less than 2 mm in diameter, contribute less than 20 per cent of the total resistance, owing to the large total cross-sectional area of airways that accommodates the flow. The low value for resistance in small airways creates difficulty in detecting their obstruction. Well-pronounced "small airway disease" can be present without any detectable increase in total airway resistance.

Several factors affect airway resistance; change in lung volume is one. As the airways form part of the elastic structure, their length and diameter vary with lung volume. At high volumes, above FRC, airway resistance changes little. However, at volumes between FRC and RV resistance increases appreciably with decrease in volume. At volumes close to RV, small airways may close completely and the resistance becomes infinite. Increase in smooth muscle tone, edema of the bronchial mucosa, and bronchial secretions are other factors that influence airway resistance.

Flow Limitation During Expiration

Airways are supported by the elastic recoil of the lung, an important factor in so-called dynamic compression of airways. During forced expiration, the lung is compressed, pleural pressure turns positive, and this in turn is transmitted to both lungs and airways, resulting in airway compression, narrowing, and increased resistance to flow with further expiratory effort. At high lung volumes, close to TLC, the high elastic recoil of the lung preserves the patency of small airways; only the main stem bronchi and the intrathoracic part of the trachea are compressed owing to their extraparenchymal location. At progressively lower lung volumes, with decrease in the elastic recoil of the lungs, the compression extends into the more peripheral airways. Thus, maximal expiratory flow is highest close to TLC, progressively decreasing as lung volume diminishes during expiration. In healthy individuals, maximal expiratory flow is about 10 L/sec close to TLC, and about 5 L/sec around FRC. In severe obstructive disease, the maximal expiratory flow rate attainable may be as low as 1 L/sec, representing the true limits of ventilation. The physiologic limitation imposed on the normal lung during expiration confers an obvious advantage in coughing. With narrowing of the airways, the linear velocity of air flow increases so that the gas exerts a greater shearing force in dislodging mucus or other particles from the bronchial walls.

QUANTITATIVE ANALYSIS OF PULMONARY GAS EXCHANGE

In the first approach, it is useful to state the obvious equalities that apply to gas exchange between lungs and atmosphere:

I. The volume of gas expired per unit of time, $\dot{V}_E$, equals the volume of inspired gas, $\dot{V}_I$, minus O_2 consumed, $\dot{V}_{O_2}$, plus CO_2 produced, $\dot{V}_{CO_2}$:

$$\dot{V}_E = \dot{V}_I - \dot{V}_{O_2} + \dot{V}_{CO_2} \tag{1}$$

II. The volume of O_2 consumed equals the volume of O_2 inspired in $\dot{V}_I$, minus the volume of O_2 expired in $\dot{V}_E$:

$$\dot{V}_{O_2} = \dot{V}_I \cdot F_{I_{O_2}} - \dot{V}_E \cdot F_{E_{O_2}} \tag{2}$$

III. The volume of CO_2 eliminated is equal to the volume of CO_2 in $\dot{V}_E$ minus the volume of CO_2 in $\dot{V}_I$:

$$\dot{V}_{CO_2} = \dot{V}_E \cdot F_{E_{CO_2}} - \dot{V}_I \cdot F_{I_{CO_2}} \tag{3}$$

When breathing room air or any other CO_2-free gas, the second term on the right side becomes zero, and:

$$\dot{V}_{CO_2} = \dot{V}_E \cdot F_{E_{CO_2}} \tag{3a}$$

These three equations implicitly contain all variables necessary in calculations relating to the composition of respiratory gas, as developed further on (gas-exchange ratio, alveolar gas, alveolar equation, and so on).

Note from (1) that $\dot{V}_E$ is not necessarily equal to $\dot{V}_I$; the two volumes will be equal only if $\dot{V}_{O_2} = \dot{V}_{CO_2}$ (see discussion of respiratory exchange ratio, R, in the following section).

IV. Nitrogen, an inert gas, is neither consumed nor produced in the body, i.e.:

$$\dot{V}_{N_2} = 0 = \dot{V}_I \cdot F_{I_{N_2}} - \dot{V}_E \cdot F_{E_{N_2}} \tag{4}$$

Therefore:

$$\dot{V}_I = \dot{V}_E \cdot F_{E_{N_2}}/F_{I_{N_2}}$$

This expression obviates the necessity of measuring both inspired and expired gas volumes. Fractional concentrations of N_2 can be measured with a nitrogen meter, or, if no "foreign" gases (such as anesthetics) are inhaled, N_2 can be derived from measurements of F_{O_2} and F_{CO_2}, since by definition: $F_{I_{N_2}} = 1 - F_{I_{O_2}} - F_{I_{CO_2}}$, and $F_{E_{N_2}} = 1 - F_{E_{O_2}} - F_{E_{CO_2}}$.

QUANTITIES OF GAS EXCHANGED

The oxygen consumption of a healthy 70 kg individual at rest and at neutral ambient temperature is about 250 ml O_2/min (STPD). The energy equivalent is about 1.2 kcal/min, or about 70 watts. At the same time, about 200 ml of CO_2/min (STPD) are produced. With fever, metabolic rate increases by 10 per cent per 1 C rise in temperature. The volume of O_2 consumed is not necessarily the same as that of CO_2 produced. Recall that, if a mole of carbohydrate is oxidized:

$$C_6H_{12}O_6 + 6\ O_2 \rightarrow 6\ CO_2 + 6\ H_2O + \text{energy};$$
$$CO_2/O_2 = 6/6 = 1$$

Oxidation of a mole of a representative fatty acid would yield:

$$C_{16}H_{32}O_2 + 23\ O_2 \rightarrow 16\ CO_2 + 16\ H_2O + \text{energy};$$
$$CO_2/O_2 = 16/23 = 0.7$$

The ratio $\dot{V}_{CO_2}/\dot{V}_{O_2}$ is called the respiratory exchange ratio (R), its value depending on the nature of "foodstuff" being oxidized in the body. R is 1.0 for carbohydrate, 0.7 for fat, and 0.8 for protein; the standard value of R on a mixed diet is 0.82. Combining the statements in (1) and (4), one can see that the "nitrogen ratio" ($F_{E_{N_2}}/F_{I_{N_2}}$) is inversely proportional to R.

RESPIRATORY DEAD SPACE AND ALVEOLAR VENTILATION

Not all the gas inhaled reaches the respiratory zone of the lungs. In addition to anatomic dead space, in disease some alveoli may be ventilated and devoid of perfusion, thus contributing to the alveolar dead space, sometimes called parallel dead space. The sum of the anatomic and alveolar dead space is called physiologic dead space, probably a misnomer as alveolar dead space is often the result of pathologic changes.

The volume of the anatomic dead space can be estimated from Radford's empirical formula: anatomic dead space (ml) = body weight (lb). About one half the anatomic dead space is located in the upper, extrathoracic airways.

Determination of the physiologic dead space can be explained by means of a model of the respiratory system (Fig. 37–5). Visualize the respiratory system as if it consisted of a single conducting tube of dead space, V_D, and an expansible volume in the respiratory zone. Upon inspiration, the first part of a tidal volume, V_T, enters the respiratory zone and instantaneously mixes by diffusion with the gas present, FRC. The first portion of the tidal volume is the effective or alveolar share, V_A. At end inspiration, the latter part of V_T occupies the conducting tube where no blood-gas exchange occurs in the dead space, V_D. During expiration, dead-space gas emerges first and the alveolar component of the tidal volume appears later. Thus, in terms of gas volumes involved:

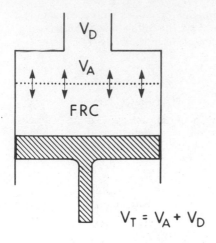

$$V_T = V_A + V_D$$

FIGURE 37–5. Model of the respiratory system to show the derivation of the Bohr formula for respiratory dead space.

$$V_T = V_D + V_A, \text{ or } V_A = V_T - V_D$$

What is the composition of the two components of the exhaled volume, V_D and V_A? The dead-space component does not exchange with blood; therefore its composition is the same as that of inspired gas. The alveolar component exchanges with blood, and its composition is a reflection of this. We shall look into its composition later. In terms of quantities of a gas that undergoes respiratory exchange (O_2, CO_2, or a "foreign" gas, x):

$V_T FE_x$	$=$	$V_D FI_x$	$+$	$V_A FA_x$
quantity of gas in total mixed volume		quantity of gas in dead-space component		quantity of gas in alveolar component

Substitute ($V_T - V_D$) for V_A, and solve for V_D:

$$V_D = V_T \frac{FE_x - FA_x}{FI_x - FA_x}.$$

Since F_x is $P_x/(P_B - P_{H_2O})$:

$$V_D = V_T \frac{PE_x - PA_x}{PI_x - PA_x}$$

This is the Bohr formula employed for determination of physiologic dead space.

The difficulty with the original Bohr formula lies in obtaining a reliable sample of alveolar gas for analysis. The Enghoff modification of the Bohr formula is based on the assumption that the partial pressure of CO_2 in alveolar gas is the same as that in arterial blood. When room air is inhaled, $PI_{CO_2} = 0$, and the equation for dead space is simplified:

$$V_D = V_T \frac{Pa_{CO_2} - PE_{CO_2}}{Pa_{CO_2}}$$

Thus, physiologic dead space, sometimes expressed as the wasted fraction of ventilation, V_D/V_T, can be simply measured by collecting mixed expired gas and measuring the partial pressure in this and in a sample of arterial blood. In normal individuals, V_D/V_T is about 0.3, so that approximately 30 per cent of ventilation is "wasted" on dead-space ventilation.

The effective or alveolar ventilation, $\dot{V}_A$, is the total minute ventilation, $\dot{V}_E$, less wasted dead space ventilation, $\dot{V}_D$:

$$\dot{V}_A = \dot{V}_E - \dot{V}_D$$

To maintain a given $\dot{V}_A$ with increase in physiologic dead space, the total ventilation, $\dot{V}_E$, has to increase. A large increase in V_D/V_T, for example, to 0.8, as sometimes seen in patients with acute respiratory insufficiency, can require very high total ventilation, over 20 L/min for adequate gas exchange.

Alveolar ventilation can be simply determined by measuring total ventilation, $\dot{V}_E$, and subtracting the wasted part (dead space times respiratory frequency). Another way of determining V_A is as follows: since $\dot{V}CO_2$ equals $\dot{V}_E \cdot FE_{CO_2}$, it also equals $\dot{V}_A \cdot FA_{CO_2}$. Thus, $\dot{V}_A = \dot{V}CO_2/FA_{CO_2}$. $\dot{V}CO_2$ can be measured in mixed expired gas ($V_E \times FE_{CO_2}$) and FA_{CO_2} derived from $PA_{CO_2} = Pa_{CO_2}$, as measured in a sample of arterial blood: $FA_{CO_2} = Pa_{CO_2}/(P_B - P_{H_2O})$. Thus

$$\dot{V}_A = \frac{\dot{V}_{CO_2}}{Pa_{CO_2}} (P_B - P_{H_2O})$$

or, since

$$\dot{V}_{CO_2} = R \cdot \dot{V}O_2,$$

$$\dot{V}_A = \frac{\dot{V}O_2}{Pa_{CO_2}} R (P_B - P_{H_2O})$$

ALVEOLAR GAS

One can visualize alveolar gas as a compartment interposed between atmospheric air and capillary blood in the lungs. Oxygen is continuously removed and CO_2 added as blood flows, whereas O_2 is supplied to alveolar gas and CO_2 is removed by the cyclic process of alveolar ventilation ($\dot{V}_A$). By means of $\dot{V}_A$, alveolar gas tends to approach the composition of inspired gas, whereas through perfusion ($\dot{Q}$) it tends to approach the gas composition of mixed venous blood, the latter determined by the cardiac output, O_2 consumption, and CO_2 production. The steady-state composition of alveolar gas is determined by the combination of $\dot{V}_A$ and $\dot{Q}$. The higher the $\dot{V}_A/\dot{Q}$ ratio, the more alveolar gas approaches inspired gas in composition; the lower the ratio, the more alveolar gas resembles the gas composition of mixed venous blood. In summary, the composition of alveolar gas is determined by ($\dot{V}_A$), the rate of $\dot{Q}$, and the composition of inspired gas and mixed venous blood.

Pulmonary ventilation is so regulated that a healthy human breathing air at sea level maintains an effective alveolar ventilation to keep PA_{CO_2} at 40 torr; PA_{O_2} is close to 100 torr, the other constituents of the alveolar gas being water vapor, 47 torr at 37 C, and N_2, adding up to P_B. Note that once a value of PA_{CO_2} has been "chosen" by the regulatory mechanisms of pulmonary ventilation, it follows from the gas exchange ratio ($\dot{V}CO_2/\dot{V}O_2$) that PA_{O_2} is also determined for any given composition of inspired gas. This is stated in the simplified alveolar equation:

$$PA_{O_2} = PI_{O_2} - PA_{CO_2}/R$$

The term PI_{O_2} can also be stated as $FI_{O_2} \cdot (P_B - P_{H_2O})$. If $R = 1$, the equation simplifies to $PA_{O_2} = PI_{O_2} - PA_{CO_2}$.

Note that the PA_{O_2} is directly related to concentration of O_2 in inspired gas (FI_{O_2}) and to barometric pressure (P_B). PA_{O_2} is less than the inspired O_2 tension in proportion to PA_{CO_2} as O_2 is removed from and CO_2 delivered to alveolar gas. The ratio of the two processes is the respiratory ratio R. PA_{CO_2}, in turn, is determined by regulation of $\dot{V}_A$.

PULMONARY VENTILATION AND METABOLIC RATE

Earlier we showed that:

$$\dot{V}_A = \frac{\dot{V}O_2}{PA_{CO_2}} R (P_B - 47)$$

By re-arrangement, to solve for $P_{A_{CO_2}}$:

$$P_{A_{CO_2}} = \frac{\dot{V}_{O_2}}{\dot{V}_A} R (P_B - 47)$$

Two important implications emerge from this relation: (1) With varying $\dot{V}_{O_2}$, as during fever or muscular activity, to maintain a constant $P_{A_{CO_2}}$, and thus a constant composition of alveolar gas, $\dot{V}_A$ must vary in precise proportion to increase in metabolic rate. For the usual values of P_B, R, and $P_{A_{CO_2}}$,

$$\dot{V}_A \text{ (L/min, STPD)} = \frac{\dot{V}_{O_2} \text{ (L/min, STPD)}}{40 \text{ torr}} \cdot 0.82 \cdot 713 \text{ torr} = 15 \cdot \dot{V}_{O_2}$$

Thus, for each liter of O_2 consumed, 15 L of $\dot{V}_A$ must be provided to maintain $P_{A_{CO_2}}$ at 40 torr. (2) At a given metabolic rate ($\dot{V}_{O_2}$), $P_{A_{CO_2}}$ is reciprocally related to effective pulmonary ventilation ($\dot{V}_A$). Thus doubling $\dot{V}_A$ will, at a given $\dot{V}_{O_2}$, halve $P_{A_{CO_2}}$, and, conversely, halving $\dot{V}_A$ will double $P_{A_{CO_2}}$. This relation is the basis for the important role the respiratory system plays in short-term adaptation to disturbances in acid-base balance. As CO_2 is an acid ($CO_2 + H_2O \rightleftarrows H_2CO_3$), lowering of P_{CO_2} by increasing $\dot{V}_A$ at a given $\dot{V}_{O_2}$ will remove H^+ from the body fluids to compensate for metabolic acidosis. Conversely, a decrease in $\dot{V}_A$ at a given $\dot{V}_{O_2}$ will increase P_{CO_2} in alveolar gas and body fluids, thus effectively adding H^+ to compensate for metabolic alkalosis. This is referred to as respiratory compensation for metabolic disturbances in acid-base balance.

If the lung were a perfect and homogeneous gas exchanger, $P_{a_{CO_2}}$ and $P_{a_{O_2}}$ in the systemic circulation would be the same as in alveolar gas. However, this is not true because of two factors: presence of physiologic right-to-left shunts — bronchial veins drain into the pulmonary veins, whereas some thebesian veins in the myocardium drain into the left heart; distribution of $\dot{V}_A$ and $\dot{Q}$ to various parts of the lungs is not uniform, producing $\dot{V}_A/\dot{Q}$ inhomogeneity reflected in the composition of alveolar gas and of pulmonary end-capillary blood. We point out later how $\dot{V}_A/\dot{Q}$ inhomogeneity produces differences between mixed alveolar gas and arterial blood.

PULMONARY CIRCULATION

The lung accommodates the cardiac output (CO); nevertheless, perfusion pressure is low. Mean pulmonary artery pressure (PAP) is normally about 15 torr, or 25/8 torr systolic/diastolic. The pressure in pulmonary veins is nearly the same as that in the left atrium, about 8 torr, in reference to atmospheric pressure. Pulmonary wedge pressure (PWP) is obtained by occluding blood flow to an arterial branch; this measures the pressure in the pulmonary capillaries and small veins, usually indistinguishable from left atrial pressure. Thus, the pressure drop across the pulmonary vascular bed is only about 7 torr, more than ten times less than the pressure gradient across the systemic circulation. Typical values for pulmonary vascular resistance (PVR) in the resting state (CO = 5 L/min), defined as the ratio of perfusion pressure to flow, would be (15 − 7) torr over 5 L/min, or 1.6 units, as compared with the systemic vascular resistance of (95 − 5)/5 = 18 units. However, because of the special structure and mechanical behavior of pulmonary vessels, PVR as defined does not provide meaningful insight into pressure-flow relations as a means of evaluating pulmonary hemodynamics, both in respect to the whole lung and especially in respect to regional perfusion.

The pulmonary arteries, like the veins, are thin walled and therefore, distensible and collapsible. Pulmonary arterioles possess an incomplete layer of smooth muscle. The capillaries form a mesh within the alveolar walls, occupying most of the alveolar surface, and their walls are collapsible. Lymphatics begin as capillaries in the bronchovascular spaces in the vicinity of respiratory bronchioles; alveolar septa contain no lymphatics.

The shape and caliber of the pulmonary vessels vary with transmural pressure, that is, the difference between pressure inside and that outside. As they are both distensible and collapsible, the vessels remain open only with positive transmural pressure, or when the pressure within the vessel is higher than in the perivascular space.

In relation to perivascular pressure, the pulmonary vessels can be divided into (a) "alveolar" vessels (capillaries, small arterioles, and venules) with perivascular pressures equal to gaseous pressure in the alveoli, which in spontaneous breathing is close to barometric pressure; and (b) "extra-alveolar" vessels (arteries and veins) that are "tethered" to the lung parenchyma, their perivascular pressures usually similar to pleural pressure. Like the pleural pressure, the perivascular pressure of extra-alveolar vessels is determined by elastic recoil of the lungs. Thus, in the erect position, the perivascular pressure of extra-alveolar vessels is more negative or subatmospheric at the apices than at the base.

Changes in lung volume exert differing effects on the two kinds of vessels: increase in lung volume, either total or regional, increases the "pull" on the walls of the tethered vessels, increases their diameters, and decreases resistance. On the other hand, the alveolar vessels are stretched and their cross-sectional area decreased by stretching the alveolar walls at high lung volume. With decrease in lung volume, the perivascular pressure of extra-alveolar vessels becomes less subatmospheric, transmural pressure is less, and resistance increases. Thus, lung volume is one determinant of the variable pulmonary vascular resistance.

Another determinant is perfusion pressure. As the pulmonary vessels are distensible, increase in perfusion pressure increases their diameters. As the vessels are also collapsible, increase in perfusion pressure recruits additional vessels, thus increasing the total cross-sectional area of the perfused vessels and decreasing the calculated PVR.

The neurogenic and humoral control of pulmonary vessels is probably of little clinical significance but is under continuing investigation. Hypoxia is an important determinant of constriction of the pulmonary resistive vessels. Hypoxia in both alveolar gas and systemic blood produces vasoconstriction and an increase in PAP. Hypoxemic influences on pulmonary vasoconstriction are augmented by both low pH and elevated Pa_{CO_2}. The mechanism of vasoconstriction probably entails a direct action on vascular smooth muscle. Presumably the usefulness of this mechanism is to divert blood from hypoventilated parts of the lung with low PA_{O_2}, thus tending to match ventilation and perfusion. In chronic hypoxemia, however, the generalized pulmonary vasoconstriction results in pulmonary hypertension and development of cor pulmonale.

REGIONAL DISTRIBUTION OF PULMONARY BLOOD FLOW

As the pulmonary circulation is a low pressure system, the hydrostatic pressure differences caused by gravity in the lung are large enough to modify effective arterial inflow pressure. Local perfusing pressure in various parts of the lungs is determined by the pressure in the main pulmonary artery (PAP) and the hydrostatic pressure difference away from the hilum. Figure 37–6 is a schematic representation of the effective pressure heads available for perfusion in the vertical lung. Pressures within the vessels decrease with height above the heart and increase below. At the apex, PAP may not be sufficient to raise blood into the apex; thus effective perfusion pressure will be less than the pressure in alveolar gas. As a result, the alveolar vessels collapse and flow ceases (Fig. 37–6, zone 1). In the normal lung with spontaneous

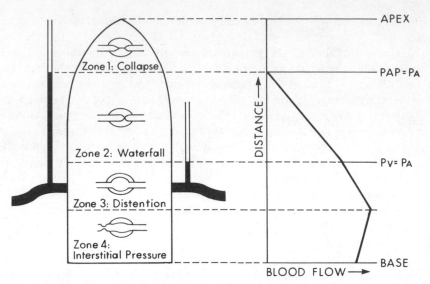

FIGURE 37–6. Schematic representation of the four zones of the lung in which different hemodynamic conditions govern blood flow. For discussion, see text. PAP, mean pulmonary arterial pressure; P_A, pressure in the alveolar gas; P_v, pulmonary venous pressure. (Redrawn with permission from Hughes JMB, Glazier JB, Maloney JE, West JB: Resp Physiol 4:58, 1968.)

breathing, a zone of no flow probably does not exist; however, if PAP is lowered, as in hemorrhage or hypotension, or if the pressure in alveolar gas is raised, as in PPV and especially with PEEP, there will be a pronounced zone 1—unperfused and ventilated—of alveolar dead space. In lower parts of the lung (zone 2) the effective inflow pressure is higher because height above the heart is less; effective inflow pressure will be higher than alveolar pressure. Pulmonary venous pressure, however, is still lower than alveolar pressure; blood flow is determined by the difference between effective inflow pressure and alveolar pressure. The change in venous pressure—unless it exceeds alveolar pressure—has no effect on local blood flow (waterfall effect). Further down the lung, venous pressure will be higher than that in alveoli (zone 3) and blood flow will be governed by the difference between effective inflow pressure—PAP now increased by the hydrostatic effect—and venous pressure. Since in zone 3 the pressure within the alveolar vessels must lie between that of arterial inflow and venous outflow, it will be higher than pressure in the alveoli; the alveolar vessels will be distended and their resistance to flow is low. Thus a gradient in local perfusion exists, with less blood flow at the apex and progressively increasing flow toward the base of the erect lung.

We have described the perfusion gradient produced by gravity in relation to variations in regional resistance of alveolar vessels. However, the true picture is more complicated, owing to the contribution of extra-alveolar vessels to local resistance to flow. As noted, the pressure about extra-alveolar vessels is influenced by lung recoil, thus depending on lung volume. In poorly inflated lung regions, as at the base, the perivascular pressure of extra-alveolar vessels can approach positive collapsing values. Transmural distending pressure is low, local resistance to flow increases, and when the lung is upright blood flow is reduced, presumably the result of this mechanism (zone 4).

In the supine position, the apex-to-base gradient of perfusion is abolished and a gradient between upper and lower parts of the lung prevails. The gradient is less pronounced as the distance between frontal and dorsal regions lessens.

FLUID EXCHANGE IN THE LUNGS

As in other vascular beds, fluid exchange across the pulmonary capillaries is governed by Starling's law. Net filtration ($\dot{n}$) is proportional to the difference between filtering and re-absorbing forces. The force of filtration is the difference between hydrostatic pressure within the pulmonary microvasculature (P_c) and hydrostatic pressure in pulmonary interstitial fluid (P_{isf}). The re-absorptive force is the difference between oncotic pressure in plasma (π_c) and that in interstitial fluid (π_{isf}):

$$\dot{n} = K \, [(P_c - P_{isf}) - (\pi_c - \pi_{isf})]$$

where K is the permeability coefficient of the capillary membrane.

In the pulmonary capillaries not all the pressures involved in the Starling equilibrium are known. The colloid-osmotic pressure of plasma protein is about 25 torr; oncotic pressure in the interstitial fluid, as estimated from protein concentration in lung lymph, is about 19 torr. This would give a net colloid osmotic pressure of about 6 torr for fluid re-absorption. Hydrostatic pressure within the capillaries must lie between that of the pulmonary arterioles and that of the left atrium. Owing to the effect of gravity on arterial inflow pressure, pressure in the arterioles, and thus in capillaries, is not uniform throughout, varying between 7 and 12 torr from apex to base of the lung, with an average of about 10 torr. The hydrostatic pressure in pulmonary interstitial fluid is not known with certainty. At present two schools of thought exist concerning its magnitude: one holds that P_{isf} is slightly positive in reference to atmospheric pressure (about 4 torr), whereas the other maintains that the pressure is distinctly subatmospheric (-2 to -4 torr). According to the first assumption, the net balance of Starling forces in the capillaries would be $(10-4) - (25-19) = 0$, and the lung should be "dry." In the second case, the balance would be $[10 - (-4) - (25 - 19)] = +8$ torr of net filtering pressure, suggesting an appreciable continuous filtration of fluid to be carried away by lymph. Indeed, recent observations in experimental animals indicate that there is continuous lymph outflow from the lungs, presumably also applicable to human lungs. Fluid formed by filtration in alveolar capillaries moves along the interstitial spaces of the alveolar septa where lymphatics are lacking, toward the perivascular and peribronchial spaces, thence absorbed into lymph capillaries. Lymph flows toward the hilum as a result of rhythmic contraction of smooth muscle in lymphatic vessels; the unidirectional propulsion of lymph results from the presence of funnel-shaped valves.

Pulmonary Edema

Interstitial fluid accumulates in the lungs when the rate of formation exceeds the transporting capacity of the lymphatic system. The latter can increase in capacity about ten times. From the preceding considerations, it is apparent that an increase in intracapillary hydrostatic pressure, a decrease in plasma colloid pressure, and an increase in permeability of capillary membrane will induce fluid accumulation if the capacity for lymphatic drainage is exceeded.

Lowering plasma oncotic pressure alone is hardly ever severe enough to cause pulmonary edema; in patients with nephrosis there may be anasarca and ascites but not pulmonary edema, in the absence of left ventricular failure. Lymphatic obstruction, as from a tumor, may cause localized edema. The most common causes of pulmonary edema, however, are an increase in intracapillary pressure (high pressure pulmonary edema), as in left ventricular failure or fluid overload, and leaky capillaries (low pressure pulmonary edema), as in septicemia, acute post-traumatic pulmonary insufficiency, or following inhalation of noxious gases. Traditionally, hypoxemia has been considered one of the causes of increased permeability of pulmonary capillaries, but there are no data to support this belief. Measurement of pulmonary wedge pressure is essential for differentiating the two kinds of edema.

Excess fluid accumulates first in perivascular and peribronchial spaces to interfere with local perfusion and ventilation. Wheezing in cardiac asthma is produced by compression of small airways by edema fluid. Compression of pulmonary vessels and small airways interferes with gas exchange, by producing $\dot{V}/\dot{Q}$ mismatch, leading to hypoxemia (low $\dot{V}/\dot{Q}$) and increased alveolar dead space (high $\dot{V}/\dot{Q}$ regions). Further accumulation of fluid propagates toward alveolar septa, lowering lung compliance and thickening the gas-exchanging membrane. Only in the final stages of fluid accumulation are the alveoli filled and the typical rales, frothy sputum, and severe hypoxemia observed.

TRANSPORT OF O_2 AND CO_2 BETWEEN LUNGS AND TISSUES

The next step in gas exchange between alveolar gas and pulmonary capillary blood is a matter of simple diffusion as molecules of O_2 and CO_2 move in the gas phase through the gas-exchanging membrane and blood.

The transfer rate of a gas by passive diffusion ($\dot{V}$, ml of gas per minute) in lungs is directly proportional to the area available for diffusion (A) and to the difference in partial pressures in the gas phase (P_A) and capillary blood (P_c), while inversely proportional to the distance over which the diffusion occurs (d). This is Fick's law of diffusion.

$$\dot{V}_{gas} = D \frac{A}{d} (P_A - P_c)$$

The diffusion coefficient (D) is characteristic for each gas. The heavier the gas molecule, the slower the movement; and the more soluble the gas in tissue water, the more rapid the diffusion. Carbon dioxide is somewhat heavier than O_2 but much more soluble in the aqueous phase of tissues, and the diffusion coefficient for CO_2 is about 20 times higher than that for O_2.

In the lungs, area and distance cannot be evaluated separately, so they are considered together and measured as the diffusing capacity for a given gas, D_L. Thus, the diffusing capacity for O_2 is:

$$D_{L_{O_2}} = \dot{V}_{O_2}/ (P_{A_{O_2}} - P\bar{c}_{O_2})$$

where $P\bar{c}_{O_2}$ is the mean partial pressure of O_2 in pulmonary capillary blood; the latter is not easily determined, so instead of measuring $D_{L_{O_2}}$, carbon monoxide is employed as a marker gas. This offers the advantage that, with the very low concentration of CO inhaled — a fraction of 1 per cent — and the avid binding of CO to hemoglobin, $P\bar{c}_{CO}$ is negligibly small. Thus, $D_{L_{CO}} = \dot{V}_{CO}/P_{A_{CO}}$. The normal value for $D_{L_{CO}}$ is 25 to 40 ml/min/torr of driving pressure.

During exercise, diffusing capacity increases two to three times owing to recruitment of alveolar vessels. In pulmonary fibrosis, diffusing capacity is decreased and values as low as 5 to 10 ml/min/torr are found in ambulatory patients. The reduction in D_L is produced by decrease in the area available for diffusion; increased thickness of the membrane is probably a minor factor, and the apparent diffusion barrier observed in diseased lungs results mainly from abnormalities of $\dot{V}/\dot{Q}$.

TRANSPORT OF O_2 IN BLOOD

After crossing the alveolar capillary membrane, O_2 is carried in blood in physical solution and in reversible combination with hemoglobin. The quantity present in solution is determined by the solubility coefficient and partial pressure (Henry's law). The

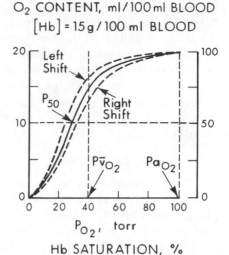

O₂ CONTENT, ml/100 ml BLOOD
$[Hb] = 15 g/100$ ml BLOOD

FIGURE 37-7. Dissociation curve of O_2 in blood. Pa_{O_2} and $P\bar{v}_{O_2}$ are the usual normal values in arterial and mixed venous blood. Note how shifts in the dissociation curve affect the saturation (and O_2 content) in the range of $P\bar{v}_{O_2}$.

P_{O_2}, torr

Hb SATURATION, %

solubility of O_2 in blood is very low, 0.003 ml O_2/100 ml blood per torr, at 37 C. With the usual Pa_{O_2} about 100 torr, only 0.3 ml of O_2 is present in solution in 100 ml of arterial blood, 0.3 vol per cent.

Oxygen combines with hemoglobin (Hb) reversibly to form oxyhemoglobin (HbO_2). At full saturation, each gram of Hb binds 1.36 ml O_2, and the oxygen capacity is the maximum that can be carried by available hemoglobin. With the usual Hb concentration of 15 gm per 100 ml, the normal O_2 capacity is 20 ml/100 ml blood. The O_2 content, or O_2 concentration (Co_2) in blood, is the sum of dissolved O_2 and that bound to Hb. Oxygen saturation of hemoglobin (So_2) is the ratio of O_2 combined with Hb over O_2 capacity, expressed as per cent. Oxygen transport is the product of oxygen content in arterial blood and the cardiac output: $Ca_{O_2} \times CO$.

Saturation of Hb with O_2 is primarily determined by Pa_{O_2}. The relation between So_2 and Pa_{O_2} is complex and best described and analyzed in graphic form, the oxygen dissociation curve (Fig. 37-7). The peculiar shape of this curve offers certain physiologic advantages. A horizontal top prevents wide fluctuations in Sa_{O_2} with changes of Po_2 normally prevailing in alveolar gas. The steep part is advantageous in unloading O_2 in tissues: a large decrease in So_2 is produced by a relatively small drop in Po_2. The location of the dissociation curve is also of importance in loading and unloading Hb as it is affected by temperature, pH, and Pco_2 (Bohr effect), and by the concentration of 2,3-diphosphoglycerate (2,3-DPG) in erythrocytes. By convention, the position of the dissociation curve is defined by the Po_2 value that produces 50 per cent saturation (P_{50}). The P_{50} of normal human Hb is 26 to 27 torr at 37 C, pH 7.40, Pco_2 40 torr, and a normal concentration of 2,3-DPG. P_{50} increases with shift to the right of the curve, or decreased affinity of Hb for O_2; with shift to the left, or increased affinity, P_{50} is lowered. With decreased affinity of Hb for O_2, unloading of O_2 in tissues is facilitated. A shift to the right is produced by increase in temperature, decrease in pH, increase in Pco_2, and increase in 2,3-DPG; opposite changes shift the curve to the left. The increase in affinity of Hb for O_2 produced by the leftward shift impedes unloading of O_2 in tissues; a lower tissue Po_2 must prevail for a given unloading of O_2 from blood.

Among other factors, the pH within erythrocytes is important in determining the concentration of 2,3-DPG: acidosis reduces and alkalosis increases 2,3-DPG levels. The shift of the curve instantaneously produced by the Bohr effect is thus counterbalanced by changes in 2,3-DPG, although on a much slower time scale—a matter of hours. Therefore, acidosis initially causes a rightward shift; however, after several days the curve shifts backward, in spite of persisting acidosis, owing to lowering of 2,3-DPG. Sudden correction of acidosis leads to a shift to the left until the level of 2,3-DPG re-adjusts to the new acid-base balance.

The amount of O_2 transported to tissues is the product of Ca_{O_2} and CO. Ca_{O_2} depends on the concentration of Hb and its saturation, the latter in turn a function of Pa_{O_2} and of the position of the Hb dissociation curve. Thus, all these variables—CO, Hb concentration, Pa_{O_2}, and the position of the dissociation curve—affect the efficiency of oxygen transport to tissues. Hypoxia can result from disturbance of any or a combination of these variables.

TRANSPORT OF CO_2

CO_2 is produced in tissues and diffuses into capillary blood, where it is present in physical solution and is also chemically bound. The solubility coefficient of CO_2 in blood is 0.03 mM/L/torr P_{CO_2}. Thus, in mixed venous blood with the usual P_{CO_2} of 46 torr, about 1.38 mM of CO_2 is physically dissolved; in arterial blood, with the usual Pa_{CO_2} of 40 torr, 1.2 mM/L of CO_2 is dissolved. Chemical binding occurs in two ways: (1) via hydration of CO_2 to H_2CO_3 and subsequent involvement in the complex process of buffering; (2) through direct reaction with NH_2 groups of proteins, to form carbamino compounds: $CO_2 + R - NH_2 \rightleftarrows R-NHCOOH$, which are fairly strong acids (pK < 6). Hemoglobin plays a primary role in transporting CO_2 in blood, both by providing most of the buffering of carbonic acid formed by hydration of CO_2 and by forming the carbamino compound, carboxyhemoglobin. In plasma, hydration of CO_2 to H_2CO_3 is a slow process; however, within erythrocytes the process is accelerated by the enzyme carbonic anhydrase. Thus, most of the H_2CO_3 and subsequent buffering and formation of HCO_3^- is provided by erythrocytes. HCO_3^- subsequently diffuses into plasma, and Cl^- diffuses into erythrocytes to maintain electric equilibrium. The reduction of HbO_2 that occurs simultaneously upon loading of blood with CO_2 enhances the capacity of Hb to form the carbamino compound carboxyhemoglobin, also causing the molecule of Hb to be a weaker acid. Both factors increase the capacity of reduced Hb to bind CO_2 (the Haldane effect). In the lungs, these processes are reversed and as Hb is oxygenated to HbO_2, CO_2 is released from both carboxy-Hb and bicarbonate.

The relation between P_{CO_2} and total content of CO_2 in blood is described by the CO_2 dissociation curve (Fig. 37–8). Unlike the dissociation curve for O_2, within the range of P_{CO_2} values present in mixed venous and arterial blood, the relation is almost linear.

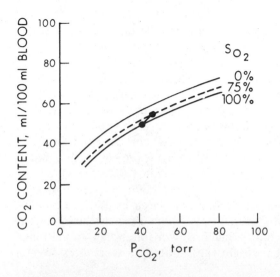

FIGURE 37–8. CO_2 dissociation curves for whole blood at 0.75 and 100 per cent oxyhemoglobin saturation (S_{O_2}). The Haldane effect between arterial and mixed venous blood is shown by the heavy straight line.

MATCHING OF VENTILATION AND PERFUSION IN LUNGS

We have stated that the composition of alveolar gas is determined by the ratio of effective pulmonary ventilation to rate of perfusion with mixed venous blood ($\dot{V}_A/\dot{Q}$), the composition of mixed venous blood and of inspired gas being additional factors. The composition of alveolar gas and of blood leaving each alveolus is determined by the local $\dot{V}/\dot{Q}$. In a normal person at rest, the lungs receive about 4 L/min of $\dot{V}_A$ and 5 L/min of blood or cardiac output ($\dot{Q}$). Thus, the overall value of $\dot{V}_A/\dot{Q}$ for the whole system is 4/5 or 0.8. If ventilation and perfusion were distributed equally to all parts of the lungs, the composition of alveolar gas and of blood leaving pulmonary capillaries would be the same in all gas-exchanging units. On the other hand, if there were units in which $\dot{V}/\dot{Q}$ was high (> 0.8), the composition of local alveolar gas would approach that of inspired gas, a low Pa_{CO_2} and high Pa_{O_2}. In ventilated alveoli with no perfusion, $\dot{V}/\dot{Q} = \infty$, thus constituting alveolar dead space. Units with low $\dot{V}/\dot{Q}$ (< 0.8) would contain alveolar gas of a composition approaching that of mixed venous blood, or high Pa_{CO_2} and low Pa_{O_2}. Perfused alveoli with no ventilation are characterized by $\dot{V}/\dot{Q} = 0$, constituting an intrapulmonary shunt or venous admixture.

In a normal, upright person with better ventilation and perfusion at the base of the lung, the gradient from apex to base is more pronounced for perfusion than for ventilation; therefore $\dot{V}/\dot{Q}$ ratios are high at the apex, about 3, and low at the base, about 0.6, with a continuum of $\dot{V}/\dot{Q}$ values along the gradient. The presence of regions with low and high $\dot{V}/\dot{Q}$ carries important consequences for efficiency of gas exchange. A simplified presentation of this intriguing problem follows. Readers interested in a more rigorous treatment are referred to West's monograph on $\dot{V}/\dot{Q}$ or to Farhi's text.

Assuming that blood leaving each alveolus is in equilibrium with Pa_{CO_2} and Pa_{O_2} within the alveolus, blood coming from alveoli with low $\dot{V}/\dot{Q}$ will have an abnormally high Pco_2 and an abnormally low Po_2, whereas blood coming from alveoli with high $\dot{V}/\dot{Q}$ will have an abnormally low Pco_2 and a high Po_2. When contingents of blood from various regions with differing $\dot{V}/\dot{Q}$ values are mixed, the *content* of O_2 and CO_2 in arterial blood will be on the weighted average of the *content* of the two gases. The resulting *partial pressures* of the two gases in mixed arterialized blood will depend on their dissociation curves. As the CO_2 dissociation curve is almost a straight line over the range of Pco_2 between 25 and 50 torr (see Fig. 37–8), a change in Pco_2 is simply proportional to change in CO_2 content. If, for instance, equal volumes of blood, one with a Pa_{CO_2} of 30 and the other of 50 torr, were mixed, the resulting Pco_2 would be 40. On the other hand, the dissociation curve of O_2 is nonlinear (see Fig. 37–7). If equal volumes of blood with a Po_2 of 50 torr, So_2 83 per cent, and 120 torr, Sa_{O_2} 99 per cent, were mixed, the resulting Sa_{O_2} is $(83 + 99)/2 = 91$, corresponding to a Po_2 of only 63 torr. The O_2 dissociation curve is flat in the range of Po_2 values over 80 torr; therefore, when breathing room air, the moderate increase in Pa_{O_2} in blood coming from regions with high $\dot{V}/\dot{Q}$ cannot compensate for the low saturation of the blood coming from regions of low $\dot{V}/\dot{Q}$. Upon inhalation of air, hypoxemia is an inevitable consequence of maldistribution of ventilation and perfusion with low $\dot{V}/\dot{Q}$ values. If inspired gas is enriched with O_2, hypoxemia can be relieved, because with a fairly high $F_{I_{O_2}}$ even poorly ventilated alveoli will fill with gas containing Pa_{O_2} high enough to saturate the blood circulating through them.

The presence of low $\dot{V}/\dot{Q}$ regions also affects elimination of CO_2. A tendency to hypercapnia in mixed arterialized blood results from admixture of blood from underventilated and overperfused regions with low $\dot{V}/\dot{Q}$. However, the increased Pa_{CO_2} drives respiration, and hypercapnia can be averted if total ventilation is increased. Owing to the linearity of the CO_2 dissociation curve, it is possible to further lower the content of CO_2 in already well-ventilated areas; however, this is at the cost of a large increase in the work of breathing.

High $\dot{V}/\dot{Q}$ regions do not cause hypoxemia; they merely increase the wasted fraction of ventilation, requiring a higher total ventilation ($\dot{V}_E$) to maintain a given $\dot{V}_A$. This, together with the increase in ventilation required to forestall hypercapnia resulting from low $\dot{V}/\dot{Q}$ regions, eventually leads to respiratory failure and CO_2 retention, when the limits of total resting ventilation are reached.

Abnormality in matching $\dot{V}$ and $\dot{Q}$ is the most common cause of hypoxemia in patients with chronic lung disease. Maldistribution is produced by regional differences in compliance and resistance to air flow, by vascular obstruction as occurs in pulmonary embolization, and by additional factors. Other common causes of hypoxemia involve alveolar hypoventilation and intrapulmonary shunting. Alveolar hypoventilation is synonymous with hypercapnia, causing hypoxemia when room air is inhaled. Hypoventilation can occur in skeletal, muscular, neuromuscular, or CNS disorders, including curarization and administration of CNS depressants, or in pulmonary disease when an increase in V_D/V_T is so high that adequate $\dot{V}_A$ is not achieved by the attainable total ventilation.

True intrapulmonary shunt, when mixed venous blood is not exposed to gas on passage through the lungs, is probably not the most important cause of hypoxemia in patients with acute respiratory failure; true venous admixture does occur with atelectasis and lung collapse. Rather, it is the $\dot{V}/\dot{Q}$ abnormality with extremely low values of $\dot{V}/\dot{Q}$ that underlines most of what is commonly called "shunt" in patients with acute respiratory distress. The magnitude of the true shunt, that is, the fraction of pulmonary blood flow completely bypassing alveolar gas, can best be evaluated after prolonged inhalation of 100 per cent O_2 to abolish the contribution of low $\dot{V}/\dot{Q}$ to hypoxemia. If a sample of mixed venous blood is then taken, the magnitude of shunt can be evaluated quantitatively; however, this is seldom justifiable in acutely ill patients because of the risk of accelerating development of atelectases in diseased lungs, caused by elimination of N_2 in alveolar gas upon inhalation of 100 per cent O_2.

REGULATION OF PULMONARY VENTILATION

The "respiratory pump," unlike the heart, has no intrinsic rhythmicity but is operated by skeletal muscles that do not contract unless stimulated through appropriate somatic innervation. The rhythmic stimuli are generated in the respiratory centers, a network of oscillator neurons located in pons and medulla. An intact efferent pathway from these centers down to the respiratory muscles is essential for spontaneous breathing.

Smooth operation of the rhythmic contraction and relaxation of respiratory muscles is achieved through various modulating reflexes, the receptors located in the lungs and chest wall. The afferent limb of reflexes originating in the lungs reaches the respiratory centers via the vagi (Hering-Breuer inflation reflex, deflation reflex). In man the function of most of these reflexes is poorly understood. The intercostal muscles and diaphragm are equipped with muscle spindles that sense the tension in muscle fibers. This reflex control of muscle tone is integrated at the spinal level, thus helping to stabilize contraction in the face of variable mechanical loads, as in changing resistance or compliance.

What is the nature of the information reaching the respiratory centers that influences rate and depth of breathing? First, many physiologic functions unrelated to the needs of steady-state gas exchange require that the normal breathing pattern be interrupted or modified. Some of these are voluntary: breath holding, voluntary hyperventilation, straining, speech, or playing a wind instrument. Others are of reflex nature: sneezing, swallowing, vomiting, and hiccoughing. These inputs originating in various parts of the CNS merely interfere with the primary function of respiratory regulation, which is to provide gas exchange. The essential input in this respect comes to respiratory centers through chemoreflexes that detect the concentration of respiratory gases in blood and other body fluids. Chemoreception for respiration customarily has been linked with the composition of arterial blood. This seems logical, as the blood is a natural link between lungs — the effector — and respiratory center — the regulator. The effect of O_2 on respiration is indeed brought about by chemical stimuli originating in arterial blood, in the carotid chemoreceptors. On the other hand, the respiratory drive owing to CO_2 and to accompanying changes in pH is not simply explained by chemical stimuli in blood. The acidity of cerebral fluids detected by central medullary chemoreceptors appears to be an important additional stimulus.

The remarkable sensitivity of respiration to CO_2 can be demonstrated by inhalation of various CO_2 mixtures. An increase in Pa_{CO_2} of 1 torr produces an increase in $\dot{V}_E$ of 2 to 3 L/min. If a reduction of Pa_{CO_2} is induced, as by means of artificial hyperventilation, ventilation may be completely suppressed temporarily; posthyperventilation apnea may be pronounced in anesthetized patients. The ventilatory response to CO_2 is reduced by CNS depressants — anesthetics, opioids, and sedatives. Also the state of wakefulness influences the respiratory response to CO_2; during sleep it is reduced.

Ondine's curse is a syndrome observed in patients after operations involving the brain stem and higher segments of the cervical cord or during bulbar poliomyelitis. Patients develop long periods of apnea; however, while awake they breathe on command. A similar phenomenon occurs with overdose of opioids. Marked insensitivity to CO_2 seems to be the underlying disturbance. Recently it has been suggested that a related disturbance is present in the "central" form of sleep apnea. It may also be responsible for some of the crib deaths of infants.

The respiratory drive derived from CO_2 is mainly detected by central medullary chemoreceptors. These receptors are exposed to cerebrospinal fluid (CSF), thus detecting the acidity of this fluid. CSF is separated from blood by the blood-brain barrier; molecular CO_2 is lipid soluble and the blood-brain barrier is freely crossed, whereas HCO_3^- is presumably regulated by active transport between blood and CSF, the functional blood-brain barrier. The pH in CSF that goes with a given CSF $[HCO_3^-]$ and Pco_2 sets the level of resting pulmonary ventilation. In metabolic acidosis, therefore, lowered CSF $[HCO_3^-]$ results in hyperventilation, thus lowering Pa_{CO_2}. In metabolic alkalosis, an increase in CSF $[HCO_3^-]$ lowers ventilation, thus producing compensatory CO_2 retention found in arterial blood. The extent of respiratory compensation for metabolic acid-base disturbances as observed in arterial blood results in changes in Pa_{CO_2} of approximately 1 torr for each mE per liter of base excess or base deficit. Thus, the physiologically normal Pa_{CO_2} in a patient with a base excess of $+10$ mE/L is maintained close to 50 torr, and with a base deficit of -10 mE/L Pa_{CO_2} is normally set close to 30 torr. In patients with chronic lung disease and CO_2 retention, the buildup of $[HCO_3^-]$ in CSF is appreciable, probably one of the factors contributing to the notorious insensitivity of these patients to increases in Pa_{CO_2}. It follows from the Henderson-Hasselbalch equation that the higher the CSF $[HCO_3^-]$, the smaller the change in pH resulting from a given increase in Pco_2 in CSF.

The effect of O_2 on respiration can be studied by inhaling abnormal concentrations of O_2. At sea level, the effect on $\dot{V}_E$ of decreasing FI_{O_2} is surprisingly small: no appreciable change in breathing is seen until about one half of the O_2 concentration in air is reached, and even at FI_{O_2} values less than 8 per cent there is a large variation in sensitivity among individuals. However, this is not a fair appraisal of the isolated effect of O_2 on respiration; as soon as respiratory rate increases, P_{CO_2} decreases, thus reducing the total respiratory drive. Still, if Pa_{CO_2} is maintained constant while inhaled O_2 is lowered (isocapnic hypoxia), the effect on ventilation is not dramatic until Pa_{O_2} values around 60 torr are reached. Thus, the bodily mechanisms for detecting O_2 lack are not very sensitive.

Hypoxemia combined with hypercapnia increases ventilation more than mere additive effects of both stimuli. This is referred to as interaction of the respiratory drives of O_2 and CO_2, but the site of interaction is not known.

Chemoreceptors detecting lack of O_2 are located in the bifurcation of the carotid arteries, the carotid bodies, and at the aortic arch or aortic chemoreceptors. The stimulus is a fall in Pa_{O_2}, not in O_2 content. Thus, anemia or poisoning with carbon monoxide does not stimulate respiration. Afferent impulses from peripheral chemoreceptors reach respiratory centers through the glossopharyngeal nerve from the carotid bodies and via the vagi from the aortic bodies. Thus the anoxic drive for respiration is of reflex nature; the direct effect of anoxia on respiratory centers is purely depressive.

Patients with chronic obstructive pulmonary disease and CO_2 retention as a result of a virtually abolished sensitivity to CO_2 depend on the coexisting hypoxemia for respiratory drive. If given high concentrations of oxygen to relieve hypoxemia while breathing spontaneously, they lose their only effective respiratory drive and may succumb to CO_2 narcosis.

Surprisingly enough, recent observations indicate that individuals who are hypoxemic from birth, such as people living at high altitudes or patients with cyanotic congenital heart disease, have very low O_2 respiratory drives. It is not clear whether this phenomenon relates to the chemoreceptors *per se* or the CNS.

RESPIRATORY FAILURE

Respiratory failure occurs when gas exchange is inadequate for metabolic needs; consequently, arterial blood gases are deranged, and this is manifested as hypoxemia alone or hypoxemia with hypercapnia.

Because the normal values for Pa_{CO_2} and Pa_{O_2} have a certain range, depending on age, concentration of O_2 in inhaled gas, acid-base balance, and other factors, it is not easy to quantify exactly the derangements in arterial blood gases that define respiratory failure. Most workers consider as indicators of respiratory failure a Pa_{O_2} lower than 60 torr at sea level while breathing room air at rest (with no abnormal intracardiac right-to-left shunt) and a Pa_{CO_2} of 50 torr or higher. However, Pa_{O_2} decreases with age and is of course affected by $F_{I_{O_2}}$. Most clinicians consider a Pa_{O_2} of 70 torr when breathing O_2 via face mask to be an indication of significant hypoxemia; those who measure alveolar-arterial (A-a) gradients in P_{O_2} during inhalation of 100 per cent O_2 consider an A-a gradient of more than 450 torr an indication of failure. Pa_{CO_2} varies with the respiratory compensation for metabolic acid-base imbalance: a Pa_{CO_2} of 50 torr in a patient with metabolic alkalosis and a base excess of +10 mE/L of several days' duration is a normal physiologic response, whereas a Pa_{CO_2} of 40 torr in a patient with metabolic acidosis and a base deficit of −10 mE/L would indeed indicate relative hypercapnia.

Hypercapnia has only one cause—alveolar hypoventilation. Hypoxemia can result from hypoventilation while breathing air, a low $F_{I_{O_2}}$, high altitude, $\dot{V}/\dot{Q}$ abnormalities, intrapulmonary shunt, and a decrease in lung diffusing capacity. A combination of these factors may also prevail.

An attempt at a clinical classification of respiratory failure is given in Table 37-1.

TABLE 37–1. Clinical Classification of Respiratory Failure

I. Acute respiratory failure with previously normal lungs:
  (a) Without initial pulmonary pathology
     (Failure of the "respiratory pump")
     Examples: myasthenia, botulism muscular paralysis, drug overdose
  (b) With pulmonary pathology
     (Failure of the "gas-exchanger")
     Examples: severe pneumonia, post-traumatic pulmonary insufficiency
II. Acute failure superimposed on chronic lung disease:
  (a) Without pre-existing CO_2 retention
     Example: bronchopneumonia in chronic pulmonary fibrosis
  (b) With chronic CO_2 retention
     Example: bronchopneumonia in COPD

The problems posed in management of various kinds of respiratory failure differ as do the underlying pathophysiologic mechanisms. With failure of the respiratory pump the principal problem is hypoventilation, usually combined with inability to protect airways and to clear bronchial secretions. Pathologic changes in the lungs can develop secondarily: aspiration, infection, atelectasis, or barotrauma as a result of mechanical ventilation. The task is to assure adequate artificial ventilation, to protect the airways, and to provide general supportive therapy including pulmonary toilet.

With failure of the gas exchanger, the initial and important problem is hypoxemia caused by $\dot{V}/\dot{Q}$ abnormalities and pulmonary shunts. Initially, PA_{CO_2} is normal or low owing to the hypoxic drive; secondarily, with increase in V_D/V_T as a result of pulmonary disease and with increase in alveolar dead space, hypoventilation and CO_2 retention may set in. The most common clinical entity in this category is the acute respiratory failure seen after trauma, burns, aspiration, shock, immune reactions to transfusions of blood, gram-negative septicemia, viral infection, and prolonged inhalation of high concentrations of O_2, among other conditions. The clinical manifestations comprise breathlessness with patchy pulmonary infiltrates that culminate in the "white" lungs seen on chest x-ray, severe hypoxemia, initially with a normal or low P_{CO_2}, and subsequent hypercapnia. The pathologic changes in the lung are not specific. Interstitial infiltrates, microemboli, and alveolitis, sometimes with formation of hyaline membranes, are seen. The main pathophysiologic disturbance is a severe reduction in lung compliance, owing to the infiltrates and increase in lung water. FRC is low, leading to closing of lung units and shunt, whereas severe $\dot{V}/\dot{Q}$ mismatch contributes to hypoxemia and produces a large alveolar dead space, the latter eventually leading to hypercapnia. The main therapeutic problems entail treatment of hypoxemia and mechanical ventilation when CO_2 elimination is inadequate.

Although it is the chest physician who sees most of the acute complications of chronic pulmonary disease, postoperative pulmonary complications are well within the anesthetist's domain. Here, the problem is usually severe hypoxemia, especially in patients already hypoxemic with chronic pulmonary fibrosis. Adequate oxygenation is mandatory. The situation differs in patients with chronic obstructive disease with CO_2 retention and hypoxemia. Here the derangement lies in the chemical regulation of respiration, with depressed sensitivity to CO_2 and dependence on hypoxic respiratory drive, together with abnormal pulmonary mechanics (increased lung compliance and airway obstruction). These patients usually reveal values for both Pa_{CO_2} and Pa_{O_2} between 50 and 60 torr and Sa_{O_2} about 80 per cent. Mechanical ventilation is to be avoided if possible because of subsequent difficulties in weaning. Oxygen therapy (see Chapter 38) with moderately increased O_2 concentrations (24 to 30 per cent) aims at relieving hypoxia by gaining somewhat on Sa_{O_2} without abolishing the hypoxemic respiratory drive.

DIAGNOSIS OF RESPIRATORY INSUFFICIENCY

The presence of conditions predisposing to respiratory insufficiency must be recognized: drug overdose, aspiration, neuromuscular dysfunction, trauma, or presence of chronic lung disease. Clinical indicators of hypoxemia and hypercapnia are sought: breathlessness with tachypnea and mental derangement are common signs of impending respiratory failure. Hypoxemia may be present without cyanosis; nevertheless, cyanosis should be looked for in the oral mucosa, so-called central cyanosis. When present, central cyanosis indicates severe hypoxemia with a Pa_{O_2} usually less than 40 torr. CO_2 retention produces few and variable clinical signs. Prominent are restlessness, followed by depression and coma. The periphery is warm and sweaty, and the pulse bounds with a rise in blood pressure owing to sympathetic stimulation. On the whole, clinical impressions of respiratory failure are unreliable and should be confirmed by measurement of arterial blood gases.

THE ROLE OF ANESTHETISTS IN RESPIRATORY CARE

In their work in the operating room, anesthetists support respiration and circulation of anesthetized patients, therefore the care of more prolonged respiratory problems is a natural extension and application of their knowledge and skills.

Because of the complexity of care for patients in acute respiratory failure, a team approach provides the best solution, involving anesthetist, surgeon, internist, pediatrician, neurologist, and microbiologist. Nursing of these patients is difficult and requires special skills, notably related to complex monitoring equipment in use. Pulmonary physiotherapy is an essential component of intensive care (see Chapter 38). As the equipment used in respiratory care is unique, proper use calls for collaboration of well-trained respiratory therapists. All these activities require unity and continuous communication among the specialists mentioned and are best organized in the setting of an intensive care unit. An efficient laboratory working around the clock is essential for measurement of arterial blood gases.

PRINCIPLES OF RESPIRATORY SUPPORT IN ACUTE PULMONARY INSUFFICIENCY

For hypercapnia, there is only one treatment — adequate ventilation. If the patient is unable to do this spontaneously, mechanical ventilatory support is provided.

Treatment of hypoxemia relies upon three principal measures: enrichment of inspired gas with O_2, fluid management to prevent and treat pulmonary edema, and mechanical measures to prevent and remedy the causes of intrapulmonary venous admixture. The latter is achieved by artificially operating the lungs at large volumes through application of positive pressure to the airways to prevent and treat atelectasis. Use of extracorporeal membrane oxygenation (ECMO) for treatment of intractable hypoxemia has not met expectations. Very high frequency ventilation (VHFV), with tidal volumes less than anatomic dead space and frequencies of 8 to 15 Hz, is presently in an experimental stage. Both the theoretical basis of gas exchange with this mode of ventilation and technical solutions are the subject of active research.

TRACHEAL INTUBATION AND TRACHEOSTOMY

The indications for tracheal intubation in patients in respiratory failure are summarized in Table 37–2. Techniques of tracheal intubation are described in Chapter 16. Nasotracheal tubes, as compared with oral tubes, are better tolerated by awake patients, can be more securely anchored, and enter the larynx at an angle that applies less pressure to the posterior wall. On the other hand, the size of the tube is limited by

TABLE 37–2. Indications for Endotracheal Intubation

I. Patency of the airway (e.g., facial burns, edema of glottis)
II. Protection from aspiration (e.g., coma, absent gag reflex)
III. Pulmonary toilet (e.g., inadequate cough)
IV. Positive pressure applied to airways
   (a) Intermittent positive-pressure ventilation (IPPV)
   (b) Continuous positive airway pressure (CPAP)
      1. spontaneous breathing with CPAP
      2. positive end-expiratory pressure (PEEP) in combination with IPPV

the diameter of the nasal passages, posing problems in suctioning and adding appreciable resistance during spontaneous breathing.

Tubes with low pressure cuffs are used for prolonged tracheal intubation because they coapt over a large tracheal surface, better stabilizing the tube, and provide a satisfactory seal while still pliable, whereas a rubber or latex tube with a rigid cuff inflates to a spherical shape; contact with the tracheal mucosa is therefore narrowly applied. When inflated to seal the airway the stiff cuff is unyielding and rigid, applying unnecessary force to the tracheal wall.

The decision to perform tracheostomy in patients needing prolonged intubation is usually postponed unless it becomes obvious that the need for control of the airways may extend over weeks. Translaryngeal intubation is maintained for two or more weeks by most clinicians. However, intubation via tracheostomy is better tolerated by awake patients, in which case tracheostomy tubes with soft cuffs are used. With respect to avoiding the damage of prolonged tracheal intubation, the only advantage of tracheostomy over translaryngeal intubation lies in consideration of laryngeal trauma, for the trachea incurs damage with both. Tracheostomy is not without risk, however, and the wound acts as a portal of entry for infection. Moreover, partial resection of the tracheal cartilage must be performed as part of the procedure. Chondromalacia is a possible complication, and fatal hemorrhage resulting from erosion of the innominate artery by a tracheostomy tube has occurred.

Once an endotracheal tube is placed, regardless of kind, a sterile technique is employed in clearing secretions. When the tube is removed, certain complications should be anticipated: after prolonged intubation laryngeal reflexes are obtunded with a high risk of aspiration. Further complications include edema and ulceration of the larynx with the translaryngeal tube and damage to the tracheal wall with both translaryngeal intubation and tracheostomy that can result in tracheoesophageal fistula or tracheal stenosis.

VENTILATORY SUPPORT

The factors are complex that lead to and ultimately precipitate respiratory failure to the extent that mechanical respiratory support is needed. To mention a few: mechanical derangements of the respiratory system, in turn increasing the work of breathing; alterations in distribution of gas flow and blood and efficiency of gas exchange; variable metabolic needs in ill patients; the state of consciousness; and the failure of chemical regulation of respiration. It is, therefore, impossible to quantify all possible derangements that ultimately call for ventilatory support. Instead, one relies on predictive indicators of need that have been empirically established as guidelines (Table 37–3).

Mechanical ventilators produce intermittent expansion of the lungs by application of positive pressure (IPPV) to the airways or by creating subatmospheric pressure around the chest wall. The prototype of negative-pressure ventilators is the tank

TABLE 37–3. Indices of Need for Ventilatory Support

	Normal Range	Ventilatory Support Indicated
I. Indices of the mechanical properties of the respiratory system and the respiratory muscles		
Vital capacity (ml/kg of body weight)*	65–75	<15
FEV_1 (ml/kg of body weight)*	50–60	<10
Inspiratory force (cm H_2O)	75–100	<25
II. Indices of adequacy of $\dot{V}_A$ and of oxygenation		
Resting respiratory rate (breath/min)	12–20	>35
Pa_{CO_2}, torr	35–45†‡	>55‡
V_D/V_T	0.25–0.40	>0.60
Pa_{O_2}, torr: breathing air	75–95	<60 torr‡
O_2 mask	variable	<70
$F_{I_{O_2}}$ 1.0	>600	<200

*In very obese patients, use "ideal" weight.
†See page 441 for modifying influence of metabolic acid-base imbalance.
‡Applies to acute elevation of Pco_2, not to patients with chronic CO_2 retention.
Modified from Pontoppidan H, Geffin B, Lowenstein E: Acute Respiratory Failure in the Adult. Boston, Little, Brown and Co, 1973.

ventilator or iron lung; cuirass ventilators are also occasionally used. The latter consist of a plastic shell that covers the anterior aspect of the thorax and abdomen, while subatmospheric pressure is intermittently applied beneath the shell. Today, practically all patients who need mechanical ventilation are treated with IPPV.

Two basic designs of positive pressure ventilators prevail: those in which a preset volume of gas is delivered, and those in which gas flow ceases when the pressure reaches a preset level. With the latter, variations in compliance or resistance of the respiratory system can result in large variations in tidal volumes delivered. Ventilators are also classified according to their capacity to control or assist respiration. With respiratory assist, the patient's inspiratory efforts initiate delivery of a tidal volume. Thus the patient's respiratory center regulates the rate of minute ventilation and Pa_{CO_2}. With controlled ventilation, the rate of delivery of the chosen tidal volumes is determined by a setting on the machine. The expiratory phase in IPPV is passive, utilizing the elastic recoil of the patient's respiratory system. It is beyond the scope of this text to enter further into details of design or operation of the ventilators available.

MANAGEMENT OF RESPIRATORY SUPPORT

In patients with stiff lungs, large tidal volumes are used — 10 ml/kg of body weight — more than twice the normal spontaneous V_T. This provides continuous "sighing" to prevent or treat the hypoxemia presumably caused by closure of lung units in association with high elastic recoil of diseased lungs. The rate of ventilation is set at 10 to 14 breaths per minute; lower frequencies are poorly tolerated by conscious patients. However, in patients with chronic obstructive lung disease in whom lung compliance is increased, large tidal volumes and a high minute ventilation are avoided. With airway obstruction and highly compliant lungs, very high FRC values can be produced and peak inspiratory volumes beyond the patient's spontaneous TLC can result, causing difficulty in weaning and resumption of spontaneous breathing. Tidal volumes of more than 600 ml are seldom used in these patients.

Depending on the need of $\dot{V}_E$ to achieve adequate $\dot{V}_A$, adjustments are made: if the setting of the machine results in hyperventilation, dead space is added to the circuit; if more ventilation is needed to maintain adequate CO_2 elimination, frequency is increased. $F_{I_{O_2}}$ is initially set high and subsequently adjusted to provide adequate oxygenation. These adjustments are evaluated by serial blood gas determinations. Humidification of inspired gas is provided (see Chapter 38).

For controlled ventilation, synchronization of the patient's breathing efforts with the machine is desirable; sedation is usually necessary. In agitated, hypoxic patients, especially in those with abnormally high respiratory drives as in pulmonary embolism, hyperammonemia, or head trauma with CNS acidosis, neuromuscular blockade with deep sedation is sometimes necessary.

While on mechanical ventilation close monitoring of the patient is essential, especially blood pressure, serial determinations of arterial blood gases, and evaluation of the effective compliance of the respiratory system. Effective compliance is the tidal volume delivered, divided by peak inspiratory pressure registered by the ventilator, influenced by both compliance and resistance to flow in the system. Obstruction of airways or decreased compliance is thus detected, as in pneumothorax or voluntary use of expiratory muscles opposing the respirator. Expired volumes are continuously monitored by a spirometer in the respiratory circuit, and alarm systems signal failure of delivery of preset tidal volumes.

Treatment of hypoxemia requires careful selection of $F_{I_{O_2}}$ to achieve adequate oxygenation. Pulmonary edema is forestalled by careful regulation of fluid balance. Bedside measurement of pressures in the pulmonary circulation with the flow-directed catheter is useful in differentiating between low pressure and high pressure edema. Selective use of diuretics in combination with intravenous colloids can produce dramatic reductions in pulmonary shunting.

The purpose of positive end-expiratory pressure (PEEP) is to counterbalance the high elastic recoil of stiff lungs and to prevent the lungs from reaching very low volumes at expiration, where closing occurs. Some ventilators offer built-in valves to provide PEEP, but PEEP can also be improvised by submerging the end of the expiratory line under water, the depth determining end-expiratory pressure. In treatment of pulmonary edema, PEEP improves gas exchange. The mechanism is thought to entail improvement of distribution of ventilation and blood flow rather than reduction of accumulated fluid. No simple rules pertain to recommending any specific level of PEEP. Each patient has to be "titrated" to achieve the desired effect of improved oxygenation while avoiding potentially toxic $F_{I_{O_2}}$ values. Increments of 5 cm H_2O PEEP are usually tried, with levels up to 15 to 20 cm H_2O routinely used.

Continuous positive pressure (CPAP or CPPB) can also be applied to the airways of spontaneously breathing patients. CPPB can be devised by submerging the expiratory line of a T-piece under water and providing a flow of inspired gas high enough to maintain positive pressure during the entire breathing cycle, including inspiration. This is facilitated by incorporating a reservoir bag at the inspiratory line. CPPB is useful in combating hypoxemia in some patients who do not require mechanical ventilation for CO_2 elimination.

The two main complications of positive airway pressure, with either IPPV or PEEP, are depression of cardiac output owing to an increase in mean intrathoracic pressure, and pulmonary barotrauma.

Depression of cardiac output is manifest as systemic hypotension and decreased urinary output. Thus, with use of PEEP, a decrease in cardiac output can reduce oxygen transport to tissues in spite of improved arterial oxygenation. Cardiovascular consequences of increased intrathoracic pressure resulting from IPPV and PEEP are complex and now under investigation. Prevention and treatment of hypovolemia are essential hemodynamic adjustments needed to maintain adequate venous return in the face of increased intrathoracic pressure.

Pulmonary barotrauma results from disruption of lung tissue as occurs when a bulla is ruptured or more commonly from local disruption of lung parenchyma, with gas entering the pulmonary interstitium and propagating along bronchovascular bundles (pulmonary interstitial emphysema), thus compressing small airways and vessels (see Chapter 33). Through these interstitial channels gas can reach the mediastinum (pneumomediastinum) and subcutaneous tissues of the neck (subcutaneous emphysema), or it can enter the retroperitoneal space. If any of the visceral or parietal coverings are disrupted, pneumothorax, pneumopericardium, or pneumoperitoneum results. Gas under positive pressure can also enter disrupted pulmonary vessels to cause air embolization.

Accumulation of secretions in the respiratory tract should be avoided. Obstruction of airways by mucus leads to maldistribution of ventilation and patchy or massive atelectases. Stagnant secretions, especially in atelectasis, provide a nidus for infection. Humidification of inspired gases, adequate fluid balance, and chest physiotherapy help to move the secretions toward the larger airways.

Weaning from the Ventilator

Indicators for weaning from the ventilator are the reverse of those that suggest the need for mechanical respiratory support (Table 37–3). In principle, mechanical indices such as vital capacity and inspiratory pressure should predict the patient who will be able to carry on adequate ventilation, whereas indices characterizing the performance of the lung, such as arterial blood gases, V_D/V_T, and shunt, should be satisfactory according to empirically established rules.

A T-piece is attached to the endotracheal tube, and humidified O_2 or air enriched with O_2 is inhaled. Attempts to wean may begin while the patient is still on PEEP; a CPPB circuit is then used in trials of spontaneous breathing. Sedation is avoided, and weaning is best carried out during the day when sufficient personnel are present. The patient is closely observed for tachypnea, tachycardia, increase in blood pressure, arrhythmias, or distress in general. If spontaneous breathing is tolerated, arterial blood gases are checked to evaluate the efficiency of gas exchange. Periods of spontaneous breathing may be short, 10 to 15 minutes, alternating with controlled ventilation, especially after long periods of mechanical ventilation. Progressively, as tolerated, spontaneous breathing is prolonged.

Intermittent mandatory ventilation (IMV) is sometimes used in the process of weaning from mechanical ventilation. Here, as opposed to the previously described technique of alternation between spontaneous breathing with a T-piece and periods on ventilatory support, the process is continuous and gradual. In principle, the endotracheal tube is attached to a T-piece and a ventilator delivers tidal volumes at a preset rate while the patient can inhale spontaneously through the inspiratory line. This allows gradual progression from complete ventilatory control by the respirator to a situation in which the patient spontaneously provides more and more of the ventilation. All the while the frequency of tidal volumes delivered by the machine is gradually lowered until weaning is complete. IMV can easily be combined with CPAP. In some patients with difficult weaning problems, IMV has been helpful.

REFERENCES

Farhi LE: Ventilation-perfusion relationship and its role in alveolar gas exchange. *In* Caro CG (ed): Advances in Respiratory Physiology. Baltimore, Williams & Wilkins Co, 1966, pp 148–197.

Fenn WO, Rahn H: Handbook of Physiology. Section 3, Respiration, Vols I and II, Washington, DC, American Physiological Society, 1964.

Hedley-Whyte J, Burgess GE III, Feeley TW, et al: Applied Physiology of Respiratory Care. Boston, Little, Brown and Co, 1976.

Hensley MJ, Fencl V: Lungs and respiration. *In* Vandam LD (ed): To Make the Patient Ready for Anesthesia. Menlo Park, CA, Addison-Wesley Co, 1980.

Murray JF: The Normal Lung. The Basis for Diagnosis and Treatment of Pulmonary Disease. Philadelphia, WB Saunders Co, 1976.

Mushin WW, Rendell-Baker L, Thompson PW, et al: Automatic Ventilation of the Lungs. 3rd ed. Oxford, Blackwell Scientific Publications, 1980.

Nunn JF: Applied Respiratory Physiology. 2nd ed. Boston, Butterworth, 1978.

Pontoppidan H, Geffin B, Lowenstein E: Acute Respiratory Failure in the Adult. Boston, Little, Brown and Co, 1973.

Pontoppidan H, Wilson RS, Rie MA, Schneider RC: Respiratory intensive care. Anesthesiology 47:96, 1977.

Shoemaker WC (ed): The Lung in the Critically Ill Patient. Baltimore, Williams & Wilkins Co., 1976.

Skillman JJ: Intensive Care. Boston, Little, Brown and Co. 1975.

Staub NC: Pulmonary edema. Physiol Rev 54:678, 1974.

Slutsky AS, Drazen MJ, Ingram RH Jr: Effective pulmonary ventilation with small-volume oscillations at high frequency. Science 209:609, 1980.

West JB: Respiratory Physiology — the Essentials. Baltimore, Williams & Wilkins Co, 1974.

West JB: Pulmonary Pathophysiology — the Essentials. Baltimore, Williams & Wilkins Co, 1977.

West JB: Ventilation/Blood Flow and Gas Exchange. 3rd ed. Oxford, Blackwell Scientific Publications, 1977.

Chapter 38

INHALATION THERAPY AND PULMONARY PHYSIOTHERAPY

The scope of what was traditionally called "Inhalation therapy" and "Chest physiotherapy" has changed over the past decade. Until the end of the 1950s, inhalation therapy meant little more than delivery of oxygen in tents, for sometimes poorly defined indications and without systematic monitoring of the effects. Then, during the 1960s, intermittent positive pressure breathing (IPPB) was also used somewhat indiscriminately, again without strictly defined indications or aims. Pulmonary physiotherapy, for many years accepted in Europe, has only recently been widely adopted in this country. Several developments account for the changes that have occurred in respiratory therapy. First, the understanding of the pathophysiology of pulmonary diseases, acute and chronic, has improved, as has understanding of the pathophysiology of the perioperative period. Second, efficient monitoring of the respiratory status of patients has been made possible by methods for routine measurement of partial pressures of O_2 and CO_2 in arterial blood. Finally, respiratory therapists are better trained and have become actively involved in dealing with critically ill patients in respiratory intensive care, which itself has undergone dramatic development over the past 15 years. Table 38–1 summarizes what may be considered the present scope of respiratory care.

TABLE 38–1. Scope of Respiratory Care

I. Respiratory Therapy
  Delivery of increased oxygen concentration in
    inspired gas
  Humidification of inspired gases
  Aerosol therapy
    Bland aerosols
    Delivery of medications
  Intensive respiratory care
    Mechanical ventilation
    Monitoring of critically ill patients
    Cardiopulmonary resuscitation
II. Pulmonary Physiotherapy
  Techniques for improved airway clearance
  Preoperative instruction and postoperative
    followup and treatment
  Other (e.g., exercise training, ventilatory
    muscle training)

TABLE 38–2. Water Vapor in Gas at Full Saturation (100 Per Cent Humidity)

Temperature		Partial Pressure (P_{H_2O})	Water Content mg H_2O/L gas
C	F	torr	at $P_B = 760$ torr
20	68.0	17.5	18.5
25	77.0	24.0	24.0
37	98.6	47.0	43.8
38	100.4	50.0	46.0
40	104.0	55.0	50.0
42	107.6	61.0	56.4

In this chapter, we shall deal with some of the topics pertinent to respiratory care outside the domain of intensive care.

PHYSICS OF WATER VAPOR

The partial pressure of water vapor (P_{H_2O}) at full saturation (100 per cent humidity) is determined solely by temperature. Table 38–2 gives P_{H_2O} values at full saturation for temperatures of interest in clinical settings. In addition, the content of water in gas (mg H_2O/L gas) is given.

When saturation of a gas with water vapor is incomplete (relative humidity less than 100 per cent), the P_{H_2O} values (and water content) are reduced in proportion to per cent humidity. For instance, at 20°C temperature and 50 per cent humidity, P_{H_2O} is 17.5 torr × 0.50 = 8.8 torr, and the content of water in the gas is 18.5 mg/L × 0.50 = 9.3 mg/L gas. For each liter of this gas inhaled, 34.5 mg of water (43.8 mg − 9.3 mg) will be vaporized from the airway mucosa in the process of complete saturation at the body temperature of 37°C.

The presence of water vapor in a gas mixture influences the partial pressure of other gases present. Partial pressure of a gas is the product of the fractional concentration of that gas (F_x) times the total (atmospheric) pressure (P_B) reduced by P_{H_2O} ($P_B - P_{H_2O}$);

$$Px = Fx \cdot (P_B - P_{H_2O})$$

Thus, room air ($F_{O_2} = 0.21$) at normal barometric pressure ($P_B = 760$ torr) and fully saturated with water vapor at 37°C has a partial pressure of oxygen (P_{O_2}) 0.21 × (760 − 47) torr = 150 torr.

OXYGEN THERAPY

The purpose of oxygen therapy is to relieve hypoxemia (decreased PaO_2). Causes of hypoxemia are listed in Table 38–3 (also see p. 443).

TABLE 38–3. Causes of Hypoxemia

I. Without abnormal (A-a)O_2 gradient
   1. Hypoventilation while inhaling room air
   2. Inhalation of abnormally low FI_{O_2} (accidental)
II. With increased (A-a)O_2 gradient
   1. Venous admixture ("shunt"; see p. 443)
   2. Mismatch of ventilation/perfusion with low
      $\dot{V}/\dot{Q}$ values (see p. 439)
   3. Decrease in lung diffusing capacity (see p. 436)

Hypoxemia can be relieved by increasing the partial pressure of oxygen in alveolar gas ($P_{A_{O_2}}$). This is evident from the simplified alveolar equation (also see p. 431):

$$P_{A_{O_2}} = P_{I_{O_2}} - P_{A_{CO_2}}/R$$

It is $P_{I_{O_2}}$ that is primarily manipulated in oxygen therapy by increasing $F_{I_{O_2}}$:

$$P_{I_{O_2}} = F_{I_{O_2}} \times (P_B - P_{H_2O})$$

It follows from the alveolar gas equation that, at a given $P_{A_{CO_2}}$ (and R, the respiratory exchange ratio, see p. 429), $P_{A_{O_2}}$ will increase in direct proportion to increase in $P_{I_{O_2}}$. At a given $P_{A_{O_2}}$, the partial pressure of oxygen in arterial blood ($P_{a_{O_2}}$) will be determined by the gradient of O_2 between alveolar gas and arterial blood (A-a)O_2]:

$$P_{a_{O_2}} = P_{A_{O_2}} - (A\text{-}a)O_2$$

TECHNIQUES FOR DELIVERING INCREASED OXYGEN CONCENTRATIONS

Few techniques for delivery of increased concentrations of oxygen to a patient's natural airway can guarantee a precise $F_{I_{O_2}}$. The reason is that many devices supply gas at a rate that is less than the patient's maximal inspiratory flow rate; room air is therefore entrained at a variable rate, diluting the nominal O_2 concentration in delivered gas. These devices are referred to as low flow, or variable, $F_{I_{O_2}}$ devices.

High Flow Techniques

Techniques are available that can deliver known and precise $F_{I_{O_2}}$, although at low to moderate concentrations. Accurate control of $F_{I_{O_2}}$ can be secured if the gas mixtures are delivered at flows equal to or greater than a patient's maximal inspiratory flow rate. Such devices usually use an oxygen-driven injector to entrain fixed proportions of room air. To prevent further room air entrainment at the airway opening, the total flow generated must be very high (over 50 L/min). Devices utilizing these techniques are referred to as high flow, or fixed, $F_{I_{O_2}}$ systems. (With tracheal intubation and a sealed airway, the nominal $F_{I_{O_2}}$, of course, is attained in the patient's respiratory system.)

Low Flow/Variable $F_{I_{O_2}}$ Systems

These devices provide inspired oxygen flows that are less than a patient's maximal inspiratory flow. Therefore, the effective $F_{I_{O_2}}$ is determined by both the oxygen delivered and the entrained room air. This mixing varies greatly with changes in the patient's tidal volume and respiratory rate. Such devices are used routinely in oxygen therapy because they are inexpensive and moderately effective in increasing $F_{I_{O_2}}$.

A nasal cannula is a small plastic device applied to the upper lip with two small prongs extending into the nares. The effective $F_{I_{O_2}}$ varies with oxygen flow rate and with the patient's breathing pattern. With oxygen flows of 0.5 to 7 L/min, the effective $F_{I_{O_2}}$ values range from 0.24 to 0.40 per cent.

Oxygen masks are available in several designs, providing for a wide range of $F_{I_{O_2}}$ values. The effective $F_{I_{O_2}}$ is determined by several factors: flow rate, mask fit, size of oxygen reservoir, and the patient's inspiratory flows. A simple device (Fig. 38–1A) is a mask with a small internal volume. The oxygen inlet is situated at the bottom, and holes in the sides allow escape of exhaled gas. The usual oxygen flow rates used with this mask are 5 to 10 L/min, resulting in effective $F_{I_{O_2}}$ values of 0.30 to 0.50.

A partial rebreathing mask (Fig. 38–1B) has a plastic bag to serve as a reservoir;

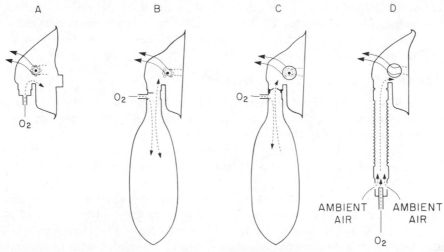

FIGURE 38–1. Oxygen masks. *A.* Simple oxygen mask. Oxygen flows directly into the mask, and exhaled gas leaves through the holes at side of mask. *B.* Partial rebreathing mask. The reservoir stores the inflowing oxygen and the initial portion of the exhaled gas (dead space gas, i.e., inspired gas); the remaining exhaled gas (alveolar gas) leaves through the holes at side of mask. *C.* Nonrebreathing mask. The addition of one-way valves prevents mixing of oxygen with exhaled gas and reduces entrainment of ambient gas. *D.* Venturi mask. Large volumes of room air are entrained by oxygen flow through an injector. $F_{I_{O_2}}$ (0.24–0.40) is determined by the bore of the injector. Stable $F_{I_{O_2}}$ values are delivered to the airway owing to the high total flow.

oxygen flows simultaneously to mask and reservoir. As there are no valves in this mask, exhaled gas (the dead-space gas, i.e., inspired gas) mixes with incoming oxygen in the reservoir. However, once the reservoir is refilled during initial exhalation, gas exhaled during the later part of expiration (alveolar gas) leaves through the ports at the side of the mask, and CO_2 rebreathing does not occur. With oxygen flow rates high enough to keep the reservoir bag inflated (greater than 10 L/min), effective $F_{I_{O_2}}$s of 0.50 to 0.65 can be achieved.

Nonrebreathing masks (Fig. 38–1*C*) offer a reservoir similar to that of the partial rebreathing mask; a one-way valve located between reservoir and mask prevents mixing of exhaled gas with incoming oxygen. The side holes in the body of the mask are replaced with exhalation valves, which lessen entrainment of room air at this location. Theoretically, effective F_{I_O} should exceed 0.90 with this mask. However, it is difficult to provide a tight enough mask fit to completely eliminate entrainment of room air.

High Flow/Fixed $F_{I_{O_2}}$ Systems

Another kind of oxygen mask is the Venturi mask (Fig. 38–1*D*). This mask utilizes the Bernoulli principle to entrain large volumes of room air (up to 100 L/min) to mix with oxygen flowing through an injector (4 to 8 L/min). The resultant mixture of gases

TABLE 38–4. **Typical Air Entrainment Ratios Used to Provide Different $F_{I_{O_2}}$**

$F_{I_{O_2}}$(%)	Oxygen Flows (L/min)	Air Entrainment (L/min)	Ratio	Total Flow (L/min)
24	2–4	50–100	1:25	52–104
28	4–6	40–60	1:10	44–66
31	6–8	56	1:7	72
35	8	40	1:5	48
40	8–12	24–36	1:3	32–44

produces stable effective $F_{I_{O_2}}$ values between 0.24 and 0.40, depending on the bore of the O_2 injector. Similar injector devices are used in various pneumatic nebulizers, which, when coupled with tracheostomy masks, T-pieces, aerosol masks, and so on, can provide fairly precise $F_{I_{O_2}}$ values (Table 38–4).

COMPLICATIONS OF OXYGEN THERAPY

1. Risk of fire and explosions. As $F_{I_{O_2}}$ is raised, the possibility of and resultant rate of combustion increase rapidly. For this reason sources of ignition must be eliminated in an oxygen-enriched atmosphere.

2. Effects on respiratory mucosa. Dry gas, including oxygen, when not properly humidified leads to decreased mucociliary clearance because of the drying effect on secretions (see p. 422).

3. Oxygen toxicity. High concentrations of oxygen can exert deleterious effects on the lung including increased alveolar capillary permeability, interstitial and alveolar edema, atelectasis, and intra-alveolar hemorrhage (see p. 443). However, the risk of oxygen toxicity certainly does not equal the dangers associated with hypoxemia.

4. Retrolental fibroplasia. This affliction occurs in premature infants who have been exposed to an excessive $F_{I_{O_2}}$ and results in proliferation of retinal vessels, intraocular hemorrhage, retinal edema and detachment, and formation of a fibrous retrolental membrane. Development of the condition is associated with a high Pa_{O_2}. Every attempt should be made, therefore, to keep the Pao_2 below 100 torr (lower, if possible) by frequent or continuous monitoring of PaO_2.

5. CO_2 retention in patients with chronic hypoxemia and deranged regulation of respiration. Patients with chronic hypoxemia may have chronically elevated $Paco_2$s, as well. Sensitivity to the CO_2 stimulus is depressed, so these patients depend on an hypoxic respiratory drive. If oxygen is administered in a concentration high enough to abolish the "hypoxic drive" for respiration, $Paco_2$ will increase (see p. 442).

HUMIDIFICATION OF GASES

For the respiratory mucosa to function properly, humidification and warming of inspired gases are necessary. This "conditioning" of inspired gas is normally accomplished in the upper airways. When the latter are bypassed and the water content of inspired gas is too low, the lower airways must provide the additional moisture. This increases the viscosity of mucosal secretions, thereby impairing mucociliary clearing function (see p. 422).

Gas reaching the alveoli is fully saturated with water vapor at body temperature. At 37°C, each liter of gas contains 43.8 mg of water vapor when fully saturated. The difference between the water content of inhaled gas and that required at the alveolar level is referred to as the "humidity deficit." A normal "conditioning system" in the upper airways makes up the deficit. However, when this system is bypassed or dry gases are inhaled, artificial humidifying devices are needed.

When dry oxygen or mixtures of oxygen and air are supplied for inhalation via natural airways, a humidifier is used to provide a water content similar to that normally present in room air. Humidifiers are devices by which the delivered dry gas is simply bubbled through water kept at room temperature in a reservoir. With usual room temperature (around 20°C) and relative humidity (30 to 45 per cent), the water content of atmospheric air is 6 to 8 mg/L. A simple bubble humidifier between gas source and patient will add 6 to 8 mg H_2O/L to elevate dry gas humidity to that of ambient air. When the upper airway is bypassed, the bubble humidifier is inadequate and the humidity deficit must be made up by more efficient means.

The simplest means of raising the level of humidity supplied by humidifiers is to heat the water (and the gas passing through the unit). The capacity of a gas to hold moisture is greatly increased when temperature is increased. At 20°C and fully saturated with water, gas contains 18.5 mg H_2O/L, but at 37°C the water content is 44 mg/L. The water in the humidifier can be heated to body temperature, but as gas travels through the delivery tubing, it cools and water "rains" out. To circumvent this problem, one can raise water temperature in the humidifier above body temperature to assure delivery of gas at body temperature at the airway opening. This, however, introduces the risk of thermal injury to the patient's airway. Systems have been devised by which the delivery tubing is heated to body temperature, thus avoiding the necessity of keeping the water at a high temperature in the humidifier.

AEROSOL THERAPY

Aerosol generators (nebulizers) increase the amount of liquid in gas by suspending small droplets in the gas stream. Two basic types of nebulizers are available: one uses a jet of gas to fracture fluid into particles, whereas the other employs a rapidly vibrating transducer to produce aerosol.

The first kind, a pneumatic nebulizer, most often utilizes the Bernoulli effect to draw fluid into a small capillary tube placed in the fluid reservoir. Once the fluid reaches the gas stream, it is broken into small particles and blown against one or more baffles, which serve to further fragment and remove large droplets. The usual output of these nebulizers is in the range of 15 to 35 mg H_2O/L gas flow. Again, as with humidifiers, one can use heat to increase the fluid output of nebulizers to a level of full saturation or supersaturation of gas. (Supersaturation occurs when the amount of water in gas is greater than that gas can hold in vapor form alone at that temperature.)

A second kind of nebulizer is of the ultrasonic variety. Sound waves are focused at the fluid surface, where they generate aerosols. The frequency of oscillation determines particle size, and the amplitude determines output. A frequency is chosen so as to produce stable particles in the size range of 1 to 10 μm. With ultrasonic nebulizers, the output can be as high as 55 mg of water per L/gas; therefore heating is not required.

BLAND AEROSOLS

Bland aerosols are commonly used for rehydration and mobilization of bronchial secretions in patients with indwelling tracheal tubes, following operation with dry anesthetic gases, and in patients with disease processes that disturb mucociliary clearance. Another indication for the use of bland aerosols is laryngeal and tracheal edema resulting from tracheal intubation. Sterile water or isotonic saline is usually delivered by aerosol.

DELIVERY OF MEDICATIONS

Many pharmacologic agents can be delivered to the tracheobronchial tree by suspension in aerosol. Some drugs, such as the bronchodilators, act much more rapidly when delivered by aerosol than when taken by mouth. Others, like mucolytics, exert a topical effect and therefore can be administered only by inhalation.

Drugs most often used via inhalation to produce bronchodilation do so by stimulating beta receptors to relax bronchial smooth muscles. Isoproterenol, once the most widely used bronchodilator, has been replaced by newer drugs that exhibit fewer cardiac side effects. Isoetharine and metaproterenol sulfate are examples.

Racemic epinephrine, a drug with fewer cardiovascular side effects than epinephrine, is useful as a topical vasoconstrictor and has been employed in treating laryngeal and tracheal edema and croup in children.

Mucolytics influence the viscosity of respiratory secretions. Acetylcysteine, the most popular mucolytic, reduces viscosity by disrupting the disulfide bonds between mucoprotein strands.

TECHNIQUES FOR ENHANCEMENT OF AIRWAY CLEARANCE

Intermittent positive pressure breathing (IPPB).   During the 1960s and early 1970s, IPPB was extensively used in the treatment of chronic lung disease. Its therapeutic value has been difficult to validate by controlled studies, and in the postoperative period its usefulness is unproved.

Incentive spirometry.   This therapy aims at preventing and treating postoperative atelectasis. A device guides the patient to inspire to a preset volume. Recent studies indicate that, in preventing and treating postoperative pulmonary complications, incentive spirometry offers no demonstrable advantage over simple encouragement of cough and deep inspiration. Other techniques attempt to encourage deep breathing (e.g., "blow bottles" or inflation of surgical gloves). With these, however, full expirations are emphasized, which, without preceding deep inhalation, are useless in preventing or treating atelectasis.

Pulmonary physical therapy (PPT).   Although adopted and accepted as a valuable therapeutic modality for many years in Europe, the method has only recently gained acceptance in the United States. Originally, PPT comprised postural drainage combined with manual percussion and vibration of the chest wall to enhance expectoration of sputum. Later on the scope of PPT was broadened to include retraining (of breathing) in patients with COPD ("diaphragmatic abdominal" and "basal costal" breathing). The value of these techniques in management of patients with stable COPD (with or without large sputum production) is not easily demonstrated. Potential benefits of specific respiratory muscle endurance training are presently the subject of active research.

In surgical patients, especially those with upper abdominal and thoracic incisions, PPT is valued by most therapists for prevention and treatment of pulmonary complications. Treatment includes teaching of relaxation, proper positioning, assisted coughing, postural drainage, and "cupping" and "tapping" of the chest. Furthermore, a preoperative pulmonary physical therapy session is advisable. Here the patient receives instruction on postoperative procedures, such as airway clearance techniques and breathing exercises; more importantly, rapport with the therapist is established. Although the results of such preoperative therapy sessions are difficult to document objectively, it is evident that a cooperative and trusting patient will be more willing to accept postoperative therapy that is sometimes painful and difficult.

APPRAISAL

Inhalation therapy and its concomitants as provided by trained respiratory therapists are accepted in the hospital community as essential for patient care. The methods employed and their putative efficacy depend in large part on a knowledge of pulmonary physiology and pathology and an understanding of the pharmacology of therapeutic agents administered and the physics of gases and vapors plus the technicality of devices employed. Although the benefits of such therapy are not easily defined in statistical terms, physicians and patients alike seem assured of its favorable effects.

REFERENCES

Egan DD: Fudamentals of Respiratory Therapy. 2nd ed. St. Louis, C V Mosby Co, 1973.

Gaskell DV, Webber BA: The Brompton Hospital Guide to Chest Physiotherapy. 2nd ed. Oxford, Blackwell Scientific Publications, 1975.

McPherson SP: Respiratory Therapy Equipment. St. Louis, C V Mosby Co, 1977.

Proceedings of the Conference on the Scientific Basis of Respiratory Therapy. Am Rev Respir Dis 110: Suppl to 6, 1974.

Sykes MK, McNicol MW, Campbell EJM: Respiratory Failure. 2nd ed. London, Blackwell Scientific Publications, 1976.

Ziment I: Respiratory Pharmacology and Therapeutics. Philadelphia, W B Saunders Co, 1978.

Appendix I

COMMON ABBREVIATIONS

a—arterial blood
A—alveolar gas
ACD—acid citrate dextrose
Ach—acetylcholine
ACTH—adrenocorticotropic hormone
ADH—antidiuretic hormone
AR—assisted respiration
ATN—acute tubular necrosis
ATP—adenosine triphosphate
B—barometric
c—capillary blood
C—concentration of gas in blood phase
CGA—Compressed Gas Association
cm—centimeter
CO—cardiac output
COPD—chronic obstructive pulmonary disease
CPAP—continuous positive airway pressure
CPK—creatine phosphokinase
CPPB—continuous positive pressure breathing
CPPV—continuous positive pressure ventilation
CR—controlled respiration
CRF—corticotropin-releasing factor
CSF—cerebrospinal fluid
CVP—central venous pressure
D—dead-space gas
D—diffusing capacity
DIC—disseminated intravascular coagulation
E—expired gas
EACA—epsilon-aminocaproic acid
ECG—electrocardiogram
EEG—electroencephalogram
EO—ethylene oxide
ER—endoplasmic reticulum
ERV—expiratory reserve volume
f—respiratory frequency
F—fractional concentration in dry gas phase
FRC—functional residual capacity
GFR—glomerular filtration rate
gm—gram

HB$_S$Ag—hepatitis B surface antigen
Hz—hertz
I—inspired gas
IC—inspiratory capacity
IPPB—intermittent positive pressure breathing
IPPV—intermittent positive pressure ventilation
IRDS—idiopathic respiratory distress syndrome
IRV—inspiratory reserve volume
kg—kilogram
kcal—kilocalorie
L—liter
LP—lumbar puncture
MAC—minimum alveolar concentration
mamp—milliampere
MAO—monoamine oxidase
mEq—milliequivalent
mg—milligram
ml—milliliter
mm—millimeter
mOsm—milliosmole
mv—millivolt
ṅ—net filtration
NE—norepinephrine
NFPA—National Fire Protection Association
opioid—a narcotic, either synthetic or opium-related
P—gas pressure
P̄—mean gas pressure
PAH—para-aminohippurate
PAP—pulmonary artery pressure
PEEP—positive end-expiratory pressure
ppm—parts per million
PPV—positive pressure ventilation
psi—pounds per square inch
PTF—post-tetanic facilitation
PVR—peripheral vascular resistance
PCWP—pulmonary capillary wedge pressure
Q̇—volume of blood
Q̇—volume of blood/unit time
R—respiratory exchange ratio

REM — rapid eye movement
RIHSA — radioactive iodinated human
        serum albumin
RPF — renal plasma flow
RV — residual volume
S — per cent saturation of hemoglobin
STPD — 0°C, 760 torr, dry
T — tidal gas
TBT — tracheobronchial toilet

TLC — total lung capacity
torr — mm Hg
μamp — microampere
μm — micrometer
v — venous blood
V — gas volume
V̇ — gas volume/unit time
VC — vital capacity

Appendix II

NUMERICAL EQUIVALENTS

Length

1 cm = 0.3937 in	1 in = 2.54 cm
1 m = 39.37 in	1 ft = 0.305 m

Volume

1 liter = 1.057 qt (US)	1 cu ft = 0.028 cu m
= 61 cu in	= 28.32 L
= 0.0353 cu ft	1 qt = 0.946 L
1 cu m = 35.26 cu ft	= 946 ml
1 ml = 0.0338 oz (Av)	1 US fluid oz = 29.57 ml
= 16.231 minims	1 minim = 0.0616 ml

Mass or Weight

1 kg = 2.205 lb	1 lb (Av) = 0.454 kg
1 gm = 0.0353 oz (Av)	1 oz (Av) = 28.35 gm
= 15.45 grains	1 grain = 0.0648 gm
1 mg = 0.0155 grains	= 64.80 mg

Force

1 dyne $= 2.24 \times 10^{-6}$ lb weight*
             $= 1.02 \times 10^{-3}$ gm weight $= 1.00 \times 10^{-2} \times m \times s^{-2}$
             $= 0.015$ grain weight
1 newton $= 10^5$ dynes   1 lb weight $= 453.59$ gm weight
             $= 0.224$ lb weight $= 4.44 \times 10^5$ dynes
             $= 101$ gm weight $= 4.44$ newtons
             $= 1573$ grain weight
             $= 0.102$ kg weight $= 1.00$ kg $\times m \times s^{-2}$
1 gm weight $= 980.665$ dynes
1 kg weight $= 9.80 \times 10^5$ dynes
             $= 9.8$ newtons

*All weights based on acceleration due to gravity of 9.8 meters/sec^2

Pressure

1 mm Hg = 0.019 lb/sq in
       = 0.133 kPa = 133.3 Pa
       = 1.35 gm/sq cm
       = 13.5 kg/sq m
       = 1333.22 dynes/sq cm
       = 133.32 newtons/sq m
   1 lb/sq in (psi) = 51.715 mm Hg
                    = 70.307 gm/sq cm
                    $= 6.8 \times 10^4$ dynes/sq cm
                    $= 6.8 \times 10^3$ newtons/sq m
                    = 703.07 kg/sq m

Pressure (Continued)

$$
\begin{aligned}
1 \text{ atm} \quad &= 760 \text{ mm Hg (Torr)} = 101.3 \text{ kPa} \\
&= 14.7 \text{ psi} \\
1 \text{ cm } H_2O &= 0.0979 \text{ kPa} \qquad = 97.9 \text{ Pa} \\
1 \text{ kPa} \quad &= 7.52 \text{ mm Hg} \qquad = 10.22 \text{ cm } H_2O \\
1 \text{ psi} \quad &= 6.89 \text{ kPa} \qquad\quad = 51.7 \text{ mm Hg}
\end{aligned}
$$

Work or Energy

$$
\begin{aligned}
1 \text{ joule} \quad &= 0.239 \text{ g-cal} \\
&= 2.39 \times 10^{-4} \text{ cal (kg)} \\
&= 9.48 \times 10^{-4} \text{ BTU} \\
&= 2.77 \times 10^{-7} \text{ kw-hr} \\
&= 1 \text{ watt-sec} \\
&= 0.62 \times 10^{19} \text{ electron volts}
\end{aligned}
$$

$$
\begin{aligned}
1 \text{ calorie} \quad &= 4.18 \text{ joules} \\
1 \text{ BTU} \quad &= 1054.8 \text{ joules} \\
\\
1 \text{ kw-hr} \quad &= 3.6 \times 10^6 \text{ joules} \\
1 \text{ watt-sec} \quad &= 1 \text{ joule} \\
1 \text{ electron volt} &= 1.6 \times 10^{-19} \text{ joules}
\end{aligned}
$$

1 curie $= 3.7 \times 10^{10}$ disintegration/sec
1 rad (radiation absorbed dose) $= 1 \times 10^{-2}$ joule/kg
1 roentgen $= 2.57 \times 10^{-4}$ coulomb/kg

Power

$$
\begin{aligned}
1 \text{ watt} &= 0.056 \text{ BTU/min} \\
&\doteq 0.00131 \text{ horse power} \\
&= 0.00134 \text{ horse power (electric)} \\
&= 0.737 \text{ ft-lb/sec} \\
&= 1 \times 10^7 \text{ ergs/sec} \\
&= 1 \text{ J} \times s^{-1} = 0.239 \text{ g-cal} \times s^{-1}
\end{aligned}
$$

$$
\begin{aligned}
1 \text{ BTU/min} \quad &= 17.58 \text{ watts} \\
1 \text{ horse power} &= 745.7 \text{ watts} \\
1 \text{ horse power (electric)} &= 746 \text{ watts} \\
1 \text{ ft-lb/sec} \quad &= 1.35 \text{ watts} \\
1 \text{ gm-cm/sec} \quad &= 9.8 \times 10^{-5} \text{ watts} \\
1 \text{ erg/sec} \quad &= 1 \times 10^{-7} \text{ watts} \\
1 \text{ cal/sec} \quad &= 4.18 \text{ watts}
\end{aligned}
$$

Temperature

$$
\begin{aligned}
\text{Temperature Fahrenheit} &= 9/5 \times C + 32 \\
\text{Temperature Centigrade} &= 5/9 \ (F - 32) \\
\text{Temperature Kelvin} \quad &= 273.15 + C
\end{aligned}
$$

Appendix III

SYSTÈME INTERNATIONAL d'UNITÉS (SI UNITS)*

Basic SI Units

Physical Quantity	Name	Symbol
Length	meter	m
Mass	kilogram	kg
Time	second	s
Electric current	ampere	A
Thermodynamic temperature	kelvin	K
Luminous intensity	candela	cd
Amount of substance	mole	mol

Derived SI Units

Quantity	SI Unit	Symbol	In Terms of Basic or Derived Units
Frequency	hertz	Hz	$1\ Hz = 1\ cycle \times s^{-1}$
Force	newton	N	$1\ N = 1\ kg \times m \times s^{-2}$
Work, energy, quantity of heat	joule	J	$1\ J = 1\ N \times m$
Power	watt	W	$1\ W = 1\ J \times s^{-1}$
Quantity of electricity	coulomb	C	$1\ C = 1\ A \times s$
Electric potential, potential difference, tension, electromotive force	volt	V	$1\ V = 1\ W \times A^{-1}$
Electric capacitance	farad	F	$1\ F = 1\ A \times s \times V^{-1}$
Electric resistance	ohm		$1\ \Omega = 1\ V \times A^{-1}$
Flux of magnetic induction, magnetic flux	weber	Wb	$1\ Wb = 1\ V \times s$
Magnetic flux density, magnetic induction	tesla	T	$1\ T = 1\ Wb \times m^{-2}$
Inductance	henry	H	$1\ H = 1\ V \times s \times A^{-1}$
Pressure	pascal	Pa	$1\ Pa = 1\ N \times m^{-2}$ $= 1\ kg \times m^{-1}s^{-2}$

Prefixes

Factor	Name	Symbol	Factor	Name	Symbol
			10^{-18}	atto-	a
			10^{-15}	femto-	f
10^{12}	tera-	T	10^{-12}	pico-	p
10^{9}	giga-	G	10^{-9}	nano-	n
10^{6}	mega-	M	10^{-6}	micro-	μ
10^{3}	kilo-	k	10^{-3}	milli-	m
10^{2}	hecto-	h	10^{-2}	centi-	c
1	deca-	da	10^{-1}	deci-	d

*SI units were adopted by the International Union of Pure and Applied Chemistry and the International Federation of Clinical Chemistry. Their use is standard in many European medical journals. Other units in common use in the United States are included in Appendix II.

BIBLIOGRAPHY

Anaesthesia and the Systeme International (SI). Anaesthesia 30:604, 1975.

Page CH, Vigoureux P: The International System of Units (SI). Washington, DC, National Bureau of Standards, Special Publication 330, 1972.

Young DS: Normal laboratory values (case records of the Massachusetts General Hospital) in SI units. N Engl J Med *292*:795, 1975.

Index

Numbers in *italics* refer to illustrations; (t) denotes tabular material.